TOOTH WHITENING TECHNIQUES

TOOTH WHITENING TECHNIQUES

Second Edition

Edited by

Linda Greenwall, BDS, MGDS RCS, MSc, MRD RCS, FFGDP (UK)
Prosthodontist and Specialist in Restorative Dentistry
Private practice, London, UK

CRC Press
Taylor & Francis Group
Boca Raton London New York

CRC Press is an imprint of the
Taylor & Francis Group, an **informa** business

CRC Press
Taylor & Francis Group
6000 Broken Sound Parkway NW, Suite 300
Boca Raton, FL 33487-2742

Printed and bound in India by Replika Press Pvt. Ltd.

Printed on acid-free paper

International Standard Book Number-13: 978-1-84214-530-2 (Hardback)

Visit the Taylor & Francis Web site at
http://www.taylorandfrancis.com

and the CRC Press Web site at
http://www.crcpress.com

CONTENTS

FOREWORD

Bleaching knowledge! How do you find it? Tray bleaching has been popular for more than 25 years, and in-office bleaching has been popular for over 125 years. There have been many articles written and opinions expressed during this time frame. There have been improvements as well as changes in both the techniques and the understanding of the process. There has been some confusing marketing as well as good advancement of the techniques by manufacturing companies and individuals. There has been good research, and not-so-good research. The challenge is how to find the most current information, and how to compare techniques and procedures. One way is to combine as many different aspects of bleaching as possible, from materials to science to techniques to marketing, into a single book. Although a book is not as current as a recent article, this approach at least addresses all the areas, questions, and concerns for the dentist or dental office to consider in a single cohesive source. That is exactly what Dr. Greenwall has been doing with this second edition of her book on bleaching.

As a pioneer in the tray bleaching era as well as a proponent of "fee for service" dentistry, Dr. Linda Greenwall has experience with many of the different techniques and has used them in her practice, and has obtained expertise from different dentists about all aspects of bleaching. Although there is seldom a single simple answer to many bleaching questions, this approach shares both her perspective and those of other experts in the field on a wide variety of bleaching or tooth whitening aspects.

This book should serve as a comprehensive reference and guideline for your practice, or a springboard to searching other sources to further your understanding of the bleaching process. I applaud Dr. Greenwall's hard work and dedication to the profession, and her work in the advancement of the safest, most conservative treatment available to change the color of your patients' teeth.

Van B. Haywood, DMD

PREFACE TO SECOND EDITION

It is now over 25 years since the introduction of the seminal paper by Van Haywood and Harald Heymann in 1989 introducing a new concept in tooth whitening. Since this introduction, there has been an explosion of literature on tooth whitening techniques. Globally, hundreds of thousands of patients have benefitted from whitened smiles with the added health benefits that whitening brings. The scientific evidence clearly shows that tooth whitening techniques can be a safe and effective treatment for patients. There is a vast body of published scientific literature that has demonstrated this and continues to demonstrate this scientifically. It is the intention of this textbook to bring you updated information on the different tooth whitening techniques using a step-by-step approach as well as clear guidance on how to deliver the treatment safely and effectively to your patients. There are new contributors to this second edition, with new photographs and many new illustrations to give clearer guidance and understanding. This edition is thus a global sharing of scientific knowledge from our contributors across the world.

As the tooth whitening industry has expanded, the tooth whitening product market has become available to consumers on the Internet and in drugstores and at beauty salons. Beauty therapists and nondentists have tried to muscle in on providing tooth whitening treatments to members of the public. Unfortunately, this has led to many controversies in the tooth whitening industry and continues to do so. The tooth whitening materials and techniques discussed in this textbook are related to those used in the dental practice that have been carefully researched for safety, efficacy, and predictability. These tooth whitening materials are to be supplied by dentists in their offices. These materials, besides being carefully regulated, have demonstrated safety and long-lasting effects. Tooth whitening is the practice of dentistry, and as such the whole dental team should be engaged in delivering efficient tooth whitening services with the appropriate training and knowledge. This textbook is intended for dentists and their dental teams to gain a deeper and broader understanding of the whole subject of tooth whitening.

Safe tooth whitening requires an understanding of the subject, a knowledge of the scientific literature, and an understanding of how to conduct an oral health evaluation and dental examination for patients wishing to lighten their teeth. As tooth whitening is now an essential part of restorative dentistry, the treatment planning for patients wishing to lighten their teeth is vitally important. Those dentists who embrace the delivery of effective tooth whitening treatments within their practices will grow their practices exponentially in the coming years. Research has also shown that 80% of patients who elect to have tooth whitening then choose to have further esthetic dentistry. This means that dentists who wish to deliver excellent whitening treatment in their practice also need to have an advanced knowledge of esthetic and restorative dentistry and how to combine whitening and esthetics within their practice, because these two subjects are closely integrated. There may be a steep learning curve for many, but it is a great journey! Although all this knowledge is important, it is also essential to know how to run and manage an effective tooth whitening program within the dental practice to deliver effective care to patients. All this is covered in this new edition.

Across the globe there is different legislation concerning tooth whitening products pertinent to each country, and each reader should ensure that he or she is fully au fait with his or her country's regulations concerning tooth whitening legislation. Whereas U.S. legislation permits higher concentrations of hydrogen peroxide to be used in power whitening, European legislation was amended and ratified by the European Council of Dentists in 2012 to restrict the use to concentrations at or below 6% hydrogen peroxide. The photographs and case illustrations in this edition mostly demonstrate the use of the whitening products at or below 6% hydrogen peroxide. Safe and effective whitening treatments can be delivered at these lower concentrations, and this is clearly illustrated in this textbook. Although advice is given herein on different concentrations of hydrogen peroxide and carbamide peroxide, practitioners should always consult their own countries' legislation for the permitted concentrations to ensure that they are in compliance.

ACKNOWLEDGMENTS

There are many people to thank for this second edition, which is an international contribution to the dental literature. Tooth whitening is now a global phenomenon, being undertaken across all corners of the world. Over the past 25 years my involvement in the subject of tooth whitening has taken me on an interesting career pathway. I began my involvement with tooth whitening when I was studying for my master's in conservative dentistry in 1990 to 1992. First, I wish to thank Dr. Van Haywood and Dr. Harald Heymann for publishing their paper on tooth whitening in 1989. Their major contribution to dentistry has had a global impact and has affected the lives of many thousands of patients worldwide. I have to thank Professor B.G.N. Smith for guidance in steering me away from the study of amalgam and toward the study and science of tooth whitening. I undertook my master's research in this subject and have been involved ever since. My first tooth bleaching textbook, the first edition of this book, was published in 2001 and received the award for the best new textbook for medicine and dentistry. I wish to thank my commissioning editor, Robert Peden, for his perseverance in steering me to complete both editions.

The challenge of writing involves finding time to write while maintaining a busy dental practicing schedule, running the dental wellness trust charity, editing the journal *Aesthetic Dentistry Today,* fulfilling the responsibilities of numerous committee appointments, and bringing up a family of four boys. I thank my husband, Dr. Henry Cohen, for his help with the children and encouragement and for his sense of humor and easygoing nature.

I thank my wonderful sons, Andrew, Joseph, Edward, and Rayno, for their love, support, and kindness and for teaching me the world through their eyes every day.

I also thank my parents for their encouragement and inspiration to follow in the family tradition—dentistry—and for their leadership. My mother's help in looking after the boys and stern guidance on many life aspects were gratefully appreciated.

I wish to thank all who have contributed to this book. Thanks go to Dr. Bruce Matis from the University of Indiana, who undertook extensive research on tetracycline discoloration; Dr. Ralph Leonard from North Carolina; Dr. Thomas Attin from Zurich; Dr. Joseph Ontiveros and Dr. Rade Paravino from the University of Texas; Dr. Marie Carmen Puy and my colleagues from the Spanish Bleaching Society; Dr. Leopoldo Fornez; Dr. Jose Amengual; and Dr. Carlos Oteo. Also, I thank Dr. Yiming Li for his contribution to the literature on safety and toxicity of the tooth whitening products; Dr. Phil Newsome for his contribution from Hong Kong; and Dr. Gerard Kugel and coworkers from Tufts University, who have contributed to the literature on tooth whitening strips and written the chapter on that subject in this book.

Thanks also go to my dental colleagues and students across the globe who have shared their knowledge and continued to question the many aspects of tooth whitening so that we can all learn and share in the dental bleaching knowledge and develop the practice of tooth whitening as it is today.

In 2008, together with colleagues, we established the British Dental Bleaching Society to be able to lobby and change the U.K. law surrounding tooth bleaching. I thank my fellow dentists on this committee: Sir Paul Beresford, Mervyn Druain, Chris Orr, James Goolnick, Martin Kelleher, Edward Lynch, Wyman Chan, and David Phillips, all of whom contributed to the discussion and amendments to lobby for changes in the U.K. law. Also, I thank Dr. Stuart Johnson for his leadership of the Council of European Dentists as Chair of the Working Group on tooth whitening during the years of major change. Although much has been accomplished, there remain some outstanding issues to be discussed, such as whitening for patients younger than 18 and the safe use of higher concentrations for chairside bleaching.

Thanks also go to Mhari Coxon from Phillips for her leadership in establishing the Tooth Whitening Information Group to help the general public in the U.K. access Safe Tooth Whitening. Thanks go to my colleagues in the dental industry, Geoff, Tom and Sam Cheetham, Lyn Chau from SDI Australia, Mike Farrow, Jayne Cahill from SDI U.K., Yann Karafka Ramon from SDI Spain, Simon Gambold from Henry Schein, Payman Langroudi from Enlighten Industries, Mike Volk from Dental Directory, David Oultram and the Butterfield Family from Optident, Dan Fischer from Ultradent who have supported my lectures, courses, teaching programs, and hands-on training programs across the globe. Thanks also to Dr. Felix Worle, Dr. Paul Wilmes, Claudia Englisch, Jana Rosenthal and the entire team at DMG, Hamburg, Germany for their support and assistance.

I also wish to thank my entire dental team for help on all aspects of this textbook. Their help is so integral in the treatment we undertake and accomplish for our patients and the management aspects of running and administrating the practice, which includes the collating of photographs and developing the paperwork we use in the practice to deliver better care. I wish to thank the administrative team, Nicola Ayo Adebanjo, Sarah O'Hara, Rachel Grosvenor, and Sarah Jewell for their dedicated hard work and friendly smiles in helping our patients and the clinical team; Diane Rochford, dental hygienist; and Alison Gaze, dental therapist. Thanks also to my specialist colleagues in our Specialist Group Practice, particularly Dr. Jude Ferreira, our endodontist.

Immense thanks, gratitude, and appreciation go to the many patients who have willingly shared their experiences on tooth whitening and allowed us to record their before and after photographs, which have contributed to this textbook. I have learned so much from them.

CONTRIBUTORS

Thomas Attin
Clinic of Preventive Dentistry, Periodontology and Cariology
Center of Dental Medicine
University of Zurich
Zurich, Switzerland

Robert W. Gerlach
Department of Prosthodontics and Operative Dentistry (Research Administration)
School of Dental Medicine
Tufts University
Boston, Massachusetts

and

Global Oral Care
The Procter & Gamble Company
Mason, Ohio

Linda Greenwall
Private practice
London, U.K.

Van B. Haywood
Department of Oral Rehabilitation
College of Dental Medicine
Georgia Regents University
Augusta, Georgia

Gerard Kugel
Department of Prosthodontics and Operative Dentistry
School of Dental Medicine
Tufts University
Boston, Massachusetts

Ralph H. Leonard, Jr.
Department of Diagnostic Sciences and General Dentistry
University of North Carolina School of Dentistry
Chapel Hill, North Carolina

Yiming Li
Restorative Dentistry
Center for Dental Research
Loma Linda University School of Dentistry
Loma Linda, California

Britta E. Magnuson
Department of Oral and Maxillofacial Pathology, Oral Medicine and Craniofacial Pain
School of Dental Medicine
Tufts University
Boston, Massachusetts

Bruce Matis
Department of Clinical Research
Indiana University School of Dentistry
Indianapolis, Indiana

Brian Millar
Restorative Dentistry and Distance Learning
King's College London Dental Institute
London, U.K.

Philip R.H. Newsome
Private practice
Hong Kong, P.R.C.

Joe C. Ontiveros
Restorative Dentistry and Prosthodontics
University of Texas Health Center at Houston
University of Texas School of Dentistry
Houston, Texas

Rade D. Paravina
Restorative Dentistry and Prosthodontics
University of Texas Health Center at Houston
University of Texas School of Dentistry
Houston, Texas

Ilan Rotstein
Endodontics, Oral and Maxillofacial Surgery and Orthodontics
Herman Ostrow School of Dentistry
University of Southern California
Los Angeles, California

1 DISCOLORATION OF TEETH

Linda Greenwall

INTRODUCTION

Tooth discoloration is a common problem leading patients to seek treatment to have the discoloration removed. People of various ages may be affected, and it can occur in both primary and secondary teeth. The etiology of dental discoloration is multifactorial, and different parts of the tooth can take up different stains. This effect is a result of the anatomy of the tooth. Intrinsic discoloration increases with increasing age and is more common in men (Eriksen and Nordbo 1978). It may affect 31% of men and 21% of women (Ness et al. 1977). The result is a complex of physical and chemical interactions with the tooth surface. The aim of this chapter is to assess the etiology of tooth discoloration and the mechanisms by which teeth stain. It is the intention of this chapter to explain the complexity of tooth discoloration.

COLOR OF NATURAL HEALTHY TEETH

Teeth are polychromatic (Louka 1989). The color varies among the gingival, incisal, and cervical areas according to the thickness, reflectance of different colors, and translucency in enamel and dentin (see Figure 1.2). The color of healthy teeth is primarily determined by the dentin and is modified by the following:

- The color of the enamel covering the crown.
- The translucency of the enamel, which varies with different degrees of calcification.
- The thickness of the enamel, which is greater at the occlusal or incisal edge of the tooth and thinner at the cervical third (Dayan et al. 1983).
- The intensity, thickness, structure of the dentin.
- Presence of secondary or tertiary dentin trauma.
- Existing restorations.

CLASSIFICATION OF DISCOLORATION

Many researchers classify staining as either extrinsic or intrinsic (Dayan et al. 1983, Hayes et al. 1986, Teo 1989). There is confusion concerning the exact definitions of these terms. Feinman et al. (1987) described extrinsic discoloration as that occurring when an agent stains or damages the enamel surface of the teeth, and intrinsic staining as occurring when internal tooth structure is penetrated by a discoloring agent. According to these definitions, the terms *staining* and *discoloration* are used synonymously. However, extrinsic staining will be defined here as staining that can be easily removed by a normal prophylactic cleaning (Dayan et al. 1983). Intrinsic staining is defined here as endogenous staining that has been incorporated into the tooth matrix and thus cannot be removed by prophylaxis.

Some discoloration is a combination of both types of staining and may be multifactorial. For example, nicotine staining on teeth is extrinsic staining that becomes intrinsic staining. The modified classification of Dzierzak (1991), Hayes et al. (1986), and Nathoo (1997) will be used as a guide. See Table 1.1.

STAINS DURING ODONTOGENESIS (PRE-ERUPTIVE)

These alter the development and appearance of the enamel and dentin on permanent teeth.

Developmentally defective enamel and dentin

Defects of enamel development (Figures 1.6A and 1.6B) can be caused by, for example, amelogenesis imperfecta (Figure 1.5), dentinogenesis imperfecta, and enamel hypoplasia. The defects in enamel are either hypocalcific or hypoplastic (Rotstein 1998). Enamel hypocalcification is a distinct brownish or whitish area found on the buccal aspects of teeth (see Figure 1.5). The enamel is well formed and the surface is intact. Many of these white and brown discolorations can be removed with whitening in combination with microabrasion (see Chapter 10). Enamel hypoplasia is developmental defective enamel. The surface of the tooth is defective and porous and may be readily discolored by materials in the oral cavity. Depending on the severity and extent of the dysplasia, the enamel surface may be whitened with varying degrees of success. Some enamel white hypoplastic lesions are due to exposure of chemicals (such as bisphenol a) peri- or postnatally (Jedeon et al. 2013).

Fluorosis

This staining is caused by excessive fluoride uptake with the developing enamel layers. The fluoride source can be from the ingestion of excessive fluoride in the drinking water or from overuse of fluoride supplements (Ismail and Hasson 2008) or fluoride toothpastes (Shannon 1978). It occurs within the superficial enamel and appears as white or brown patches of irregular shape and form (Figure 1.7A). The acquisition of stain, however, is posteruptive. The teeth are not discolored on eruption, but because the surface is porous they gradually absorb the colored chemicals present in the oral cavity (Rotstein 1998). Staining caused by fluorosis manifests in three different ways: as simple fluorosis, opaque fluorosis, or fluorosis with pitting (Nathoo and Gaffar 1995). Simple fluorosis appears as brown pigmentation on a smooth enamel surface, whereas opaque

Table 1.1 Etiology of tooth discoloration

Extrinsic stains

- Plaque (Figure 1.26), chromogenic bacteria, surface protein denaturation
- Mouthwashes (e.g., chlorhexidine)
- Beverages (tea [Figure 1.28], coffee [Figures 1.27 and 1.31], red wine, cola)
- Foods (curry, cooking oils and fried foods [Figure 1.33], foods with colorings, berries, beetroot)
- Illness
- Antibiotics (erythromycin [Figure 1.29], amoxicillins [Figures 1.6A and 1.30])
- Iron supplements (Figures 1.34)

Intrinsic stains

Pre-eruptive

Disease

- Hematologic diseases (Figure 1.15)
- Liver diseases
- Diseases of enamel and dentin (Figure 1.5)

Medication

- Tetracycline stains (Figures 1.8–1.10)
- Other antibiotics
- Fluorosis stains (Figure 1.7)

Posteruptive

- Trauma (Figure 1.4), intrapulpal hemorrhage (Figure 1.14A), pulp necrosis (Figure 1.15B)
- Primary and secondary caries (Figure 1.27) and erosion, buccal (Figure 1.36) and palatal (Figures 1.22–1.24, 1.38)
- Dental restorative materials (Figures 1.17 and 1.18), endodontic materials (Figure 1.4, lower right incisor tooth)
- Aging (Figure 1.25)
- Smoking (Figures 1.33 and 1.35)
- Chemicals
- Some foodstuffs (long-term use causes deeper intrinsic staining)
- Minocycline (Figure 1.12)
- Tetracycline (Figure 1.37)
- Functional and parafunctional changes (Figure 1.25)

fluorosis appears as gray or white flecks on the tooth surface (Figure 1.7B). Fluorosis with pitting occurs as defects in the enamel surface, and the color appears to be darker.

Stannous fluoride treatment causes discoloration by reactions of the tooth with the tin ion (Shannon 1978). No intraoral discolorations occur from topical use of fluoride at low concentrations. The severity and degree of staining are directly related to the amount of fluoride ingested during odontogenesis.

Tetracycline

Tetracycline is a broad-spectrum bacteriostatic antibiotic (van der Bijl and Ptitgoi-Aron 1995) that is used to treat a variety of infections. The tetracycline antibiotics are a group of related compounds that are effective against gram-negative and gram-positive bacteria. It is well known that the administration of tetracycline during odontogenesis causes unsightly discoloration of both primary and secondary dentitions (Thomas and Denny 2014). The discoloration varies according to the type of tetracycline used (Table 1.2). The staining effects are a result of chelation of the tetracycline molecule with calcium ions in hydroxyapatite crystals, primarily in the dentin (Swift 1988). The tetracycline is incorporated into the enamel and dentin. The chelated molecule arrives at the mineralizing predentin–dentin junction via the terminal capillaries of the dental pulp (Patel et al. 1998). The brown discoloration is a result of photooxidation, which occurs on exposure of the tooth to light.

Table 1.2 Tetracycline stains

Drug	*Color stain on teeth*
Chlortetracycline (Aureomycin)	Gray-brown
Demethylchlortetracycline (Ledermycin)	Yellow
Oxytetracycline (Terramycin)	Yellow—lowest amount
Tetracycline (Achromycin)	Yellow
Doxycycline (Vibramycin)	No reported changes
Minocycline	Black

Adapted from Hayes et al. 1986.

The staining can be classified according to the developmental stage, banding, and color (Jordan and Boksman 1984):

- *First-degree* (mild) tetracycline staining is yellow to gray, which is uniformly spread through the tooth. There is no banding (see Figure 1.8).
- *Second-degree* (moderate) staining (Figure 1.9) is yellow-brown to dark gray.
- *Third-degree* (severe) staining is blue-gray or black and is accompanied by significant banding across the tooth (see Figure 1.10).
- *Fourth-degree* (intractable) staining has been suggested by Feinman et al. (1987), designated for those stains that are so dark that whitening is ineffective (see Figures 1.11 and 1.12).

All degrees of stain become more intense on chronic exposure to artificial light and sunlight. The severity of pigmentation depends on three factors: time and duration of administration, the type of tetracycline administered, and the dosage (Dayan et al. 1983, Shearer 1991).

First- or second-degree staining is normally amenable to whitening treatments (Haywood 1997). Prolonged home whitening has been reported in the literature to be successful for tetracycline staining. This may take 3–6 months or longer (see Figure 1.13). The whitening material penetrates into the dentin structure of the tooth and causes a permanent color change in the dentin (McCaslin et al. 1999).

Illness and trauma during tooth formation

The effects of illness, trauma, and medication (e.g., porphyria, infant jaundice, vitamin deficiency, phenylketonuria, hematologic anemia) are cumulative, creating stains and defects that cannot be altered by whitening. Staining may result from hematologic disorders such as erythroblastosis fetalis (Atasu et al. 1998), porphyria, phenylketonuria, hemolytic anemia, sickle cell anemia, and thalassemia. Because the coagulation system is affected, discoloration occurs as a result of the presence of blood within the dentinal tubules (Nathoo 1997). Bilirubinemia in patients with liver dysfunction can cause bilirubin pigmentation in deciduous teeth (Watanabe et al. 1999). These disorders can result in molar incisor hypoplasia, which reflects as white spots and white marks on the central incisors and the first permanent molars.

Stains after odontogenesis (posteruptive)

Minocycline

Minocycline is a semisynthetic second-generation tetracycline derivative (Goldstein 1998) that is often used for acne treatment. It is a broad-spectrum antibiotic that is highly plasma bound and lipophilic (McKenna et al. 1999). It is bacteriostatic and produces greater antimicrobial activity than tetracycline or its analogues (Salman et al. 1985). The drug is used to treat acne and various infections. Its lipophilicity facilitates penetration into body fluids, and after oral administration the minocycline concentration in saliva is 30–60% of the serum concentration (McKenna et al. 1999). In addition, minocycline hydrochloride has been shown to cause pigmentation of a variety of tissues including skin, thyroid, nails, sclera, teeth, conjunctiva, and bone. Adult-onset tooth discoloration after long-term ingestion of tetracycline and minocycline has also been reported (Sánchez et al. 2004). The remarkable side effect of minocycline on the oral cavity is the singular occurrence of "black bones," "black or green roots," and a blue-gray to gray darkening of the crowns of permanent teeth. The prevalence of tetracycline and minocycline staining is 3–6% (Sánchez et al. 2004).

Minocycline is absorbed from the gastrointestinal tract and combines poorly with calcium. See Table 1.3.

Adolescents and adults who take the drug are at risk for developing intrinsic staining on their teeth, gingivae, oral mucosa, and bones (Bowles and Bokmeyer 1997). It causes tooth discoloration by chelating with iron to form insoluble complexes. It is also thought that the discoloration may be a result of its forming a complex with secondary dentin (Salman et al. 1985). The discoloration does not resolve after discontinuation of therapy. The resultant staining is normally milder than that from tetracycline and may be amenable to whitening and lightening, although this is case specific. In a study examining 17 discolored third molars under fluorescent microscopy, Antonini and Luder (2011) found that when acne was treated between 15 and 22 years of age, only the roots of the third molars displayed annular discolorations, which seemed to result from the incorporation of tetracyclines into dentin, whereas fine fluorescent incremental lines in root cementum were too thin to be apparent clinically. Three accidentally removed interradicular bony septa revealed that tetracyclines incorporated into alveolar bone remained there for about 2 years, but thereafter disappeared as a result of physiologic remodeling.

Table 1.3 Tooth discoloration: causes and colors

Cause	*Color*
Extrinsic discoloration	
Cigarettes, pipes, cigars, chewing tobacco	Yellow-brown to black (Figure 1.39)
Marijuana	Dark-brown to black rings
Coffee, tea, foods	Brown to black
Poor oral hygiene	Yellow or brown shades
Chromogenic bacteria and plaque	Green
Extrinsic and intrinsic discoloration	
Fluorosis	White, yellow, brown, orange, gray, or black
Aging	Yellow to orange
Intrinsic discoloration	
Genetic conditions (e.g., amelogenesis imperfecta)	Brown, black
Systemic conditions—for example:	
Jaundice	Blue-green or brown
Porphyria	Purple-brown
Medications during tooth development (e.g., tetracycline, fluoride)	Brown, gray, or black
Body byproducts—for example:	
Bilirubin	Blue-green, brown
Hemoglobin	Gray, black (Figure 1.15)
Pulp changes	
Trauma	Yellow, orange, purple, gray
Intrapulpal hemorrhage (Figure 1.14B)	Gray, brown
Pulp canal obliteration	Yellow
Pulp necrosis (Figure 1.15B)	Yellow, brown, black
With hemorrhage	Gray, black
Without hemorrhage	Yellow, gray-brown
Iatrogenic causes	
Trauma during pulp extirpation	Gray, black
Tissue remnants in pulp chamber	Brown, gray, black
Inappropriate design of access cavity (traps pulp chromophore materials inside the pulp chamber)	Yellow, gray (Plotino et al. 2008)
Products of tissue decomposition	Yellow, brown, gray
Restorative dental materials	Brown, gray amalgam (Figures 1.17, 1.18, and 1.19), black
Endodontic materials (cement and gutta percha)	Gray, black

Adapted from Abbott 1997, with permission.

Pulpal changes

Pulp necrosis

Pulp necrosis can be the result of bacterial, mechanical, or chemical irritation to the pulp. Substances can enter the dentinal tubules and cause the teeth to discolor. These teeth will require endodontic treatment before whitening, the latter using the intracoronal method (see Chapter 8) or the outside-inside technique (see Chapter 15). See Table 1.4.

Intrapulpal hemorrhage caused by trauma

Accidental injury to the tooth can cause pulpal and dentinal degenerative changes that alter the color of the teeth

Table 1.4 Mechanisms that cause nonvital teeth to discolor

- Tissue degradation during the necrotic process (Baratieri et al. 1995).
- Trauma causing rupture of blood vessels. This results in hemolysis of red blood cells, which release hemoglobin and hematin derivatives. Iron in red blood cells may be aspirated into dentinal tubules. This may also occur if there is uncontrolled hemorrhage during endodontic treatment.
- Intracanal medications such as phenolics and iodoform-based medications can cause gradual discoloration. The dentin is penetrated, causing oxidation.
- Silver points may corrode inside the root canal.
- Coronally placed leaking restorative materials.
- Endodontic cement.
- Inadequate coronal access leaves pulp remnants and necrotic tissue in the pulp chamber.
- Contamination of the pulp cavity during endodontics.
- Insufficient irrigation and debridement.

Table 1.5 Discoloration caused by endodontic sealer

Endodontic sealer	*Color*
Grossman's cement, zinc oxide eugenol, Endomethasone and N^2	Orange-red
Diaket, Tubli-Seal	Mild pink
AH26	Gray
Riebler's paste	Dark red

Adapted from van der Burgt et al. 1986a.

(see Figure 1.14). Pulpal hemorrhage may occur, giving the tooth a gray, nonvital appearance (Nathanson and Parra 1987). The discoloration is a result of the hemorrhage, which causes lysis of red blood cells. Blood disintegration products such as iron sulfides enter the dentin tubules and discolor the surrounding dentin, which causes discoloration of the tooth (Baratieri et al. 1995). Sometimes the tooth can recover from such an episode (Marin et al. 1997) and the discoloration can reverse naturally without whitening. These discolored teeth should be vitality tested, because those that are still vital (see Chapter 4) can be successfully whitened using the home whitening technique (see Chapter 5).

Dentin hypercalcification

Dentin hypercalcification results when there is excessive irregular dentin in the pulp chamber and canal walls. There may be a temporary disruption in blood supply followed by the disruption of odontoblasts (Rotstein 1998). Irregular dentin is laid down in the walls of the pulp chamber. There is gradual decrease in the translucency of these teeth, which results in a yellowish or yellow-brown discoloration (Figure 1.20). These teeth can be whitened with good results (see Chapter 9).

Dental caries

Dental caries (both primary and secondary) may confer a discolored appearance (Kleter 1998) around areas of bacterial stagnation (see Figure 1.15), or leaking restorations. Arrested caries has a brown discoloration (Figure 1.27) because the breakdown products react with decalcified dentin (Eriksen and Nordbo 1978); this is similar to the discoloration of the pellicle.

Restorative materials and dental procedures

Eugenol causes an orange-yellow stain. Endodontic materials (such as silver points and silver-containing root canal cements) and pulpal remnants may cause a gray or pink appearance. Darkening of tooth crowns after root canal treatment has been attributed to the use of discoloring endodontic materials (Krastl et al. 2013) such as those containing silver as a constituent part of the endodontic sealer. A study by van der Burgt et al. (1986a) showed that all endodontic sealers tested caused discoloration in the dentin (see Table 1.5), whereas there was no penetration into the enamel. This discoloration is visible 3 weeks after application of the endodontic sealer (van der Burgt 1986b). However, the currently available root canal materials show only scarce or no evidence with regard to their staining ability. Endodontic therapy should not focus solely on biologic and functional aspects; esthetic considerations should be taken into account as well (Krastl et al. 2013).

Silver amalgam may cause the tooth to take on a gray appearance because silver salts are incorporated into the dentinal tubules. Discoloration in the tooth may be a result of the physical presence of the amalgam (Figures 1.17 and 1.18), corrosion products, or secondary caries (Kidd et al. 1995). Color change alone next to the margin of a restoration should not trigger replacement (Kidd et al. 1995). A leaking composite restoration (Figures 1.18 and 1.19) can cause the tooth to appear more yellow (Kidd 1991). Several types of stain adjacent to tooth-colored restorations are recognized by clinicians. Open margins may allow chemicals to enter and discolor the underlying dentin (Rotstein 1998). There may also be white or brown spots of secondary caries (Figure 1.24). Metal pins and prefabricated posts, when placed in the anterior teeth, can become visible under composite restorations. This causes discoloration of these teeth. Removal of these pins and replacement of leaking restorations is indicated.

Aging

Color changes in the teeth result from surface and subsurface changes (Solheim 1988). The degree of manifestation is related to tooth anatomy, structural hardness, and the amount of use and abuse. The following factors are encountered with increasing age:

- *Enamel changes.* There may be both thinning and texture changes (Morley 1997; Figure 1.20).
- *Dentin deposition.* Secondary and tertiary dentin deposition, pulp stones, and dentin aging all cause the tooth to appear darker (Figure 1.28).
- *Salivary changes.* Salivary content and composition may change with advancing age (Solheim 1988). Whitening treatment is normally successful in this age group provided there is sufficient enamel available to whiten.

Functional and parafunctional changes

Tooth wear may give a darker appearance to the teeth because of the loss of tooth surface (Smith and Knight 1984).

- *Erosion* is the progressive loss of hard dental tissues by a chemical process not involving bacterial action (Watson and Tulloch 1985, Bishop et al. 1997). This dissolution of enamel by acid causes the tooth to appear discolored (Shaw and Smith 1999; Figures 1.23 and 1.24) because the dentin is more yellow in color (Figure 1.36).
- *Attrition* is defined as wear of the occlusal surfaces or proximal surfaces of the tooth caused by mastication or contact between occluding surfaces (Watson and Tulloch, 1985) (Figure 1.25). It affects the occlusal and incisal surfaces (Bishop et al. 1997).
- *Abrasion* is defined as the loss by wear of tooth substance or a restoration by factors other than tooth contact (Watson and Tulloch 1985; Figures 1.37 and 1.38). It is usually caused by abnormal rubbing of a nondental object such as a pipe, hairclip, or musical instrument. It is often caused by overly vigorous tooth brushing (Bishop et al. 1997). This loss of enamel causes exposure of dentin, which makes the tooth appear more yellow.

Function and parafunction may cause loss of the incisal edges and exposure of underlying dentin, which is susceptible to color change from absorption and deposition of reparative dentin (Figures 1.36 and 1.38). Fracture lines develop as white cracks but darken on exposure to absorptive surface stains (Figure 1.35). Changes in color and texture affect the color and light reflectiveness.

Daily acquired stains

Daily acquired stains are typical of the extrinsic stains. They cause superficial color changes, which are removed by prophylaxis.

- *Plaque.* Pellicle and calculus on the surface of the tooth can give it a yellow appearance (Figure 1.26).
- *Tobacco use.* The products of tobacco dissolve in the saliva and lower its pH, facilitating penetration of pits and fissures (Dayan et al. 1983). This gives the tooth a brown or black appearance (Figures 1.27 and 1.39).
- *Food and beverages.* Consumption of food and drink such as coffee (Figure 1.27), tea (Figure 1.28), red wine and berries (Faunce 1983), curry, and colas results in surface and absorptive staining.
- *Poor oral hygiene.* Poor oral hygiene (Dayan et al. 1983) may result in green, black-brown, and orange staining (Figures 1.15B and 1.26), which is produced by chromogenic bacteria. These deposits are normally seen in children and are found on the buccal surfaces of maxillary teeth (Eriksen and Nordbo 1978).
- *Good oral hygiene.* A black type of staining can often occur in children. It is normally found in patients with good oral hygiene and can be highly retentive, particularly around the cervical margins of the teeth (Eriksen and Nordbo 1978). It sometimes occurs in patients who follow Mediterranean diets.
- *Swimmer's calculus.* This is a yellow to dark-brown stain that occurs on the facial and lingual or palatal surfaces of the anterior teeth of patients who swim and train extensively. Both primary and secondary dentitions are affected. It appears that prolonged exposure to pool water can cause stains to develop on swimmers' teeth. The stains can be accompanied by gingivitis (Rose and Carey 1995). The stains are easily removed with professional oral prophylaxis. However, some teeth can be discolored by long-term swimming in a swimming pool with high levels of acidic chlorine.

Chemicals

Chlorhexidine

Mouthwash containing chlorhexidine causes superficial black and brown staining of the teeth (Addy and Moran 1985, Addy et al. 1985a, 1985b, Leard and Addy 1997, Eley 1999). The staining is enhanced in the presence of tea and coffee. It may be related to the precipitation of chromogenic dietary factors onto the teeth and mucous membranes (Addy et al. 1985b). It is probable that the associated cationic group attaches chlorhexidine to the tooth, whereas the other cationic group producing the bactericidal effect can attach the dietary factors, such as gallic acid derivatives (polyphenols) found in foods and beverages such as tea and coffee and tannins from wine to the molecule and hence to the tooth surface (Leard and Addy 1997, Eley 1999).

Metals

Metals such as copper, nickel, and iron can cause staining of teeth. Copper ions, when they occur in the water in certain areas, can cause staining of teeth. Workers in the copper and nickel industries have also shown green staining on the teeth (Donoghue and Ferguson 1996). The combination of plaque occurring around metallic orthodontic brackets can cause green line staining. Excessive iron intake can cause cervical staining, usually dark-brown or black in color. The taking of iron supplements (Figure 1.34) can cause black staining of the teeth and tongue (Addy et al. 1985a); black stains have also been noted on the teeth of ironworkers.

Tannins and chromogens

Some stains are easier to remove by whitening than others. Different stains require different approaches to removal (Nathoo 1997). Biologic and environmental variables affect the tenacity of the different stains. Tannin stains from tea and coffee are more tenacious and may take three or four power whitening sessions or a longer period of home whitening to remove. Tannins are composed of polyphenols such as catechins and leucoanthocyanins, and it is the gallic acid derivatives in the polyphenols that cause the yellow-brown stain. The tannins may also act as stain promotors (Eriksen and Nordbo 1978; Figure 1.28).

Classifications

Extrinsic stain can be classified as either metallic or nonmetallic. However, this classification does not explain the mechanism of discoloration, and because staining is multifactorial, not all metals cause discoloration. Nathoo (1997) has proposed a classification based on the chemistry of the discoloration. This theoretic classification does not explain stains on teeth that start off as extrinsic stain and become intrinsic stain, such as nicotine staining; however, it is worth setting out in what follows as an explanation of extrinsic staining alone.

The deposition of extrinsic stain depends on the attraction of materials to the tooth surface (Nathoo and Gaffar 1995). The attraction forces include long-range interactive forces such as electrostatic and van der Waals forces and short-range interactions such as hydration forces, hydrophobic interactions, dipole-dipole forces, and hydrogen bonds (Nathoo 1997). These chemical attractive forces allow the chromogen (colored material) and prechromogen (colorless material) to approach the tooth surface and determine if adhesion will occur. The chromogens penetrate into the enamel.

- *N1-type dental stain* (direct dental stain): The chromogen binds to the tooth surface to cause tooth discoloration. The color of the chromogen is similar to that of the dental stain. Examples of these direct dental stains are the bacterial adhesion to the pellicle and formation of salivary pellicle (Eriksen et al. 1985) experienced with tea, coffee, wine, and metals (Figure 1.31). These materials generate color owing to the presence of conjugated double bonds and are thought to interact with the tooth surface via an ion exchange mechanism. Enamel that is bathed in saliva has a negative charge, which is counterbalanced by the Stern layer or hydration layer. The metal ions in this Stern layer are responsible for staining. These stains can be prevented by good oral hygiene and can be easily removed with prophylaxis paste or toothpaste.
- *N2-type dental stain* (direct dental stain): The chromogen changes color after binding to the tooth. Examples of this stain are food that has aged and the age-related formation of yellowish discoloration on the interproximal or gingival areas and increases in brown pellicle (Figure 1.27). N1-type food stains are known to darken to N2-type stains. N2 stains are more difficult to remove and may require professional cleaning.
- *N3-type dental stain* (indirect dental stain): The prechromogen binds to the tooth and undergoes a chemical reaction to cause a stain. The chromogenic material of chlorhexidine stain contains furfurals and furfuraldehydes. These compounds are intermediate products of a series of rearrangement reactions between sugars and amino acids termed the Maillard nonenzymatic browning reaction (Eriksen et al. 1985). Examples of this include browning of foods that are high in carbohydrates and sugars, such as apples and potatoes (Figures 1.31 [coffee stain] and 1.33 [food stain causing a browning reaction]). Cooking oils also can cause browning of teeth. Furfurals are also found in baked products and fruit. Dental stain from therapeutic agents such as stannous fluoride can also be classified as N3-type stains. Discoloration is caused by a redox reaction between stannous ions and the sulfhydryl groups in the pellicle proteins. These are the most difficult stains to remove and would probably require oxygenating agents such as carbamide peroxide.

It may be that tea and coffee in the freshly prepared state cause more staining of teeth and dental restorations than instant brands (Rosen et al. 1989). Tea stains glass ionomer restorations more than coffee does (Rosen et al. 1989), and chlorhexidine in combination with tea may cause more staining than in combination with coffee.

CONCLUSION

Before commencement of whitening treatment, it is essential to question the patient to determine the cause of the discoloration. In some instances, there may be a multifactorial component; the discoloration can be a result of the accumulation of stain, aging, and dietary factors over many years.

REFERENCES

Antonini LG, Luder HU. (2011) Discoloration of teeth from tetracyclines—even today? *Schweiz Monatsschr Zahnmed* **121**(5):414–31.

Abbott PV. (1997) Aesthetic considerations in endodontics: internal bleaching. *Pract Periodont Aesthet Dent* **9**(7):833–40.

Addy M, Moran J. (1985) Extrinsic tooth discoloration by metals and chlorhexidine. 2. Clinical staining produced by chlorhexidine, iron and tea. *Br Dent J* **159**:331–4.

Addy M, Moran J, Griffiths AA, Wills Wood NJ. (1985a) Extrinsic tooth discoloration by metals and chlorhexidine. 1. Surface protein denaturation or dietary precipitation? *Br Dent J* **159**:281–5.

Addy M, Moran J, Newcombe R, Warren P. (1985b) The comparative tea staining of phenolic, chlorhexidine and anti-adhesive mouthrinses. *J Clin Periodontol* **22**:923–8.

Atasu M, Genc A, Ercalik S. (1998) Enamel hypoplasia and essential staining of teeth from erythroblastosis fetalis. *J Clin Pediatr Dent* **22**(3):249–52.

Baratieri LN, Ritter AV, Monteiro S, de Andrada MAC. (1995) Non-vital tooth bleaching: guidelines for the clinician. *Quintessence Int* **26**(9):597–608.

Bishop K, Kelleher M, Briggs P, Joshi R. (1997) Wear now? An update on the etiology of tooth wear. *Quintessence Int* **28**(5):305–13.

Bowles WH, Bokmeyer TJ. (1997) Staining of adult teeth by minocycline: binding of minocycline by specific proteins. *J Esthet Dent* **9**(1):30–4.

Dayan D, Heifferman A, Gorski M, Beigleiter A. (1983) Tooth discoloration—extrinsic and intrinsic factors. *Quintessence Int* **12**(14):1–5.

Donoghue AM, Ferguson MM. (1996) Superficial copper staining of teeth in a brass foundry worker. *Occup Med (Lond)* **46**(3):233–4.

Dzierzak J. (1991) Factors which cause tooth colour change. *Pract Periodont Aesthet Dent* **3**(2):15–20.

Eley BM. (1999) Antibacterial agents in the control of supragingival plaque—a review. *Br Dent J* **186**:286–96.

Eriksen HM, Nordbo H. (1978) Extrinsic discoloration of teeth. *J Clin Periodontol* **5**:229–36.

Eriksen HM, Nordbo H, Kantanen H, Ellingsen OO. (1985) Chemical plaque control and extrinsic tooth discoloration. A review of possible mechanisms. *J Clin Periodontol* 12:345–50.

Faunce F. (1983) Management of discoloured teeth. *Dent Clin North Am* **27**(4):657–5.

Feinman RA, Goldstein RE, Garber DA. (1987) *Bleaching teeth*. Quintessence: Chicago.

Goldstein RE. (1998) Bleaching discoloured teeth. In *Esthetics in dentistry*, 2nd edn. Vol 1: *Principles, communications, treatment methods*. BC Decker: London, 245–76.

Greenwall LH. (1992) The effects of carbamide peroxide on tooth colour and structures: an *in vitro* investigation. MSc thesis, University of London.

Hayes PA, Full C, Pinkham J. (1986) The etiology and treatment of intrinsic discolorations. *J Can Dent Assoc* **52**:217–20.

Haywood VB. (1997) Extended bleaching of tetracycline-stained teeth: a case report. *Contemp Esthet Restor Pract* **1**(1):14–21.

Ismail AI, Hasson H. (2008) Fluoride supplements, dental caries and fluorosis: a systematic review. *J Am Dent Assoc* **139**(11):1457–68.

Jedeon K, De la Dure-Molla M, Brookes SJ, Loiodice S. (2013) Enamel defects reflect perinatal exposure to bisphenol A. Am J Pathol **183**(1):108–18.

Jordan RE, Boksman L. (1984) Conservative vital bleaching treatment of discoloured dentition. *Compend Contin Educ Dent* **V**(10):803–7.

Kidd EA. (1991) The caries status of tooth-coloured restorations with marginal stain. *Br Dent J* **171**:241–3.

Kidd EA, Joyston-Bechal S, Beighton D. (1995) Marginal ditching and staining as a predictor of secondary caries around amalgam restorations: a clinical and microbiological study. *J Dent Res* **74**(5):1206–11.

Kleter GA. (1998) Discoloration of dental carious lesions (a review). *Arch Oral Biol* **43**(8):629–32.

Krastl G, Allgayer N, Lenherr P, Filippi A. (2013). Tooth discoloration induced by endodontic materials: a literature review. *Dent Traumatol* **29**(1):2–7.

Leard A, Addy M. (1997) The propensity of different brands of tea and coffee to cause staining associated with chlorhexidine. *J Clin Periodontol* **24**:115–18.

Louka AN. (1989) Esthetic treatment of anterior teeth. *J Can Dent Assoc* **55**(1):29–32.

Love RM, Chandler NP. (1996) A scanning electron and confocal laser microscope investigation of tetracycline-affected human dentine. *Int Endodont J* **29**:376–81.

Marin PD, Bartold PM, Hiethersay GS. (1997) Tooth discoloration by blood: an in-vitro histochemical study. *Endodont Dent Traumatol* **13**:132–8.

McCaslin A, Haywood VB, Potter BJ, Dickinson GL. (1999) Assessing dentin color changes from Nightguard Vital Bleaching. *J Am Dent Assoc* 130:1485–90.

McKenna BE, Lamely PJ, Kennedy JG, Batten J. (1999) Minocycline-induced staining of the adult permanent dentition: a review of the literature and report of a case. *Dent Update* **24**(4):160–2.

Morley J. (1997) The esthetics of anterior tooth aging. *Curr Opin Cosmet Dent* **4**:35–9.

Nathanson D and Para C. (1987) Bleaching vital teeth: a review and clinical study. *Compendium* **8**(7):490–2, 494, 496–7.

Nathoo SA. (1997) The chemistry and mechanisms of extrinsic and intrinsic discoloration. *J Am Dent Assoc* Suppl; **128**(4):6S–10S.

Nathoo SA, Gaffar A. (1995) Studies on dental stains induced by antibacterial agents and rational approaches for bleaching dental stains. *Adv Dent Res* **9**(4):462–70.

Ness L, Rosenkrans Dde L, Welford JF. (1977) An epidemiologic study of factors affecting extrinsic staining of teeth in an English population. *Community Dent Oral Epidemiol* **5**:55–60.

Patel K, Cheshire D, Vance A. (1998) Oral and systemic effects of prolonged minocycline therapy. *Br Dent J* **185**(11/12):560–2.

Plotino G, Buono L, Grande NM, Pameiger CH. (2008) Non-vital tooth bleaching: a review of the literature and clinical procedure. *J Endodont* **34**(4):394-407.

Rose KJ, Carey CM. (1995) Intensive swimming: can it affect your patients' smiles? *J Am Dent Assoc* **126**:1402–6.

Rosen M, Christelis A, Bow P, Cohen J. (1989) Glass ionomers and discoloration: a comparative study of the effects of tea and coffee on three brands of glass ionomer dental cement. *J Dent Assoc South Africa* **44**:333–6.

Rotstein I. (1998) Bleaching nonvital and vital discolored teeth. In Cohen S, Burns RC, editors. *Pathways of the pulp*, 7th edn. Mosby: St Louis, 674.

Sánchez AR, Rogers RS 3rd, Sheridan PJ. (2004). Tetracycline and other tetracycline-derivative staining of the teeth and oral cavity. *Int J Dermatol* **43**(10):709–15.

Salman RA, Salman GD, Glickman RS, Super DG. (1985) Minocycline induced pigmentation of the oral cavity. *J Oral Med* **40**(3):154–7.

Shannon IL. (1978) Stannous fluoride: does it stain teeth? How does it react with tooth surfaces? A review. *Gen Dent* **26**(5):64–71.

Shaw L, Smith AJ. (1999) Dental erosion—the problem and some practical solutions. *Br Dent J* **186**(3):115–18.

Shearer AC. (1991) External bleaching of teeth. *Dent Update* **18**(7):289–91.

Smith BG, Knight JK. (1984) An index for measuring the wear of teeth. *Br Dent J* 156(4):435–8.

Solheim (1988) Dental colour as indicator of age. *Gerodontics* **4**:114–18.

Swift EJ. (1988) A method for bleaching discoloured vital teeth. *Quintessence Int* **19**(9):607–11.

Teo CS. (1989) Management of tooth discoloration. *Acta Med Singapore* **18**(5):585–90.

Thomas MS, Denny C (2014) Medication-related tooth-discoloration: a review. *Dent Update* **41**(5):440–2, 445–7.

van der Bijl P, Ptitgoi-Aron G. (1995) Tetracyclines and calcified tissues. *Ann Dent* **54**(1/2):69–72.

van der Burgt TP, Eronat C, Plasschaert AJ. (1986a) Staining patterns in teeth discoloured by endodontic sealers. *J Endodont* **12**(5):187–91.

van der Burgt TP, Mullaney TP, Plasschaert AJ. (1986b) Tooth discoloration induced by endodontic sealers. *Oral Surg Oral Med Oral Pathol* **61:**84–9.

Watanabe K, Shibata T, Kurosawa T, Morisaki I. (1999) Bilirubin pigmentation of human teeth caused by hyperbilirubinemia. *J Oral Pathol Med* **28**(3):128–30.

Watson IB, Tulloch EN. (1985) Clinical assessment of cases of tooth surface loss. *Br Dent J* **159**:144–8.

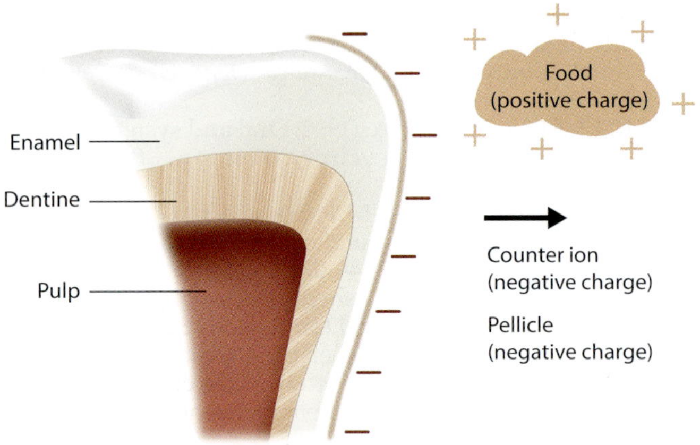

Figure 1.1

Nathoo classification Nl-type mechanism: binding of food substances via ion exchange.

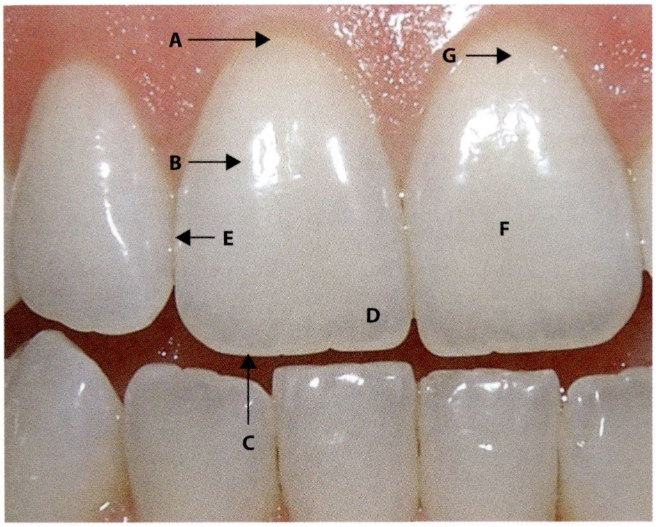

(A)

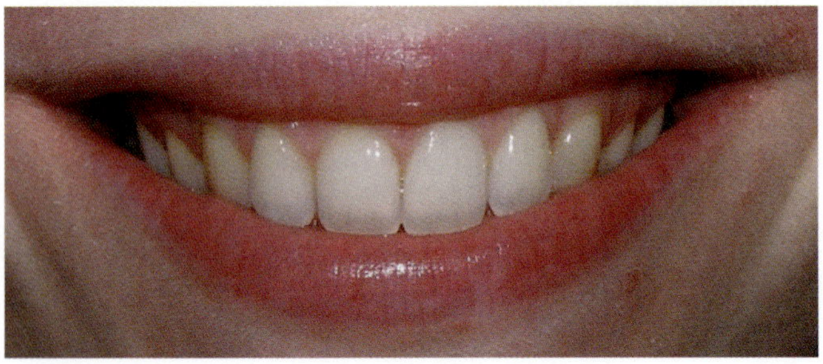

(B)

Figure 1.2

(A) The color of natural healthy teeth of a young person showing incisal translucency and healthy gingivae. *A,* The cervical margin; *B,* the body of the tooth; *C,* the incisal tip; *D,* translucency; *E,* the interproximal areas; *F,* the enamel; *G,* the dentin. (B) The color of natural healthy teeth, seen in conjunction with the lips and skin.

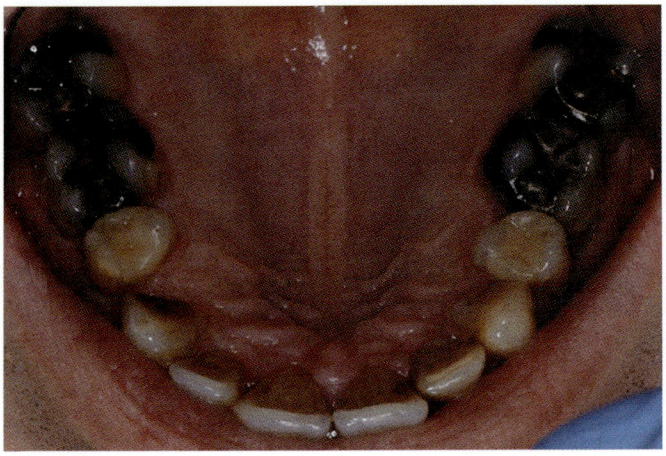

Figure 1.3

Discoloration of multiple restorations. Palatal view of stained restorations is shown. The effect of large amalgam restorations, old stained composite restorations, and extrinsic stain on the palatal aspects of the anterior teeth caused by heavy coffee consumption and poor oral hygiene.

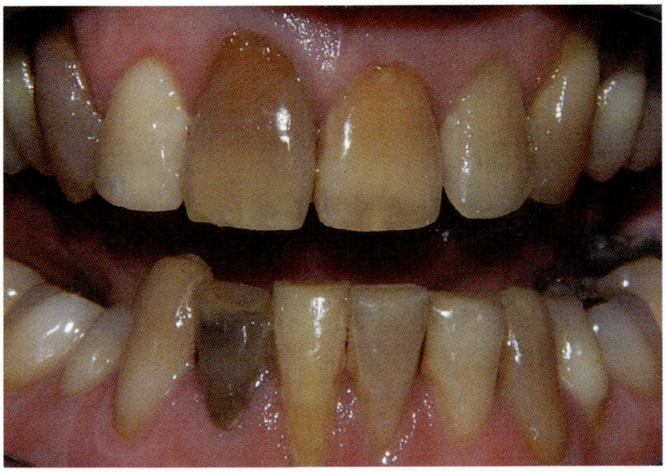

(A)

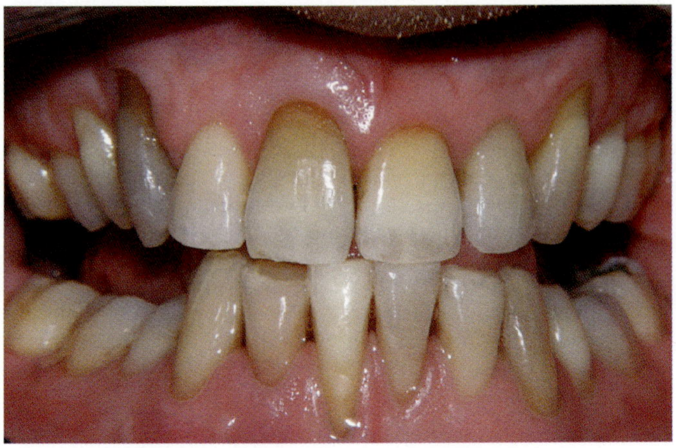

(B)

Figure 1.4

(A) Multiple colors of discoloration on the upper anterior teeth as a result of trauma and surgery. This patient had a maxillary osteotomy. (B) The result after whitening with 10% carbamide peroxide in the trays. The lower second incisor was treated with the sealed-in whitening technique using 16% carbamide peroxide.

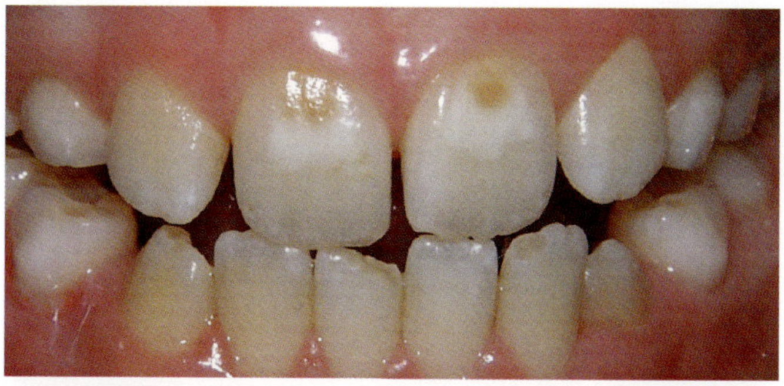

Figure 1.5

Enamel hypocalcification: white and brown spots on the facial surfaces of the upper central incisors.

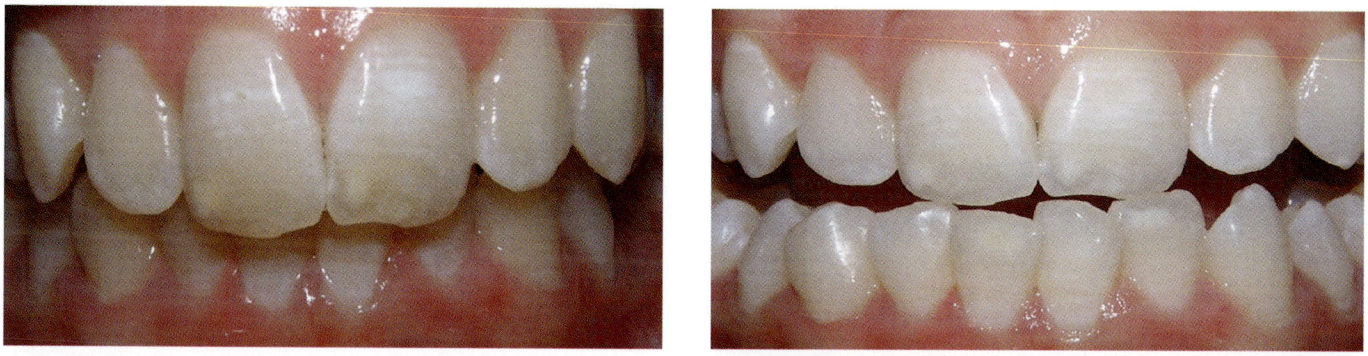

(A) (B)

Figure 1.6

(A) White developmental lines: patient has white lines on the centrals and laterals. This may have been caused by a high fever during chronologic tooth development. There is a temporary disruption in the enamel formation. The patient had taken Amoxil antibiotic. (B) After whitening with 10% carbamide peroxide, the teeth have been whitened and the white lines are less noticeable.

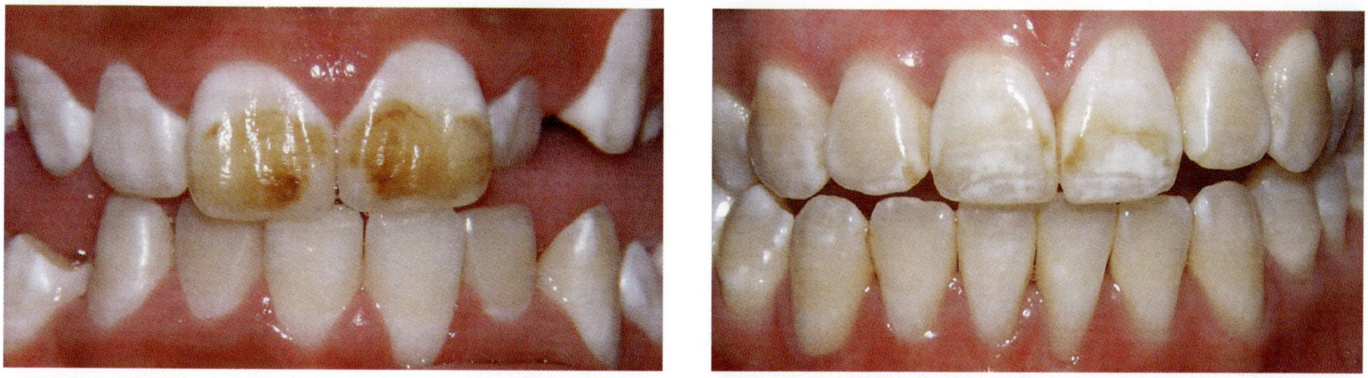

(A) (B)

Figure 1.7

(A) Generalized fluorosis, which had discolored further over time, in an 11-year-old girl, especially on the upper central incisor teeth. (B) Intermediate case of fluorosis affecting the upper central incisors. Brown and white discoloration present on more teeth.

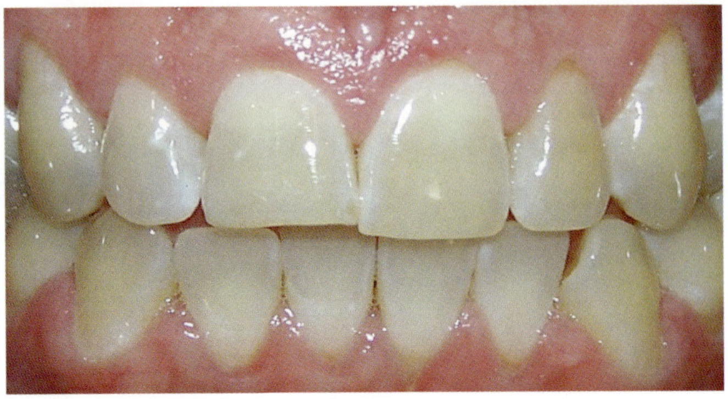

(A)

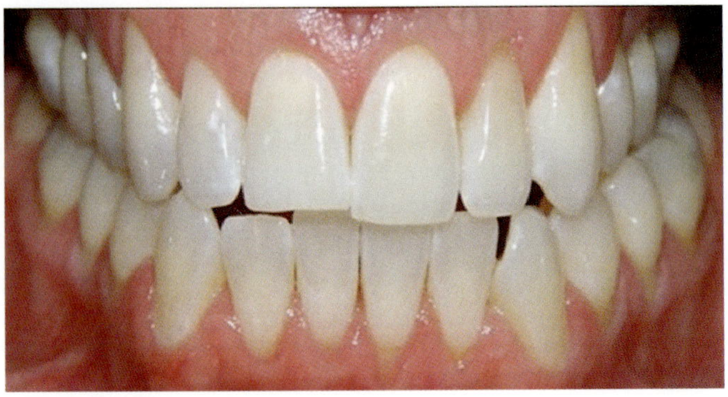

(B)

Figure 1.8

(A) Tetracycline staining. First-degree tetracycline staining without banding. This is amenable with whitening. This level shows a basic gray shade to the teeth. (B) The result after whitening of the teeth for 6 weeks with 10% carbamide peroxide.

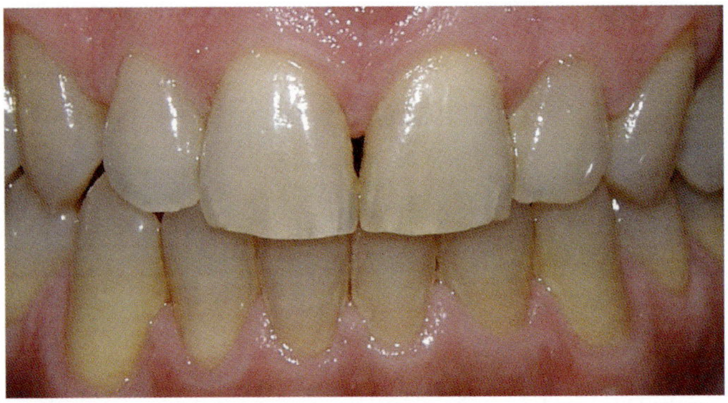

Figure 1.9

Tetracycline staining. Second-degree staining shows stronger staining with a more yellow-gray appearance and banding at the cervical margin. This is amendable with whitening, although it may take longer.

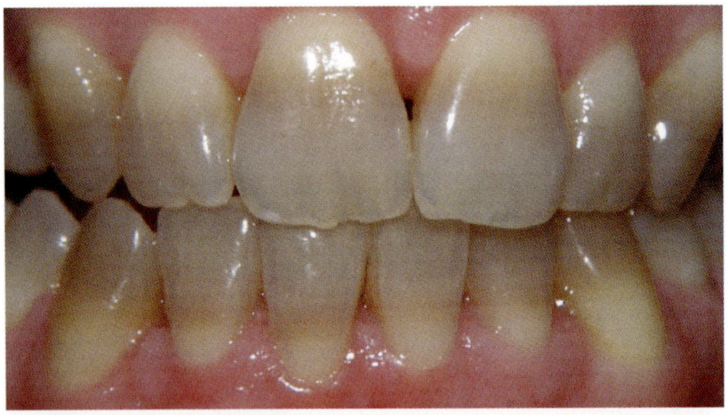

(A)

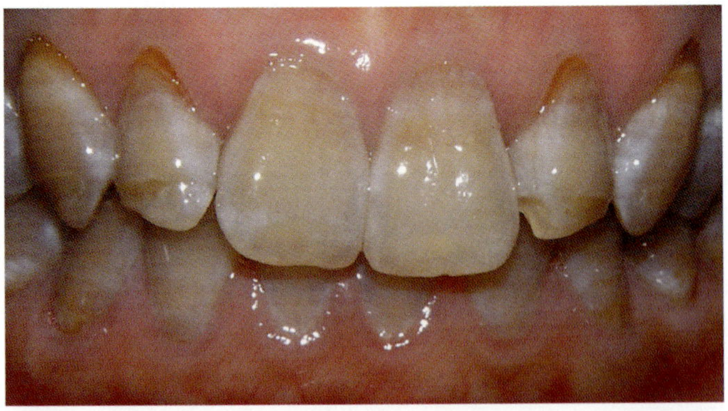

(C)

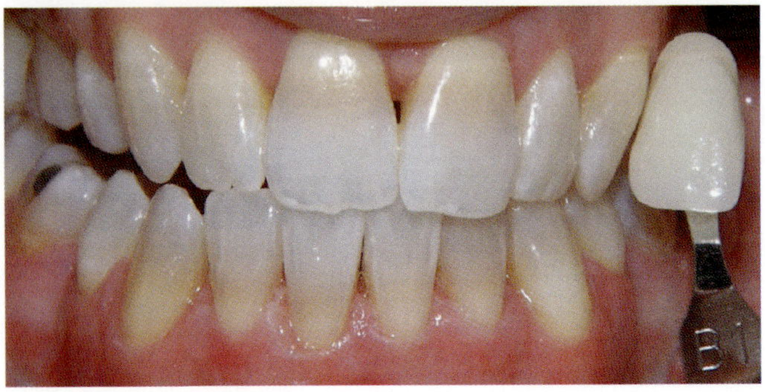

(B)

Figure 1.10

(A) Third-degree tetracycline staining: banding with gray-blue staining. This may be amendable with whitening, but patients have to be aware that it may take up to 6 months to achieve satisfactory lightening. The banding present may not necessarily disappear with whitening. (B) Result after 3 months of whitening a case of type 3 tetracycline staining. (C) Third-degree tetracycline discoloration in combination with enamel hypoplasia. In addition to the tetracycline discoloration, this patient has defects of the enamel formation on the upper lateral incisor teeth and the lower premolar teeth, as well as cervical resorption showing an orange banding at this area.

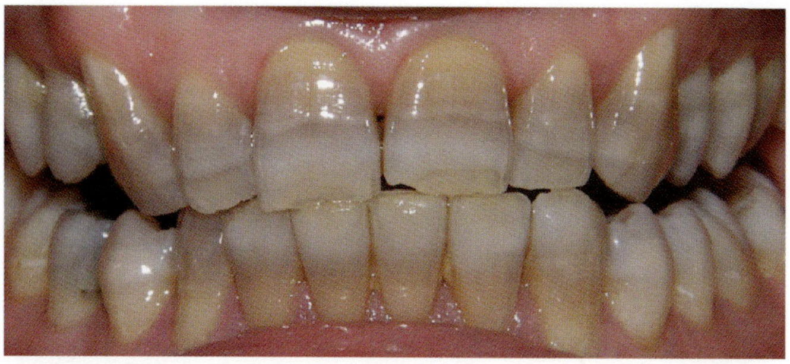

Figure 1.11

Fourth-degree tetracycline staining. Fourth-degree banding shows the different banding of yellow, gray, and blue. It is more severe and demarcated.

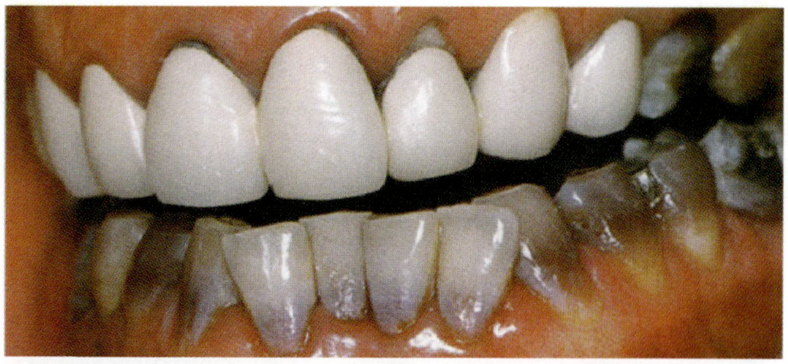

Figure 1.12

Fourth-degree staining. The discoloration is so dark that it may not respond to whitening. In this case the patient had had the upper teeth crowned 21 years previously. Besides crowning of the teeth, the other realistic treatment options available at that time were intentional endodontic treatment and intracoronal whitening. There are now additional more conservative options, which would include whitening followed by porcelain laminate veneers. Whitening treatment can always be discussed with the patient. In this case, the worst that could happen is no change in color, but it is worth a try. Gingival recession has occurred around the crown margins, and there are areas of cervical decay. These restorations will need replacement.

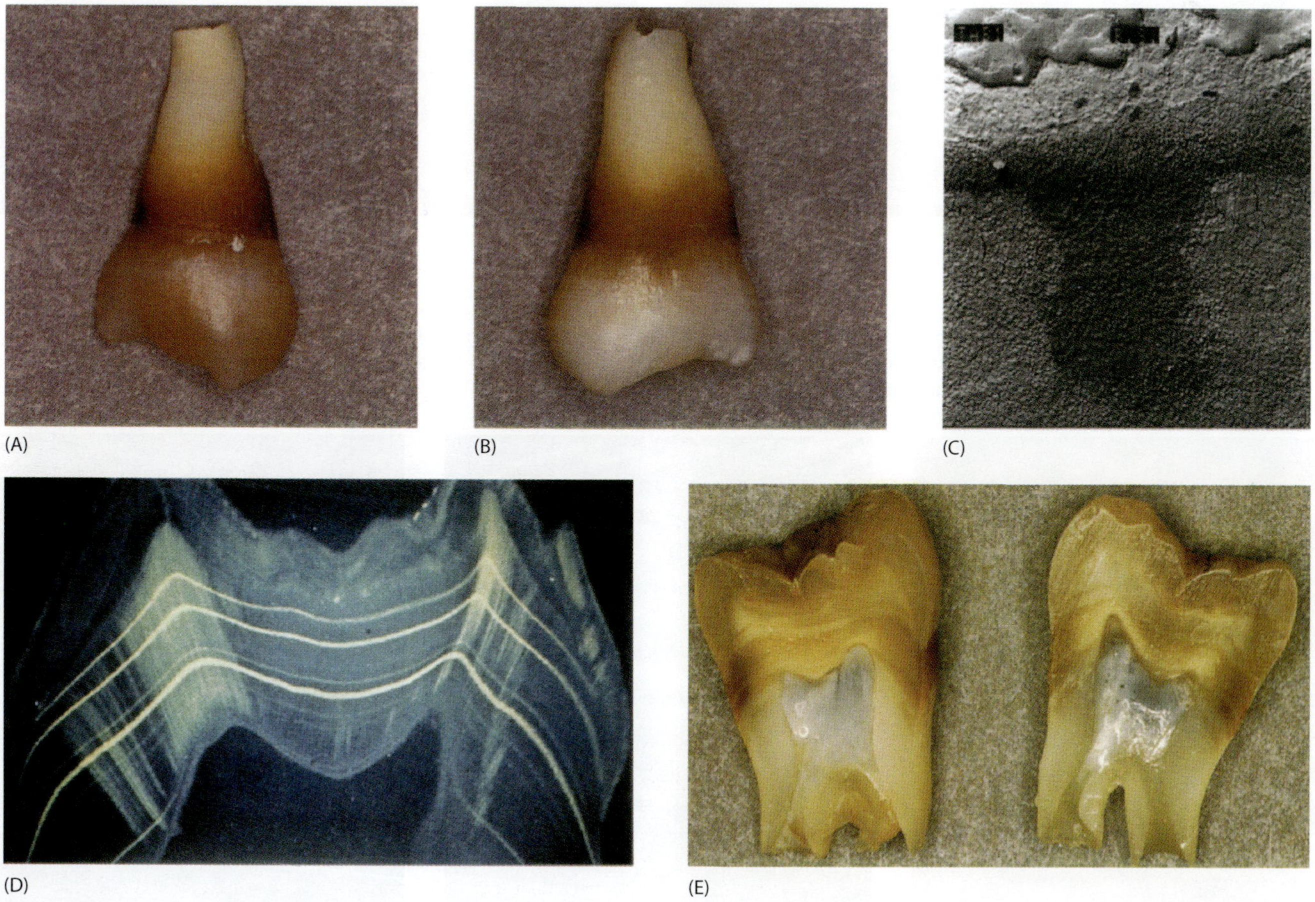

Figure 1.13

Tetracycline staining on extracted teeth. (A) Characteristic banding on the teeth that occurs through the dentin. (B) This experimental tooth has been successfully lightened using a 10% carbamide peroxide material. (From Greenwall 1992.) (C) A scanning electron microscope view of the banded area of the tetracycline-stained tooth at the junction of the enamel and the dentin (×120). The dentin in the affected band appears different from the surrounding dentin. The mineralizing front of the unaffected dentin is normal in appearance. The mineralizing front of the tetracycline-affected dentin band is devoid of calcospherite formation. (From Love and Chandler 1996.) There are many surface defects. (D) Under fluorescent light the banding of tetracycline teeth becomes visible in the dentin layers. (Courtesy of Dr. I. Rotstein.) (E) A tetracycline tooth in section showing the characteristic banding.

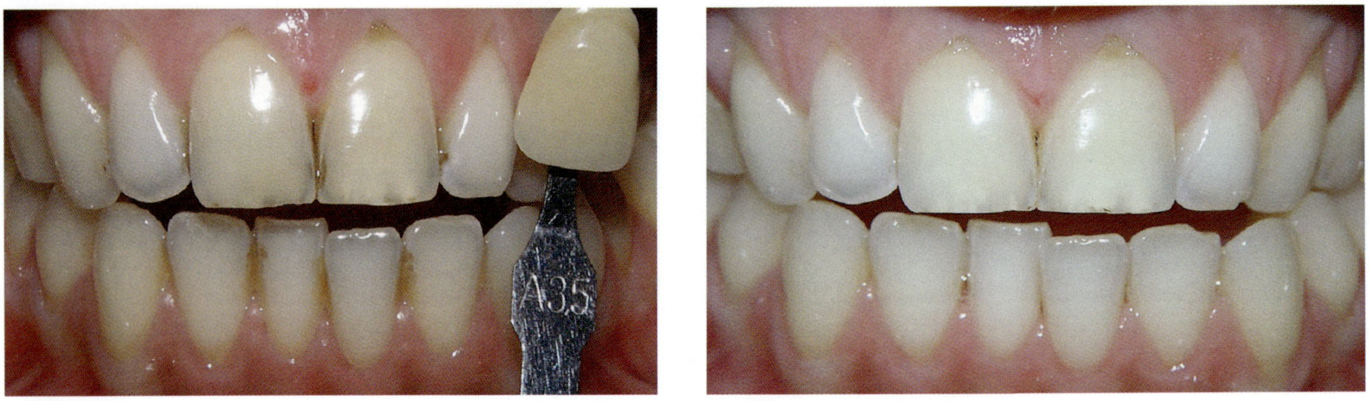

(A) (B)

Figure 1.14

(A) Pulpal changes. Different shade of teeth as a result of trauma to the central incisors, which display calcific metamorphosis. The upper central incisors are darker than the adjacent teeth. (B) Result after whitening: central incisors are darker than the other teeth because of trauma. Window whitening tray is made to whiten central teeth, then full tray is used to whiten the rest to blend in.

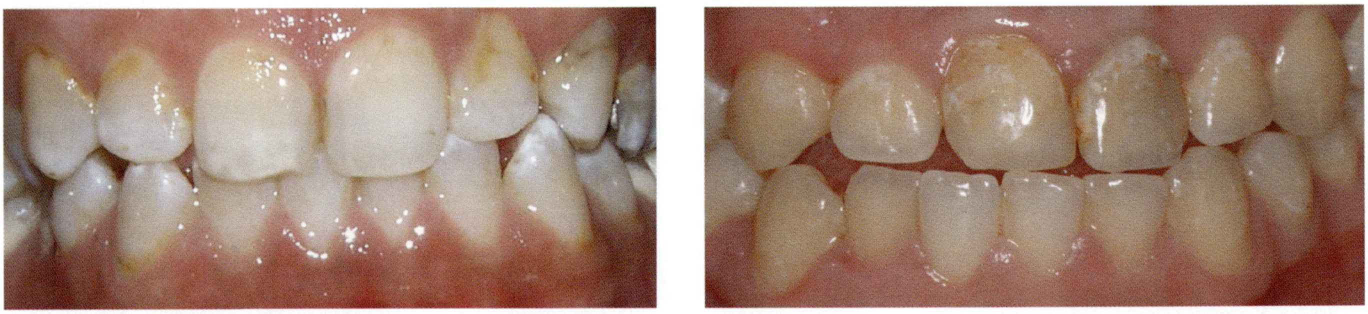

(A) (B)

Figure 1.15

(A) Patient with hemophilia. This patient has stained teeth and precarious lesions owing to poor oral hygiene. (B) Patient with white and brown staining. The teeth have brown and yellow staining owing to early root decay and poor oral hygiene. There is decalcification present, including in the upper left central incisor, which is nonvital.

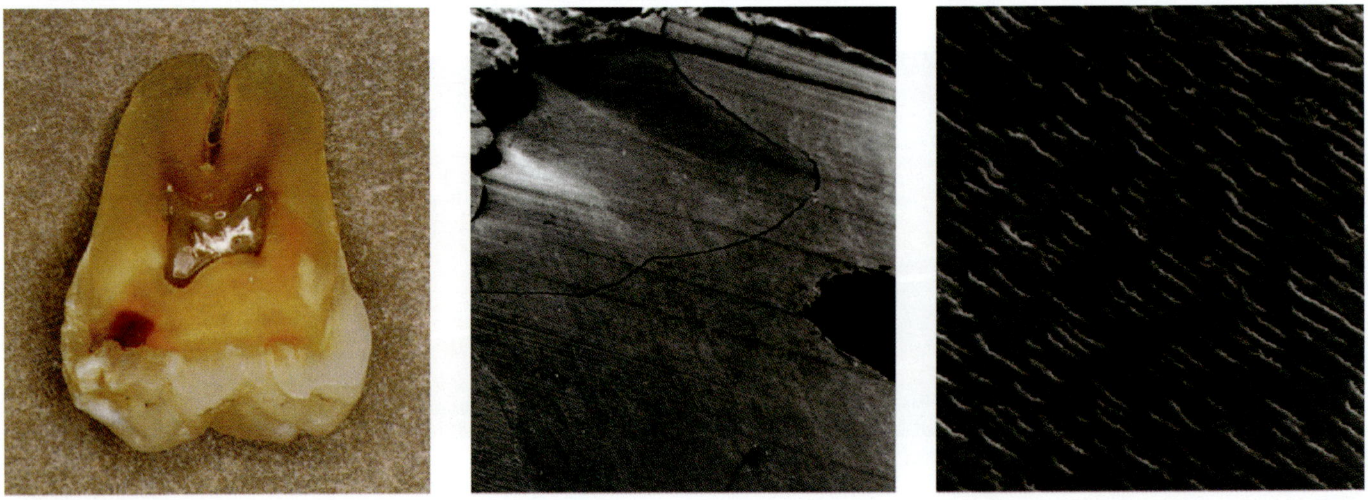

(A) (B) (C)

Figure 1.16

Dental caries. (A) Tooth in longitudinal sections exposing a primary lesion within the dentin layers. The caries is stained brown and has a white edge. The brown discoloration may be a result of the initial products of the Maillard reaction, which is formed in the carious lesion (Kleter 1998). The carious lesion can take up food dyes, making it become brown in color, and metal ions, which make it black. (B) Scanning electron micrograph of the carious lesion showing the shallow lesion (×40). (C) Scanning electron micrograph of the dentin showing the cleansing effect of the whitening material on the caries.

continued on next page

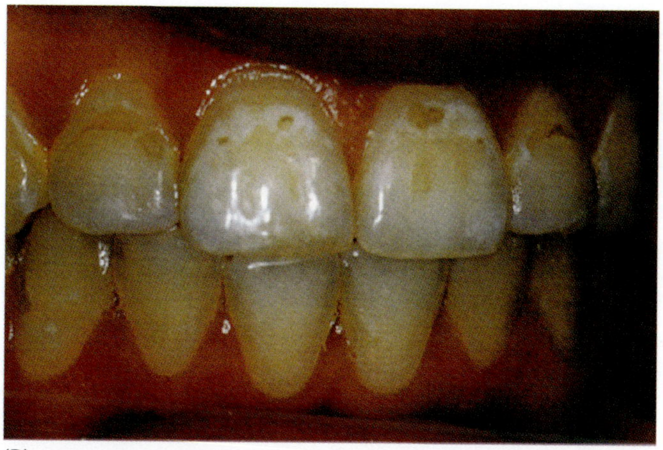

(D)

Figure 1.16 continued

(D) This patient has brown staining that developed around orthodontic bands.

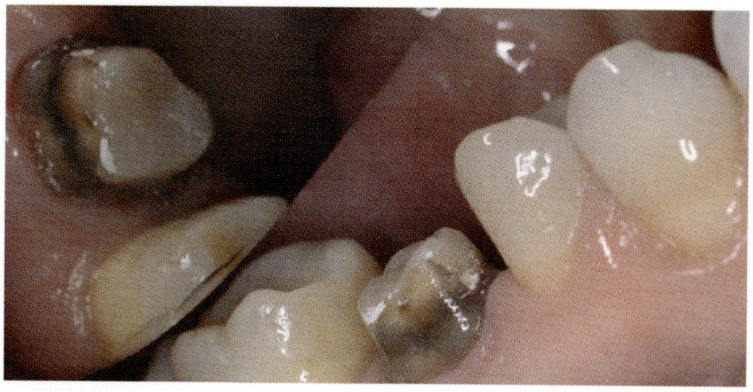

Figure 1.17

Amalgam staining. Lower first molar demonstrates blue staining caused by large previous amalgam restorations.

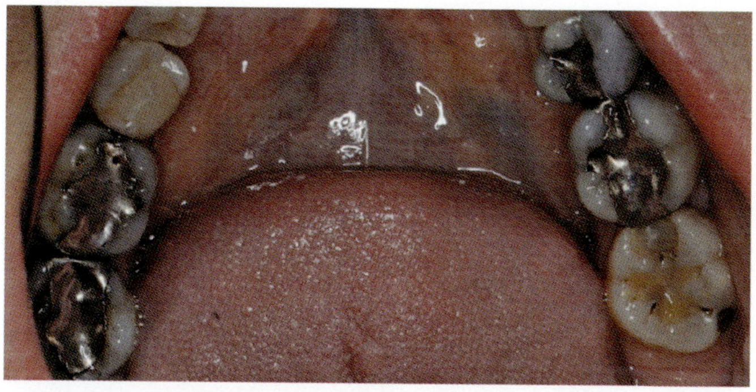

Figure 1.18

Amalgam staining. Multiple posterior restorations have been present for many years and caused the teeth to discolor.

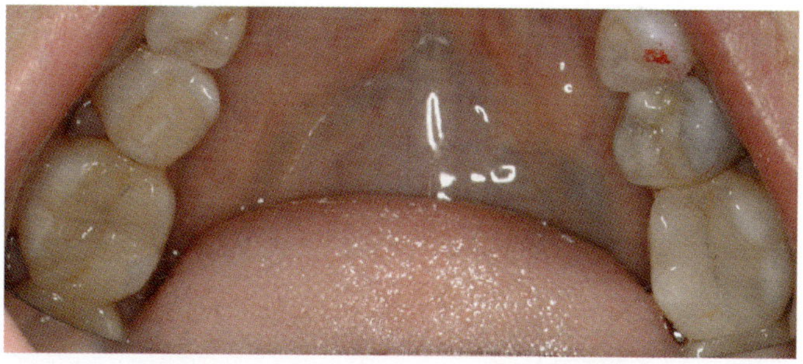

Figure 1.19

Results after replacement of the amalgam restorations with porcelain inlays and crowns.

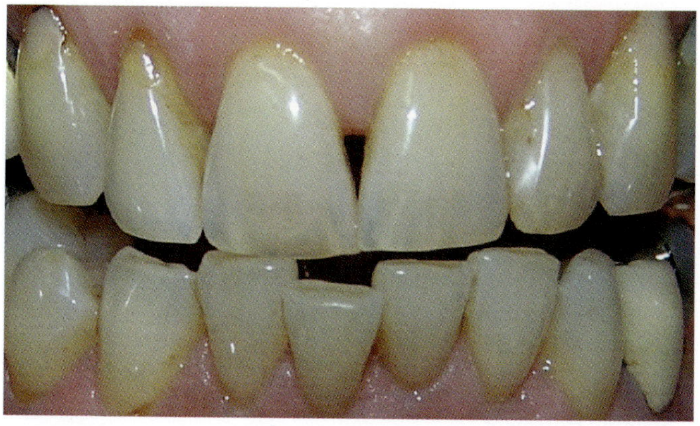

Figure 1.20

Aging enamel. The patient has color changes caused by thinning enamel and root caries developing on the upper right canine tooth.

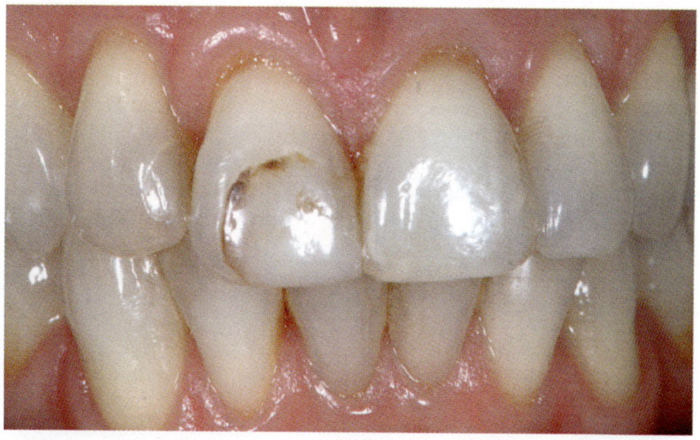

Figure 1.21

A leaking composite restoration caused by poor oral hygiene and restoration overhang. This discoloration was removed by reshaping the excess composite restoration and repolishing the edges of the restoration to a smooth luster.

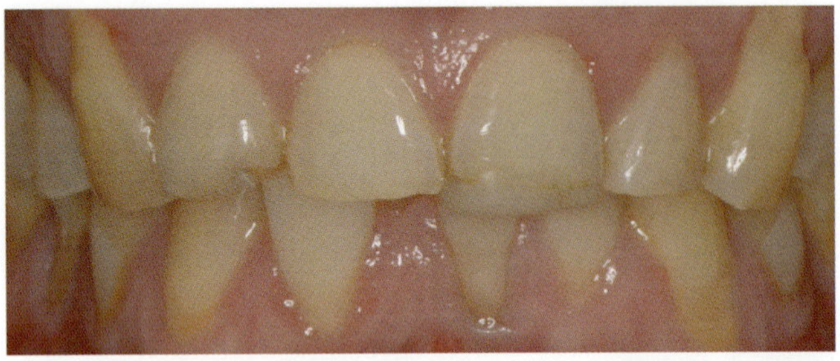

Figure 1.22

The appearance of the teeth of a patient with gastric reflux. The teeth are crowded and the incisal edges are uneven owing to the erosion and wear on the teeth. The teeth are discolored to a yellow shade.

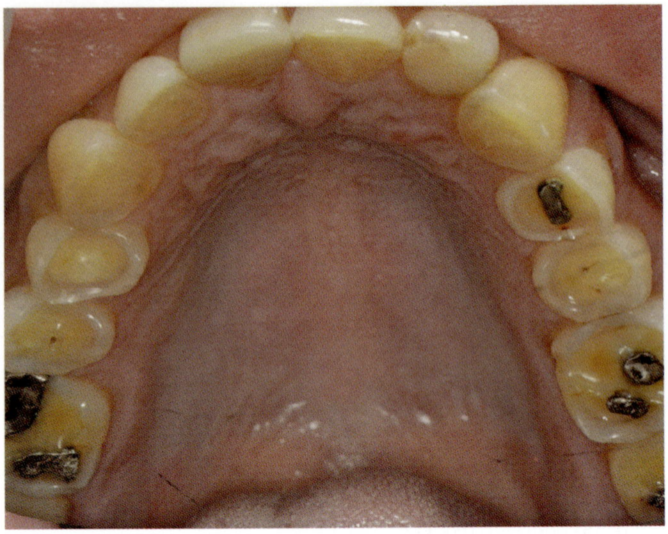

Figure 1.23

Palatal mirror view of the teeth showing erosion of enamel and exposure of dentin, which has a yellow appearance.

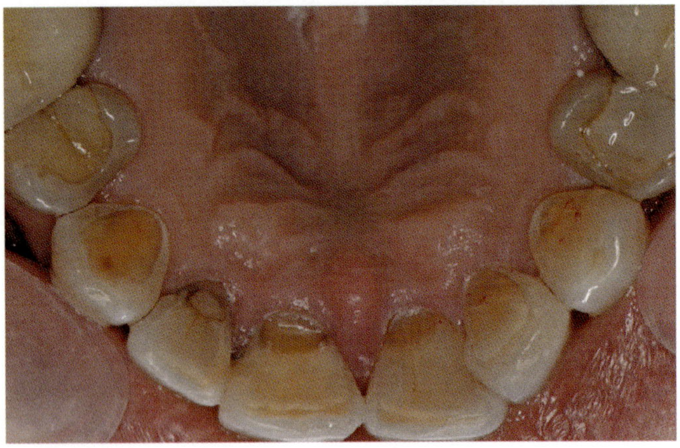

Figure 1.24

Combination of attrition and erosion on upper palatal surfaces of the anterior teeth. The patient had whitened the teeth first, and this palatal view shows the appearance of the attrition on the palatal surfaces. The patient has a very deep bite. The treatment for this patient involved six palatal composite veneers that were made by the dental technician then cemented onto these palatal areas to prevent further damage to the teeth. The bite was opened 2 mm immediately, and these veneers acted as a type of Dahl appliance. The patient reported that he accommodated the new changes in the bite within a period of 10 days.

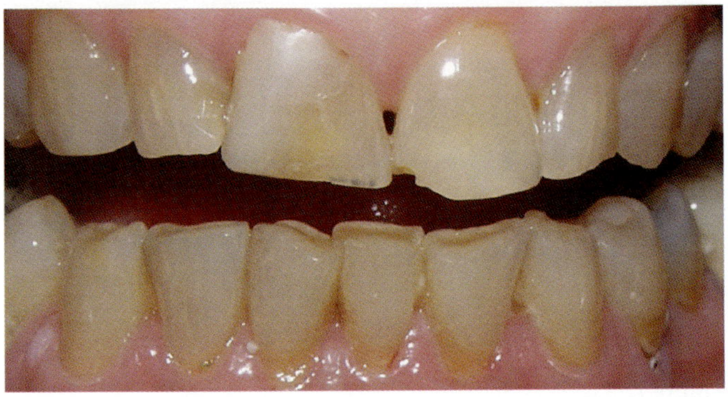

Figure 1.25

Parafunctional changes have caused loss of incisal edges. White fracture lines are present. There is a corner missing on the upper left central incisor tooth. The lower incisors show attrition and wear of the incisal edges.

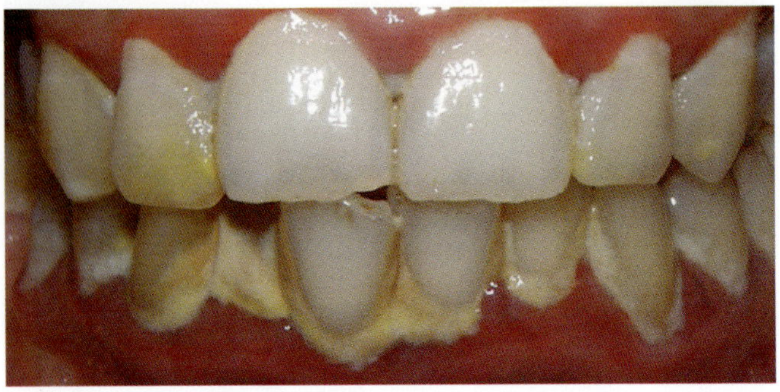

Figure 1.26

Large buildup of plaque and tartar as a result of poor oral hygiene. This will not be removed with brushing. Extensive deep cleaning appointments and oral hygiene education on brushing techniques with the hygienist are required. Good home care is essential to prevent further buildup. This patient also wished to whiten her teeth. Oral hygiene and periodontal treatment were undertaken first, before any whitening treatment.

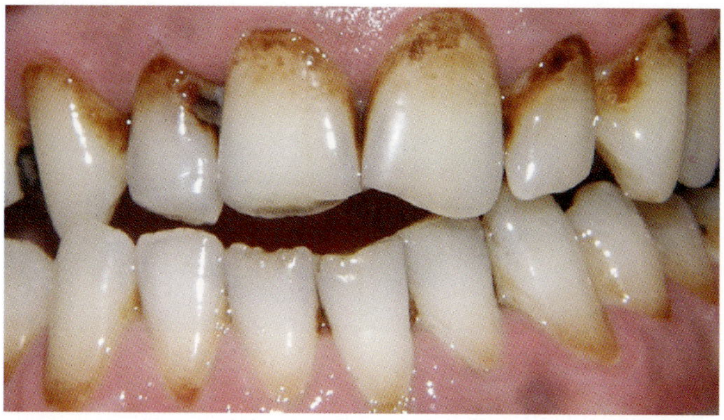

Figure 1.27

Coffee staining on teeth: patient drinks five or more cups per day, smokes cigars, and has root caries at the cervical area of his anterior teeth and poor oral hygiene.

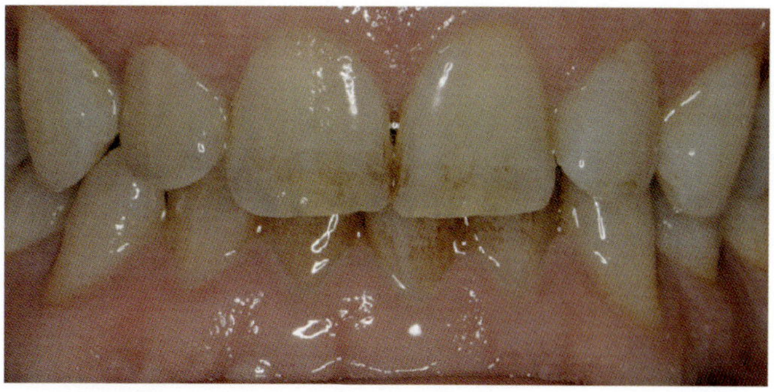

Figure 1.28

Patient has four cups of black tea per day.

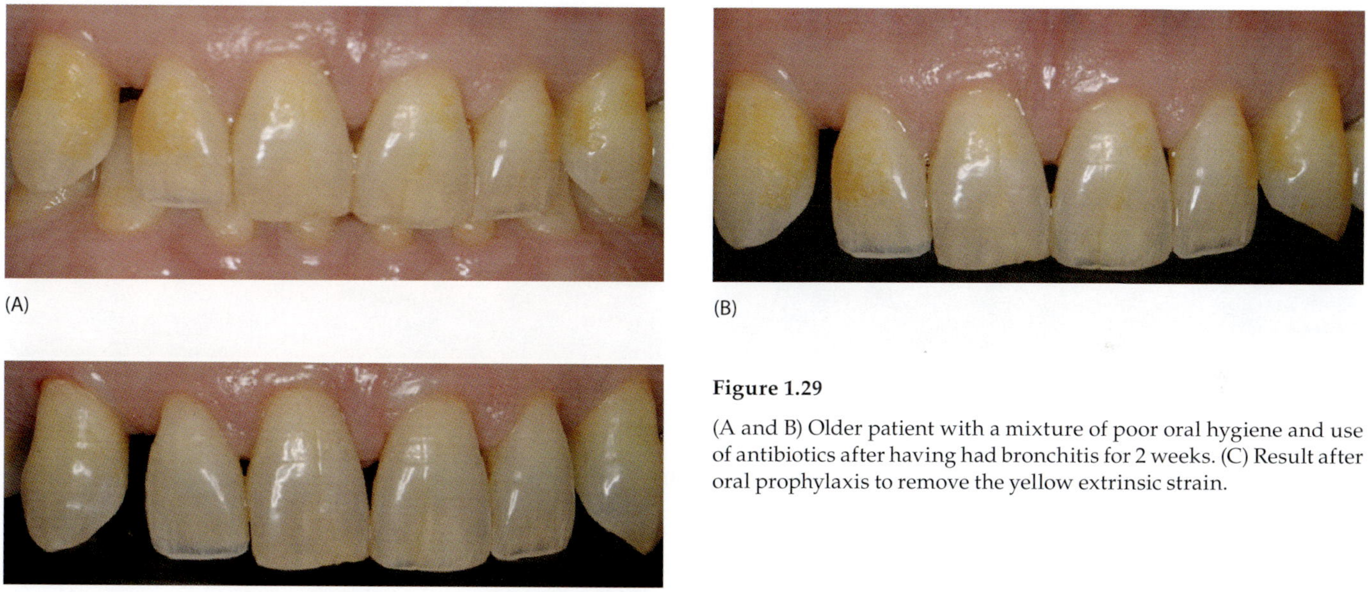

(A)

(B)

(C)

Figure 1.29

(A and B) Older patient with a mixture of poor oral hygiene and use of antibiotics after having had bronchitis for 2 weeks. (C) Result after oral prophylaxis to remove the yellow extrinsic strain.

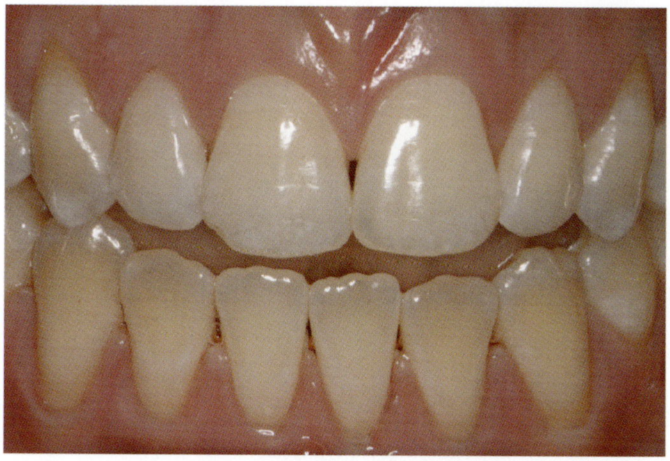

Figure 1.30

This younger patient's teeth started to discolor after a course of intravenous antibiotics and a change in medical history.

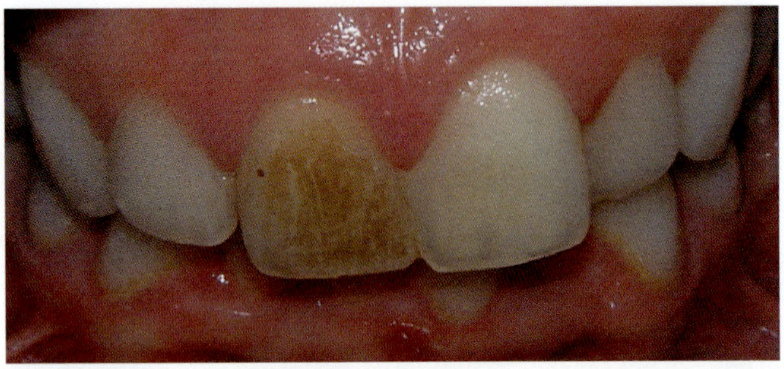

Figure 1.31

Coffee staining imposed on top of a discolored nonvital anterior tooth. The nonvital tooth was then whitened.

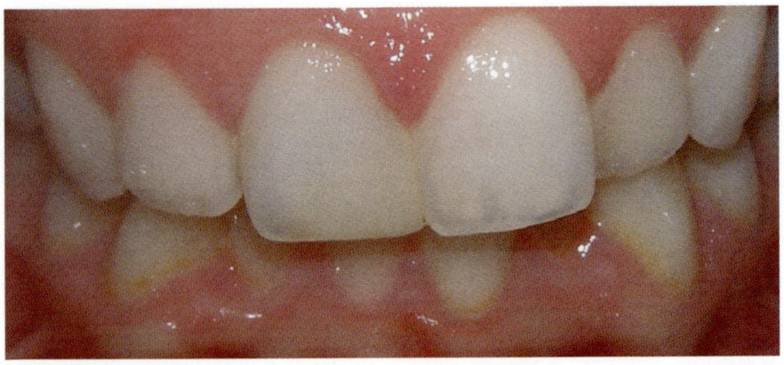

Figure 1.32

The nonvital tooth was whitened internally using 20% carbamide peroxide, and the extrinsic staining removed with prophylaxis.

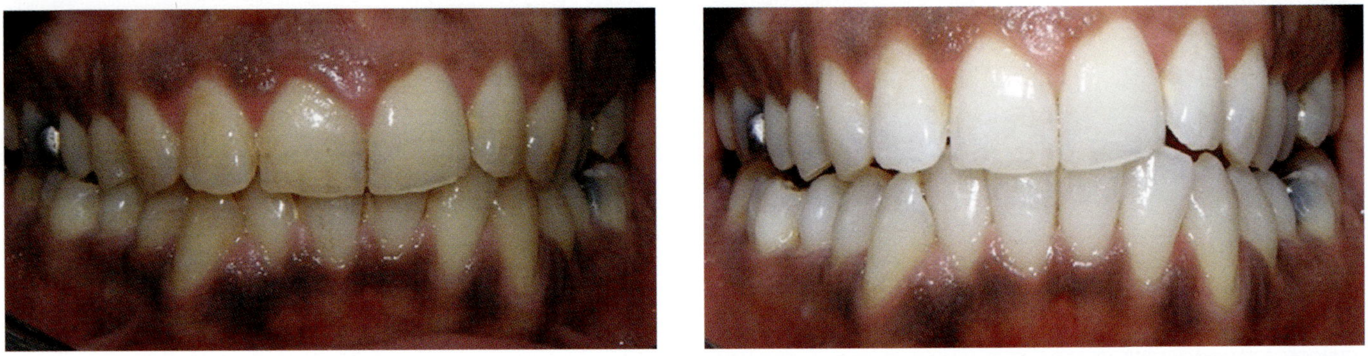

(A) (B)

Figure 1.33

(A) Patient's diet consists of fried food; he smokes 10 cigarettes per day. (B) Result after home whitening using 10% carbamide peroxide whitening for 6 weeks.

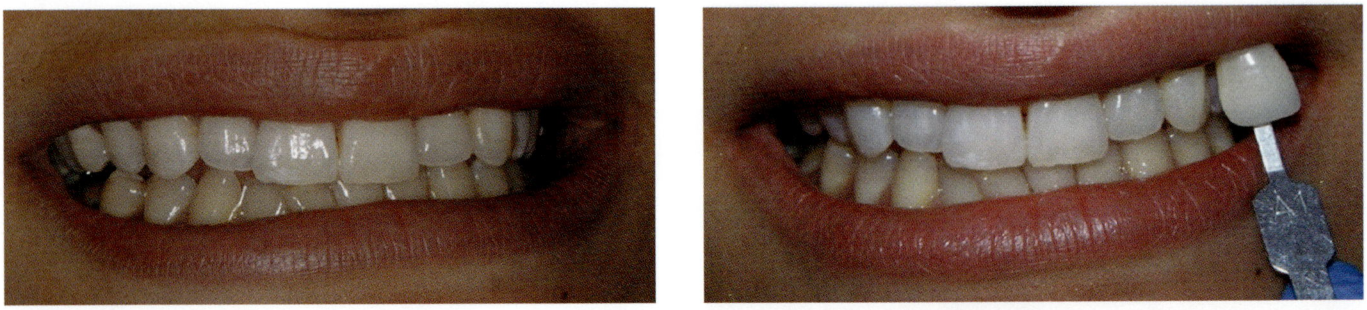

(A) (B)

Figure 1.34

(A) Patient took iron tablets for 3 years because of a complex medical history after trauma. The intake of iron tablets resulted in the teeth developing a gray discoloration, particularly noticeable on the lower incisor teeth. (B) Result after whitening for 6 weeks.

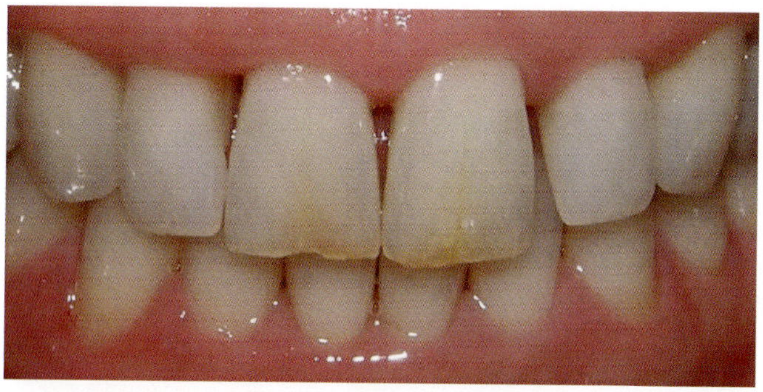

Figure 1.35

Dark crack lines remain after whitening. This patient smoked and had brown lines present on the teeth. After whitening the brown crack lines changed to orange.

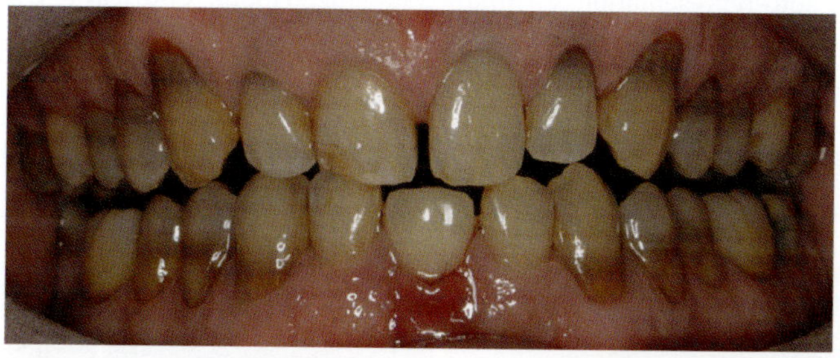

Figure 1.37

Patient with numerous problems: tetracycline staining, peri-implantitis of the lower central incisor implant, and abrasion lesions. There are numerous abrasion lesions on the lower premolar teeth, which were filled in with glass ionomer restorations.

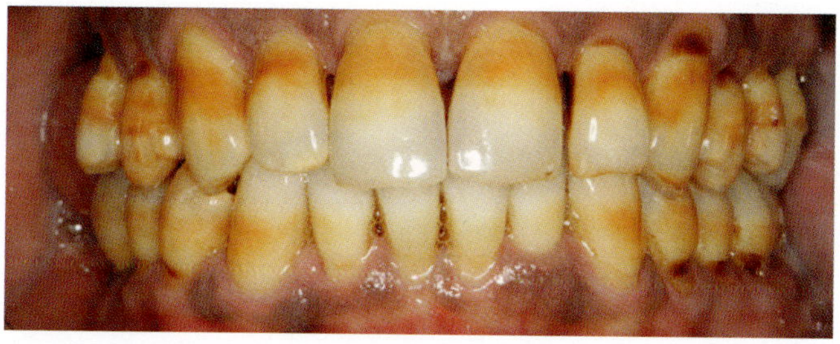

Figure 1.39

Quat discoloration. This type of discoloration is caused by a type of chewing tobacco. (With permission from Dr. Nils Calcar.)

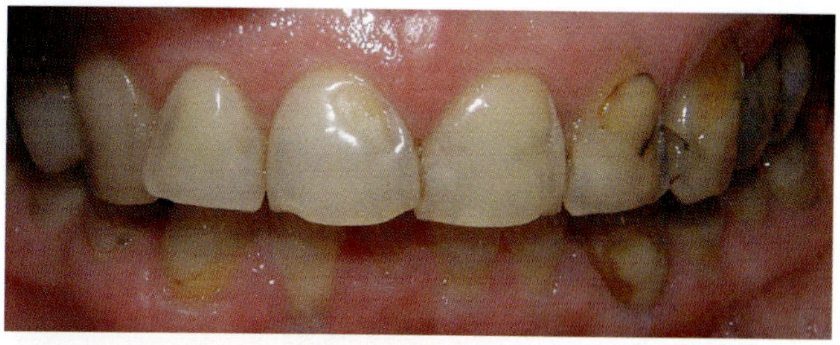

Figure 1.36

Wear and erosion on the buccal surface of the upper left lateral and canine tooth. These teeth are not suitable for whitening because there is insufficient enamel present.

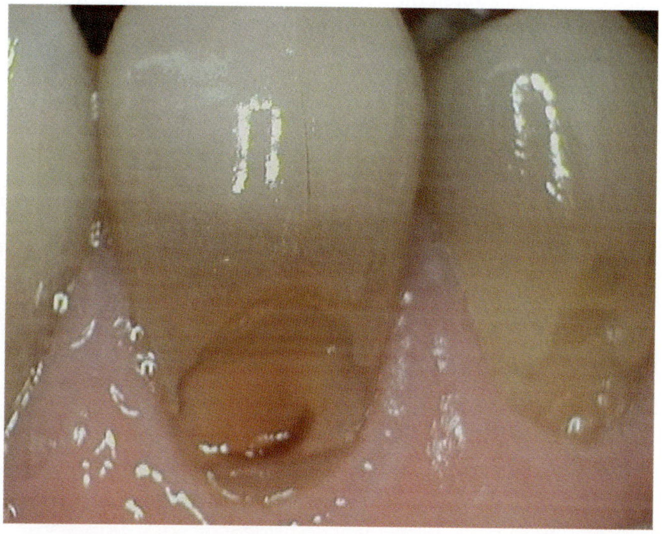

Figure 1.38

The cervical of the tooth surface loss that may be attributable to erosion, attrition, and abrasion.

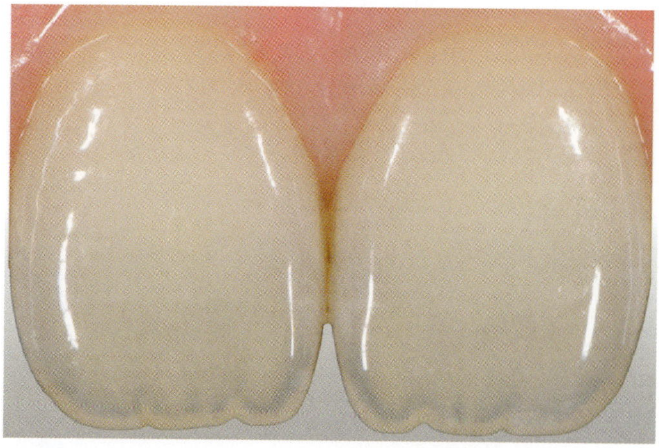

Figure 1.40

Photo-representation of natural teeth: two central incisors. (Courtesy of Dr. Carlos Oteo.)

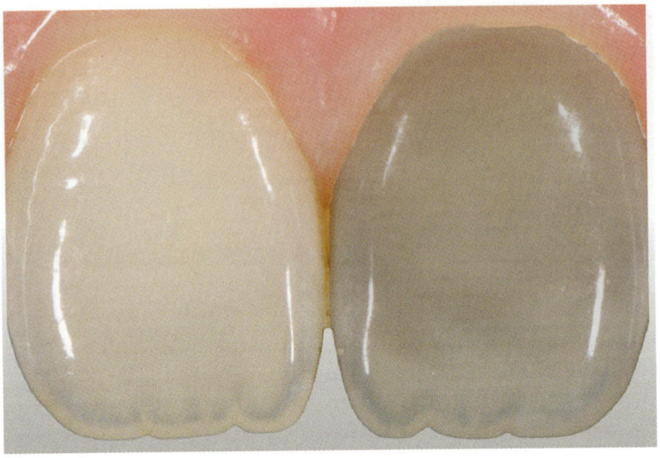

Figure 1.41

Photo-representation of the discoloration that can occur to nonvital tooth after root canal treatment. (Courtesy of Dr. Carlos Oteo.)

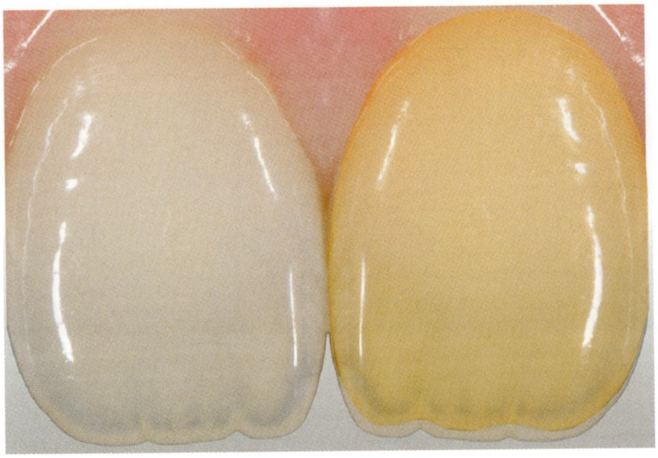

Figure 1.42

Photo-representation of a mildly traumatized tooth. (Courtesy of Dr. Carlos Oteo.)

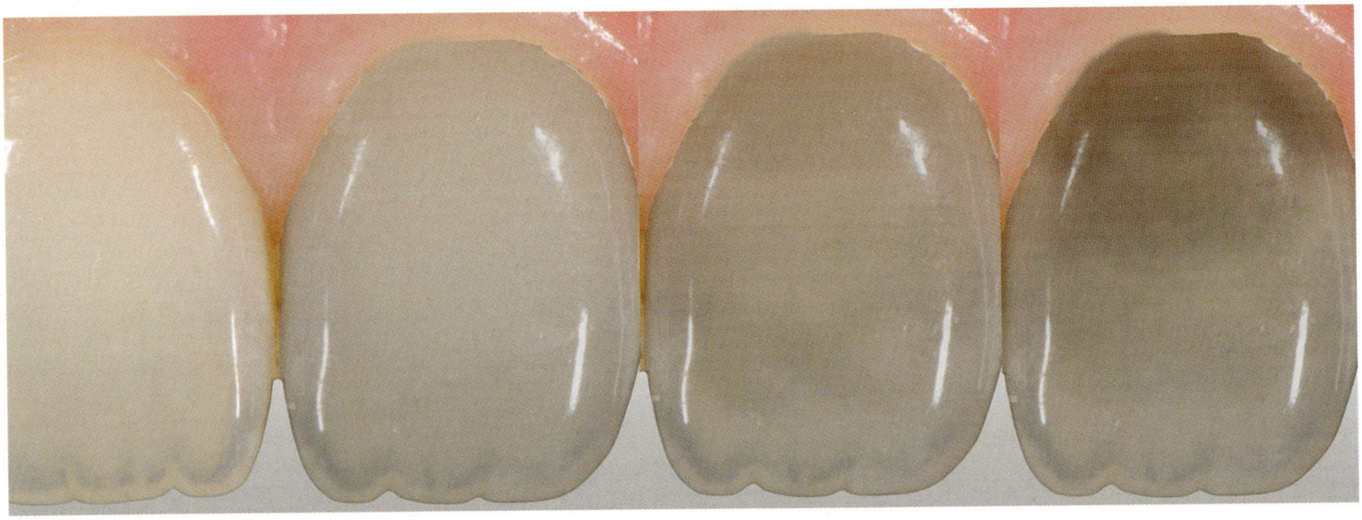

Figure 1.43

Representation of the stages of progressive discoloration that follow root canal treatment or tetracycline staining. (Courtesy of Dr. Carlos Oteo.)

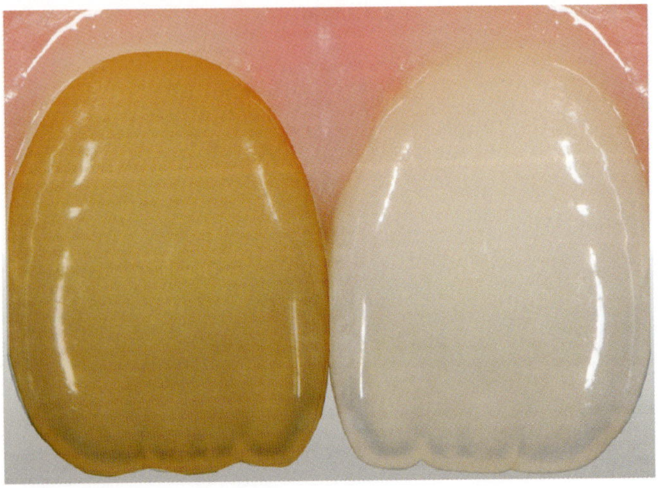

Figure 1.44

Rrepresentation of the discoloration that is possible after major trauma or root canal treatment with bleeding or decay. (Courtesy of Dr. Carlos Oteo.)

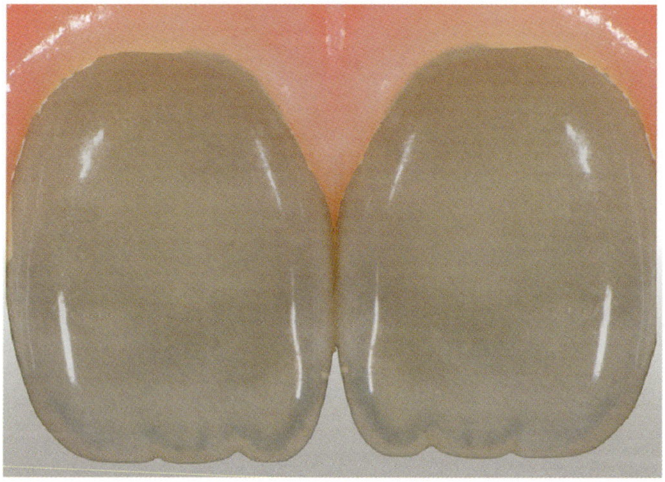

Figure 1.45

Representation of the discoloration that is possible from genetics, absorptive stain, or iron or medication such as tetracycline. (Courtesy of Dr. Carlos Oteo.)

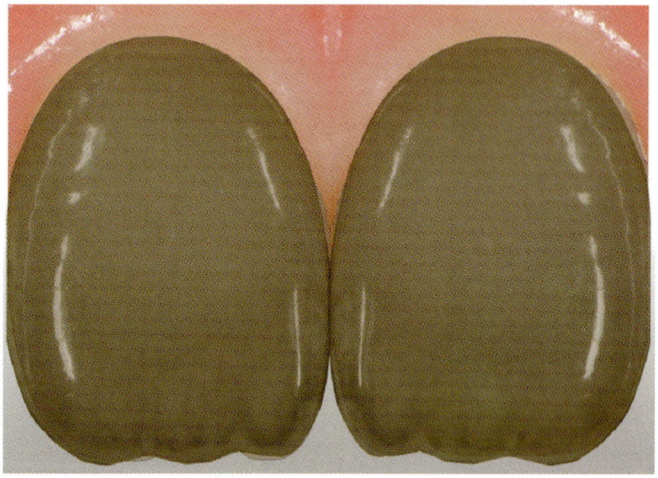

Figure 1.46

Representation of the discoloration that is possible from congenital blood disease such as porphyria. (Courtesy of Dr. Carlos Oteo.)

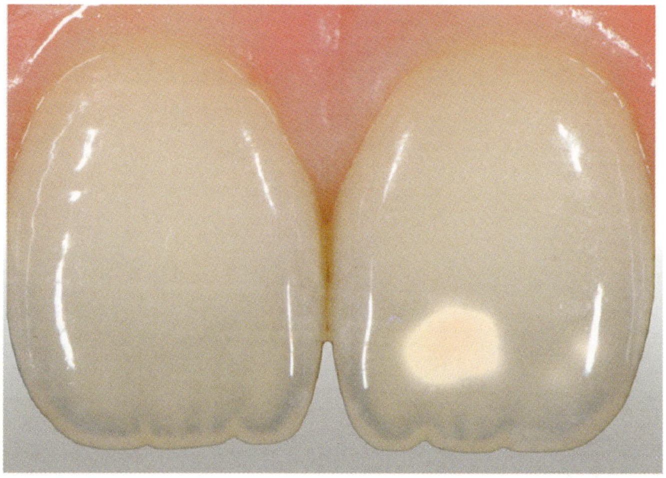

Figure 1.47

Representation of one major and two minor white opacities that are possible after trauma, associated perinatal medical history, high fever, or medication such as tetracycline or excess fluoride (see Chapter 10). (Courtesy of Dr. Carlos Oteo.)

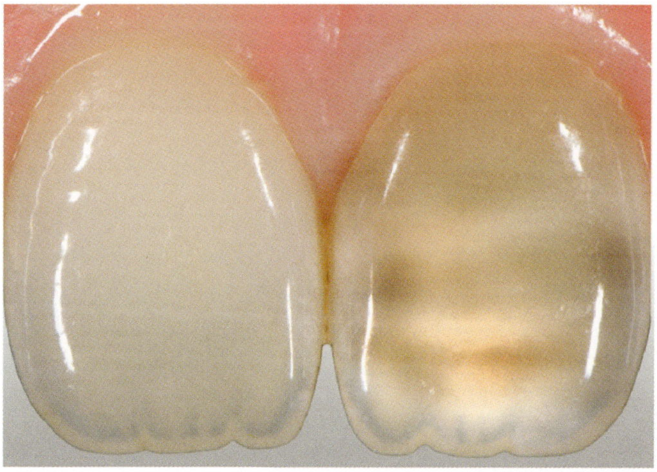

Figure 1.48

Representation of discoloration bands possible from medication such as tetracycline or excess fluoride (see Chapter 10). (Courtesy of Dr. Carlos Oteo.)

2 THE SCIENCE OF TOOTH WHITENING

Linda Greenwall

INTRODUCTION

Over the past 25 years there has been an explosion in research on tooth whitening and the science behind the process of whitening, including its effectiveness (Table 2.1).

There are still many aspects that have not been researched, and some of these are discussed in this chapter. The purpose of this chapter is to understand the scientific basis behind the tooth whitening treatments available and how the whitening gels whiten the teeth.

HOW DOES WHITENING WORK?

The chemical reaction

Whitening agents mainly consist of hydrogen peroxide. The empirical formula for hydrogen peroxide is H_2O_2. The structural formula is HO–OH (Kelleher 2008). The whitening agents act by a redox reaction with the discolored substrate. When the whitening agent is placed onto the teeth, reactive oxygen is released; the discolored substrate is chemically reduced and transformed into a colorless material (McEvoy 1989). The oxidation reaction occurs when the peroxide diffuses through the dentin structure and into the peritubular dentin (Chng et al. 2005). See Figure 2.1.

The enamel can be considered a semipermeable membrane because it allows the permeation of the whitening gel through the tooth. The surface area of the enamel is important. The active mechanism of whitening agents mainly depends on a complex oxidation reaction, which releases oxygen and other free radicals. The oxygen and free radicals establish their primary mechanism of action in tooth whitening by penetrating through the porosities of the enamel prism to the dentin (Han et al. 2014).

The whitening gel moves from the enamel to the dentin and into the pulp within 5 to 15 minutes of gel application (see Figures 2.1 and 2.2). The whitening gel also penetrates into the weakest part of the tooth, which is a crack (Kwon et al. 2012) or an area of demineralization or hypomineralization, such as a white spot. Patients should be warned that white spots on the tooth get whiter during the initial whitening process (see Figure 2.7).

Minoux and Serfaty recognized that in-office tooth whitening is a very complex process that depends on several factors, including (1) the pH of the whitening agent, (2) the method of application and thickness of the whitening agent applied to the enamel, (3) the fluctuation of light irradiation, (4) the length of photoactivation, (5) tooth size, and (6) selective absorption of the wavelength of light.

HOW DOES WHITENING AFFECT THE ORAL ENVIRONMENT?

Oral health benefits of whitening teeth

It has been shown that whitening teeth improves the oral health of the mouth. This has long been known; the first whitening material, a hydrogen peroxide mouthwash (Peroxyl), was first used to heal gingivae that were swollen after braces (see Figure 2.3) (Haywood 1990).

In this context, it should also be mentioned that salivary proteins adsorbed onto the surfaces of composite materials decrease after whitening with peroxide-containing agents, which is suggested to have an influence on bacterial adhesion of cariogenic bacteria, such as *Streptococcus sobrinus* and *Streptococcus mutans*, but not *Actinomyces viscosus* (Steinberg et al. 1999).

HOW DO THE TOOTH WHITENING GELS WORK ON THE TOOTH? HOW DOES IT GET WHITER?

The tooth whitening gels in the form of hydrogen peroxide were originally used as treatments to reduce the swelling of the gingivae after orthodontic treatment. An orthodontist, Bill Klausmier, noted that when the gingivae were swollen after removal of the orthodontic brackets, the use of glyoxide mouthwash 3% in the retainers resolved the gingival inflammation. The hydrogen peroxide worked by oxygenating the gingival crevice and helping to reduce the inflammation. Hydrogen peroxide rapidly breaks down into water and oxygen; the oxygen is the active ingredient. It travels into the gingival crevicular fluid and diffuses into the gingival margin and into the tooth. The appearance of oxygen bubbles at the gingival margin gives an indication that the hydrogen peroxide is being activated to break down into oxygen and water, and on contact with the tooth the gel becomes activated and starts to penetrate through the tooth. The surface contact area is important. There is discussion about the shortest contact time to produce the quickest effect. The oxygen penetrates into the enamel, the dentin, and the pulp within 5 to 15 minutes of gel application. The oxygen then moves into the pigment molecules that

Table 2.1 Changes in tooth whitening over the last 25 years

Social attitudes	
	• Increased patient expectations
	• Whiter teeth sought
	• Philosophy of perfection
	• More difficult discolorations
	• No age restrictions for older patients
	• Age limit for patients under 18
	• Whitening maintenance
	• Whitening for life
	• "Bleachorexics" and "bleachoholics"
Technical innovations	
	• Two-week tray use
	• Extended tray use
	• Changes in tray design
	• Use with aligners
	• Therapeutic uses
	• Whitening strips
	• Take-home gels
	• Soothers, potassium nitrate, fluoride, and amorphous calcium phosphate (ACP)
	• Concentrations of materials
	• Power gels
	• Light versus no light
	• Heat versus no heat
	• Lasers
	• Ozone

are embedded in the dentin. These yellow pigment molecules become white pigment molecules. The process removes the color from the tooth, which is lightened (see Figure 2.10). The oxygen remains in the tooth for a period of 2 weeks while the gel is continually applied. Oxygen is liberated and whitens the tooth. The appearance of the oxygen makes the tooth appear lighter and whiter.

Whitening penetration: the direction of the whitening process

The whitening gel travels into the weakest part of the tooth first. In some instances this can be straight into a crack in the tooth. This was demonstrated in a study by Kwon and colleagues (2012), in which the tooth was stained with rhodamine B dye to assess the pathway of the discoloration and the pathway of the whitening gel. It was noted that the process of discoloration is the same as the process of the whitening gel; it follows the direction of the dentin tubules, the odontoblasts, and the peritubular dentin. It was also noted that the whitening process is multidirectional. Although it appears that the whitening starts from the incisal tip, first it penetrates the tooth in a three-dimensional way, referred to as *multidirectional penetration*. Often it may appear that the incisal tip is lightening first (see Figure 2.10) and then the whiteness moves up the tooth toward the neck of the tooth. The upper teeth appear to whiten more quickly than the lower teeth.

Into the pulp

It is known that the whitening gel penetrates into the nerve within 5 to 15 minutes of gel application. The higher the concentration of hydrogen peroxide, the faster the gel moves into the tooth. This factor also depends on the permeability of the teeth and the tooth anatomy. A recent study assessed vascular permeability in rats (Ferreira et al. 2013) and found that hydrogen peroxide tooth whitening can induce an increase in vascular permeability in rat incisors. Importantly, this increase is more dependent on the length of the whitening procedure than on the concentration of the whitening agent.

In power whitening using higher concentrations of hydrogen peroxide, the whitening penetration into the pulp may occur more quickly depending on the concentration used and the contact time during which the whitening gel stays on the labial surface of the tooth. An in vitro study (Marson et al. 2015) on bovine teeth assessed the effects of different concentrations of hydrogen peroxide on the tooth (Opalescence Xtra Boost, 38%; White Gold In-Office, 35%; Whiteness HP Blue, 35%; Whiteness HP Maxx, 35%; and Lase Peroxide Sensy, 35%). The results showed that all products significantly reduced the concentration of H_2O_2 activates by 45 minutes; however, it was also shown that increasing the time the product remained on the tooth surface enhanced the penetration of H_2O_2. The researchers concluded that the whitening gels retained substantial concentrations of H_2O_2 after 45 minutes of application, and the penetration of hydrogen peroxide was time dependent.

Whitening of lower teeth

The whitening of the lower teeth may occur more slowly because the sublingual salivary glands may wash out or reduce the effect of the whitening gel. Often on the lower canines there is a snow-capped appearance—a clear demarcation that occurs between the tip of the tooth, which is white, and the rest of the tooth, which has yet to whiten or "catch up." The whitening in this situation needs to continue, and it may be 3 weeks before the whole tooth is completely white.

Gingival margins and root dentin

Gingival areas on cervical dentin do not whiten to the same effect. This is because at the gingival level there is reduced enamel thickness, and where there is gingival recession present the root appears more yellow. It is important to warn the patient that this area may not whiten to the full extent. There is debate as to whether extending the whitening tray over the gingival area to the extent of the gingival recession and onto the full extent of the exposed root will help to whiten this area fully. The root dentin will never whiten fully. The root dentin will lighten, but it will not be completely white. It is unrealistic to expect this, and this should be carefully explained to the patient. There are many different tray designs to address this issue, and although many manufacturers have trademarks and patents on the whitening tray design and where to finish the scalloped margin—whether to the edge of the tooth, beyond the tooth onto the gingivae, or 1 mm above the gingivae—the root has not shown a perfect white shade. Some studies have shown that the last 1 mm can be cut off the whitening tray to reduce sensitivity, and this has made no difference to the final whitening effect. Some gingival margins can become irritated from too much gel in this area. Whitening treatments were observed to reduce background luminescence of enamel, dentinoenamel junction (DEJ), and dentin in a study using confocal laser scanning microscopy (Götz et al. 2007).

WHICH TOOTH WHITENS THE QUICKEST?

The science of whitening has shown that the movement of the whitening agent is directly related to the anatomy and internal structure of the tooth. Young teeth will whiten more quickly because of the structure of the tubules and the enamel (see Figure 2.2). Even though they have much larger pulps, this does not necessarily make them more susceptible to sensitivity. Older patients can whiten their teeth as well. There is no upper age limit. Whitening will take longer in older patients because of the secondary and tertiary dentin that has been laid down over the years.

Studies have shown that the fastest teeth to whiten are the upper lateral incisors. This is because of the anatomy of the lateral incisor teeth. In patients with Class II division 2 malocclusion, when the lateral incisors move forward it is more noticeable that these teeth are whitening more quickly. Upper canines take the longest to whiten because these teeth are situated in the corners of the arch and are responsible for guiding the movement of the rest of the teeth, so they have the longest roots and more and thicker dentin. These upper canines are often much darker and more yellow than the rest of the teeth. Therefore when planning whitening with a patient, it is essential to demonstrate that the upper canines are darker and will take longer to whiten than the adjacent teeth. The central incisors are the baseline to assess the whitening in full; the upper centrals, when whitened, should match each other exactly.

The whitening potential of a tooth

Although there is very little research on whitening potential, it is my observation that sufficient whitening needs to be undertaken to reach the whitening potential of the tooth. The protocols and staging of home whitening treatment have been listed below on the treatment sequence are listed in Chapter 5. If these steps are followed, the full whitening potential of the tooth will be reached.

Whitening potential can be assessed by the dehydration pattern of the tooth. As the tooth dehydrates, the dehydration effect and the pattern of dehydration can be noted; this will give some indication of the whitening potential of the tooth. When power whitening is used, the higher concentration materials can penetrate the tooth more quickly. The higher the concentration of the hydrogen peroxide, the faster the process of the whitening and the greater the sensitivity. In a study to assess two power whitening techniques in vitro, Kwon and colleagues (2012) noted that there was no difference between the conventional whitening technique and the assisted or sealed whitening technique with regard to the color change measurements (ΔL, Δa, Δb, ΔE); however, there was significantly greater hydrogen peroxide penetration in the conventional whitening group ($P < .05$). Another study showed that the amount of hydrogen peroxide penetrating into the pulp chamber varied with the presence of calcium, the whitening protocol, and the product used (Mena-Serrano et al. 2015). The hydrogen peroxide concentration did not affect the hydrogen peroxide inside the pulp chamber, but the presence of calcium significantly reduced it ($P < .0001$).

Hydrogen peroxide–only products or day products liberate all their oxygen within 30 to 60 minutes, whereas carbamide peroxide materials liberate their oxygen over a prolonged period of time such as a sustained release over 2–10 hours. The hydrogen peroxide may increase dentin permeability (Berger et al. 2013).

The dehydration factor of the tooth is related to the whitening potential of the tooth

The way that the tooth will whiten will be determined by the anatomy of the tooth (the distribution of the dentin tubules and enamel prisms; Figure 2.2), the amount of enamel and dentin on the teeth, tooth genetics, white spots and defects that are present on the tooth, any restorations, the etiology of the discoloration, and the age of the patient. However, dehydration is also a factor: When a tooth dehydrates, it dehydrates in the weaker parts (such as white spots and markings) more quickly. Younger teeth also dehydrate more quickly, and older teeth take longer to dehydrate. This is normally particularly noticeable when isolation of the teeth is undertaken such as for power whitening. As the tooth dehydrates, when the isolation material is placed on the lips and the mucosa, the whitening effect will follow the same pattern as the dehydration. This can help determine the whitening effect.

Some patients who have a short lip have a dehydration line on the tooth. They display more tooth when the lip is at rest. This can result in an uneven shade of the tooth because it can dehydrate over time; the enamel becomes thinner and the dentin becomes thicker. Patients who display this should be warned that when the tooth lightens, the dehydration line may not disappear and the teeth will have a two-tone effect after whitening.

This concept is not fully discussed in the literature, and further research is needed. The dehydration of a tooth is also a major factor in sensitivity (Kugel and Ferreira 2005), but its exact role needs further research.

Using the white of the eye (sclera) as a reference point

It has been suggested that the sclera of the eye be used as shade assessment for the amount of whitening that can be achieved (see Figure 2.12). Although there is not much research on this aspect, Haywood has suggested that the sclera be used as a baseline reference point. When patients are having multiple assessments to evaluate the whiteness of the tooth, the sclera assessment can help to determine where the patients are on the whiteness scale as a background comparison and whether further whitening can be achieved. Although the shade is measured from a shade guide and the changes noted, the best method is to use the sclera as a background to fully understand whether the tooth can be whitened further.

"BLEACHOREXIC" OR "BLEACHOHOLIC"?

Some patients develop a syndrome wherein they continually seek whiter and whiter teeth beyond the point at which no further whitening will develop. Patients become extreme with their obsession to seek a whiter shade of the teeth to achieve a "megawatt smile." This can lead to overwhitening and daily whitening over a period of many years. This amount of whitening can be excessive. For a tooth that has experienced severe trauma, it is not known whether whitening for a period of many years may exacerbate the trauma, leading to resorption (see Figure 2.11); there is no evidence in the literature demonstrating this.

Some patients purchase whitening products on the Internet. This can lead to severe erosion damage because many of these products are unregulated and harmful to the teeth as a result of their acidic nature. For patients with constant daily use of whitening gel, the term that should be used is "bleachoholic," but the term "bleachorexic" is more commonly used.

Some of these patients travel from dentist to dentist to try to seek perfection in tooth whitening and the whitest shade of tooth, a syndrome documented by several authors. This syndrome is similar to other body dysmorphic syndromes and also affects patients with full dentures. Such a patient may arrive with multiple sets of dentures but still request that additional whitening trays be made. The patient may flatter the dentist on his or her clinical skills. This is a psychological ploy to entice the dentist into performing further whitening treatment.

Using the sclerae of the eyes and the shade of the teeth, the dentist can detect these bleachorexic patients very easily: the shade of their teeth is brilliant white—whiter than the whites of their eyes. It is important to explain to patients that there is a limit to the extent of whitening that can be achieved, and once this has been reached no further whitening is possible. Although these patients may be able to purchase whitening products on the Internet, they like to purchase the whitening gel from the dentist. The guidance is clear: dentists and their teams cannot hand out whitening gel at every appointment; with each cycle of whitening treatment an examination is needed first, followed by careful monitoring of the patient and assessment of side effects.

Many of these patients make their own concoctions of whitening gels with ingredients such as baking soda and bicarbonate of soda. There are many discussions on the Internet about how to make whitening treatments at home, but these are dangerous and unresearched and have not been tested for safety. In a recent study (Kwon et al. 2015) numerous types of whitening agents were tested for effective lightening in vitro. Using different shade assessment tools, the examiners evaluated the efficacy of do-it-yourself (DIY) whitening as compared with conventional tooth whitening modalities. Extracted human molars (120) were randomly distributed to six groups (n = 20). Whitening was performed according to manufacturer's directions for over-the-counter, dentist-dispensed for home use, and in-office whitening products. DIY whitening consisted of a strawberry and baking soda mix. In addition, negative and positive controls were used.

Evaluators used the Vita classical (VC) shade guide and Vita Bleachedguide 3D-Master shade guide with interpolated numbers (BGi) for visual assessment at baseline and 1 week, 1 month, and 3 months after whitening. Statistical analysis showed that the DIY whitening gel exhibited lower color change compared with other whitening groups at all time points ($P < .05$). There was very good agreement between evaluators with VC and BGi at each time point. Both shade guides were related with each other and strongly related to instrumental measurements ($P < .05$). The conclusions demonstrated that the DIY whitening material was the least effective whitening modality. This study can be discussed with patients who attempt to whiten using home preparations that they have made themselves.

WHITENING FOR PATIENTS YOUNGER THAN 18

Legislation in Europe has recommended that no whitening be undertaken for patients younger than 18 years. However, literature assessment shows that whitening for patients younger than 18 is safe and appropriate under certain conditions. There needs to be a specific disease of enamel or dentin present, such as amelogenesis imperfecta or molar incisor hypoplasia. It was first thought that it was unsafe to whiten the teeth of patients younger than 18 because of their large pulps, but the research has shown that this is not the case. For nonvital teeth in patients younger than 18, it is essential that the nonvital area be assessed as symptom free, that the endodontic treatment has been satisfactory in the obturation, and that there are no radiolucencies present on the nonvital tooth (see Figure 2.12).

CONCLUSION

The science of whitening has advanced sufficiently to demonstrate that whitening teeth is safe, effective, and predictable.

REFERENCES

Benetti AR, Valera MC, Mancini MN, Miranda CB. (2004) In vitro penetration of bleaching agents into the pulp chamber. *Int Endod J* **37**(2):120–4.

Berger SB, Tabchoury CP, Ambrosano GM, Giannini M. (2013) Hydrogen peroxide penetration into the pulp chamber and dental permeability after bleaching. *Gen Dent* **61**(3): e21–5.

Chng HK, Ramli HN, Yap AU, Lim CT. (2005) Effect of hydrogen on intertubular dentine. *J Dent* **33**(5):363–9.

Ferreira VG, Nabeshima CK, Marques MM, Paris AF. (2013) Tooth bleaching induces changes in the vascular permeability of rat incisor pulps. *Am J Dent* **26**(5):298–300.

Götz H, Klukowska MA, Duschner H, White DJ. (2007) Physical, morphological, and micro-Raman chemical studies on bleaching strip effects on enamel, coronal dentin, and root dentin. *J Clin Dent. 2007;***18**(4):112-9

Greenwall LH. (2014). Therapeutic aesthetics. *Aesth Dent Today* May: 9–12.

Han Y, Mo S, Jiang L, Zhu Y. (2014) Effects of antioxidants on the microleakage of composite resin restorations after external tooth bleaching. *Eur J Dent* **8**(2):147–53.

Hasson H, Ismail AI, Neiva G. (2006). Home-based chemically-induced whitening of teeth in adults. *Cochrane Database Syst Rev* 4:CD006202.

Haywood VB. (1990) Overview and status of mouthguard bleaching. *J Esthet Dent* **3**(5):157–61.

Haywood VB. (1999) Current status and recommendations for dentist-prescribed, at-home tooth whitening. *Contemp Esthet Restor Pract* **3**(suppl 1):2–9.

http://abcnews.go.com/Lifestyle/bleachorexia-dentist-warns-dangers-overbleaching-teeth/story?id=27125341. (Accessed March 28, 2016)

Kelleher MG. (2008) *Dental bleaching.* Quintessence Publishing: New Malden, UK.

Kugel G, Ferreira S. (2005) The art and science of tooth whitening. *J Mass Dent Soc* **53**(4):34–7.

Kwon S, Meharry M, Oyoyo U, Li Y. (2015) Efficacy of do-it-yourself whitening as compared to conventional tooth whitening modalities: an in vitro study. *Oper Dent* 40(1):E21–7.

Kwon SR, Wertz PW, Li Y, Chan DC. (2012) Penetration pattern of rhodamine dyes into enamel and dentin: confocal laser microscopy observation. *Int J Cosmet Sci* **34**(1):97–101.

Kwon SR, Wertz PW, Dawson DV, Cobb DS. (2013) The relationship of hydrogen peroxide exposure protocol to bleaching efficacy. *Oper Dent* **38**(2):177–85.

Marson F, Gonçalves R, Silva C, Cintra L. (2015) Penetration of hydrogen peroxide and degradation rate of different bleaching products. *Oper Dent* **40**(1):72–9.

McEvoy SA. (1989) Chemical agents for removing intrinsic stains from vital teeth. Part II. Current techniques and their clinical application. *Quintessence Int* 20(6) 379–84.

Mena-Serrano A, Parreiras S, Nascimento ED, Borges C. (2014) Effects of the concentration and composition of in-office bleaching gels on hydrogen peroxide penetration into the pulp chamber. *Oper Dent* **40**(2):E76–82.

Minoux M, Serfaty R. (2008) Vital tooth bleaching: biologic adverse effects—a review. *Quintessence Int* **39**(8):645–59.

Steinberg D, Mor C, Dogan H, Zacks B, Rotstein I. (1999) Effect of salivary biofilm on the adherence of oral bacteria to bleached and non-bleached restorative material. *Dent Mater* **15**(1):14–20.

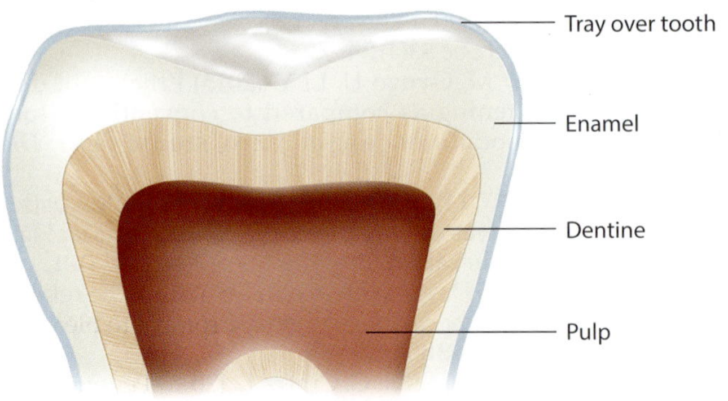

Figure 2.1

Cross section through the tooth showing the whitening tray over the tooth; the anatomy of the tooth affects the transmission of the whitening gel and how quickly or slowly the gel will move through the tooth. (Reproduced from Greenwall 2014 with permission.)

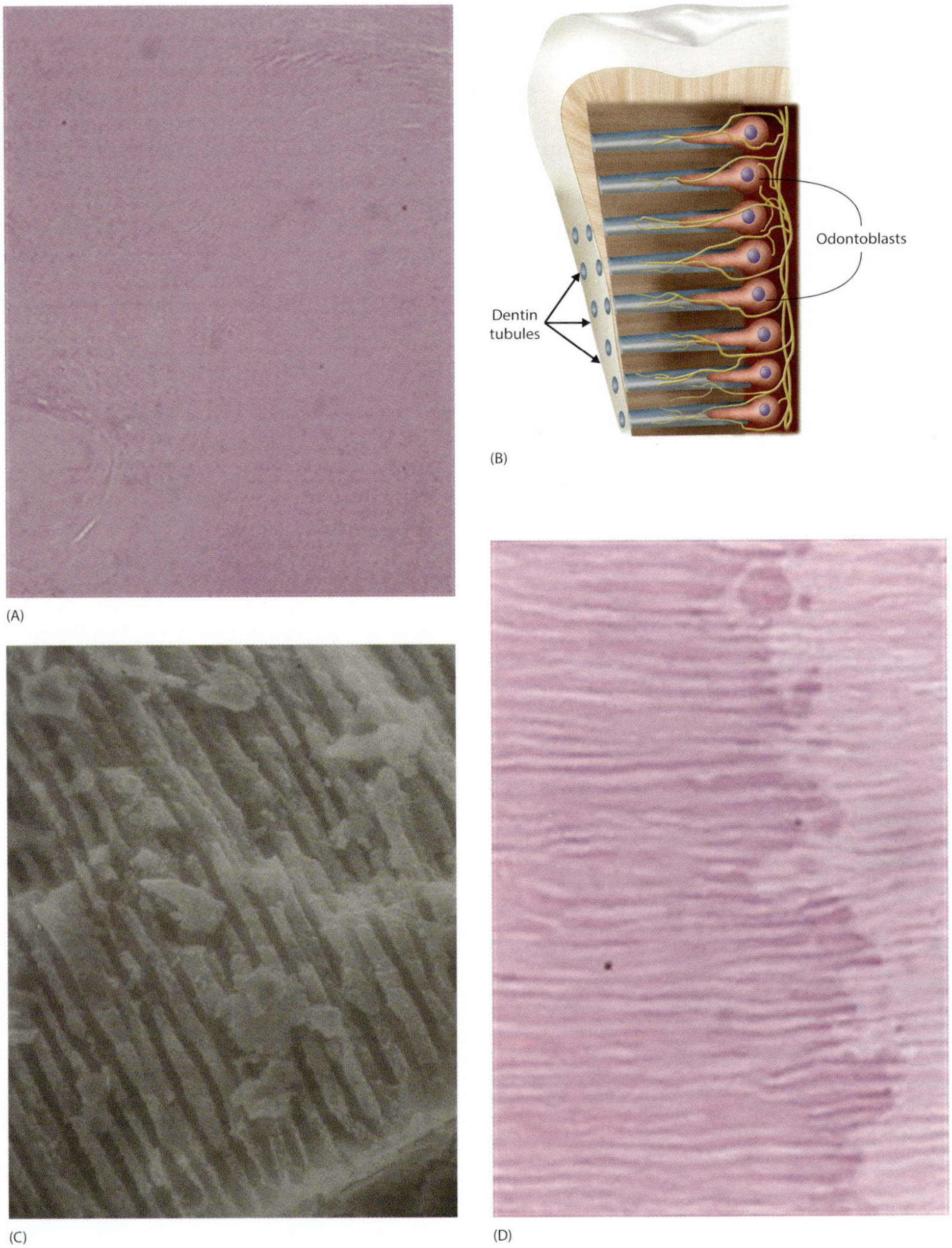

Figure 2.2

The gel travels from the enamel through the dentin (A); through the dentin tubules (B); and into the peritubular dentin (C) and the predentin (D).

continued on the next page

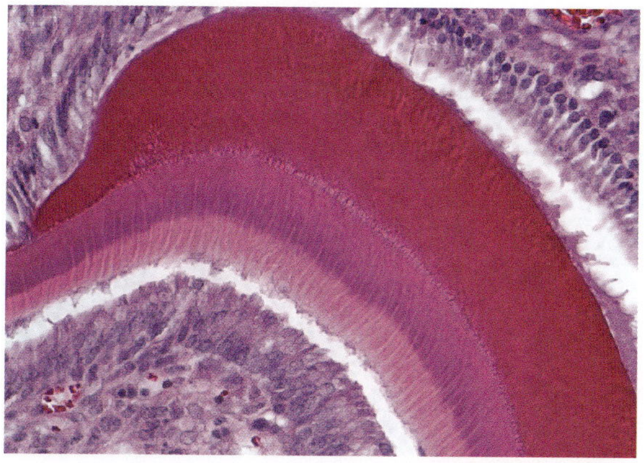

(E)

Figure 2.2 continued

(E) Young dentin formation and more open tubules allow the whitening gel to penetrate more quickly.

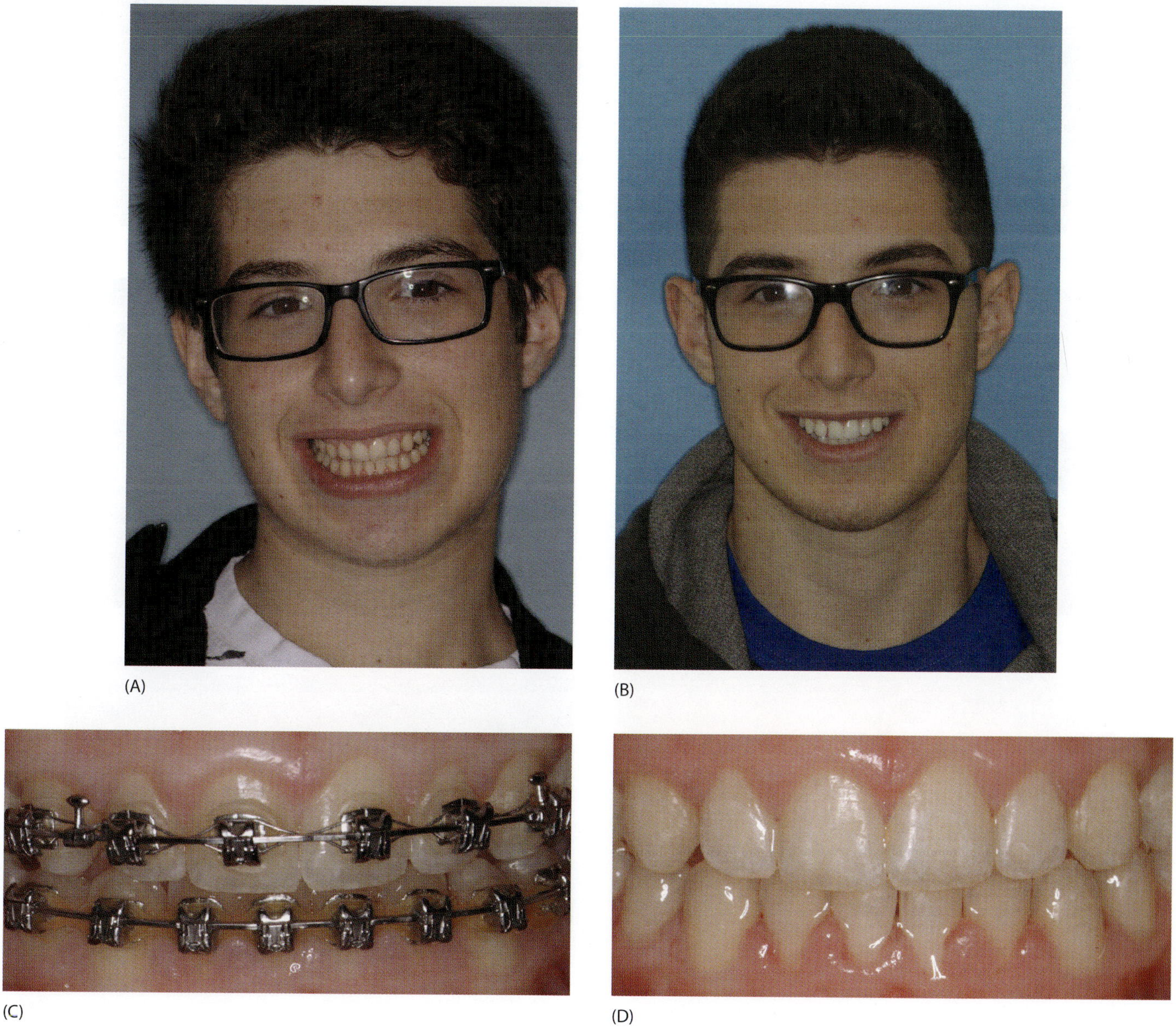

Figure 2.3

(A) Patient was age 15 when he had his orthodontic braces removed. (B) Portrait view of patient after whitening. (C) Braces positioned on the teeth. (D) When the braces were removed, the gingivae were swollen.

continued on the next page

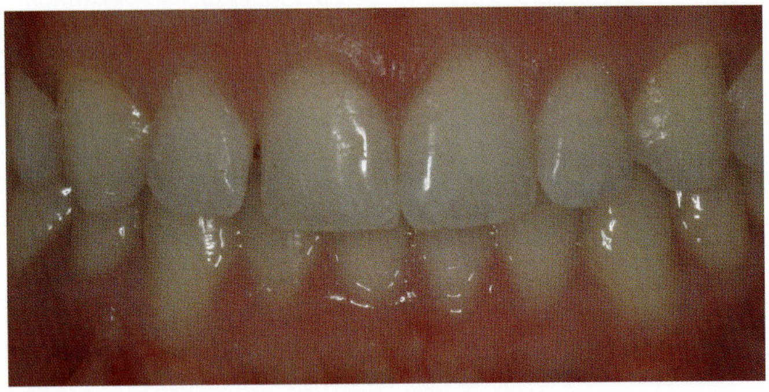

(E)

Figure 2.3 continued

(E) The result after whitening. The gingival swelling resolved after completion of the whitening treatment. (However, the patient did not wear his retainer sufficiently, which resulted in a diastema opening up at the upper right lateral position.)

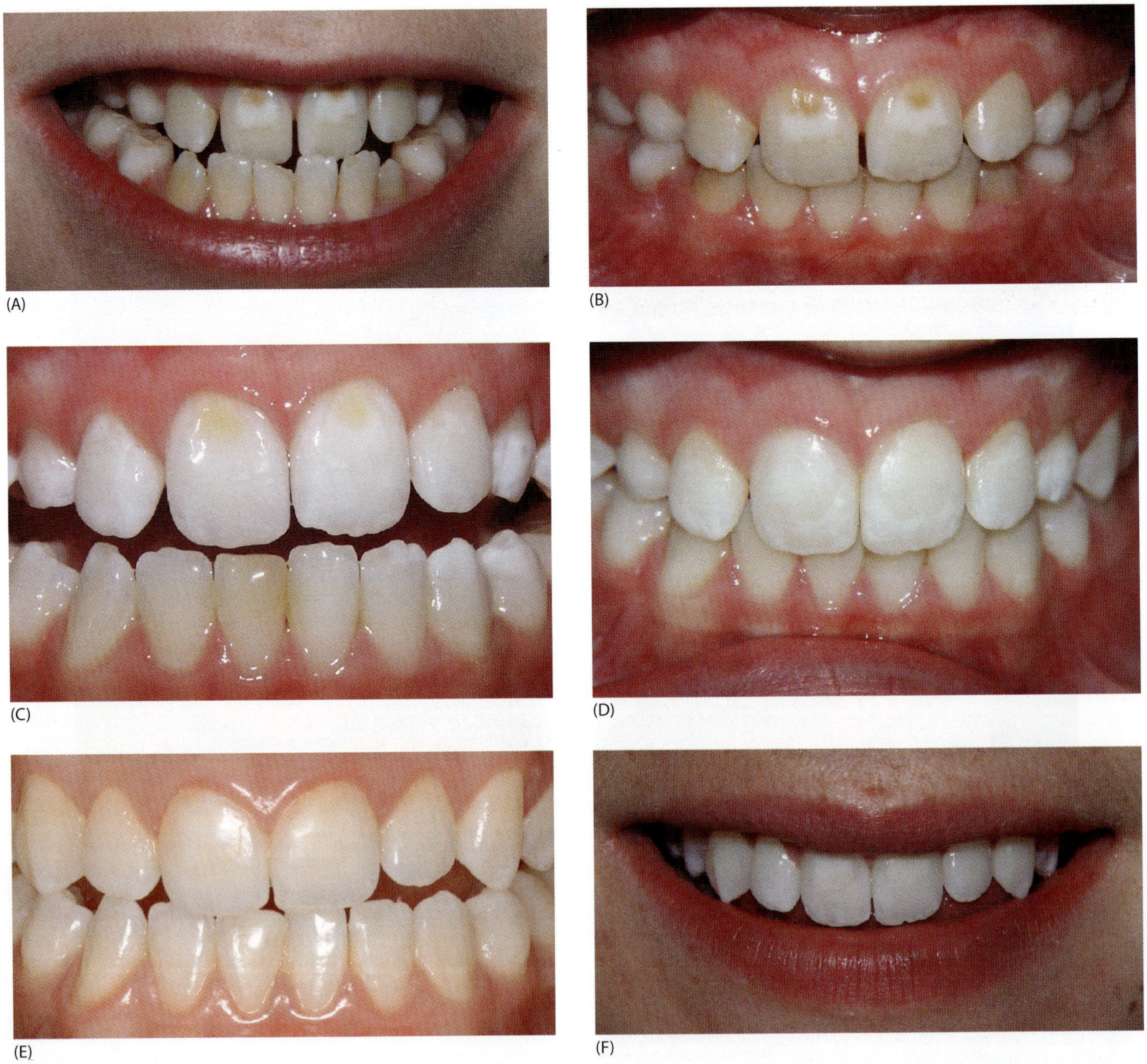

Figure 2.4

(A and B) The appearance of the teeth of a young girl age 10. She was concerned about the appearance of her upper central incisors. The teeth had enamel defects and deficiencies resulting in brown and white discoloration patches. (C and D) Appearance of the teeth after whitening during the mixed dentition stage at age 11. The teeth were then microabraded to reduce the appearance of the white marks, and the initial defects were covered with composite bonding. When the permanent canines erupted, these teeth erupted at shade A3.5. These canines were then whitened at age 14 so that all the teeth were an even A1 shade. (E and F) Postwhitening appearance of the teeth at age 15 years.

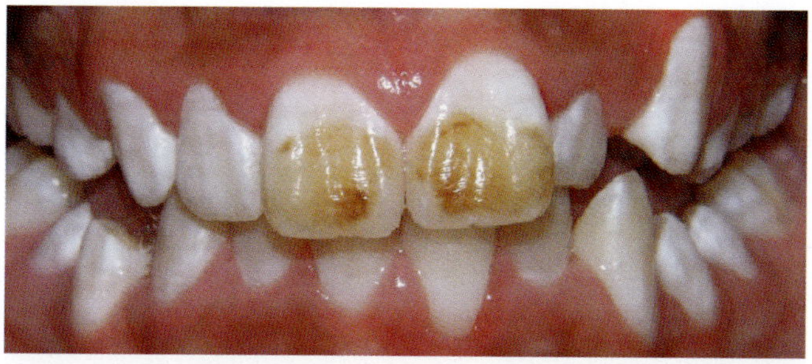

(A)

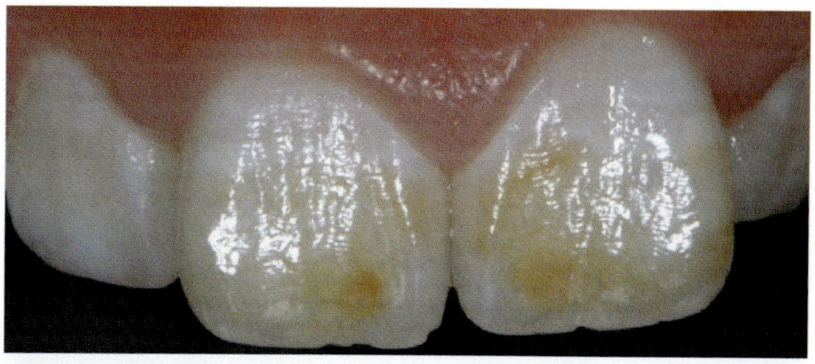

(B)

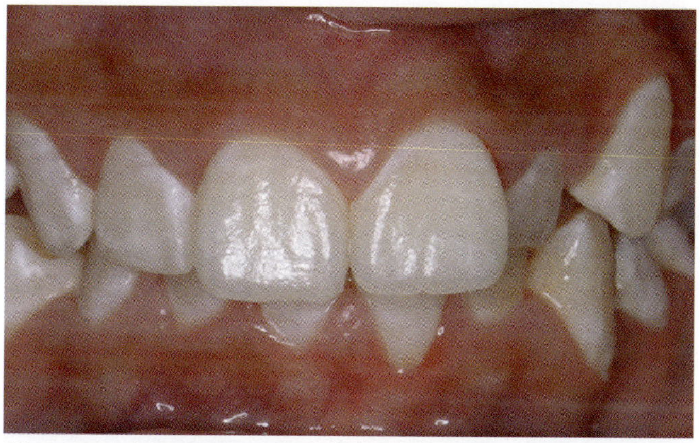

(C)

Figure 2.5

(A) Appearance of brown discoloration of the upper central incisors of an 11-year-old. The diagnosis is fluorosis. It was in the best interest of the patient to whiten her teeth. This process took a period of 8 weeks to remove the brown discoloration from the teeth. (B) Appearance after 3 weeks. (C) Appearance of the teeth after 8 weeks of whitening the upper central incisors.

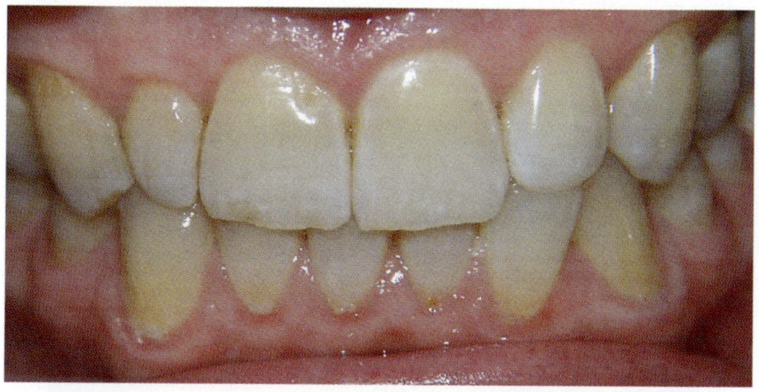

(A)

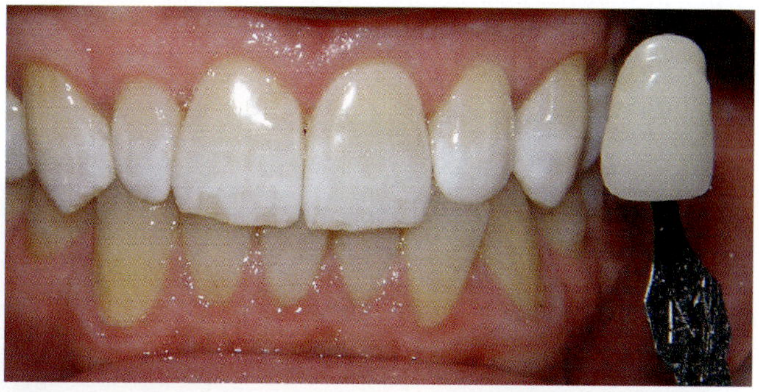

(B)

Figure 2.6

(A) This patient had faint white markings on the tips of the central incisors. (B) Appearance of the teeth 2 weeks after whitening just the upper teeth. The appearance is called the splodge effect. The whitening is uneven and the teeth appearance a little mottled. It is important to reassure the patient that this effect is transient and that the patient should continue to whiten the teeth until they appear more even in shade.

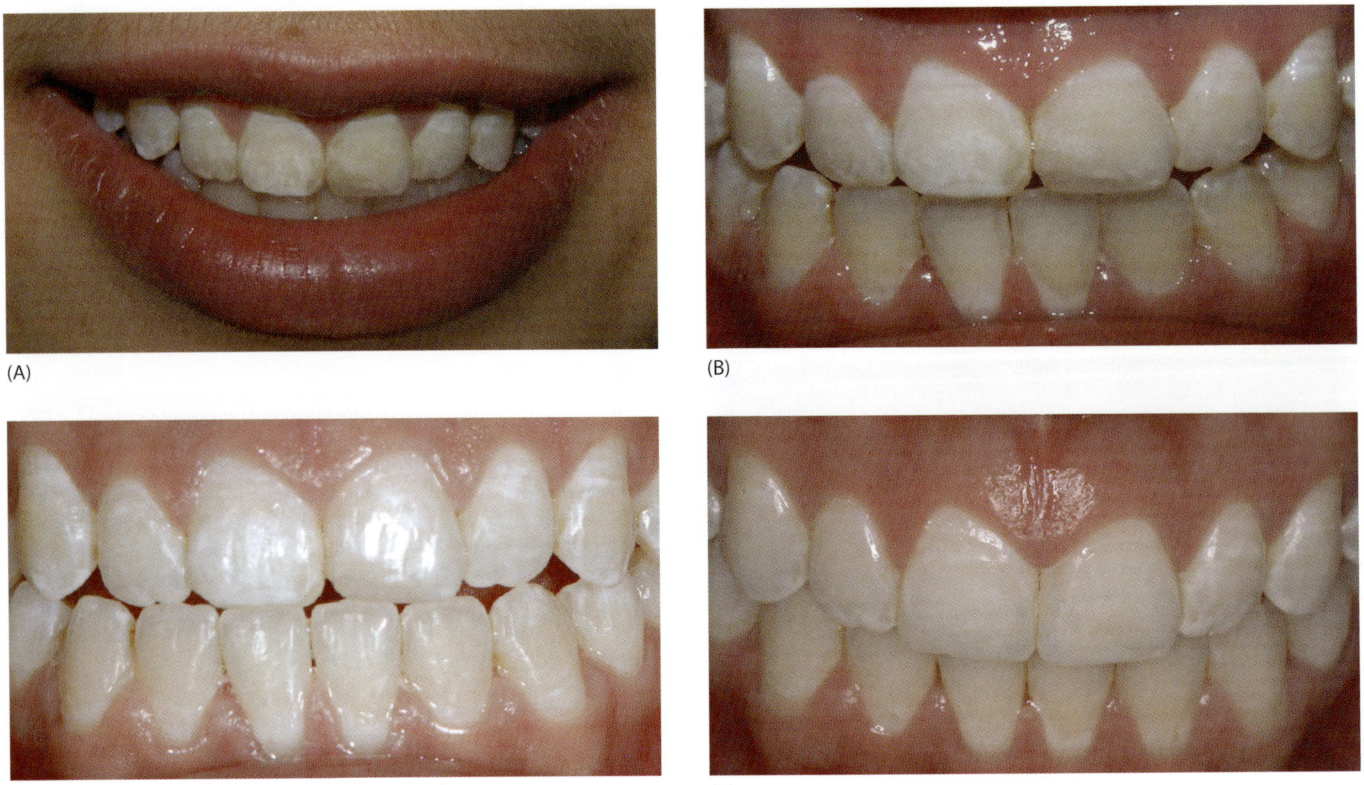

(A) (B) (C) (D)

Figure 2.7

(A) Smile view and (B) retracted appearance of the teeth of a 17-year-old girl with mild fluorosis and a class 4 fracture on the teeth. The upper teeth were whitened first, then the lower teeth. After a period of 2 weeks the class 4 restoration was redone using a more esthetic dentin whitened shade to better blend into the tooth. (C) Result after whitening. The colors are lightened, but white markings are more evident on the teeth. (D) Completed case after microabrasion and bonding.

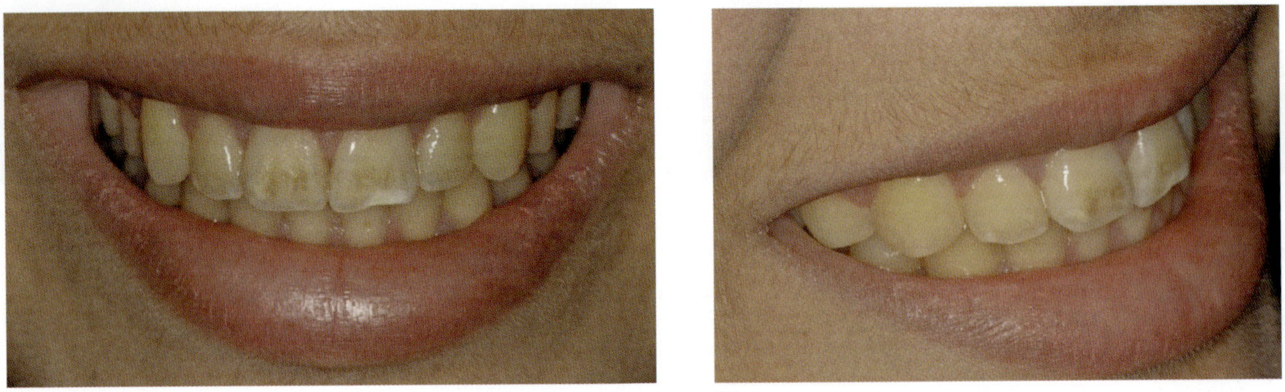

(A) (B)

Figure 2.8

(A-C) Tooth discoloration of a patient with a mild form of molar incisor hypoplasia. The teeth have a yellow discoloration, and the specific markings are present on the upper left central incisor and the molar teeth. The treatment plan included professional prophylaxis treatment followed by home whitening and icon resin infiltration.

continued on the next page

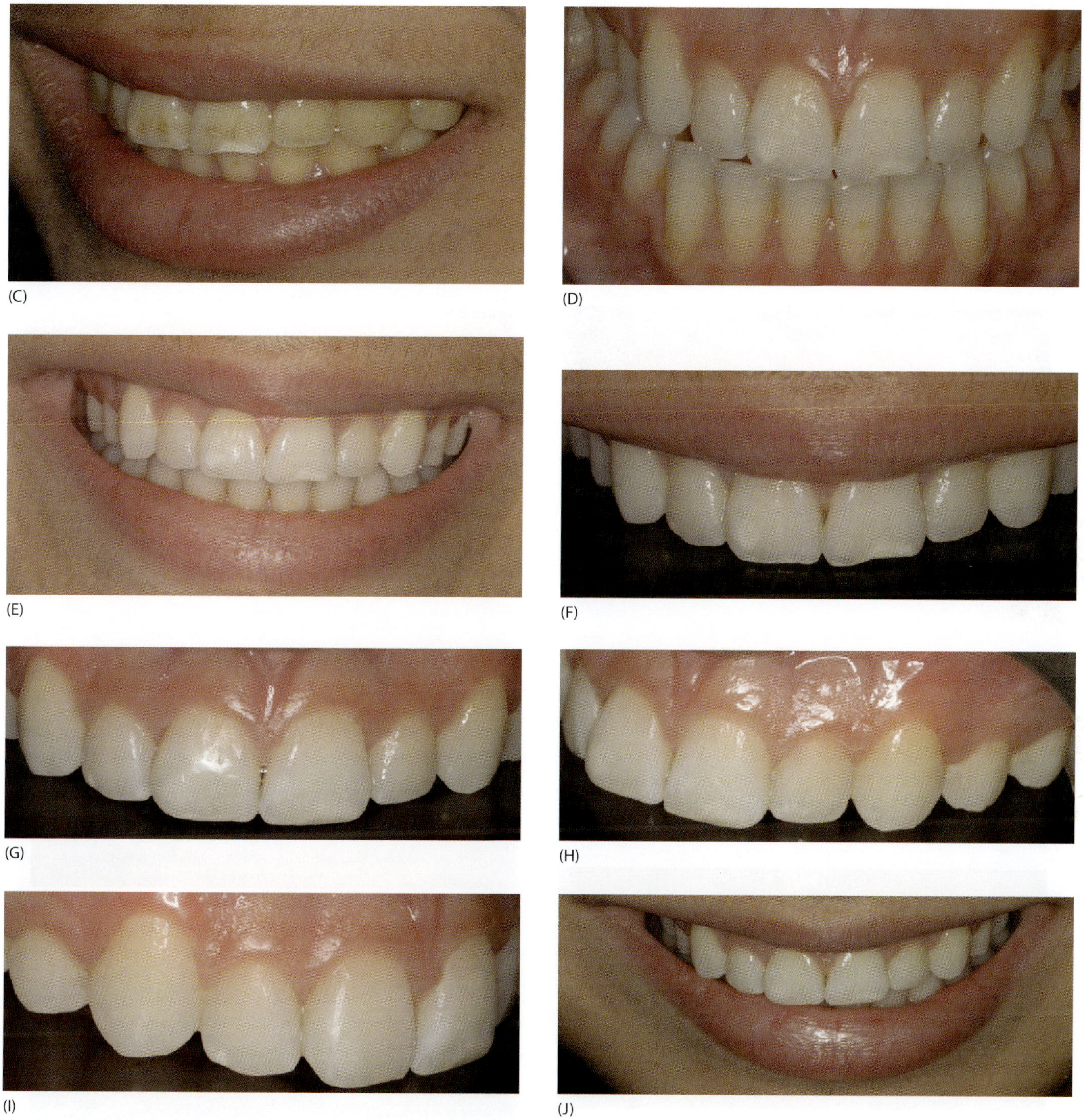

(C) (D) (E) (F) (G) (H) (I) (J)

Figure 2.8 continued

(A-C) Tooth discoloration of a patient with a mild form of molar incisor hypoplasia. The teeth have a yellow discoloration, and the specific markings are present on the upper left central incisor and the molar teeth. The treatment plan included professional prophylaxis treatment followed by home whitening and icon resin infiltration. (D-J) Appearance of the teeth after whitening, resin infiltration, and composite bonding with whitening agent shade composite.

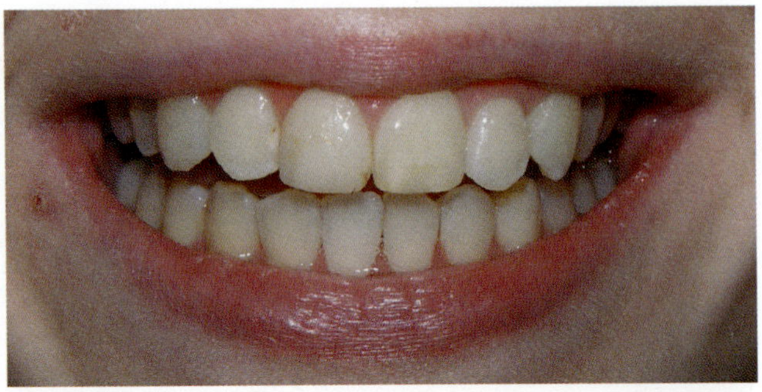
(A)

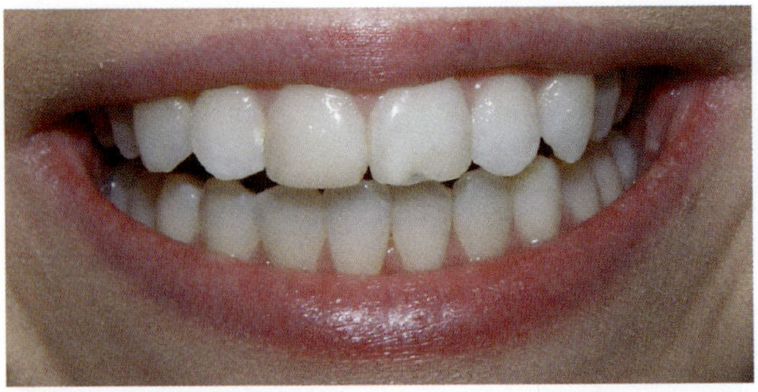
(B)

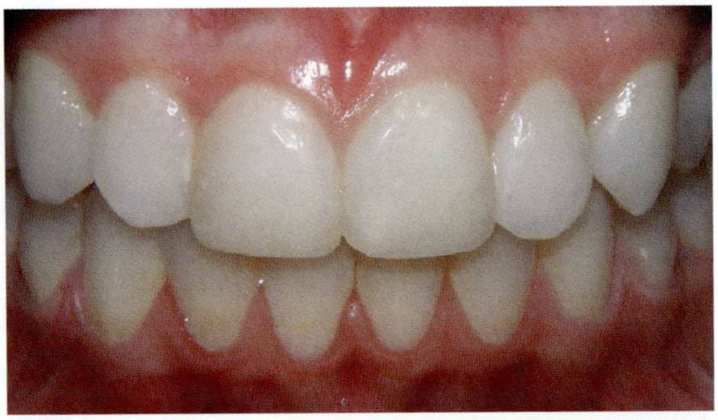
(C)

Figure 2.9

(A) Postoperative appearance of the teeth of a teenager who had just completed orthodontic treatment. This patient had experienced mild trauma to her upper central incisor teeth. The teeth were more yellow because of the previous trauma experience. (B) Appearance after completion of whitening treatment. (C) Appearance of the teeth after the completion of direct bonding onto the upper central incisor teeth.

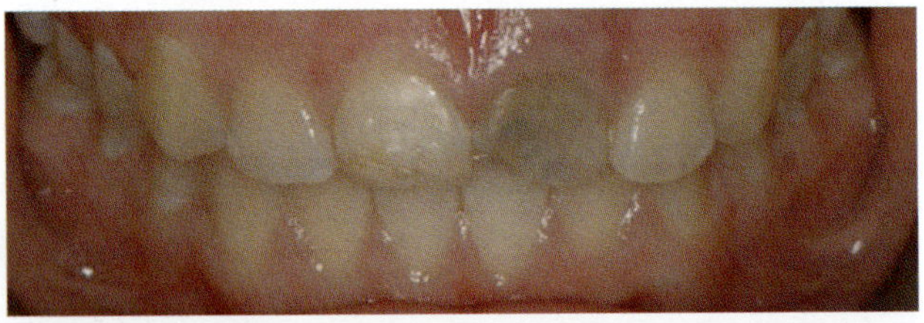
(A)

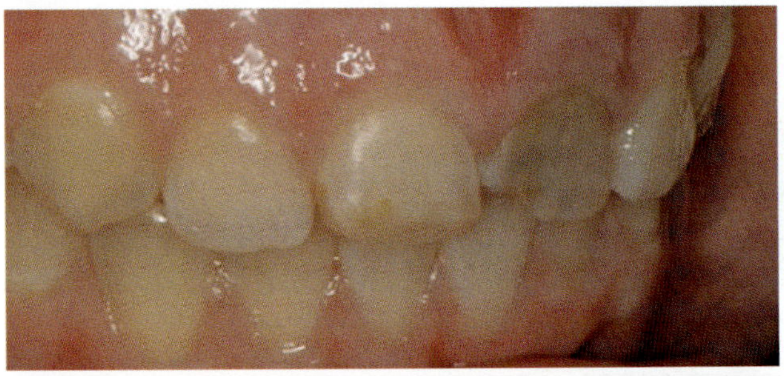
(B)

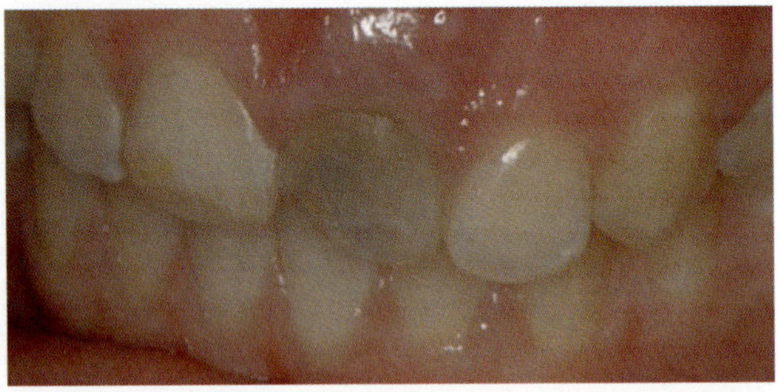
(C)

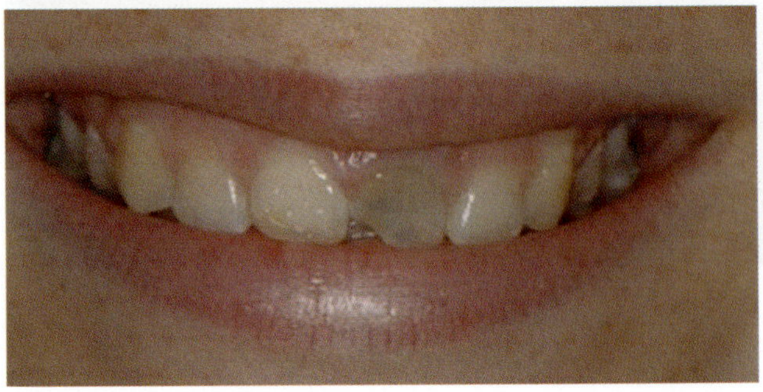
(D)

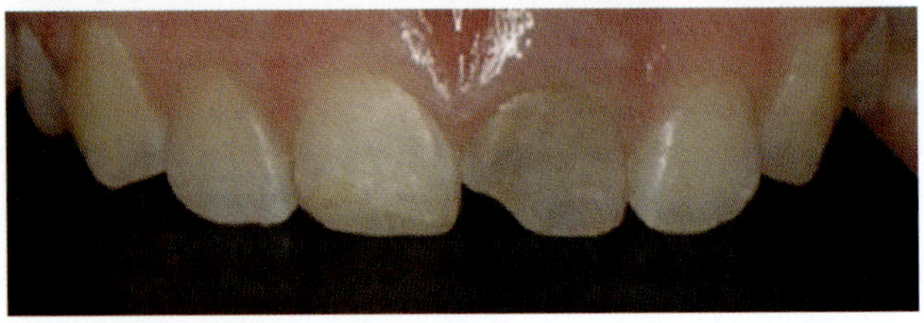
(E)

Figure 2.10

(A–E) This patient, age 11, was referred for whitening treatment because of a discolored upper left central incisor. The patient had fallen directly onto her front tooth at age 7, which had traumatized it. The tooth had previously undergone two root canal treatments; the last material used was mineral trioxide aggregate (MTA). The patient and her mother gave a history of pus pouring from the buccal and lingual area on a regular basis, despite numerous courses of broad-spectrum antibiotics. *continued on the next page*

3 TOOTH WHITENING MATERIALS

Linda Greenwall

INTRODUCTION

In the quarter century since the introduction of tooth whitening materials, there have been numerous modifications and improvements. We are currently using third-generation home whitening materials. The first-generation materials were in liquid form. These materials leaked out of the trays and needed continual replenishment over time, hence the use of reservoirs in the whitening trays. The second-generation materials were more viscous and in gel form. This viscosity allows the retention and adherence of the gel. The second-generation materials varied in concentrations of active ingredients and were known as either night products or day products. The third-generation materials differ in their concentration and incorporate soothers such as potassium nitrate, fluoride, and amorphous calcium phosphate (ACP). In general, quality control by the manufacturers and dental companies has improved, together with changes in the packaging, containers, and patient instructions, to make these products more patient-friendly. New legislation requires that tooth whitening syringes be labeled for specific use as a tooth whitening product, and in Europe they are not to be used in patients younger than 18.

Over the last 200 years, numerous attempts have been made to whiten teeth using all types of chemicals. The most effective products have been hydrogen peroxide and carbamide peroxide. These materials have different properties. This chapter will discuss the different materials that are used for tooth whitening treatments (Tables 3.1 and 3.2). Several other products that have been used for tooth whitening are discussed briefly.

THE CHEMISTRY OF WHITENING MATERIALS

Carbamide peroxide

Carbamide peroxide ($CH_6N_2O_3$) in a 10% gel formulation is the most commonly used home whitening material. The material is normally supplied in a syringe for ease of application, although some products are supplied in blister packs (see Figures 3.23–3.25). This breaks down to a 3.35% solution of hydrogen peroxide (H_2O_2) and a 6.65% solution of urea (CH_4N_2O). Fifteen percent and 20% solutions of carbamide peroxide are also available for dentist-supervised home whitening procedures. The 15% carbamide peroxide solution (CPS) yields 5.4% hydrogen peroxide, and the 20% solution yields 7% hydrogen peroxide (Fasanaro 1992) (Table 3.3).

A 35% carbamide peroxide gel is available as Quickstart (DenMat, Lompoc, CA) and 45% gel as Opalescence Quick (Ultradent Products, South Jordan, UT). These are used in an in-office procedure to enhance and accelerate the whitening process. The patient can see immediate results and is then motivated to continue the whitening treatment with 10% carbamide peroxide at home. This 35% gel yields 10% hydrogen peroxide. It can cause soft tissue damage and so should be used with a rubber dam or soft tissue protectant. The higher the concentration of materials, the faster the speed of action and the greater the likelihood of sensitivity (Table 3.4).

Hydrogen peroxide

Most of the whitening agents contain hydrogen peroxide in some form. The hydrogen peroxide breaks down into water and oxygen. It is the oxygen molecules that penetrate the tooth and liberate the pigment molecule, causing the tooth to whiten. (see Figures 3.1, 3.2, and 3.5).

The chemical hydrogen peroxide has been used for over 200 years to whiten teeth. Originally it was used as a liquid, applied directly onto a toothbrush, or as a cleansing agent in mouthwash form; now it is used in a gel formula to lengthen and preserve its short shelf life. Hydrogen peroxide is used in all types of whitening procedures—in office, chairside, and home whitening.

Thickening agents

Carbopol (carboxypolymethylene)

Carbopol is a polyacrylic acid polymer. Concentrations range from 0.5–1.5%. Trolamine, which is a neutralizing agent, is often added to Carbopol to reduce the pH of the gels to 5–7.

1. The solutions containing Carbopol (e.g., Opalescence [Ultradent Products]) release oxygen slowly, whereas those without it are fast oxygen-releasing solutions. The rate of oxygenation affects the frequency of solution replacement during whitening treatment. The fast oxygen-releasing solutions release a maximal amount of oxygen in less than 1 hour; the slow solutions require 2–3 hours for maximal oxygen release, but remain active for up to 10 hours (Matis et al. 1999).

Table 3.1 Chemistry of whitening products

Dentist supplied

- Hydrogen peroxide (HP); concentrations range from 3–35%
- Carbamide peroxide (CPS); concentrations range from 10–35% (see Figure 3.22)
- Enzymatic whitening products, which contain 3% CPS and lactoperoxidase to enhance the whitening effect

Alternative whitening products

- Sodium perborate (not permitted to be used in Europe)
- Sodium bicarbonate (used by nondental cosmetic whitening companies)
- Chlorine dioxide (used by nondental companies)

Table 3.2 Constituents of the whitening gels

- Carbamide peroxide
- Hydrogen peroxide and sodium hydroxide (Li 1998)
- Sodium perborate (on its own or included in other preparations)
- Thickening agent—Carbopol or Polyox
- Urea
- Vehicle—glycerin, dentifrice, glycol
- Surfactant and pigment dispersants
- Preservatives
- Flavorings
- Desensitizers
  - Fluoride
  - Potassium nitrate
  - Amorphous calcium phosphate (ACP) and casein phosphopeptide (CPP)
  - Others
    - Bioactive glass (e.g., calcium sodium phosphosilicate)
    - Calcium compounds (e.g., calcium carbonate, arginine)
    - Nano-hydroxyapatite

Table 3.3 Concentrations of different whitening gels

Hydrogen peroxide	*Carbamide peroxide*	
3.35%	10%	6.65% Urea, carbon dioxide, and ammonia
5.4%	15%	
6%	16%	
7%	20%	
10%	33.36%	

Adapted from Fasanaro 1992.

2. Carbopol enhances the viscosity of the whitening material. The thixotropic nature of Carbopol allows better retention of the slow-releasing gel in the tray. Less whitening material is required for treatment (approximately 29 mL per arch). The viscosity also improves adherence to the tooth. The currently available formula of Opalescence has more Carbopol than previously.

Table 3.4 Carbamide peroxide whitening products

10%

Pola Night (SDI)
Opalescence (Ultradent)
White Dental Beauty (Optident)
Optident
NiteWhite (Philips)
Perfect Bleach (Voco)
Evolution (Enlighten)
Illuminé (Dentsply)

15%

Illuminé Office (Dentsply)

16%

Pola Night (SDI)
Opalescence PF (Ultradent)
NiteWhite (Ultradent)
Evolution (Enlighten)

17%

Perfect Bleach (Voco)

20%

Opalescence Night White (Ultradent)
Pola Zing (SDI)

3. Carbopol retards the effervescence because it retards the rate of oxygen release. The thicker products stay on the teeth to provide the necessary time for the carbamide peroxide to diffuse into the tooth.
4. The increased viscosity seems to prevent the saliva from breaking down the hydrogen peroxide, which might achieve more effective results according to Haywood (1991b). The partial diffusion into the enamel may also allow the tooth to be whitened more effectively deeper within its enamel and dentin layers (Garber et al. 1991).

Polyox

Polyox (Union Carbide, Houston, TX) is the thickener used in the Colgate Platinum system. The composition of the Polyox is a trade secret (Oliver and Haywood 1999). The additive influences the activity of the material and the tray design.

Urea

Urea occurs naturally in the body. It is produced in the salivary glands and is present in saliva and the gingival crevicular fluid (Moss 1999). Urea breaks down to ammonia and carbon dioxide either spontaneously or through bacterial metabolism. The effect on the pH depends on the concentration of the urea and the duration of its application.

Urea is used in whitening kits to do the following:

- Stabilize the hydrogen peroxide (Christensen 1997). It provides a loose association with the hydrogen peroxide, which is easily broken down.

- Elevate the pH of the solution.
- Enhance other desirable qualities, such as anticariogenic effects, saliva stimulation, and wound healing properties (Archambault 1990).

Vehicle

Glycerin

Carbamide peroxide is formulated with a glycerin base, which enhances the viscosity of the preparation and ease of manipulation. However, this may dehydrate the tooth. Many dentists have reported that the tooth seems to lose its translucent appearance; this may be caused by dehydration. The dehydrating effect and the swallowing of the glycerin in the solution may be responsible for the sore throat that is sometimes reported as a side effect when these agents are used.

Glycol

This is anhydrous glycerin.

Surfactant and pigment dispersants

The surfactant functions as a surface wetting agent, which allows the hydrogen peroxide to diffuse across the gel–tooth boundary. A pigment dispersant keeps pigments in suspension (as in commercial water softeners). Gels with surfactant or pigment dispersants may be more effective than those without them (Feinman et al. 1991, Garber et al. 1991). This may result in a more active gel, and dentists who prescribe these particular kits (Nu-Smile and Brite Smile) should caution their patients to adhere to the manufacturers' suggested wearing time (Feinman et al. 1991).

Preservatives

Methyl, propylparaben, and sodium benzoate are commonly used as preservative substances. They have the ability to prevent bacterial growth in whitening materials (Alqahtani 2014).

Many of the gels contain a preservative such as citroxain, phosphoric acids, citric acid, or sodium stannate. These preservatives sequestrate transitional metals such as iron, copper, and magnesium, which accelerate the breakdown of hydrogen peroxide. These acid solutions give the gels greater durability and stability. They therefore have a mildly acidic pH.

Flavorings

Flavorings are used in whitening materials to improve the taste of the material, add to the selection of whitening agents, and improve acceptability of the product to the patient (e.g., melon and mint). Many agents also contain sodium saccharine, a sweetener.

Desensitizers

For an in-depth discussion, see Chapter 20).

1. Fluoride.
2. Potassium nitrate.
3. ACP (as in ACP–casein phosphopeptide [CPP] formulations).
4. Others, used in desensitizing toothpastes—many are recommended for use during whitening.

OVER-THE-COUNTER WHITENING PRODUCTS

Many over-the-counter (OTC) whitening-associated products have been introduced over the last 20 years.

Whitening-associated products are normally used to provide improved oral hygiene for removal of extrinsic stains, with some whitening maintenance to retain the white color. They are used as low-cost alternatives for whitening maintenance (Demarco et al. 2009).

These products include the following:

1. Whitening kits
2. Whitening maintenance kits (lower strength products)
3. Whitening mouthwash
4. Whitening toothpaste
5. Desensitizing whitening toothpaste
6. Whitening chewing gum
7. Whitening floss
8. Paint-on applicators

Such products, sold as cosmetics, have escaped rigorous legislation in the United States, the United Kingdom, and Europe. They are freely available through pharmacies, stores, mail order, and the Internet. Despite discussions with Internet mail order companies, these products are unregulated and are available to consumers. This has caused problems for patients and also for dentists, who should be monitoring whitening procedures carefully. There are many variations of these OTC materials (see Chapter 14).

The OTC kits contain the following:

1. Acid rinse. This is usually citric or phosphoric acid, which may be harmful to the dentition because continued rinsing may cause tooth erosion. The potential for misuse may be considerable (Jay, 1990). The pH of this rinse is between 1 and 2.
2. Whitening gel. This gel, applied for 2 minutes, has an acidic pH.
3. Postwhitening "polishing cream." This is an abrasive toothpaste containing titanium dioxide, which may give a temporary painted-white appearance. The efficacy and structural effects of these systems have not been evaluated in the literature.

H_2O_2 Strip System

The hydrogen peroxide strip system is a trayless whitening system that does not require any prefabrication or gel loading. The delivery system is a thin strip precoated with an adhesive 5.3% hydrogen peroxide gel (Haywood 2000, personal communication; Sagel et al. 2000). The backing is peeled off and the strip is placed directly on the facial and buccal surfaces of the six anterior teeth.

Each strip is worn for 30 minutes, removed, and discarded, and the procedure is performed twice a day for 14 days. The manufacturers (Procter & Gamble, Cincinnati, OH) claim that the strip holds the gel in place to whiten the teeth both extrinsically and intrinsically and provides a uniform controlled application of gel. The material was initially supplied to dentists and is now available OTC.

Problems with over-the-counter whitening kits

Cubbon and Ore (1991) reported that the overuse of OTC whitening agents caused erosion of the labial surfaces of the teeth, dissolution of the enamel, and loss of anatomy. The exposed dentin appeared darker than the remaining enamel, and patients overused this agent to reachieve the "white" tooth color. Dentists should be aware of these hazards when questioning patients who show evidence of tooth erosion of unknown cause (see Figure 3.3).

Patients may misdiagnose and self-prescribe whitening treatment, which may be inappropriate for their dental condition. A patient may have pulpal pathology that could be exacerbated by this treatment. In addition, a patient determined to speed up the whitening action may be overzealous in use of the product. Such abuse may lead to further problems and sensitivity (Fischer 2000a, 2000b).

SODIUM PERBORATE

Sodium perborate powder has long been used as a whitening agent. It was often used on its own as a cleansing agent and as a mouthwash (Bocasan, Oral-B, Procter & Gamble). It was used in combination with hydrogen peroxide owing to its synergistic effect to speed up the reaction of the oxidation. In 1965, Nutting and Poe recommended its use in internal whitening in combination with 35% hydrogen peroxide to be sealed inside the root canal. The effect of combining these two products was to create 50% hydrogen peroxide, which is very strong, to seal inside a nonvital tooth. In recent years, Internet suppliers of tooth whitening products were supplying it as a "safe" option because it was considered to contain no hydrogen peroxide, and so it was in effect below the "official legal" whitening limit. However, in the breakdown process of the sodium perborate, hydrogen peroxide is released. It is thus important to look at the chemistry.

Materials containing sodium perborate are Vitint System (Dental Partners, Rotterdam, the Netherlands) and Opalescence SP (Ultradent Products). The gel interacts with the moist tooth structure and is activated. The oxygen complex interacts with the tooth structure and saturates and changes the amino acids and double bonds of oxygen, which are responsible for tooth discoloration. However, sodium perborate breaks down to release hydrogen peroxide.

Chemistry of sodium perborate

There are two main forms of sodium perborate (A. Pala 2014, personal communication): monohydrate (empirical formula $NaBO3{\cdot}H2O$, molecular weight 99.81) and tetrahydrate (empirical formula $NaBO3{\cdot}4H2O$, molecular weight 153.81).

1. Sodium perborate is not simply a mixture of sodium metaborate and hydrogen peroxide, but rather an entirely different molecule with its own chemical properties.
2. Sodium perborate's whitening-oxidizing capacity increases with temperature. It works best at temperatures over 55°C.
3. As a whitening agent, sodium perborate is used with organic activators such as tetraacetylethylenediamine (TAED) to allow the use of sodium perborate at lower temperatures. In these cases peracetic acid is formed as an intermediate compound. Moreover, sodium perborate is stabilized with complex ethylenediaminetetraacetic acid (EDTA) in such a way that it is not broken down by ions. Caution should be taken to avoid addition of these chemicals to commercial preparations intended for tooth whitening.
4. The whitening activity of perborates is probably a result of the presence of not only perhydroxyl anion (HO2)–, but also the peroxoborate anion.
5. Sodium perborate has been banned in Europe for use in tooth whitening because it is considered to be fetotoxic and cytotoxic. The European Commission's Scientific Committee on Consumer Safety is of the opinion that sodium perborate and perboric acid can be considered as "hydrogen peroxide"–releasing substances and thus are covered by entry 12 of Annex III of the Cosmetics Directive 76/768/EEC (Council of European Dentists 2014).

MECHANISM OF WHITENING ACTION

Enamel should be considered a semipermeable membrane (Figure 3.15). Peroxide solutions flow freely through the enamel and dentin and into the pulp owing to the porosity and permeability of these structures (McEvoy 1989). The free movement is caused by the relatively low molecular weight of the peroxide molecule (see Figure 3.4) and the penetrating nature of the oxygen and superoxide radicals. It is difficult to set up barriers to prevent the rapid penetration.

The hydrogen peroxide acts as an oxygenator and an oxidant. Its whitening effect has been attributed to both these qualities, although the exact mechanism of action is not fully understood. In general, however, the hydrogen peroxide oxidizes the pigments in the tooth. The yellow pigments (xanthopterin) are oxidized to white pigments (leucopterin) (see Figures 3.1, 3.2, and 3.5). The oxidants react with the chromophores, which are the color radicals, to cleave the double bonds. The hydrogen peroxide must be in situ long enough and frequently enough to release the pigment molecules from the tooth by oxidation.

Carbamide peroxide is a bifunctional derivative of carbonic acid. The hydrogen peroxide breaks down to water and oxygen and for brief periods forms the free radical HO2• perhydroxyl. The free radical is very reactive and has great oxidative power.

- It can break up a large macromolecular stain into smaller stain molecules, which are expelled to the surface by diffusion.
- It can attach to inorganic structure and protein matrix (Fasanaro 1992).
- It can oxidize tooth discoloration.

Carbamide peroxide eventually breaks down to water, oxygen, urea, carbon dioxide, and ammonia (Figure 3.8).

Relative merits of H_2O_2 versus carbamide peroxide systems

Both systems contain hydrogen peroxide and work well. It appears that the H_2O_2 system may be faster than the CPS (Frysh et al. 1991), with a faster treatment and exposure time. Concentration of the hydrogen peroxide is determined by the teeth, not by the soft tissues, because the hydrogen peroxide solution contains mucous membrane protectant. However, there is no scientific literature about this, and these are purely manufacturers' claims. The H_2O_2 systems are aqueous gel based, whereas the CPS systems are anhydrous gel based. Dehydration of the hard tissue is less likely to occur with hydrogen peroxide treatment. The CPS systems whiten more slowly and need longer exposure times (see Figure 3.9). This is because of the presence and contact of Carbopol, which is a slow-release oxygen agent. The urea that is present in the gels assists with wound healing and contains a soft tissue protectant.

Movement of carbamide peroxide solution

The CPS moves freely through the tooth in a multidirectional manner. It can laterally diffuse through the tooth and into the pulp within 5–15 minutes. This means that the CPS can be applied palatally to the tooth surface to whiten the color beneath labially placed veneers. The transient pulpal sensitivity that some patients experience may be related to the rapid movement of urea and oxygen through the teeth (Haywood and Heymann 1991).

The whitening effect can be detected around the edges of the incisal area and in the incisal corners. It appears that lateral incisors take up the whitening product most quickly. Upper canines appear to be the slowest to lighten. This is because of the anatomy of the enamel and dentin microstructure. Upper teeth whiten more quickly and have fewer side effects than lower teeth.

Whitening on lower teeth can be slower. A demarcation line may be detected on lower canines, also referred to as a "snow-capped appearance," during the first few days of the treatment. This effect is most commonly noticed on lower canines, and patients are often concerned that their teeth are whitening unevenly. They can be reassured that this demarcation line usually fades after a few days of further whitening treatment. An in vitro study was undertaken by Oliver and Haywood (1999) to see whether the use of shortened dental trays could cause a demarcation line, but this proved negative and the teeth whitened evenly.

Treatment timing

There is no significant difference in the whitening efficacy of different concentrations of the material used during whitening treatments. At the end of treatment, it is not possible to know which concentration of whitening gel was used. However, studies have shown that the higher concentration materials may whiten teeth faster. An in vitro study by Leonard, Sharma, and Haywood (1998b) showed that a 16% solution of highly viscous materials (NiteWhite) successfully obtained a two-unit shade change more quickly than 5% and 10%. However, at the end of the 2-week trial period, there were no statistically significant differences among the 5%, 10%, or 16% solutions. A lower concentration of carbamide peroxide will also work, but it will take longer. The researchers observed that canines responded better to a 16% solution than did the central and lateral teeth. This would be beneficial for dentists who are treating an isolated dark tooth or darker canines (Leonard 1998).

Preferred regimens

Most of the suggested whitening times are for either overnight use or daytime use, depending on the product. Carbamide peroxide home whitening products are recommended to be used overnight. If the patient cannot manage overnight use, then 2–3 hours is recommended in the evening. This is related to the whitening potential of the Carbopol slow-release oxygen agents, which can remain active for 10 hours during the whitening treatment (Matis et al. 1999).

In a randomized double-blind clinical trial, Cibirka and colleagues (1999) tested two different 10% carbamide peroxide materials used overnight for 2 weeks to whiten the upper teeth; the results showed a significant degree of lightening. There was no significant difference between the two materials tested, which were Opalescence and NiteWhite. In another clinical evaluation of two carbamide peroxide agents, both caused the teeth to lighten (Heymann et al. 1998). The latter author made the comment that the actual treatment time may not represent the active concentration time because the carbamide peroxide is decomposing relatively rapidly in the initial phase of any treatment.

Thirty-eight patients participated in a Nightguard whitening study using two first-generation whitening materials. Participants were instructed to wear the guard at night or during the day for 2–4 hours for 6 weeks of total treatment time. Haywood et al. (1994) reported that 92% experienced successful lightening of their teeth. There were several categories of patients: (1) aging patients with inherent discoloration, (2) patients with trauma, (3) patients with fluorosis, and (4) patients with tetracycline staining. Of the first category, 100% of patients experienced tooth lightening compared with 80% of those with brown fluorosis and 75% of the tetracycline patients. Successful results could be seen within 20 hours of treatment.

The application technique relies on the mouthguard to keep the whitening agent in contact with the tooth so that the whitening product can penetrate through the enamel. The whitening process is thus dependent on the time for which the whitening agent is in contact with the tooth. It was noted that the more times the whitening tray was replenished, the greater the likelihood of sensitivity. Increase in the incidence of sensitivity was noted when the whitening technique was used twice per day rather than once per day (Leonard 1998).

Using Opalescence whitening material, Matis and coworkers (1999) have shown that carbamide peroxide degrades in an exponential manner after the first hour and that the degradation rate is higher in areas closer to the tooth structure. After 2 hours, 50% of the active ingredient of the whitening material was available and 10% was still available after 10 hours (Matis et al. 1999; see Figures 3.8 and 3.9). Longer treatment times may thus be advisable—that is, the agent needs to be active for extended periods of time; to get maximum use out of the whitening agent, it is preferable to sleep with the tray in position. The whitening potential of a material is thus an important factor to consider. Once this level has been determined, tray wearing times can be scientifically calculated.

Patients who have tetracycline staining may need to whiten their teeth for 3, 6, or 9 months or longer to achieve successful lightening. With extension of the treatment time, the efficacy rate for patients with tetracycline staining improved to 90% (Haywood et al. 1997).

Table 3.5 lists the properties of the ideal whitening agent, and Table 3.6 summarizes the factors affecting the rate of color change.

Effects on enamel

Surface texture

Most scanning electron microscopy studies of enamel surfaces treated with CPS whitening agents have shown little or no change in morphology (see Figures 3.16–3.18).

Table 3.5 Properties of the ideal whitening agent

The ideal whitening agent should:

- Be easy to apply to the teeth for maximum patient compliance.
- Be nonacidic (have a neutral pH).
- Lighten the teeth successfully and efficiently.
- Remain in contact with oral tissues for short periods.
- Have an adjustable peroxide concentration.
- Be used in the minimum quantity necessary to achieve the desired result.
- Be nonirritating.
- Not dehydrate the oral tissues or teeth.
- Not cause damage to the teeth or the enamel to be etched.

Table 3.6 Factors affecting rate of color change

- Frequency with which solutions are changed
- Amount of time for which the whitening agent is in contact with the tooth
- Viscosity of the material
- Rate of oxygen release
- Original shade and condition of the tooth
- Location and depth of discoloration (Howard 1992)
- Degradation rate of the material (Matis et al. 1999)

It is thought that the enamel surface remains intact and unaffected by the CPS and the whitening process (Haywood et al. 1991). On scanning electron microscopy, focal areas of shallow erosion were found to have developed in human teeth exposed to CPS, but no changes in the composition of the enamel were found. One study testing 16% and 35% CPS, however, reported significant changes in the enamel, including loss of the aprismatic layer, exposure and demineralization of enamel prisms, and pitting (Bitter 1995).

Surface hardness and wear resistance

Enamel surface hardness is apparently unaffected by the whitening agent (Zalkind et al. 1996, Kelleher and Roe 1999). However, a study using a whitening/remineralization cycle showed that 10% carbamide peroxide treatment significantly decreased enamel hardness. The application of fluoride improved remineralization of enamel. The reduction of hardness may reflect the loss of mineral from enamel, which could also result in reduced wear resistance (Seghi and Denry 1992). The researchers also showed that there was a change in the fracture toughness of the enamel (McCracken and Haywood 1996). Whitening may reduce the hardness of the enamel surface, and that may be more readily detected with instrumented low-load testing systems. This hardness reduction may arise as a result of degradation or denaturation of enamel matrix proteins by the peroxide oxidation (Elfallah and Swain 2013).

Enamel microhardness

A systematic review conducted by Attin showed interesting results. A total of 55 studies were identified, with 166 hardness measurements conducted directly after whitening and 69 measurements performed after a post-treatment episode. Directly after whitening, 84 treatments (51%) showed microhardness reduction compared with baseline, whereas 82 (49%) did not. After the post-treatment episode, 20 treatments (29%) showed hardness reduction and 49 (71%) did not. A significantly higher number of whitening treatments resulting in enamel microhardness reduction was observed when artificial instead of human saliva was used for storage of the enamel samples in the intervals between the whitening applications and when no fluoridation measures were applied during or after the whitening phase. Significantly, in those studies that simulated the intraoral conditions as closely as possible, the risk of enamel microhardness decrease as a result of whitening treatments seems to have been reduced. Nevertheless, more in situ and in vivo studies are needed to verify this observation (Attin et al. 2009).

Chemical composition

There may be loss of organic components from treated enamel surfaces—carbon, hydrocarbon, and tertiary amine groups replaced by oxygen, calcium, and phosphorus. The calcium/phosphate ratio of dentin was significantly decreased by whitening with 30% hydrogen peroxide and 10% carbamide peroxide in a study by Rotstein and colleagues (1996). In a study by McCracken and Haywood (1996), teeth exposed to CPS for 6 hours lost an average of 1.06 $\mu g/mm^2$ of calcium. This amount was significantly greater than in controls. However, this amount is small and the results may not be clinically significant. Drinking one can of a cola drink produced a comparable calcium loss of about 1 $\mu g/mm^2$. These results are consistent with calcium loss from enamel after 2-min exposures to carbonated cola, orange juice, apple juice, or diet carbonated cola (Grobler et al. 1990). The potential for remineralization occurs in vivo and may counteract these effects, but these have not been studied for CPS yet.

Some of the OTC whitening agents have a very low pH (5.6), and this may cause erosion of the enamel. The toothpaste provided with the kit may be abrasive to the tooth surface (Jay 1990). There is the potential side effect that the teeth can be etch-whitened (Bartlett and Walmsley 1991).

Effects on dentin

Tooth color is primarily determined by the dentin and can be changed by whitening treatments. In an in vitro study (McCaslin et al. 1999) using 10% carbamide peroxide placed directly onto the enamel to validate the color change in dentin and to assess whether dentin changed uniformly, it was noted that a color change occurred throughout the dentin and the color change was uniform.

Dentin bonding may be altered after whitening (Della Bona et al. 1992) and the smear layer may be removed (Hunsaker et al. 1990). The bonding between glass ionomer and dentin may also be affected (Titley et al. 1991). This may be a result of the precipitate of hydrogen peroxide and collagen that forms on the cut dentin surface after tooth whitening. It is suggested that adhesive dentistry be delayed for 2 weeks after whitening (Powell and Bales, 1991). (See further discussion later.)

Effects on pulp

Pulp penetration during whitening varies significantly among commercial 10% carbamide peroxide whitening products (Thitinanthapan et al. 1999), which may result in different levels of tooth sensitivity or whitening efficacy. Pulp penetration can occur within 5–15 minutes according to studies by Cooper et al. (1992). The potential for pulpal damage thus exists as a result of enamel and dentin penetration (Powell and Bales 1991). There appears to be less penetration into the pulp from carbamide peroxide than from hydrogen peroxide. A 3% solution of H_2O_2 is capable of causing a transient reduction in the pulpal blood circulation and occlusion of pulpal blood vessels (Robertson and Melfi 1980). The sensitivity is transient and lasts only for the duration of the whitening treatment (Basting et al. 2012). There is no long-lasting sensitivity.

Although the pulp is highly resilient to indirect insult from restorative materials, there is a danger that patients who are overzealous to achieve faster whitening may cause undesirable consequences (Minoux and Serfaty 2008). The most common side effect experienced by patients using the home whitening technique is transient, mild temperature sensitivity (Heymann et al. 1998) during the first hour after treatment. The sensitivity appears to be dose related rather than pH related. In a study by Scherer et al. (1991) the patients who experienced transient tooth hypersensitivity after week 2 had overloaded their trays. The studies appear to support the clinical observation that controlled home whitening is safe to the pulp (Li 1998, Kelleher and Roe 1999).

An evidence-based evaluation (Cochrane review by Hasson et al. 2006) that assessed 416 articles on tooth whitening noted that strips (5.5% to 6.5% hydrogen peroxide) are more effective than gel in tray with 10% carbamide peroxide (mean difference 1.82; 95% confidence interval [CI] 0.26–3.38). Mild to moderate tooth sensitivity and gingival irritation were the most common side effects. The whitening strips and products with high concentrations of hydrogen peroxide caused more users to report tooth sensitivity. There is evidence that whitening products work when compared with placebo or /no treatment. Hasson et al. (2006) concluded that there are differences in efficacy among the products, mainly resulting from the levels of the active ingredients, hydrogen peroxide and carbamide peroxide. All trials were, however, short term, and most were judged to be at high risk of bias and were either sponsored or conducted by the manufacturers.

Effects on cementum

It appears from recent studies that the cementum is not affected by the materials used for home whitening (Rotstein and Friedman 1991, Murphy et al, 1992). A study by Scherer et al. (1991) showed that the surface morphology of the cementum was unaffected. Cervical resorption (Latcham 1986, Madison and Walton 1990) and external root resorption (Cvek and Lindvall 1985) have been reported in teeth whitened by the internal whitening technique using 35% hydrogen peroxide. In the latter study most of the teeth were associated with previous trauma, and it is not known whether the trauma predisposed the tooth to the resorption or whether it was caused by the effects of the whitening agent. pH measurements of the root surface have demonstrated cervical resorption occurring in those teeth that were not previously traumatized.

Whiter, brighter, or lighter?

The penetration of oxygen inside the tooth gives the tooth a whiter appearance. When the oxygen becomes saturated inside the tooth, it appears bright. Two weeks after termination of whitening, the tooth appears less bright because the oxygen is dissipating from the tooth, and the shade settles to the lighter shade. There may be a decrease in the translucency of the tooth. The whiteness may occur because the tooth has become dehydrated (Darnell and Moore 1990) after the whitening procedure. This may be a transient effect. It is not apparent what effect or combination of effects is occurring. A brightness index derived from computer analysis of digitized images may be useful for monitoring effectiveness of whitening (Bentley et al. 1999).

PATIENT RESPONSE TO HOME WHITENING

Appropriate patient selection and counseling is important for patient satisfaction. In a longitudinal study by Haywood et al. (1994), at 1.5 years after treatment 74% of patients who had responded to home whitening were satisfied with the shade of their teeth. At 3 years after treatment 62% were satisfied with their color. At 7 years after treatment of the same patient pool, 35% were satisfied with the color of their teeth. No one reported reversion to the original shade (Leonard et al. 1998a).

Patient perceptions of the whitening technique are positive. Ninety-five per cent of patients are genuinely glad they went through the procedure and 97% recommended the procedure to their friends (Leonard 1998). Of the patients surveyed in the latter study, 87% said they would undergo whitening again.

COLOR REGRESSION AND SHADE RELAPSE

Once whitening has been terminated, a slight relapse in color occurs over the following 2 weeks. It has been hypothesized that the tooth is filled with oxygen from the oxidative process and this changes the optical qualities of the tooth to appear more opaque. After 2 weeks, the oxygen has dissipated and the tooth demonstrates the actual lightened shade. Patients should be informed of this phenomenon because they tend to think that the whitening is regressing; in reality the teeth are equilibrating to the new actual shade (Haywood 1999b). Color regression occurred within the first month after whitening in a study by Matis and coworkers (1998).

The process of color regression toward darker shades is poorly described and understood in the literature (Heymann et al. 1998), but is thought to be the opposite of the whitening procedure. Regression occurs over a longer period because some of the previously oxidized substances may become chemically reduced and cause the tooth to reflect the old discoloration or the enamel may become remineralized with the staining molecule of the original stain (Lyons and Ng 1998).

A clinical trial (Leonard et al. 1999) evaluating color stability after 54 months of tetracycline-stained teeth that were treated with 10% carbamide peroxide and extended whitening times showed that it is possible for the color to remain stable for 54 months after whitening treatment. The color stability may be related to the extended treatment time of 6 months. This is the longest post-treatment clinical study published. No patient felt the need to have the teeth re-treated as a result of color regression.

A 4% color regression after 6 months has been reported in nonvital whitening (Ho and Goerig 1989). The considerable application time with home whitening techniques may explain the minimal color regression reported. Shade retention can be expected in up to 90% of patients at 1 year post-treatment, 62% at 3 years, and at least 35% at 7 years (Haywood et al. 1994). Patients in the latter study rewhitened on average at 25 months. The shade never reverts to the original shade.

The success rate for home whitening using a viscous whitening material for 7–10 days is about 95% (Haywood et al. 1994). With changes to the treatment time and/or concentration of the whitening material, the success rate for tetracycline-stained teeth is 90%.

Response of the stains to whitening

The initial color of the affected teeth seems to determine the success or failure of the technique (Arens 1989). It appears that the lighter the tooth, the easier it is to whiten. Yellow stains are the easiest to whiten. Less responsive stains in order of decreasing responsiveness are light gray (see Figures 3.10 and 3.11), light brown (see Figure 3.1), dark yellow, dark brown, gray, and black (Swift 1988). Length of whitening time is an important predictor of success in teeth that have fluorosis staining (Seale and Thrash 1985). Seale and Thrash suggested that because of increased porosity, younger teeth would be easier to whiten than older ones (see Figure 3.2). Older teeth, because of the more complex dentin structure, take longer to lighten (see Figures 3.1, 3.10, and 3.11). The whitening period may need to be extended to 6–10 weeks to achieve significant lightening. Some parts of the tooth may be difficult to whiten. A dark black crack line on the central incisors caused by grinding and smoking may not be lightened with whitening (see Figure 3.12). Teeth with extreme wear and older yellow teeth may take longer to whiten. Although patients with severe wear on their teeth may request whitening, further restorative dentistry may be more appropriate. Whitening may be the beginning of the treatment plan, and then further restorative dentistry may need to be carried out (see Figure 3.14). Erosive dentin lesions may not whiten sufficiently, and it may be inappropriate to whiten areas of deep erosion. Other restorative treatment may be more appropriate for these patients (see Figure 3.15).

EFFECTS ON RESTORATIVE MATERIALS

Initially, no effects on restorative materials were reported (Haywood et al. 1991c). Recent studies have shown that surface effects may occur on existing restorative materials (such as composites, glass ionomers and, luting cements). A recent in vitro study of the effects of carbamide peroxide on provisional crowns showed that an orange discoloration occurred with provisional materials containing methacrylate (Robinson et al. 1997). Amalgams may appear to become greenish during the whitening treatment because of the copper inside the amalgam.

Bond strength to enamel

Whitening is frequently used in combination with other forms of restorative dentistry that require bonding to enamel. These procedures may include replacement of existing restorations to improve shade matching, diastema closure, and placement of veneers (see Chapter 15). All these techniques rely on adequate adhesion of the composite to the enamel. Any factor compromising adhesion can affect the aesthetics and longevity of the bonded restoration (Cvitko et al. 1991).

As we have seen, whitening with peroxide reduces the bond strength of enamel by about 20% in the immediate effect. Studies by Torneck et al. (1991) have shown that there is a reduced bond strength of composite to enamel immediately after whitening with a 35% solution of hydrogen peroxide. However, the bond strength will improve if etching and bonding are delayed for 1–2 weeks postwhitening (Titley et al. 1991, Godwin et al. 1992). Waiting 2 weeks will also allow the color to stabilize. Hydrogen peroxide appears to change the surface chemistry. Resin tags in whitened enamel are less numerous, less defined, and shorter than those in unwhitened enamel (Titley et al. 1991). The residual oxygen in the whitened tooth surface also inhibits the polymerization of the composite resin (McGuckin et al. 1991) and disrupts the surface (Haywood 1999a).

Studies using 10% CPS also showed that the bond strength of composite to etched enamel was reduced (Cvitko et al. 1991). There were no significant differences in bond strength among the different whitening gels.

The reduced bond strength is transient; it diminishes after 24 hours and disappears after 1 week (Della Bona et al. 1992). The use of topical fluoride after whitening may help to regain the bond strength (Haywood 1991c). The use of acetone- or alcohol-based adhesive systems or roughening the surface may counteract these effects of peroxides on bond strength. More conservative enamel removal may be sufficient to counteract these effects, but further research is needed. Internal whitening of endodontically treated teeth has been shown to result in greater leakage of composite restorations immediately after completion of internal whitening (Barkhorder et al. 1997). It may be more appropriate to wait for 2 weeks before placing the composite restoration and to place a glass ionomer restoration directly into the access cavity immediately after completion of the whitening treatment to prevent the reduction in bond strength.

However, recent studies have shown that application of ascorbic acid in a gel form for 60 minutes may improve the bond strength with immediate effect (Kaya et al. 2008). Miranda et al. (2013) showed that compromised bond strength to whitened enamel was immediately restored with the application of antioxidant gel sodium ascorbate and exposure to human saliva in situ for at least 7 days. Best results were obtained with exposure to human saliva in situ for 14 days. Treatment with sodium ascorbate gel for 60 minutes may be recommended if patients cannot wait for at least 7 days for adhesive techniques to be performed. However, clinically this may be difficult to achieve because patients may not tolerate the application of ascorbic acid to the teeth for such a long period of time. This effect of the acid needs further research to ensure that there is no permanent erosive effect on the teeth.

Composite material

Reports on the effects of whitening on composite resins are conflicting. Some studies have shown that composites are unaffected by CPS (Haywood et al. 1991, Baughan et al. 1992, Machida et al. 1992). Others have shown that surface hardness is altered (Bailey and Swift 1991, Friend et al. 1991), and another study showed that surface hardness was unaffected by whitening (Nathoo et al. 1994). Surface roughening and etching may occur (Singleton and Wagner, 1992) and tensile strength is affected (Cullen et al. 1993). However, these effects are unlikely to be clinically significant (Swift 1998).

Haywood and Heymann (1991) have noted no significant color changes other than the removal of extrinsic stains around existing restorations. The effect is primarily the superficial cleansing of the restoration and a lightening of the underlying tooth structure and not an intrinsic color change of the restorative material itself. Whitening has been shown to increase the micro-leakage of existing restorations. Restorations may need to be replaced after whitening owing to the color change in the tooth.

Amalgam restorations

Although there have been few reports of effects on amalgam restorations, studies (Hummert et al. 1992) suggest that there may be significantly more mercury released from amalgam restorations during the whitening procedure. Rotstein and coworkers (1997) found than 4–30 times as much mercury was released from amalgams in vitro compared to saline controls. Further clarification of this is required. It appears that prolonged treatment with whitening agents may cause microstructural changes in amalgam surfaces and this may possibly increase exposure of patients to toxic byproducts (Rotstein et al. 1997). Existing amalgams may change color from black to silver (see Figure 3.19). This effect is dependent on the type of dental amalgam used (Rotstein 1999, personal communication). However, not all combinations of amalgam and whitening agents result in higher mercury levels. Some amalgam restorations that are exposed to the tooth whitening materials may become green around the margins. This may be a result of the copper content of the amalgam (Haywood 2007).

Other materials

Fired porcelain showed a slight change after being immersed in the whitening gels for three 2-hour periods a day for 5 weeks (Hunsaker et al. 1990). No effect on gold has been reported. Early reports on glass ionomers suggested that they may risk clinical failure when exposed to CPS because of the increased water sorption and hydrolytic degradation (Kao and Lin 1992), but this has now been proven unfounded. There appears to be an alteration in the matrix of the glass ionomer (Jefferson et al. 1991). Other luting cements may also be affected. Analysis by scanning electron microscopy has revealed erosion of the matrix of the luting cement, and there was some degree of crystalline formation (Jefferson et al. 1991) of the zinc phosphate cement.

Provisional restorations such as those using intermediate restorative material (IRM) may be affected by hydrogen peroxide (see Figures 3.20 and 3.21). Macroscopically, IRM exposed to hydrogen peroxide appears cracked and swollen, whereas carbamide peroxide does not appear to have an effect. Provisional crowns made from methyl methacrylate may discolor and turn orange. Polycarbonate crowns and bis-acryl composite temporary materials do not discolor (Robinson et al. 1997).

OTHER PROPERTIES OF CARBAMIDE PEROXIDE

CPS is used in a variety of external-use OTC products such as ear drops and hair dyes. Patients with known sensitivity or allergy to any of the ingredients should not use the whitening agent. Allergic symptoms have been reported, such as swelling of the lips (Goldstein and Garber 1995).

Oral uses and effects

Carbamide peroxide also has an antibacterial effect (Gugan et al. 1996; see section on therapeutic aesthetics). It reduces plaque adherence and accumulation and therefore has been used for treatment of periodontitis, oral hygiene (Stindt and Quenette 1989), reduction of gingivitis, reduction of caries rate, and aphthous ulceration (Tse et al. 1991). It has been used since 1960 for oral wound debridement (Fasanaro 1992). CPS has been incorporated into a chewing gum with inhibition of plaque formation (Moss 1999). It has also been tried for treatment of recurrent herpes labialis. It has been tested for use as an irrigant or lubricant in root canals and as an adjunctive to sodium hypochlorite (Stindt and Quenette 1989). It was also used for post-operative rinsing after tooth extraction. The studies using CPS have shown promising results.

Systemic side effects carbamide peroxide

The only systemic effects that have been reported have been one case that produced a mild laxative effect, and mild gastric irritation reported by some patients who are using the treatment for whitening of tetracycline discoloration.

Owing to the possibility of overuse of CPS by the patient at home, it is prudent to ensure that the patient follows the prescribed regimen for tray wearing. Encourage the patient to refrain from smoking during treatment (Larson 1990). Dentists should encourage their patients to stop smoking for general health improvement and to enroll in a smoking cessation program. This would reduce the associated staining.

There is also the possibility of an allergy to the whitening materials or to the tray plastic material. One patient experienced allergies to the preservative in the whitening tray. This patient experienced swelling of the face 1 week after whitening the upper teeth when she began to whiten the lower teeth. Whitening was terminated at that point with immediate effect. Occasionally an allergy to hydrogen peroxide may be noted. This is very rare. There is no known cross-reaction between the hydrogen peroxide materials used for highlighting hair and tooth whitening materials. Table 3.7 lists the possible side effects.

The majority of the literature and research indicates that the use of 10% carbamide peroxide for dentist-monitored home whitening is an effective and safe way to lighten discolored teeth (see Figure 3.1).

WHITENING TOOTHPASTES

Toothpastes have become more specialized and sophisticated in the last decade (Koertge et al. 1998) with many designed to perform either therapeutic or cosmetic functions. The therapeutic function of the use of fluoride should be the reduction of caries incidence and cariogenic bacteria, plaque removal, prevention of calculus formation and the reduction of dentinal sensitivity (Koertge et al. 1998). Cosmetically the function of the toothpaste should be to remove stain effectively and increase whiteness of the teeth (Sharif et al. 2000).

The introduction of whitening toothpastes has been very rapid. There has not been that much clinical research conducted on these products, which concerned the American Dental Association Council on Therapeutics (1994). There are many questions about these products, particularly whether they are effective at maintaining a white smile after whitening and delay the color regression. The whitening toothpastes seem effective at removing surface stains on the teeth and may be useful to reduce extrinsic stains that occur from tea and coffee. They may be used to maintain white teeth after whitening.

Table 3.8 shows a classification of whitening toothpastes according to their mechanism of action (Haywood 1996).

More abrasive than usual

The abrasive toothpastes try to remove the surface staining by 'sanding' the teeth. The paste toothpaste is more abrasive than the gel toothpaste. The overzealous use of abrasive toothpaste will cause the removal of enamel as

Table 3.7 Possible side effects of whitening agents

Gingivae

- Tissue sloughing
- Gingival irritation
- Gingival ulceration
- Change in gingival texture
- Gingival soreness
- Whitening of the maxillary papillae
- Possible gingival irritation if the tray is overextended
- Possible opening of the black triangles and enlargement of black spaces

Teeth

External effects

- Uneven, incomplete whitening, streaky appearance
- White spots or banding within the tooth may be more noticeable
- A demarcation line may be visible between the color on the incisal tip and the cervical neck
- Snow-capped appearance on the lower incisors as a result of slower whitening

Internal effects

Pulp

- Transient thermal sensitivity
- Flare-up of an existing quiescent apical area

Oral mucosa

- Sore throat
- Unpleasant taste
- Burning palate
- Pain and sensitivity
- Ulceration
- Soft tissue lacerations

Other

- Irritation of the tongue from rough edges of the whitening tray
- Mild laxative effect
- Gastric irritation
- Allergy, facial swelling or petechiae on face and neck

well as the stain. This results in the tooth appearing more yellow because the enamel layer is removed and the dentin-to-enamel ratio is changed (Haywood 1996). The combination of a hard toothbrush and an abrasive toothpaste has been recognized as creating further tooth wear problems.

Chemical removal of surface pellicle

These toothpastes act to remove the surface pellicle, which houses the surface stain. They act in a similar manner to the tartar control toothpastes, which aim to prevent the buildup of tartar. Although these toothpastes may be effective for stain reduction, they do not change the internal color of the teeth (Haywood 1996).

Some products in this category contain titanium dioxide, a white pigment found in paint. It acts by entering the surface irregularities of the tooth (Haywood 1995b) and gives the illusion of whitened teeth. Only a surface phenomenon, titanium dioxide does not penetrate internally and thus does not modify the internal color or whiten teeth. Other ingredients include tetrasodium pyrophosphate for the soothing effect on the teeth as well as sodium lauryl sulphate for the foaming capability and hydrated silica.

Table 3.8 Classification of whitening toothpastes

1. More abrasive than usual
2. Chemical removal of surface pellicle
3. Toothpastes containing peroxides
4. Toothpastes containing desensitizers: fluoride, strontium chloride, potassium nitrates, calcium compounds, nanohydroxyapatites
5. Toothpastes containing arginine and proactive glass such as NovaMin
6. Toothpastes containing bicarbonates (e.g., Colgate Sensitive Pro Relief)
7. Toothpastes containing enzymes, e.g., lactoperoxidase (White Kin, Spain, UK, Germany)
8. Toothpastes with multiple ingredients such as triclosan

Toothpastes containing peroxides

This type of toothpaste may contain hydrogen peroxide, calcium peroxide, sodium percarbonate or carbamide peroxide as an active ingredient to lighten teeth. Some of the toothpastes contain the same concentration of peroxide as the home whitening agents, whereas other toothpastes contain hydrogen peroxide in very low concentration (a 1.5% concentration may be too low to exert a whitening effect). The mechanism of application does not seem sufficient to warrant a significant amount of tooth lightening. However, long-term use of peroxide-containing toothpastes has the potential to make some changes, but there is a question about their safety (Haywood 1996). They act to remove the discoloration of surface staining and possibly also have some chemical effects (Lynch et al. 1998).

Toothpaste containing 1% hydrogen peroxide

Studies have shown that a toothpaste containing 1% hydrogen peroxide can be effective in whitening teeth.

Prophylaxis paste containing hydrogen peroxide

There are prophylaxis pastes on the market that contain hydrogen peroxide, such as Peroxide Prophy Paste (Challenge Products, Osage Beach, MO). These products are supposed to lighten while the teeth are cleaned during a professional prophylaxis by the hygienist. A preliminary in vitro study to assess the effect on lightening of teeth by comparing a regular prophylaxis paste with the paste containing hydrogen peroxide did show more lightening than with the regular prophylaxis paste (Bowles et al. 1997). It appears that the paste containing hydrogen peroxide lightens teeth by both chemical and abrasive action (Bowles et al. 1997).

Desensitizing whitening toothpastes

There are many new whitening toothpastes such as NovaMin that are designed specifically for patients undergoing tooth whitening. They contain potassium nitrate and a bioactive glass, calcium sodium phosphosilicate (Gillam and Talioti 2014). Potassium nitrate was added to block the nerve impulses and reduce general sensitivity and sensitivity caused by whitening. Haywood (2007) showed that brushing with potassium nitrate–containing toothpaste for 2 weeks significantly reduced sensitivity.

Toothpastes containing bioactive glass

NovaMin has been mentioned already; another such product is Regenerate. These are used for desensitizing the teeth before, during, and after whitening, but also for strengthening the enamel. This is useful for many patients who have erosion from acid loss.

Toothpastes containing sodium bicarbonate

The small particle size of sodium bicarbonate may allow the material to penetrate into the enamel and clean inaccessible areas (Kleber et al. 1998). An in vitro study showed that brushing with a bicarbonate toothpaste has the potential to cause tooth lightening. However, the whitening ability of sodium bicarbonate appears to be dependent on the concentration of sodium bicarbonate, up to a threshold concentration (over 45%). A product with 65% concentration may also contain other ingredients such as sodium lauryl sulfate which may facilitate stain removal by sodium bicarbonate. A randomized, controlled 6-week clinical trial to determine the effectiveness and safety of a whitening dentifrice containing sodium bicarbonate in removing extrinsic tooth stain and whitening teeth was conducted by Ghassemi and coworkers in 2012. The subjects brushed with bicarbonate toothpaste. An additional 2-week exploratory study was conducted to determine whether the whitening or stain-prevention activity of the dentifrice would persist after cessation of use. In the first study (Phase I), 146 qualifying subjects were randomly assigned to either a sodium bicarbonate whitening dentifrice group (Arm & Hammer Advance White Extreme Whitening Toothpaste with Baking Soda and Peroxide) or a silica-based negative-control dentifrice group, and brushed twice daily with their assigned dentifrice for 6 weeks. Tooth shade on the labial surfaces of the eight incisors was assessed using a Vita classical shade guide, and extrinsic tooth stain was scored using a Modified Lobene Stain Index (MLSI) at baseline, week 4, and week 6. In Phase II (after the week 6 examination), volunteers from the Arm & Hammer whitening dentifrice group were randomly assigned to continue using the whitening dentifrice or to use the negative-control dentifrice twice daily for 2 weeks. The 6-week shade and stain index scores served as the baseline for this exploratory phase and were rescored after 2 weeks. The results showed that the whitening dentifrice tested was effective for removing extrinsic tooth stain and whitening teeth. Although the results also suggest that this dentifrice may have stain-prevention activity that persists after cessation of product use, such activity would need to be confirmed with further studies.

Toothpastes containing enzymes

There are toothpastes that contain enzymes to enhance tooth whitening. This process is called enzymatic whitening. The program involves the use of lactoperoxidase to whiten teeth in combination with a 3% carbamide peroxide material (Forner 2012). The enzymes act as catalysts by decreasing the activation energy of the whitening reactions or by generating hydrogen peroxide in situ, thereby enabling a reduction in peroxide concentration and in the risk of toxic effects.

Other enzymes, such as bromelain and papain, remove the pellicle layer and slow the development of plaque on the surface layer. The enzymes are incorporated into toothpastes to activate or accelerate the whitening potential of the toothpaste.

Toothpastes with multiple components

Some of the whitening toothpastes contain up to 20 ingredients, of which 14 are said to be active. Some also contain two or more oxidizing agents. A spray product for mouth freshening contains the same ingredients in liquid form.

Fluoride toothpastes containing the antibacterial chemical triclosan and a copolymer that aids in retention of the agent during rinsing appears to reduce plaque formation, caries, gingival inflammation, and bleeding (Riley and Lamont 2013). This will enhance the therapeutic use of the whitening agents to encourage improvement of the overall oral health of the mouth. Analysis of 14,835 participants across 30 studies found that after 6 months of using triclosan–copolymer fluoride toothpaste there was a 22% reduction in plaque and gingivitis, a 48% reduction in bleeding gums, and a 5% reduction in caries. Triclosan fights the bacteria in plaque and reduces the swelling of the gingivae.

CLINICAL STUDIES

In a clinical study to assess the stabilizing effects of two toothpastes, 30 patients who had had their teeth lightened were randomly assigned to two groups to test two whitening toothpastes (Matis 1998). The results after 3 months showed that the toothpaste containing 10% carbamide peroxide was able to stabilize the tooth lightening effect of the whitening gel better than the toothpaste containing 3% hydrogen peroxide. However, the hydrogen peroxide had a lower tooth sensitivity rating.

Another randomized, double-blind clinical study by Koertge et al. 1998 evaluated the ability of a bicarbonate-containing whitening toothpaste to reduce existing levels of stain and increase whiteness of teeth as compared with a regular silica-based toothpaste. Results showed that although the whiteness was increased with the bicarbonate-containing toothpaste, the stain removal potential

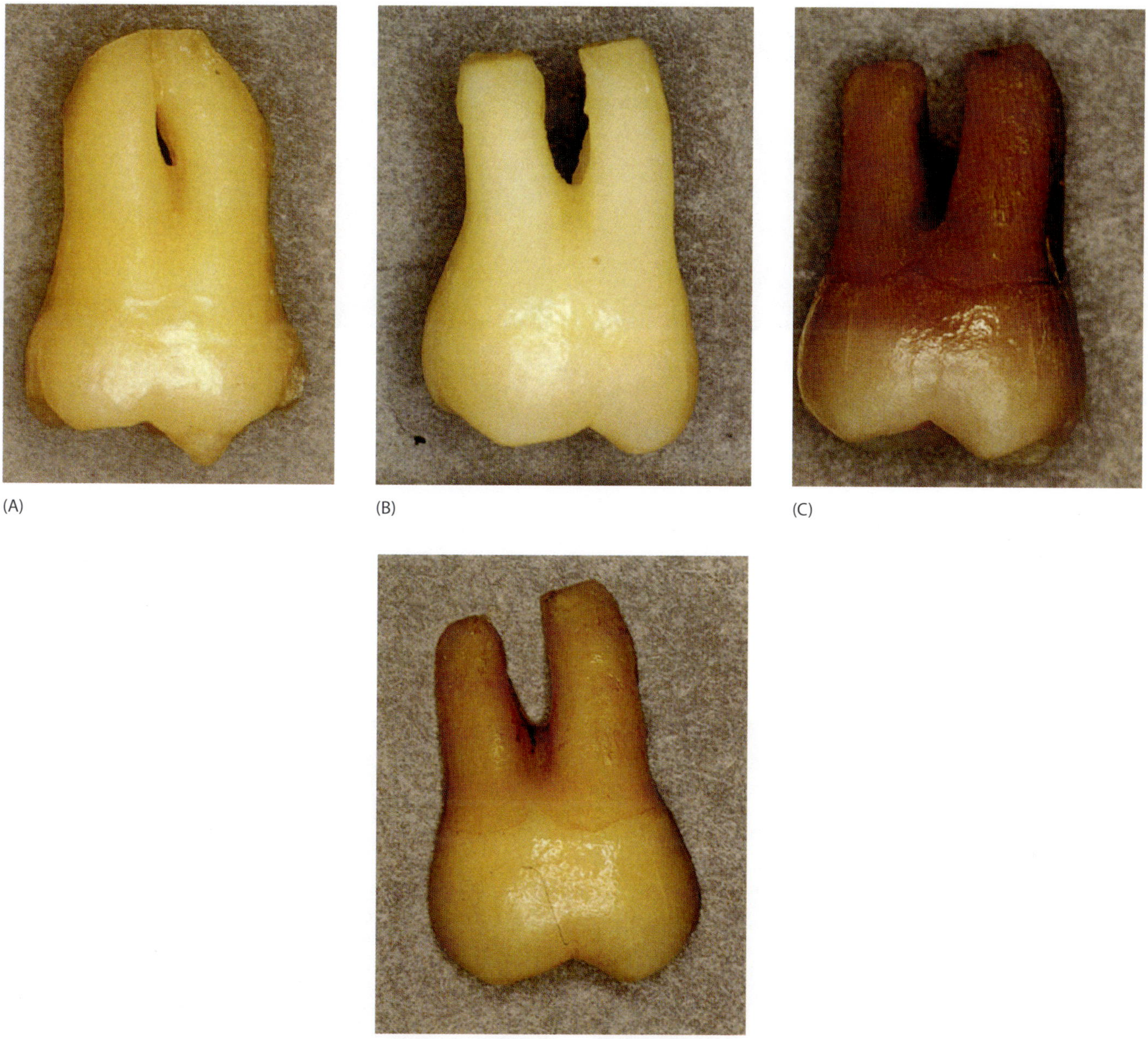

(A) (B) (C)

(D)

Figure 3.1

(A) An experimental design for testing the whitening material was devised. Teeth were discolored artificially by spinning blood into them. The color and appearance of a tooth is shown before whitening with the over-the-counter kit. (From Greenwall 1992a.) (B) After the discoloration by blood pigment, the tooth was sectioned and stored in artificial saliva. The appearance of the tooth after 3 days of whitening. Note that although the whitening material is placed onto the enamel surface only, the root surface is also getting lighter. (C) The appearance of the tooth after 7 days. (D) The appearance of the tooth after 28 days. Note that the apex of the root has also lightened.

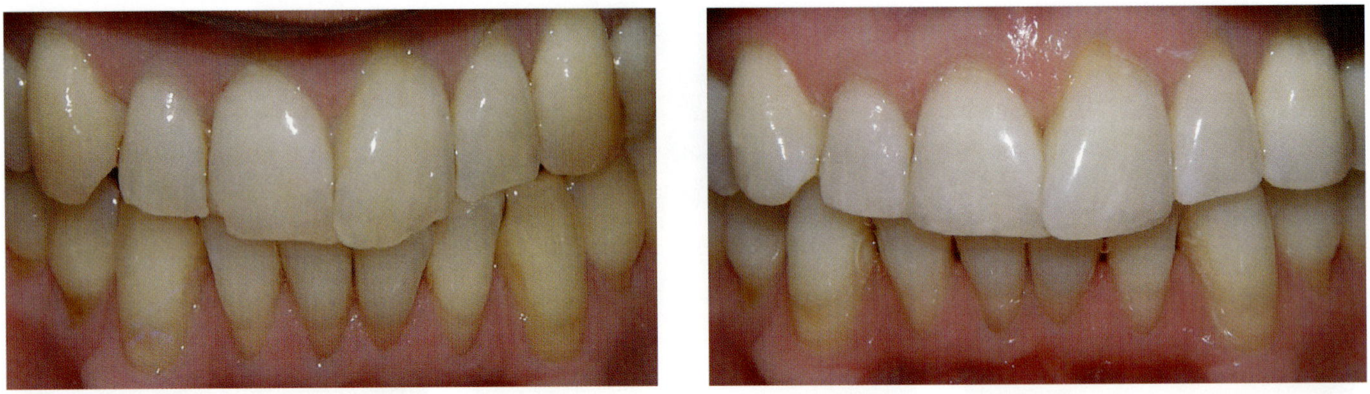

(A) (B)

Figure 3.2

(A) This middle-aged male patient had generalized discoloration with brown discoloration concentrated in his canine teeth. (B) Home whitening was undertaken using 10% carbamide peroxide in a whitening tray. Patient started with the upper tray first, followed by whitening of the lower teeth using the same technique.

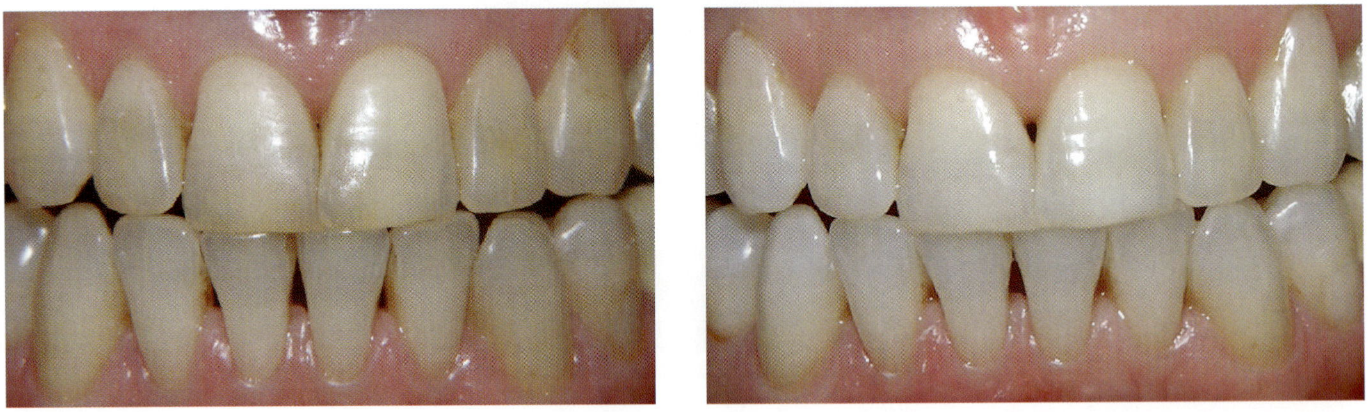

(A) (B)

Figure 3.3

(A) Appearance of teeth after undertaking whitening with a beauty therapist. The product used was 0.5% chlorine dioxide. The aftereffects were that the teeth became sensitive, the enamel lost its luster, and the enamel felt rough and picked up further stain. (B) Emergency treatment consisted of desensitization using an immediate dentin sealer such as HurriSeal (Beutlich Pharmaceuticals, Patterson Dental and distributed in the United Kingdom by Enlighten Smiles). This was followed by direct application of a dentin bonding agent. Once the sensitivity was reduced, the teeth were whitened using 10% carbamide peroxide with trays at home. The teeth were then polished and reglazed with bonding agent to restore the natural enamel luster.

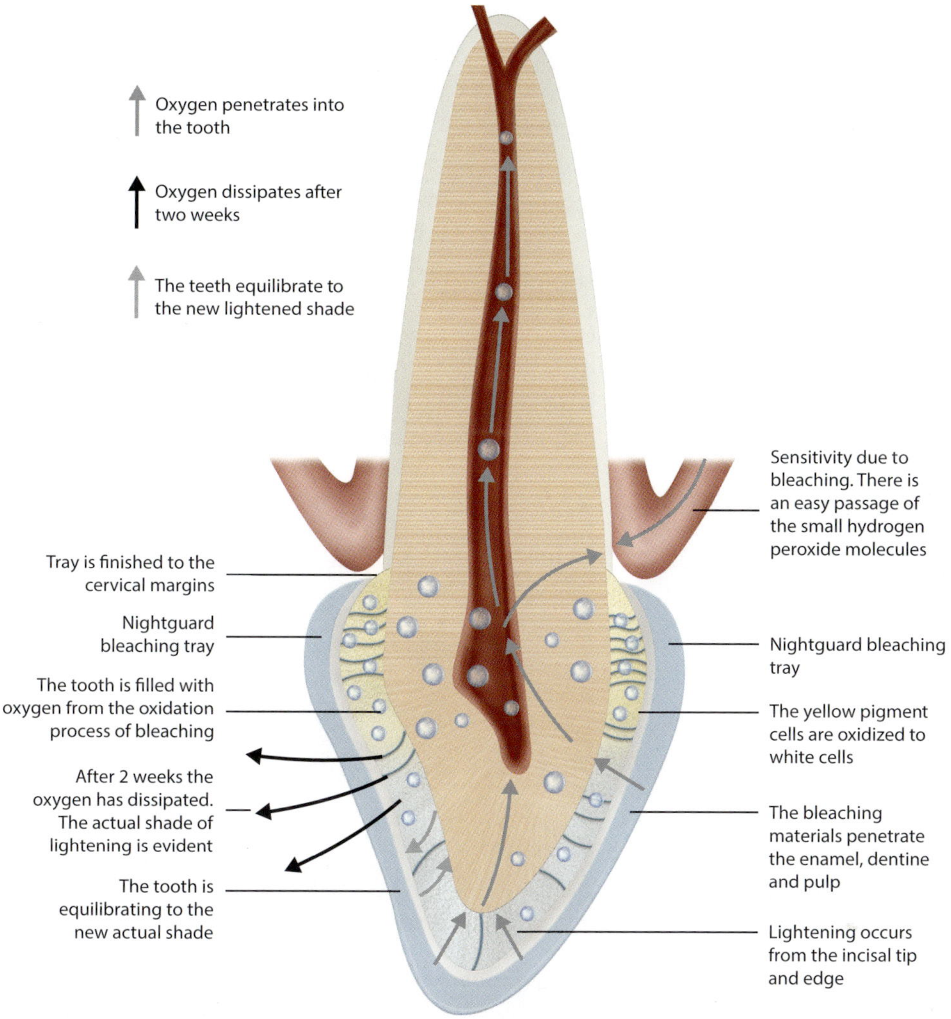

(A)

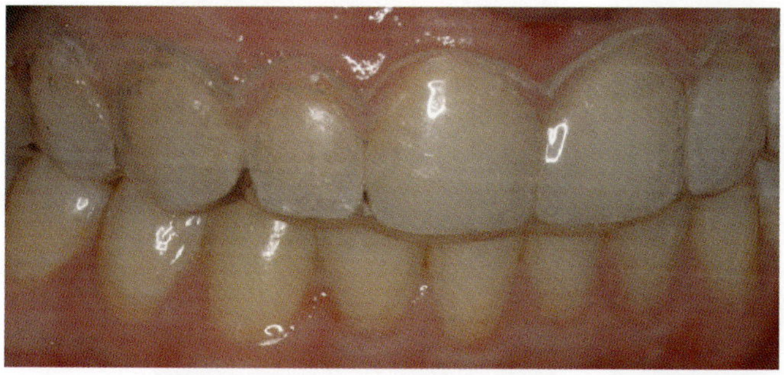

(B)

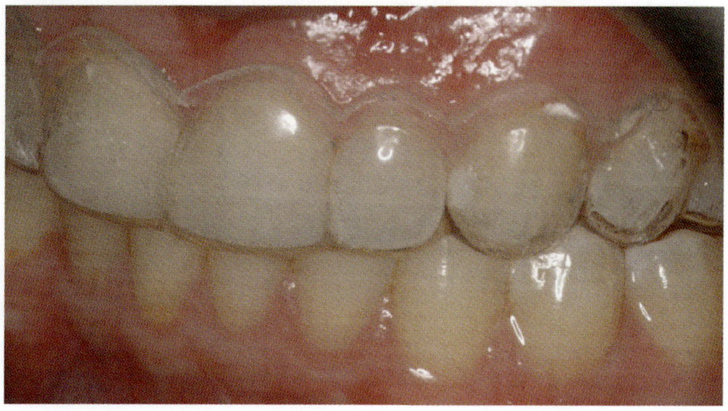

(C)

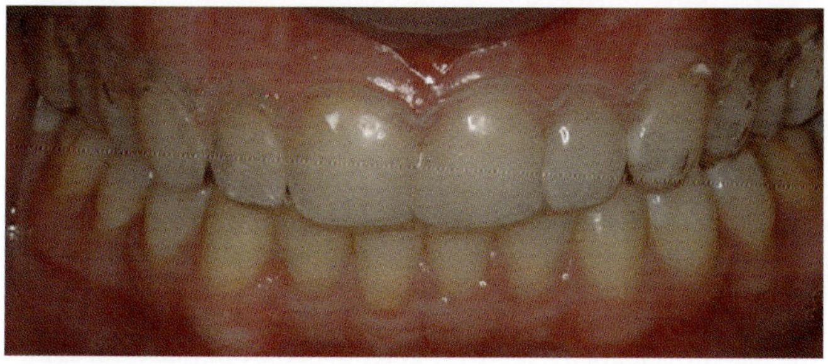

(D)

Figure 3.4

(A) Movement of the carbamide through the tooth. (B) Appearance of the upper whitening tray with the gel inside as it appears on the teeth from the right side. (C) Upper whitening tray on the teeth from the left side. (D) Upper whitening tray on the teeth. The tray fits well and extends 0.5 mm over the gingivae. There are bubbles appearing as the material becomes activated in the presence of saliva.

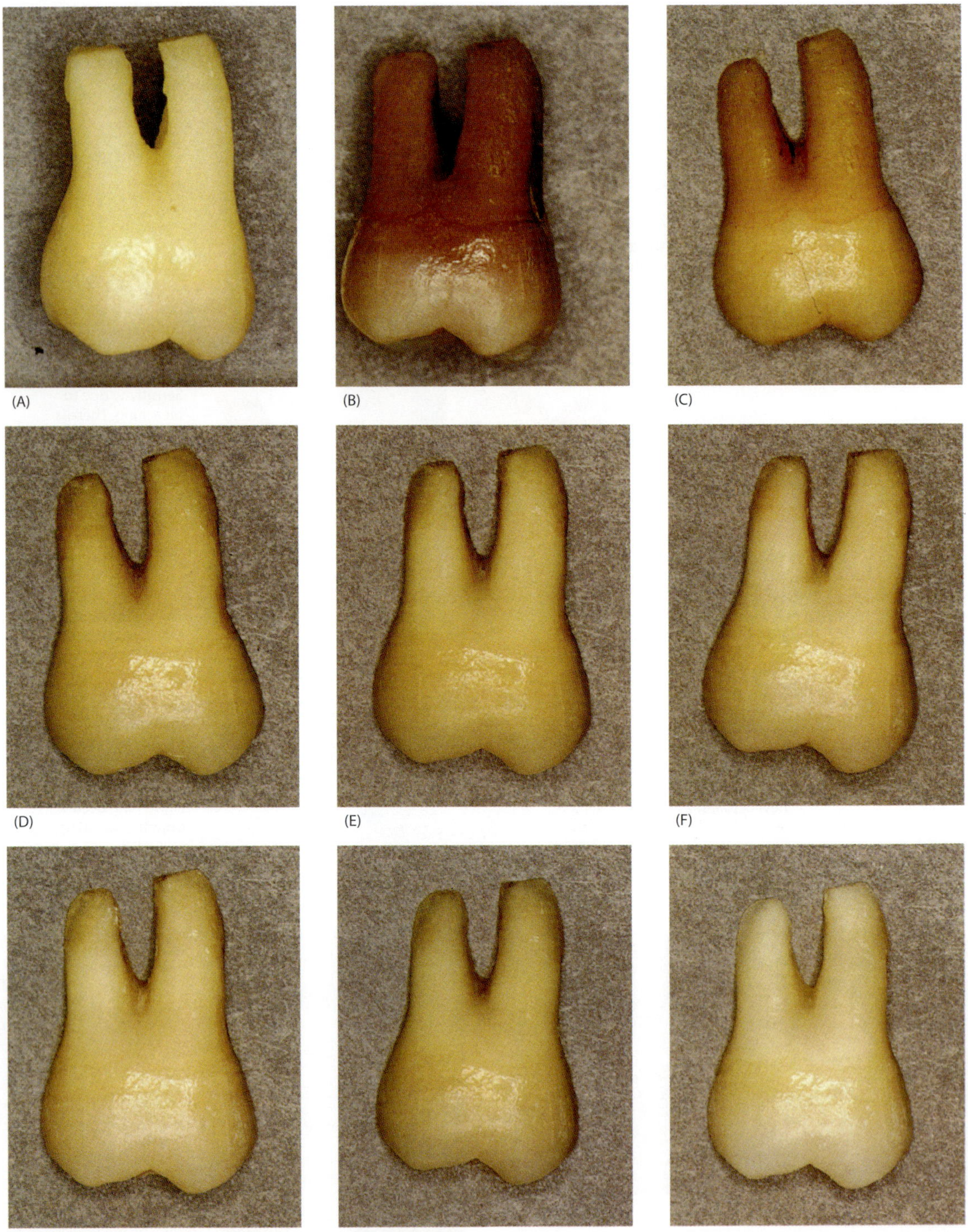

(A) (B) (C) (D) (E) (F) (G) (H) (I)

Figure 3.5

Teeth were discolored artificially in vitro using the same technique as described in Figure 3.1 (Greenwall 1992a). The teeth were stored in artificial saliva when not being whitened. The whitening treatment was undertaken for two 90-minute sessions per day. After the first session, new whitening material was placed on the teeth. The specimen was treated with Rembrandt Lighten (10% carbamide peroxide solution). The photo sequence demonstrates the lightening process as it took place. At the end of 28 days, the color was lighter than the original color before whitening, as assessed by a panel of four independent assessors. (A) The color of the tooth before whitening. (B) The appearance of the tooth immediately after blood discoloration. (C) The appearance of the tooth after sectioning and bathing in artificial saliva. (D) The appearance of the tooth after 90 minutes of whitening treatment with Rembrandt Lighten. (E) The appearance of the tooth after 3 hours of whitening treatment. (F) The appearance of the tooth after 3 days of whitening treatment. (G) The result after 7 days of whitening treatment. (H) The result after 14 days of whitening treatment. (I) The result after 28 days of whitening treatment. Note that the color of the tooth is lighter than the original color before whitening treatment commenced.

4 TREATMENT PLANNING FOR SUCCESSFUL WHITENING

Linda Greenwall

INTRODUCTION

Planning is essential for whitening treatment because tooth whitening is normally the beginning of the esthetic journey. The dentist needs to prepare a thorough treatment plan for the patient who wants to undertake tooth whitening. It is essential to take time to plan the treatment carefully and to fully explain the options for whitening and any necessary treatment that needs to be undertaken before whitening. When the mouth is assessed for whitening, the basic goals of health improvement and health sustainability should be addressed first. Several considerations need to be taken into account. Because 80% of patients who have had tooth whitening choose to undergo further esthetic or restorative dentistry after whitening, it is essential to plan comprehensively for the patient.

Before assessing the patient, it is important that the dentist understands what the patient needs and wants in terms of dental and oral health. Ask the new patient, "What are your hopes and aspirations for your mouth?" Patients may have specific concerns about the appearance of their teeth that they wish to discuss. Although some patients may not have considered this before, many patients have a dental "wish list" of improvements that they would like to make. When they visit the dentist, they may request specific esthetic improvements.

For most patients, this question has not been asked. It is important to wait a few moments after asking so that the patient has time to think and respond. Allow ample time during the appointment interview for the patient to express thoughts and concerns. When discussing tooth whitening, ask the patient about the shade of white that he or she wishes to achieve. Although there are many shades of white to select, most patients request a natural enhancement of their existing shade. If the patient requests extreme whiteness, the request may be unrealistic. It is essential at this stage to understand whether the patient's requests are realistic or unrealistic.

This chapter outlines what is required for a thorough examination for whitening and describes how to undertake a whitening treatment plan and how to plan further esthetic treatment to follow whitening. This chapter also demonstrates methods of gathering useful information about patients, emphasizing the importance of medical and dental histories. Patient communication, methods for undertaking a smile analysis, management of patients' expectations, informed consent, and fee planning for whitening treatment are discussed. Examples of questionnaires and forms are provided, which can be used in the information-gathering process.

PATIENT COMMUNICATION

Although tooth whitening is an elective esthetic treatment, it also has essential therapeutic benefits; these are discussed in Chapter 24. Before undertaking any esthetic treatment, it is essential that excellent and clear communication be established with the patient. It is essential for the dentist to understand exactly what the patient is requesting, in order to understand the patient's concerns about his or her tooth discoloration and esthetic needs. Beauty is an abstract and subjective concept, but an essential and ineradicable part of human nature (Etcoff 1999). Culture, age, gender, and time can influence perception of beauty. Because of this subjectivity, it is extremely important to establish good communication between the dentist and patient early, so that both can work toward the same goals. Excellent communication leads to treatment acceptance (Jameson 1994). To provide informed consent, the patient needs to understand the benefits and risks and advantages and disadvantages of treatment; the issues associated with not going ahead with treatment; and the importance of each treatment option that is available. Risks and benefits of the treatment need to be discussed before it commences. This is particularly important when the patient's expectations exceed the reality of what is possible to achieve. Studies have shown significant differences between dentists' and patients' preferences for esthetic dentistry (Brisman 1980).

A questionnaire can be used to evaluate the patient's hopes and aspirations for his or her smile (see Figure 4.1). The questionnaire can include questions regarding the patient's self-perception of teeth and smile. Questions should be open-ended, allowing the patient to talk and express any concerns. Patients can be asked about shape, positioning, color, and proportion of teeth. The information gathered will establish a base from which the clinician can interact, communicate, and evaluate the patient's problems.

The individuality of each case makes esthetic decisions more difficult, but also more interesting and challenging. Patients should be educated and questioned regarding their expectations and perceived final outcome. Before tooth whitening can be undertaken, it is essential to start with a comprehensive dental and oral health evaluation. It is useful to gather information with a checklist so that all the information that is necessary is received.

New patient checklist (see Table 4.1)

As with any new patient consultation, it is important to obtain or perform the following:

- Consent to undertake an examination.
- Medical history.
- Previous dental history: patient's attitude toward dentistry, patient's previous experiences, patient's expectations.
- Extraoral examination: in addition to assessing for pathology and temporomandibular joint dysfunction, it is essential to do a smile analysis.
- Intraoral examination.
  - Soft tissue examination: tongue, palate, and cheek mucosa
  - Dental examination
  - Periodontal examination
  - Occlusal examination
  - Assessment of temporomandibular joint function
  - Special tests: vitality tests
- Other information:
  - Study models
  - Face-bow records
  - Articulated study models with a diagnostic wax-up if necessary
  - Photography
  - Intraoral camera shots
- Digital radiographs

Medical history

The patient's medical history should be carefully assessed. Previous history of chronic illness and long-term use of antibiotics—such as minocycline for acne treatment or other antibiotics for chronic infections or perinatal infection—may lead to discoloration of teeth (Antonini and Luder 2011). Individuals who were born prematurely may develop molar incisor hypoplasia (MIH) or multiple white spots on the teeth. A specific whitening questionnaire should be filled out with the patient (see Figure 4.2). Patients' smoking habits need to be assessed. Patients should not smoke and whiten their teeth. It is essential for those patients who smoke to stop or at least to reduce the amount they are smoking before whitening is undertaken. This can sometimes be used as an incentive for patients to stop smoking altogether.

Allergies to plastic, peroxide, or any of the other ingredients of the whitening system should be noted. Patients' current medications need to be recorded on the medical history sheet, especially those preparations that cause a dry mouth such as antihistamines. Patients taking hormones sometimes have an exaggerated gingival response. Patients who are pregnant or breastfeeding should be excluded from whitening procedures because there is lack of information concerning possible effects on the developing fetus (Haywood 1995a).

The medical history needs to be stable, and patients with chronic diseases such as ulcerative colitis need to have clearance from their medical doctor before undertaking treatment. Patients undergoing chemotherapy should be in a stable condition before commencing whitening treatment and may need to get clearance from their medical doctor. Patients need to be checked for lichen planus before whitening because in some patients the lichen planus may flare up during the whitening process.

Table 4.1 Stages of new patient assessment

New patient interview
• Hopes and aspirations
• Listening skills
• Empathy
Medical history
• Dental history
• Dental issues and checklist
Intraoral examination
• Radiologic investigation
• Intraoral camera shots
• Clinical photography
• Study casts
Timing?
• Schedule next appointment for a treatment planning discussion

Dental history

The etiology of the discoloration needs to be assessed because different causes (e.g., caries, internal resorption, external cervical resorption, trauma, medication) necessitate different treatments. It is important to assess dental trauma that the patient has experienced that may affect the long-term prognosis of a tooth and the outcome of the whitening treatment. Severe trauma can lead to both internal and external cervical resorption (Patel et al. 2009). There is insufficient research at present linking home whitening treatments with promotion or exacerbation of resorption.

Extrinsic staining can usually be easily removed with a good dental cleaning and prophylaxis. Establish whether new patients are regular dental attenders or those who visit the dentist only when they have pain; the latter type of patient may not comply with home whitening instructions and may not follow the whitening program or return for review appointments when requested.

SMILE ANALYSIS AND ESTHETICS

What makes a beautiful smile? One definition is one in which the size, position, and color of the teeth are in harmony and the teeth are in proportion and in relative symmetry with one another and with the elements that frame them. Analysis, by definition, means reduction of the component parts to discover the interrelationships (Ricketts 1968). The components of a smile consist of the facial components (the facial features, tooth visibility, age, upper lip curvature, negative space, smile symmetry, and occlusal line) as well as the dental components (the dental midline, axial alignment, tooth arrangement, gradation, shape of the teeth, contact points, and gingival morphology and contour) and the physical components (Rufenacht 1990). The teeth are only part of a greater picture that must be viewed within the frame of the gingival soft tissue, the interarch dark space, the lips (Moskowitz and Nayyar 1995), and the face (Paletz et al. 1994).

Whitening teeth alone may not solve patients' esthetic requirements (see Figures 4.10 and 4.17). A smile analysis should be conducted before whitening and should be included in the treatment planning stages (Table 4.2). Smile analysis sheets can be used to determine the smile requirements and the patient's needs (see Figures 4.4 and 4.5). There are many factors to consider when conducting a smile analysis: the shape and length of the teeth, the lip line, the smile line, and the occlusal relationship of the teeth. Each element is an important feature, but all these features are interwoven to create esthetic harmony (Moskowitz and Nayyar 1995).

Table 4.2 Treatment planning checklist

Stage 1—Emergency treatment: elimination of pain

- Dressings for broken fillings
- Emergency relief of pain; emergency root canal therapy
- Root treatment of any undiagnosed periapical areas before any whitening treatment is undertaken
- Extractions
- Control of infections
- Discussion of possible treatment options, treatment implications, financial arrangements

Stage 2—Elimination of active disease and achievement of oral stability: disease control

Periodontal

- Assessment with indices
- Oral hygiene instruction
- Scaling and prophylaxis
- Root surface debridement (root planning and curettage)
- Surgery
- Other treatment

Caries control

- Use of fluorides: topical applications, mouthwash
- Dietary counselling

Provisional restorations and simple restorations

- Intracoronal restorations: glass ionomers, composites, amalgams
- Extracoronal restorations: provisional veneers, crowns, bridges, prostheses

Table 4.2 Continued

- Root canal treatment
- Extractions: routine, surgical
- Occlusal analysis and adjustment
- Orthodontics
- Referral for advice or treatment
- Other treatment: whitening considered after elimination of active disease

Tooth wear management

- Deep cervical lesions: may require glass ionomer restorations for a well-fitting tray to be made

Stage 3—Definitive restorations: once oral stability has been achieved

- Monitor periodontium
- Monitor caries (inactive lesions)
- Record indices as applicable
- Assess long-term implications with patient (costs, ability to maintain)
- Periodontal: monitoring, crown lengthening, other
- Whitening
- Definitive restorations:
  - Veneers and laminates
  - Crowns
  - Bridges
  - Prosthesis
- Orthodontics
- Implant fixture placement
- Oral surgery
- Other (including post-treatment photographs)

Stage 4—Maintenance and monitoring at monthly intervals

- Record indices
- Check radiographs
- Review preventive advice: dietary assessment, oral hygiene instruction, fluoride applications
- Oral prophylaxis
- Repeat aspects of stages 2 and if applicable (such as implant abutment connection and implant prosthesis)

Treatment planning time

- Plan time for treatment planning—assess radiographs and photographs and patient's concerns.
- Prepare written treatment plan; financial responsibilities discussed with the patient at the face-to-face treatment planning discussion.
- Obtain signed financial responsibility form and payment plan.
- Consent form to be signed by patient after explanations of risks, benefits, advantages, and disadvantages.
- Administration:
  - Estimated laboratory bill, laboratory work to be returned on time
  - Total time estimated
  - Appointments scheduled accordingly
  - Total fees earned

Adapted from Eaton and Nathan 1998, with permission.

The components of a smile

The appearance of a smile involves the relationships among the three primary components (Garber and Salama 1996).

The teeth

- The shade and shape.
- Position, length, and axial alignment.
- The tooth surface characteristics and morphology.
- The shade and shape of the opposing dentition.
- The occlusion and occlusal line.
- The dental midline—an imaginary line that separates the two central incisors.
- The surface texture (e.g., perikymata, stippling, rippling). The surface texture will not change with whitening.

The lip framework

- The lip line—the amount of tooth exposed during a smile.
- The smile line—a hypothetical curved line drawn along the edges of the four anterior maxillary teeth that should run parallel with the curvature of the inner border of the lower lip (Rufenacht 1990).
- The upper lip curvature—the position of the upper lip height relative to the teeth.
- Negative space—the dark space that appears between the jaws between laughter and talking.
- The smile symmetry—the symmetric placement of the corners of the mouth in the vertical plane (see Figure 4.7B).

The gingival scaffold

- The gingival height of contour.
- Appearance of the gingival tissues.
- Symmetry of the heights of the central incisors (see Figure 4.7).
- Incisal and gingival embrasures.

The golden proportion

Artists, mathematicians, and philosophers have long been preoccupied with the relationship between beauty and harmony. Harmony in proportion has been regarded as the essential esthetic principle. A simple but profound mathematical ratio (the discovery of which has been attributed to Pythagoras) appears frequently in nature—1:1.618 (Levin 1978). Levin has designed a golden mean gauge in the same proportion (see Figure 4.7). He discovered that the relationship between the widths of the central and lateral incisors were in the golden proportion and that the lateral negative space was in the golden proportion of one-half the width of the anterior segment. This golden mean gauge can help assess the harmony of the face and can help to determine the relationships of the teeth to the lips and to the face and of the teeth to one another. This gauge can help with planning treatment and lengths and shape of teeth for veneers after whitening.

What is an ideal smile?

Photographs of fashion models in the media demonstrate many "ideal" smiles. The smile should be harmonious (see Figure 4.7).

The ideal smile is considered to have the following characteristics:

- Bright (Philips 1996)
- Vigorous
- Youthful, regardless of age (Moskowitz and Nayyar 1995)
- Symmetric teeth
- Showing natural teeth
- White to light tooth shade (Dunn et al. 1996)
- Healthy gingival color, harmony, and form (Garber and Salama 1996)
- Gingival line following upper lip contour
- Incisal edge following lower lip contour

Tooth shade was the most important factor in a study conducted by Dunn et al. (1996) to assess patients' perceptions of dental attractiveness. This was followed in sequence by natural (unrestored) tooth appearance and the number of teeth showing. Whitening is thus an attractive, simple option to lighten the appearance of natural teeth.

Intraoral examination

The existing condition of the teeth and periodontium needs to be examined before whitening. Defective restorations are noted; these need to be discussed with patients before whitening. The teeth are assessed for the following:

- *Thickness of the enamel.*
- *Existing gingival or cervical recession.*
- *Existing sensitivity before whitening,* which needs to be noted on the patient's dental chart.
- *The translucency of the teeth.* Translucent teeth still retain their "blackish" look after whitening (Haywood 1995a). Patients need to be told of this effect to avoid disappointment. Most patients are so happy with their new whiter smile that the existing translucency is of no concern.
- *White spots or opacities.* These do not disappear during whitening and in the early stages of whitening may become more visible. Patients need to be warned about this.
- *Teeth that are banded* because of tetracycline staining or desiccation will retain their banded appearance after whitening. These aspects need to be discussed with patients before whitening so the patient is not disappointed with the result.
- *Gingivitis.* Although whitening teeth improves gingival health, whitening treatment should not be attempted on teeth with surrounding gingivitis or more severe gingival problems (Small 1998).

- *Dehydration line.* As patients age, if they have a high lip line with a short lip, the lower half of the incisal tip may appear darker. This is because as the patient ages the enamel becomes thinner and the dentin becomes thicker with the laying down of tertiary dentin, allowing the tooth to become age-yellowed. Many patients are concerned about the dehydration line. Patients should be warned that when the teeth whiten, they do not whiten in an even band and can become lighter with a two-toned effect.
- Dark crack lines should be assessed prior to whitening and the patient should be told that the dark crack lines (often due to smoking and/or grinding teeth) will not disappear with whitening treatment.

Special tests

- *Vitality testing* of all teeth to be whitened should be undertaken. This can be done using heat or cold temperature testing or electric pulp testers. All test results need to be recorded in the patient's record.
- *Radiographs.* Recent radiographs need to be used to check for pathology or existing decay of all teeth. A single screening anterior periapical radiograph can be taken with the aid of a beam-aiming device (see Figure 4.12). However, it is better to have full-mouth periapical radiographs of all teeth to be whitened to ensure there is no previous or existing pathology. Problems have arisen when dentists have not taken an anterior periapical radiograph before whitening. Teeth with existing periapical pathology can develop exacerbations that may be difficult to treat endodontically. Single dark teeth may be nonvital, and these need to be checked before commencement of whitening treatment. The rule is that a periapical radiograph of all discolored teeth should be taken.
- *Digital intraoral photographs* of each individual tooth, outlining decay, cracks, defects, and problems, are very useful to assess the condition of the tooth and the restoration before whitening.
- *Diagnostic wax-up.* Sometimes it may be necessary to take study models and have the dental technician make a diagnostic wax-up of how the teeth will appear after the total treatment, because whitening treatment may be followed by porcelain laminate veneers, direct composite bonding, or opening of the vertical dimension with composite bonding or inlays or onlays. The diagnostic wax-up will help the patient to visualize the final result before treatment commences (see Figure 4.10).

Patients with existing restorations in esthetic areas

It is essential to warn patients with existing matching anterior composite restorations that because the shade of the teeth will change, new composite restorations using a lighter shade composite may be required after whitening. The actual composite restorations do not change color. Sometimes composite restorations that have a black edge around them appear whiter because the black edge disappears. Teeth with caries or defective, discolored anterior restorations can be repaired after whitening. The cariostatic action of the whitening material will stop any progression of the lesion during whitening. Patients should be aware that the restorations can be replaced 2 weeks after the termination of the treatment, because bond strengths to enamel are weakened during whitening.

Patients' expectations

It is fundamental before commencement of any whitening procedure that the patient's expectations are assessed. A patient who expects pure white teeth is seldom satisfied (Haywood 1995a). Normally a color change of two shades occurs; this can be demonstrated on a porcelain shade guide before whitening. Patients need to be made aware that some teeth may not whiten and some teeth do not whiten evenly. Darker teeth take longer to whiten. Older patients' teeth respond well to whitening, although the root surfaces do not whiten as well. It takes longer for older patients' teeth to whiten. The timing and sequencing of appointments for older patients will be different than for younger patients or those with a lighter shade to start. Patients should be warned of these factors before commencement of whitening, and of the fact that additional bonding procedures may be necessary to place composites at the neck of the roots (Table 4.3).

DENTAL PHOTOGRAPHY FOR TOOTH WHITENING

It is essential to take photographs in a standard way for treatment planning for whitening. It is essential that the photographs are of excellent quality and standardized and that clear before and after shots are achieved. Digital photographs are easy to standardize and crop, and very quickly a library of before and after pictures can be collected. Photographs should also be taken during the whitening treatment. Patients often forget how dark or discolored the teeth were before commencing treatment and may be dissatisfied if they do not notice further shade changes. It helps to photograph the teeth with the baseline porcelain shade tab so that the patients can appreciate the degree of color change when they see the

Table 4.3 Factors that affect the amount of lightening

- The existing color of the teeth
- How often the trays are replenished and the solutions are changed
- The time for which the whitening materials are in contact with the teeth
- The concentration of the whitening material
- The rate of oxygen release (different in carbamide peroxide [night] gels versus hydrogen peroxide [day only] gels)
- The nature of the discoloration (e.g., tetracycline staining)

color change on the guide. That is why it is usually best to whiten only one arch at a time—so that a direct color comparison can be made. Normally the upper arch is whitened first because patients notice this more. Lower teeth take longer to whiten, and often the lower canine may have a snow-capped appearance as the whitening starts from the tip of the tooth.

Photographs to be taken for whitening

Before treatment

1. Portrait view with the patient smiling
2. Smile view
3. Smile view with standardized shade tab opposite the upper left canine tooth
4. Retracted view
5. Retracted view with shade tab in the same position
6. Anterior retracted view with a black piece of paper blocking the lower teeth

For Class II teeth, lower teeth should be protruded forward so that the upper and lower teeth are visible.

During and after treatment

1. Portrait view with the patient smiling
2. Smile view
3. Smile view with standardized shade tab opposite the upper left canine tooth
4. Retracted view
5. Retracted view with shade tab in the same position
6. Anterior retracted view with a black piece of paper blocking the lower teeth

For Class II teeth, lower teeth should be protruded forward so that the upper and lower teeth are visible.

Photographing teeth during whitening

It is often difficult to photograph and capture the slight differences of the shade changes during the whitening treatment. There are many reasons for this.

- The lighting in the room may not be adequate.
- The reflectance of the operating light may distort the color change.
- It is often difficult to record the same patient at the same distance so that the teeth appear the same size, with the same exposure.
- Metamerism (differences in the spectral characteristics of light reflected from natural teeth) may play a part.
- The flash of the camera may not fire at the same rate.

Photographs should include a shade tab (see Figure 4.9) that closely matches the baseline color of the teeth. The entire sequence of photographs should include this shade tab in the same position, normally using the upper left canine tooth as a reference. Often the color of the porcelain shade tab appears different because of variations in the reflecting light.

TREATMENT PLANNING DISCUSSION AND INFORMED CONSENT

Before any dental treatment is begun, it is essential to have a treatment planning discussion with the patient. During this appointment the patient's clinical situation can be discussed with the patient. The patient is given a tour of the mouth on the computer screen, which may include digital dental photographs, intraoral digital photographs, the patient's digital radiographs, study models, diagnostic wax-ups, or digital images of the possible outcome. The treatment can be explained and discussed, as well as treatment sequencing and any further treatment that may be required. Tooth whitening may not solve the patient's esthetic requirements completely, and all associated and additional treatments need to be fully discussed with the patient. At this time the patient can have the opportunity to ask further questions and gain clarification of what is involved in the proposed treatment, particularly regarding the dentist-prescribed home whitening treatment. It is prudent to give the patient an informed consent form to sign. The benefits and risks need to be discussed as well as the advantages, disadvantages, and alternatives to whitening and other treatment options (see Figure 4.15). Two copies should be signed; one is given to the patient and one is kept with the patient's dental records. Any expected or possible side effects need to be mentioned.

Success rates of whitening

Although whitening teeth as a dental treatment is now more predictable than ever, there is still no guarantee that the teeth will whiten to a lighter shade. The only way of knowing whether teeth will respond is to undertake the treatment. Further treatment, such as composite bonding, porcelain laminates, or full crowns, may be required to achieve an excellent smile (see Figure 4.19).

The success rates of whitening have been published by numerous researchers. However, the success rates vary and there are numerous reasons for these differences. Patients often ask about success rates, and it is important to discuss these and be realistic with patients before treating their teeth (Haywood 1995b). Not all teeth are responsive to treatment and not all teeth respond at the same rate. Some patients' teeth can whiten to the lightest shade on the shade guide, whereas others respond with a slight degree of lightening. The patient's smile, though, often appears brighter, and this is an added benefit.

Shade assessment and selection

There are many ways to select the correct shade before whitening. The study of color and shade selection is a vast subject in itself and is not discussed in depth here. Proprietary shade guides are normally used to determine the preoperative shade. There can be variation among the individual shade guides (Miller 1987). Some whitening kits have their own customized shade guides, which can be used by dentists and patients as a reference. However, small changes in shade may be difficult to discern using these guides. Determination of the correct shade before, during, and after whitening is easier when the shade tabs are arranged according to value, not hue (see Figure 4.14). This helps particularly well when assessing small changes in color after a few days of whitening. A study trying to assess the viewer's perceived arrangement of value showed that none of the observers was able to arrange the shades as per the manufacturer's recommendations (Geary and Kinirons 1999). They also showed that some color differences encountered by observers may be too small to be noticed. New whitening shade guides (Paravino et al. 2007) have been developed specifically for assessing the changes in whiteness during treatment. The shades are arranged by value in half increments with a gray background to help the viewer discern these changes in shade.

Selecting the appropriate shade has always been difficult because it is dependent on so many factors. Shade selection is often subjective. Some examination rooms are fitted with special color-corrected bulbs in their fluorescent lights to help with shade determination.

Factors involved in shade determination

The following factors determine shade value:

- The amount of natural light in the area where the shade is taken.
- The hue of the tooth color (yellow or blue range).
- The value of the color (i.e., the lightness and brightness).
- Chroma: the strength or weakness of the color.

There are three dimensions of color: hue, chroma, and value (Miller 1987). Hue is the pigment—most commonly called the color. Chroma denotes the strength or concentration of a hue and may also be referred as the color saturation. Value is the relative whiteness or blackness of a color and is a qualitative assessment of the gray component. Value is independent of hue or chroma; in dental shade matching, it is the most important of the three dimensions of color. Value should be selected first. Rearrangement of the color guide from the lightest to the darkest shade is recommended to avoid distractions. Hue selection should be undertaken next. The basic hue can be best seen in the middle and cervical thirds. Chroma variations can be perceived within the same tooth. The cervical third usually has a higher chroma and a more saturated hue than the middle third. The incisal third often has a lower value when compared with the middle and cervical thirds.

There have been great technical improvements to help dentists select shades. One innovation is the 3D-Master shade system (Vita, Bad Säckingen, Germany). It is claimed that the systematic arrangement of the tabs within the guide in three-dimensional color space is designed to cover almost the complete range of naturally occurring shades. User instructions on shade-taking protocol recommend determination of each of the three elements separately. The initial step is the evaluation of color value from five shades covering the lightest to darkest. This should be beneficial for assessing changes in shade that occur during whitening.

Because some teeth can whiten beyond the color of the normal Vita shade guide, the manufacturers have introduced lighter porcelains to match the shade of the whitened teeth. There are many new whitening shade guides because teeth have whitened beyond the original lightest shade (B1). These shades are called OM1, OM2, and OM3. This helps in the communication and treatment planning stage to show what may be possible. Some patients may not want the very whitest shade because they do not think it looks natural. Overwhitened teeth may take on a very white, opaque appearance.

After the shade has been selected, a decision must be made regarding whether the discoloration or change in color can be corrected. A guideline mentioned by Haywood (1999) states that if the sclera (white of the eye) is lighter than the existing shade of the teeth, the teeth can usually be lightened. If the color of the teeth is lighter than the sclera, it is probably going to be more difficult to achieve successful tooth whitening.

Planning fees for whitening treatment

It is essential during treatment planning that the correct fees for whitening treatment are planned and assessed. Careful treatment planning includes careful planning of fees. Careful planning involves all members of the dental team and particularly the team members responsible for scheduling appointments and fee collection (Jameson 1996). Problems with patients can arise if the correct fees are not quoted before commencement of treatment. Some dentists quote a separate fee per arch; the first arch is normally more expensive than the second arch because it takes longer to assess and plan the first arch. Normally the upper arch is treated first.

Factors affecting the level of fees

- Darker teeth will take longer to whiten. Thus they will require more whitening material. Should fees be assessed per arch or per the amount of materials used?
- Patients who sleep with the trays in the mouth may require less whitening material (one application) than those who use the trays during the day (one or two applications).
- Tetracycline-stained teeth will require extended treatment times and thus use more material. These patients should be charged for the additional amount of whitening material used. This can be arranged as a monthly fee whereby they have an assessment and collect new material. Fees can be charged per visit, plus the whitening materials, rather than per arch.
- Patients who wear a partial denture will require two whitening trays, one to wear during the day and one for nighttime use, and should be charged accordingly.
- Patients who have a single dark tooth should have two whitening trays made, one with a window cut adjacent to the dark tooth on each side and one full arch tray.
- Fees should be quoted per arch, assuming a certain amount of whitening material is used. If the patient

requires double this amount to whiten the teeth, charges should be calculated accordingly.

- Fees will vary depending on the whitening material used. Some are more expensive than others. Some products include the fee for making the whitening trays in the whole kit; thus the cost to the dentist will be less.
- Fees should be planned and discussed. Written estimates should be given to patients who will require additional treatment—for example, the cost of replacing anterior composites to change them to a lighter shade, or placement of porcelain veneers or crowns on certain teeth.
- Patients should sign a consent form before treatment commences. They should consent to the whitening treatment and they should be aware of the full treatment plan prior to commencing treatment.

Benefits of quoting fees per arch

- Once the upper arch is whitened, the patient may be satisfied with the result and not wish to continue to the lower teeth.
- If one arch does not whiten or does not lighten satisfactorily, the fee for the other arch is avoided (Haywood 1995b).
- If one arch will lighten, the other arch will lighten, although the lower arch does not lighten as well as the upper arch.

The Dentist's Costs

1. Surgery time; examination and discussion with the patient, impression taking; checking the fit of the trays; review and assessment time (three to five appointments).
2. Laboratory costs for making the whitening trays.
3. Material costs: whitening material, whitening toothpaste, appliance case.
4. Photography costs: developing of film or digital imaging.
5. Indirect costs of marketing the whitening techniques to new and existing patients.
6. Overhead costs: running a surgery and employing staff.

A rider clause should be included on the estimate sheet to ensure that the patient is made aware of the following:

- The full fee is due at the impression appointment.
- Fees cannot be waived if the treatment is voluntarily discontinued or discontinued because of side effects.
- There will be a replacement fee if the appliance is lost, worn out, or damaged.
- Further treatments may be necessary, and these will be discussed with the patient before commencing.
- Separate fees will be quoted for in-office and power whitening treatments.

Setting the appropriate fees for whitening treatment within the practice is essential to the survival and profit of the dental practice (Lund 1997). Misunderstanding can be averted through correct treatment planning, consent, and appropriate fees for treatment. Most dentists enjoy providing whitening treatments for their patients because it is rewarding to see patients who are delighted with their whitened teeth and improved self-esteem (Small 1998).

REFERENCES

Antonini LG, Luder HU. (2011) Discoloration of teeth from tetracyclines—even today? *Schweiz Monatsschr Zahnmed* **121**(5):414–31.

Brisman AS. (1980) Esthetics: a comparison of dentists' and patients' concepts. *J Am Dent Assoc* **100**:345–52.

Dunn WJ, Murchison DF, Broome JC. (1996) Esthetics: patients perceptions of dental attractiveness. *J Prosthodont* **5**(3):166–71.

Eaton K, Nathan K. (1998) The MGDS examination: a systemic approach. 3. Part 2 of the examination: diagnosis, treatment planning, execution of treatment, maintenance and appraisal, writing-up log diaries. *Prim Dent Care* **5**(3):113–18.

Etcoff N. (1999) *Survival of the prettiest: the science of beauty.* Doubleday: New York.

Garber DA, Salama M. (1996) The aesthetic smile: diagnosis and treatment. *Periodontology 2000* **11**:18–28.

Geary LJ, Kinirons MJ. (1999) Use of a common shade guide to test the perception of differences in the shades and values by members of the dental team. *Prim Dent Care* **6**(3):107–110.

Goldstein RE. (1998) *Esthetics in dentistry*, 2nd edn. Vol 1: *Principles, communications, treatment methods.* BC Decker: London.

Greenwall LH, Jameson C. (2012) *Success strategies in aesthetic dentistry.* Quintessence Publications: London.

Haywood VB. (1995a) An examination for Nightguard Vital Bleaching. *Esthet Dent Update* **6**(2):51–2.

Haywood VB. (1995b) Nightguard Vital Bleaching: information and consent form. *Esthet Dent Update* **6**(5):130–2.

Haywood VB. (1999) Current status and recommendations for dentist-prescribed, at-home tooth whitening. *Contemp Esthet Restor Pract* **3**(Suppl 1):2–9.

Jameson C. (1994) *Great communication = great production.* Pennwell Publishing: Tulsa, Oklahoma.

Jameson C. (1996) *Collect what you produce.* Pennwell Publishing: Tulsa, Oklahoma.

Klaff D. (1999) Aesthetic dentistry for the millennium. *Restor Aesthet Pracy* **1**(1):98–104.

Korson D. (1990) *Natural ceramics.* Quintessence Publishing: Chicago.

Levin EI. (1978) Dental esthetics and the golden proportion. *J Prosthet Dent* **40**:244–52.

Lund P. (1997). *Building the happiness-centred business*, 2nd edn. Solutions Press: Capalaba, Australia.

McClean JW. (1979) *The science and art of dental ceramics*, Volume 1. Quintessence Publishing: Chicago.

Miller L. (1987) Organizing colour in dentistry. *J Am Dent Assoc* (Special issue): 26E–40E.

Miller LL. (1994) Shade selection. *J Esthet Dent* **6**:47–60.

Morris RM. (1999) *Strategies in dental diagnosis and treatment planning.* Martin Dunitz: London.

Moskowitz ME, Nayyar A. (1995) Determinants of dental aesthetics: a rational for smile analysis and treatment. *Compend Contin Educ Dent* **16**(12):1164–86.

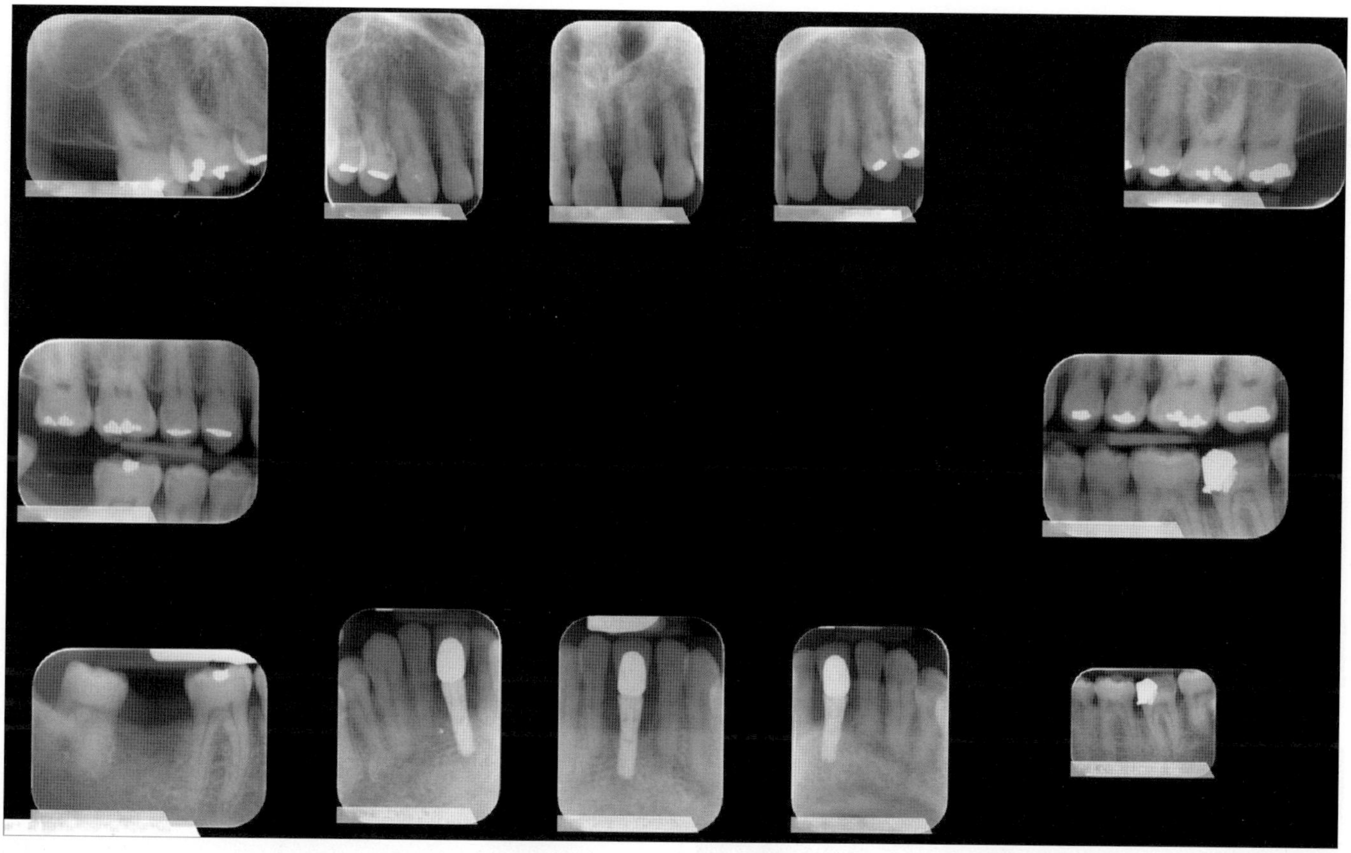

Figure 4.8

Full-mouth radiographic investigation. This patient had deep tetracycline staining and complex restorative problems. The patient's presenting feature was peri-implantitis of the lower right central incisor, which needed immediate management. In addition, the lower left second molar was fractured, requiring restorative treatment. Once these factors and the periodontal issues were addressed, whitening treatment could be planned.

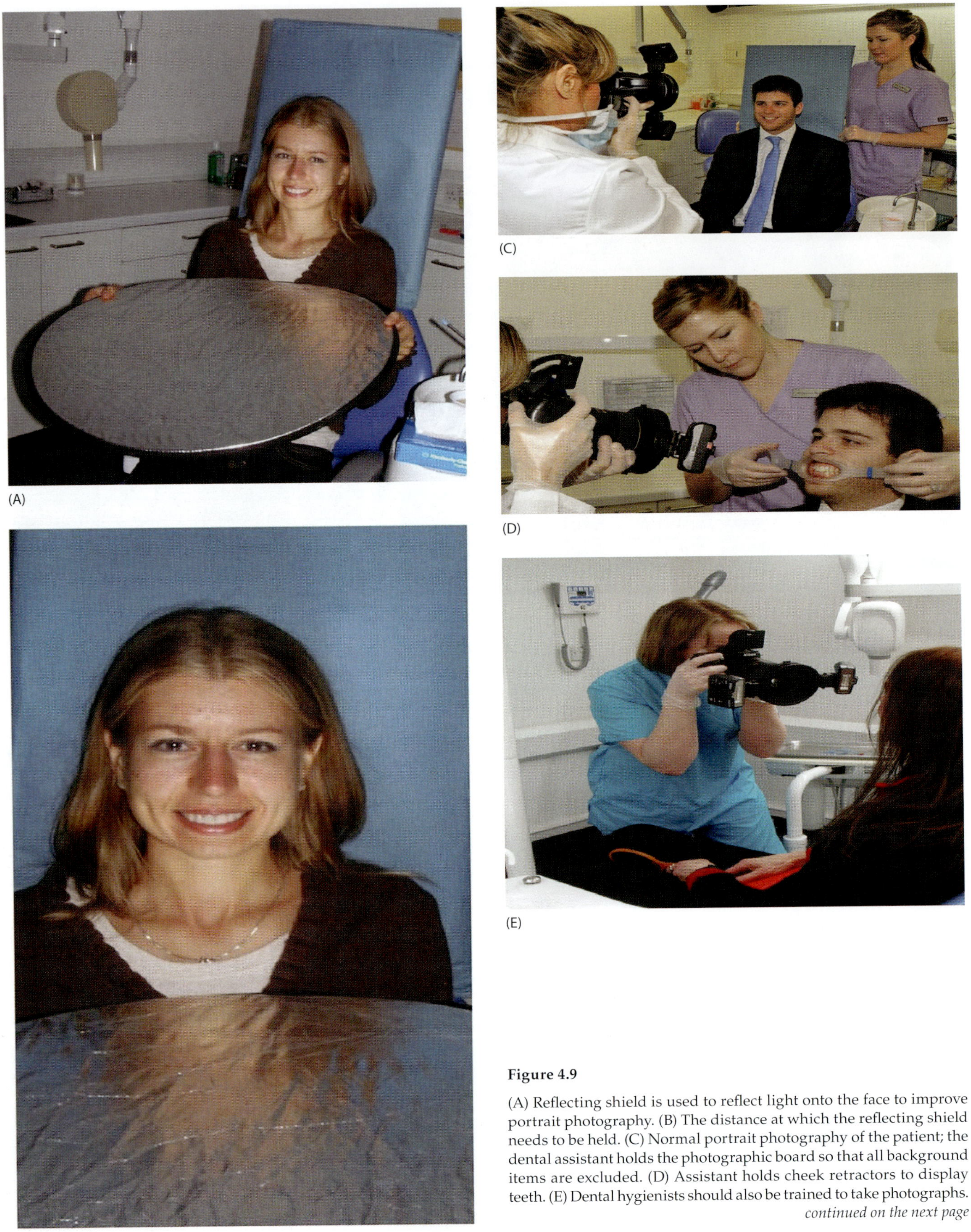

(A) (B) (C) (D) (E)

Figure 4.9

(A) Reflecting shield is used to reflect light onto the face to improve portrait photography. (B) The distance at which the reflecting shield needs to be held. (C) Normal portrait photography of the patient; the dental assistant holds the photographic board so that all background items are excluded. (D) Assistant holds cheek retractors to display teeth. (E) Dental hygienists should also be trained to take photographs.

continued on the next page

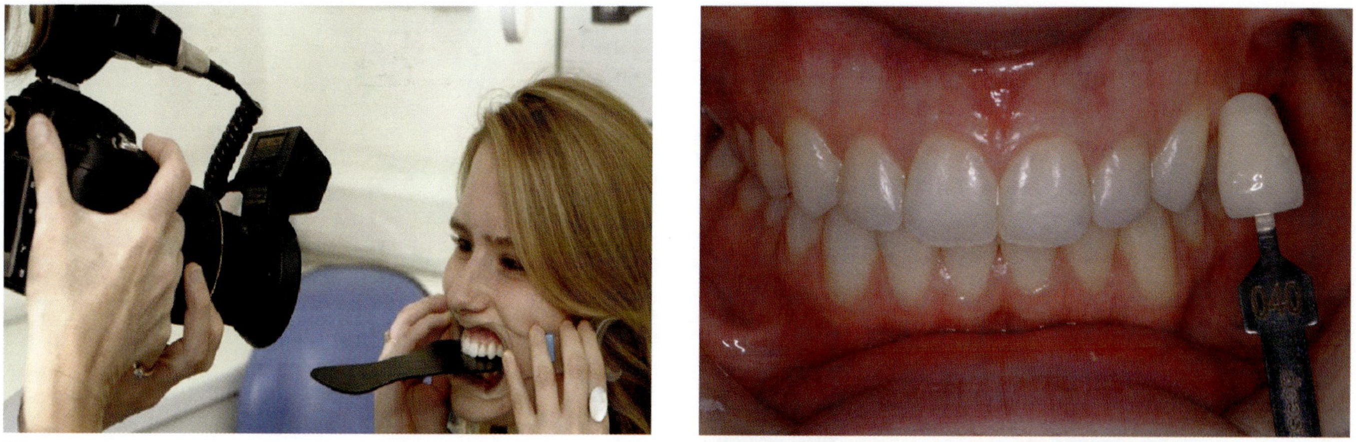

(F) (G)

Figure 4.9 continued

(F) Patient bites on black contrast material; the neutral background helps determine shade. (G) Taking pictures with the shade tab.

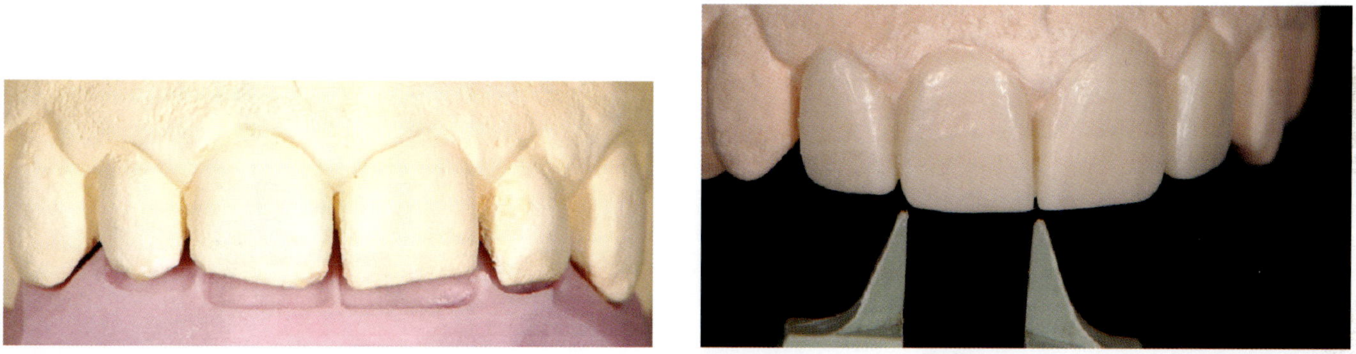

(A) (B)

Figure 4.10

(A) Whitening alone would not solve the patient's esthetic dilemma of spaces between the teeth and uneven shapes and lengths. (B) Diagnostic wax-up to illustrate the ideal proportions of what can be achieved for the patient with direct composites or veneers.

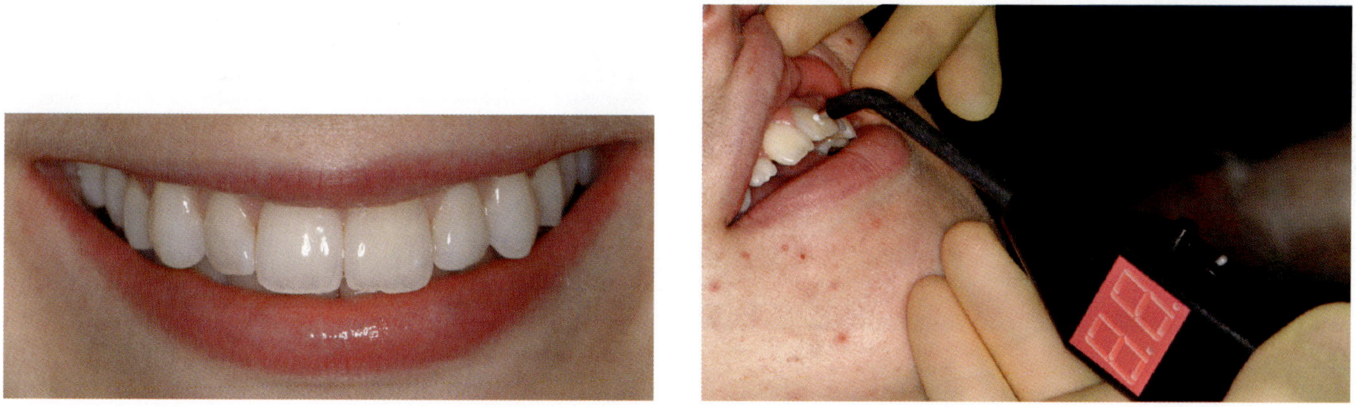

(A) (B)

Figure 4.11

(A) Natural translucency of central incisors, a feature of youthful teeth. The upper left central incisor appears slightly more yellow than the corresponding upper right tooth and therefore may require testing of the pulp. (B) Testing the vitality of the tooth with an electric pulp tester.

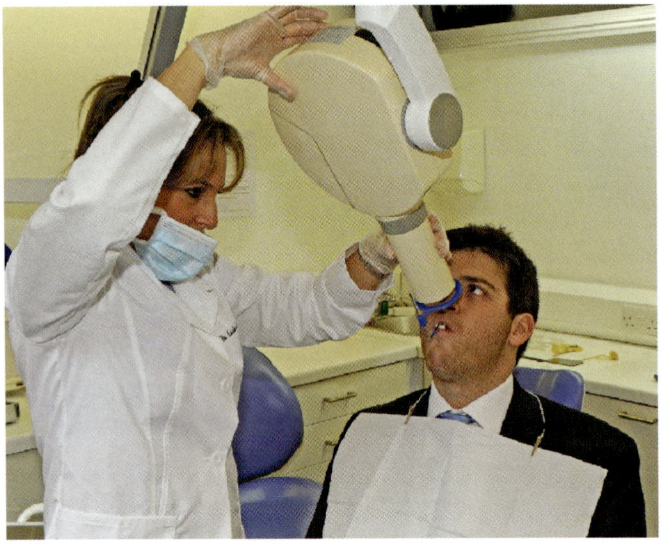

Figure 4.12

Taking an anterior radiograph with a beam-aiming device.

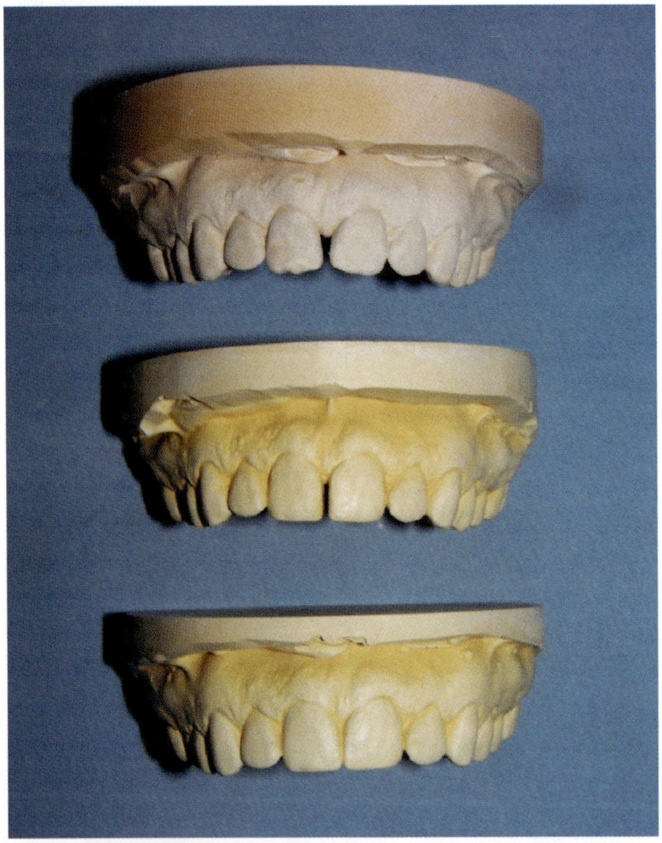

Figure 4.13

Diagnostic wax-ups to show the patient the options for closing the midline diastema (top, existing; middle, partial closure; bottom, complete closure).

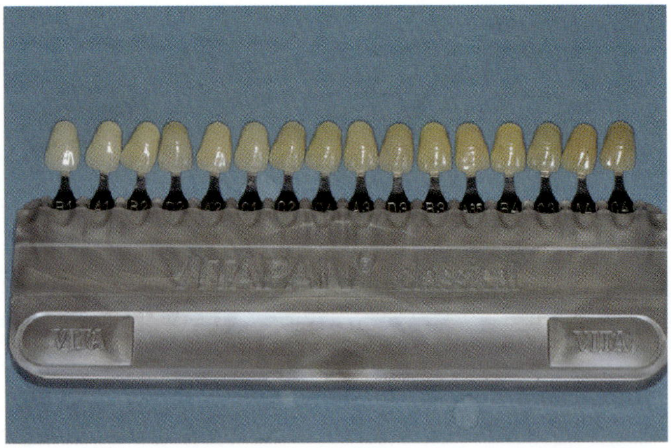

(A)

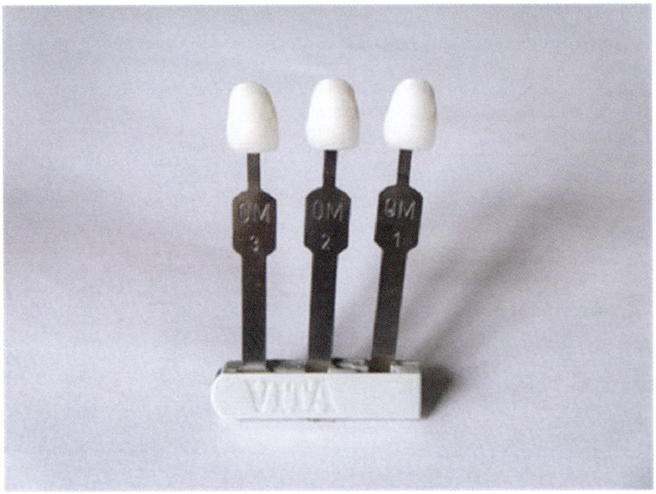

(B)

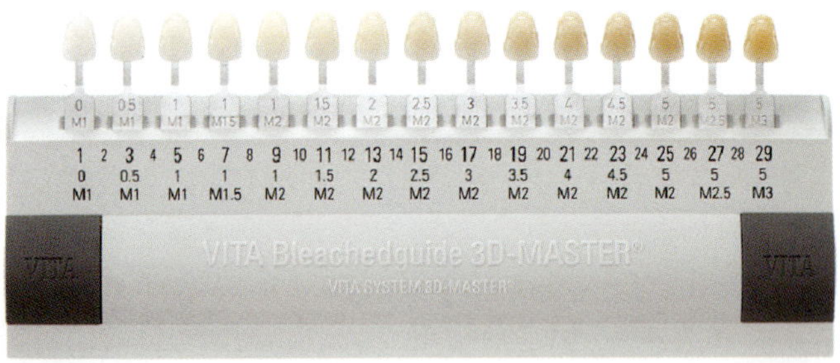

(C)

Figure 4.14

(A) Shade selection according to VitaPan classical shade guide, showing value and not hue. (B) Latest whitening shade guide introduced because shades of teeth have become much whiter. (C) Recent Vita Bleachedguide 3D-Master shade guide showing the value shades from light to dark; this allows for easier comparison of whiteness.

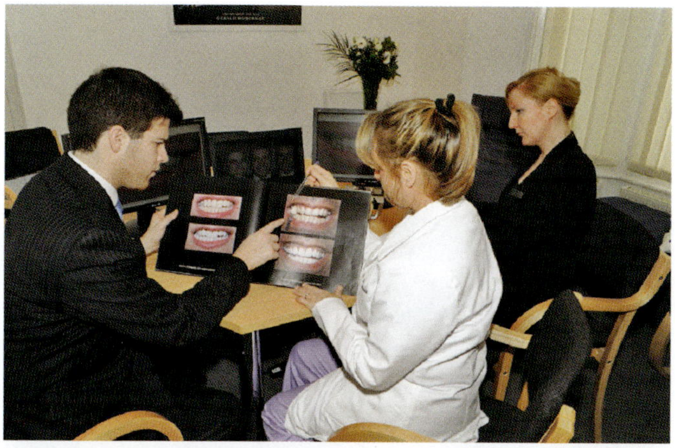

(A)

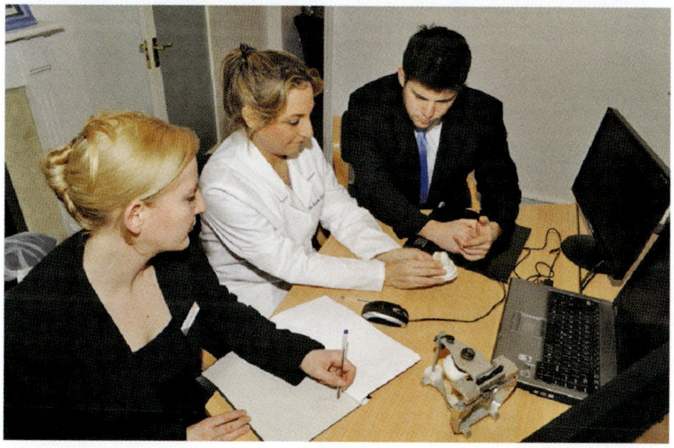

(B)

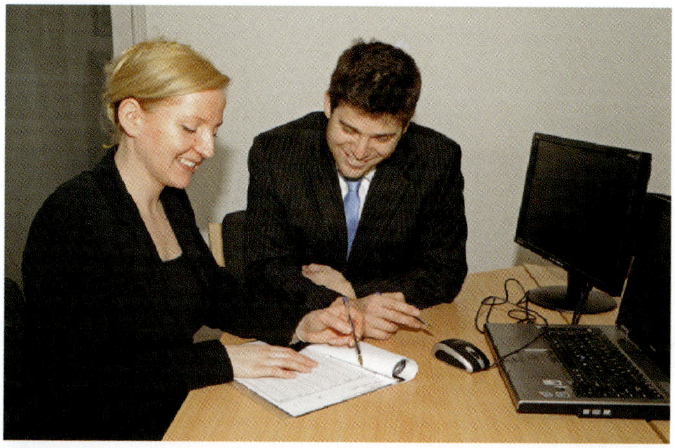

(C)

Figure 4.15

(A) Sitting down with the treatment coordinator and planning the patient's treatment. (B) Going through the treatment plan and options: dentist, patient, and treatment coordinator. (C) Treatment coordinator getting signed consent and going through financing options.

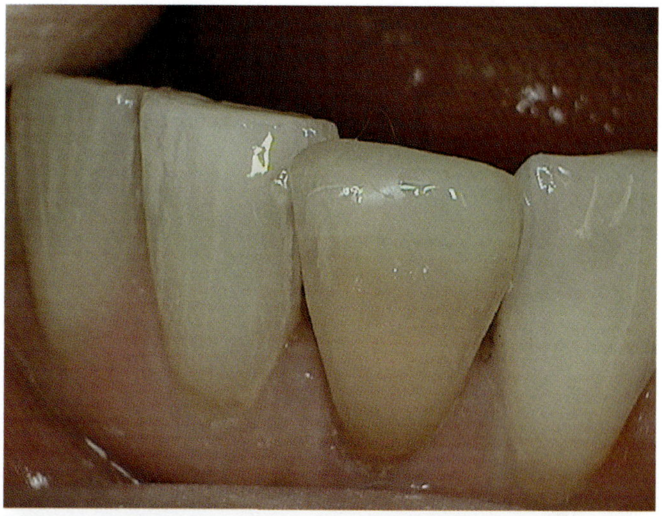

(A)

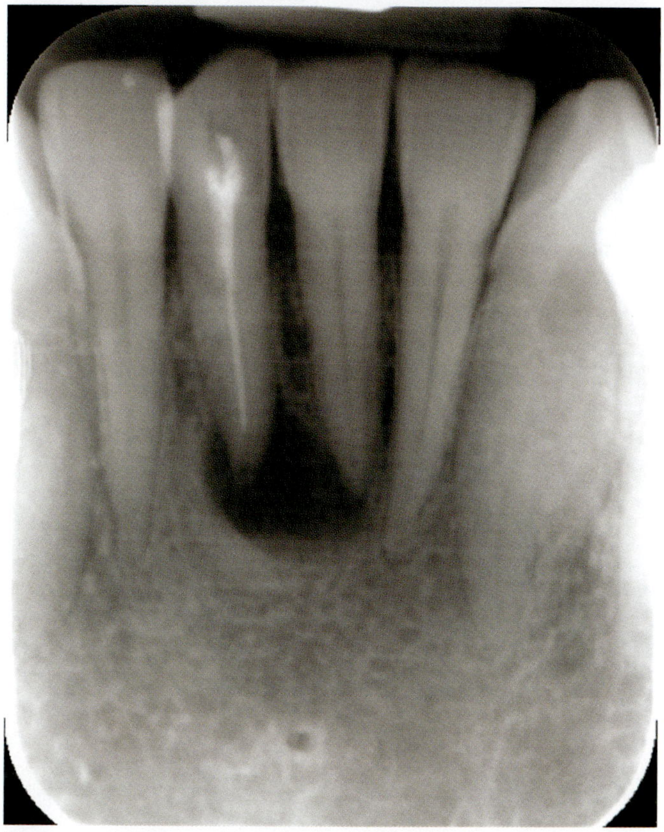

(B)

Figure 4.16

(A) Intraoral digital photograph showing discolored lower incisor tooth. (B) Radiograph shows large cyst associated with discoloration of right central incisor; no whitening could be undertaken because disease was present. *continued on the next page*

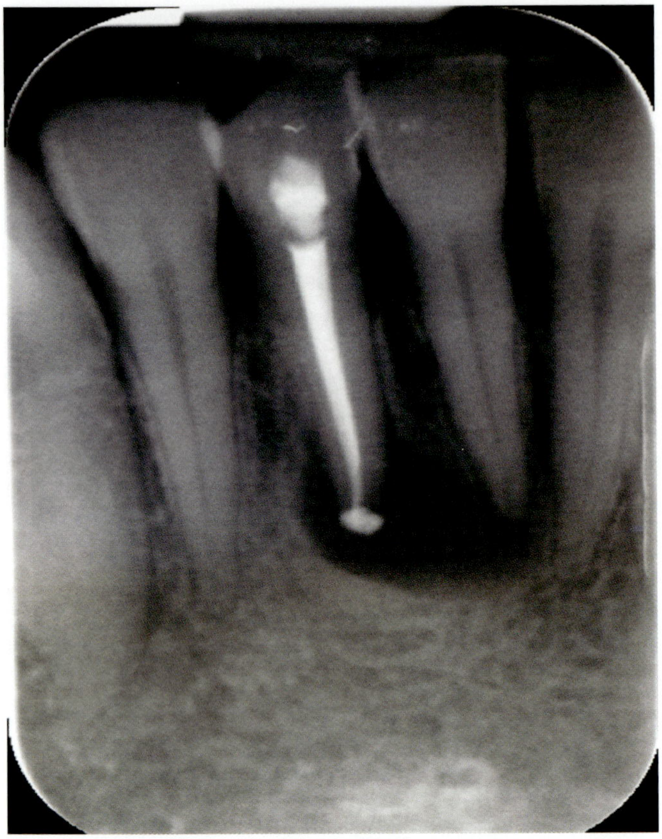

(C)

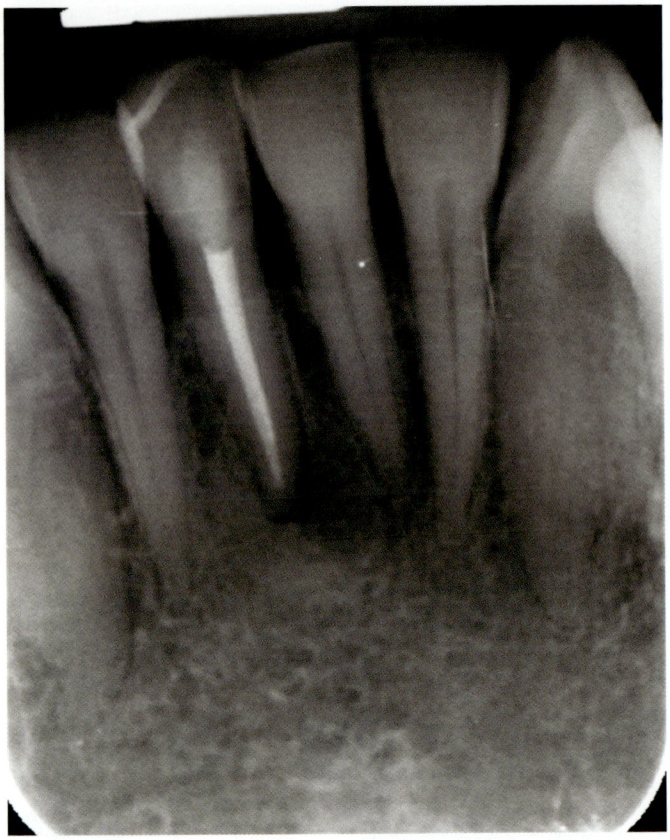

(D)

Figure 4.16 continued

(C) Result after root canal treatment. (D) Final healed stage at which whitening treatment could be commenced.

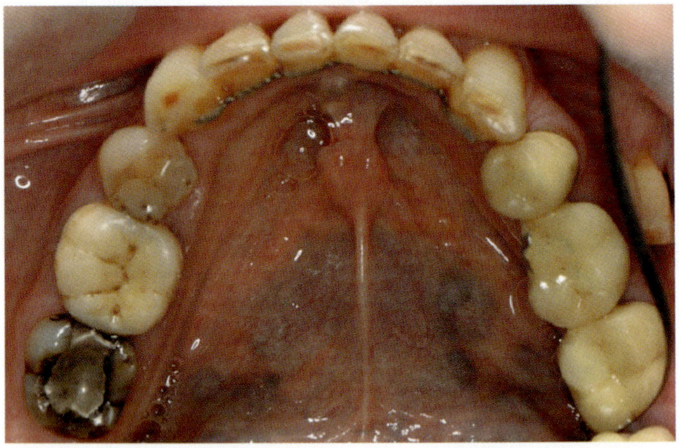

(A)

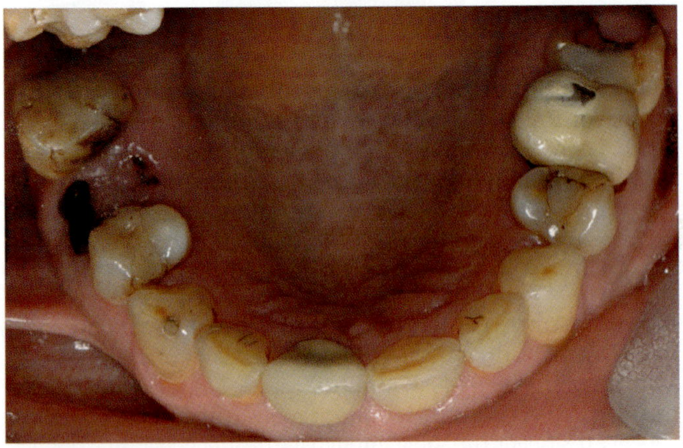

(B)

Figure 4.17

A patient with complex restorative needs: a loose crown on upper right first molar; lower right first molar crown has decay. Detailed evaluation is essential with treatment planning before any whitening treatment can be commenced. (A and B) Presenting photographs of upper and lower teeth.

continued on the next page

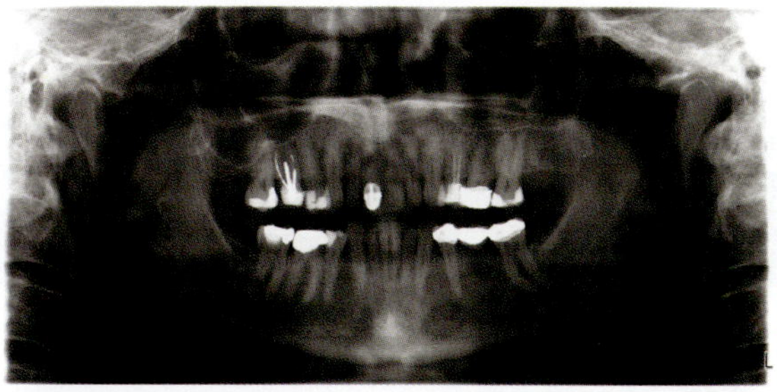

(C)

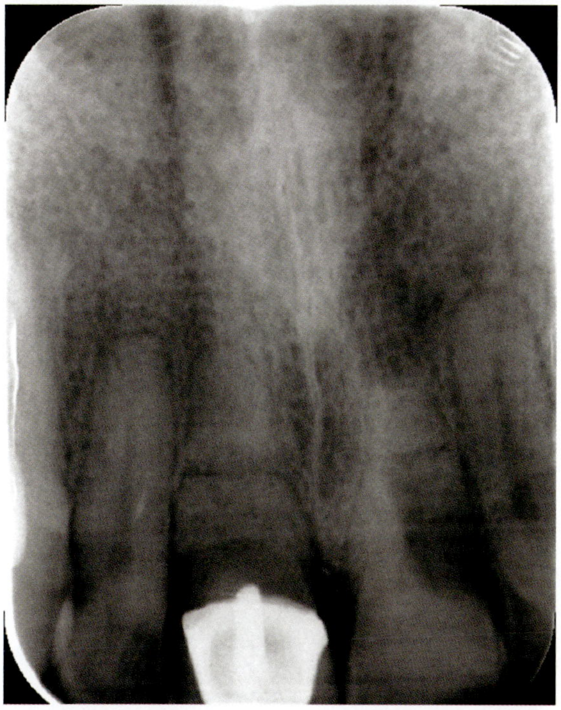

(D)

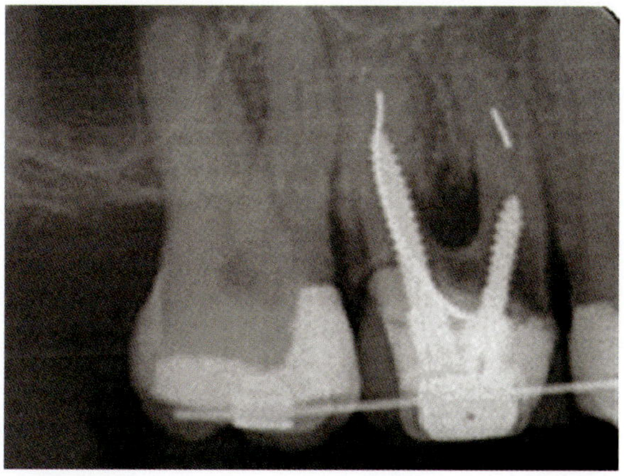

(E)

Figure 4.17 continued

(C) Panoramic radiograph. (D) Periapical radiograph of upper central incisors, which the patient wanted to whiten, showing that both are fractured and there is external resorption in the upper left central such that no whitening can be undertaken in these teeth. This detail was not evident in the panoramic radiograph. (E) Subsequent deterioration of the upper right first molar with decay present. Extraction was necessary.

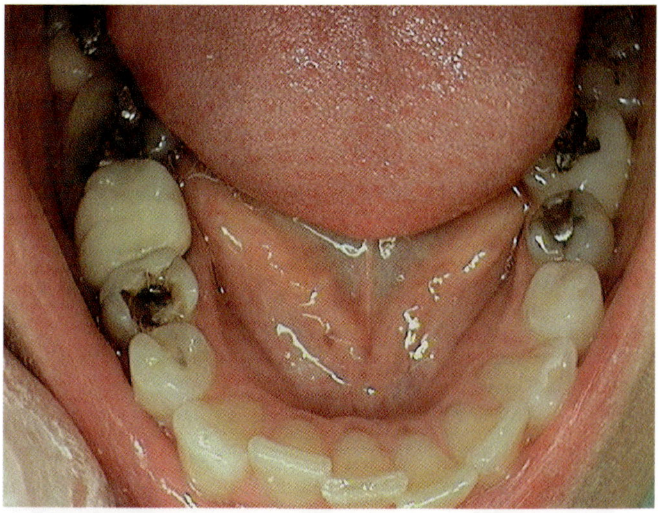

Figure 4.18

Fractured restoration on lower right second premolar, which should be treated before whitening by placing a temporary restoration.

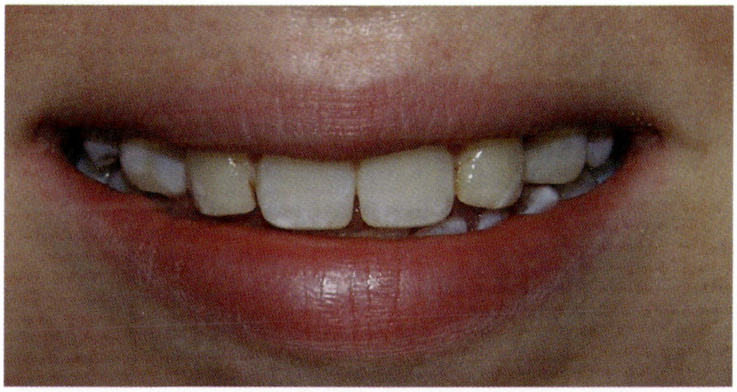

(A)

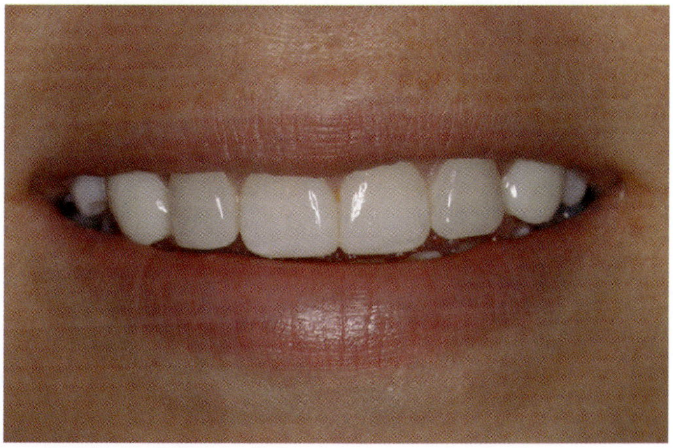

(B)

Figure 4.19

(A) Missing lateral incisor teeth; the canines were previously bonded to give the appearance of incisors. There are multiple discolorations present. Detailed treatment planning is essential so that all options can be discussed. (B) Final result after whitening and bonding; preformed composite veneers were placed on both canines to give the appearance of lateral incisors.

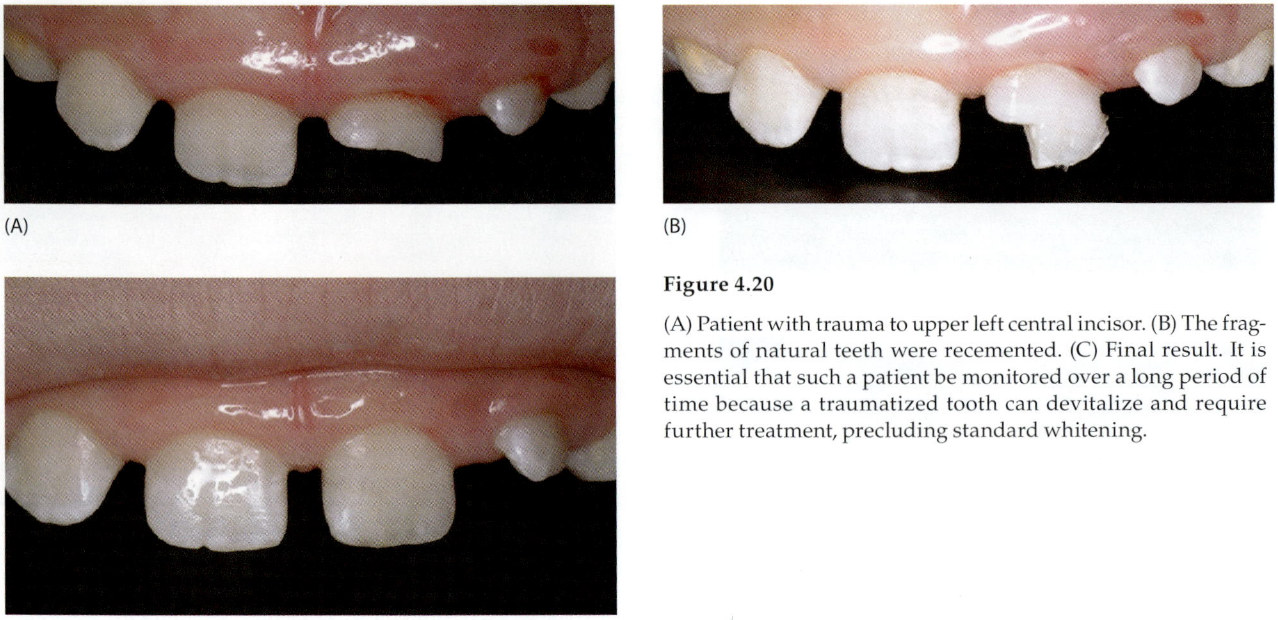

(A)

(B)

(C)

Figure 4.20

(A) Patient with trauma to upper left central incisor. (B) The fragments of natural teeth were recemented. (C) Final result. It is essential that such a patient be monitored over a long period of time because a traumatized tooth can devitalize and require further treatment, precluding standard whitening.

5 THE HOME WHITENING TECHNIQUE

Linda Greenwall

INTRODUCTION

Home whitening is a simple technique whereby, after an initial consultation with the dentist, a mouthguard or tray is made for the patient to whiten the teeth at home. The patient is given the tooth whitening materials (normally 10% carbamide peroxide) to take home, together with a detailed whitening protocol. The patient applies the whitening material to the tray. The tray with the material is worn for several hours during the day or at night depending on the patient's schedule, while the teeth lighten. It is a predictable technique and has a success rate of 98% for non–tetracycline-stained teeth and 86% for tetracycline-stained teeth (Leonard 2000). The introduction of Nightguard Vital Bleaching in 1989 revolutionized whitening technology; the technique was simple, and dentists could provide treatment easily for patients. The overall cost was reduced and the technique has become extremely popular, enabling millions of people around the world to benefit from whitening treatment. It is the aim of this chapter to describe the home whitening technique and protocol in detail, so that successful whitening treatments can be achieved.

Terminology

Many names have been used for home whitening. The original term used was "Nightguard Vital Bleaching," because patients whitened the teeth at night while they slept with the tray in their mouths (Haywood and Heymann 1989). "Home whitening," some may argue, does not distinguish the procedure from that performed by patients who buy the over-the-counter kits and self-prescribe the whitening treatments. However, the term will be used for simplicity. Names associated with home whitening include the following:

- Nightguard Vital Bleaching.
- Matrix bleaching.
- Dentist-assisted or dentist-prescribed home-applied whitening.
- Dentist-supervised at-home whitening.
- At-home whitening.

THE PROS AND CONS OF HOME WHITENING

Advantages

- It is simple and fast for patients to use (Christensen 1997).
- It is simple for dentists to monitor without extended clinical time.
- It is cost-effective (Greenwall 1992).
- The laboratory fees for making the whitening tray are not high.
- It is not usually a painful procedure.
- Patients can whiten their teeth at their convenience, according to their personal schedule.
- Patients can see the results relatively quickly.
- Patients are normally delighted with the result!

Disadvantages

- Patients need to participate actively in their treatment (Miller 1999).
- The color change is dependent on the amount of time that the trays are worn. If patients do not wear the whitening agent in the trays for the specified amount of time, changes in tooth lightening will be slow.
- Some patients cannot be bothered with applying the whitening agent in the trays every day. The dropout rate for home whitening may be as much as 50% according to anecdotal feedback (Miller 1999). Some patients may need further motivation and encouragement to continue whitening through use of an office-assisted program or power whitening.
- The system may be open to abuse by use of excessive amounts of whitening agent for too many hours per day (Garber 1997).
- It is difficult for patients who gag easily to tolerate the whitening trays in the mouth.

Indications for use

Home whitening (Greenwall 1999b) can be used for the following:

- Mild generalized staining (combination of factors [Greenwall 1992]; see Figures 5.10A–G).
- Age-yellowing discoloration (see Figures 5.24A–C).
- Mild tetracycline staining.
- Very mild fluorosis (brown or white) (see Figures 5.10A–G).
- Acquired superficial staining.
- Stains from smoking tobacco (see Figure 5.20A–C).
- Absorptive and penetration stains (tea and coffee; see Figure 5.22A).
- Color change related to pulpal trauma or necrosis.
- Patients who desire a minimal amount of dental treatment to achieve a color shift (see Figures 5.19A–G).
- Young patients with an inherited gray or yellow hue to the teeth who are unhappy about this (see Figures 5.18A and 5.18B).

Contraindications to use

There are many contraindications to home whitening (Greenwall 1999b). Home whitening agents should not be used in the following situations:

- Severe tetracycline staining.
- Severe pitting hypoplasia.
- Severe fluorosis stain.
- Discolorations in the adolescent patient with large pulps (Haywood 1995).
- Patients with unrealistic expectations about the anticipated esthetic result (Wise 1995).
- Teeth with inadequate or defective existing restorations (these should be temporarily blocked before whitening).
- Teeth with tooth surface loss from attrition, abrasion, and severe erosion.
- Teeth with insufficient enamel to respond to whitening (i.e., pitted teeth, defective enamel); however, this might be acceptable because it is the dentin that is important for determining the shade color (Bentley et al. 1999).
- Teeth with deep and surface cracks and fracture lines (see Figure 5.22A).
- Teeth with large anterior restorations that have existing sensitivity.
- Teeth with pathology such as a periapical radiolucency.
- Teeth that are fractured or misaligned may be better treated with other treatments such as porcelain veneers or orthodontics. Further treatment may be necessary.
- Patients who demonstrate a lack of compliance through inability or unwillingness to wear appliance for the required time (Garber et al. 1991).
- Patients who are pregnant or lactating—at this stage, the effect of the whitening agent on development of the fetus is unknown (Garber et al. 1991).
- Patients who smoke—patients cannot smoke and whiten their teeth at the same time because this may enhance the carcinogenic effect of the smoking (see Figure 5.20).
- Teeth exhibiting extreme sensitivity to heat, cold, touch, and sweetness.

Although the last point is not strictly a contraindication, whitening teeth can sometimes cause transient sensitivity. It may be better to treat the sensitivity first with fluoride applications, a bonding agent, or a bonded restoration before whitening. It may also be necessary to protect any erosion or abrasion area (Greenwall 1999a).

Alternatives

The alternatives to home whitening may involve the following:

- In-office whitening, such as power or laser whitening.
- Porcelain veneers (see Figures 5.17A and 5.17B).
- Composite veneers.
- Composite bonding.
- Crowns: all-porcelain crowns or porcelain-bonded-to-metal crowns.
- Further restorations.
- Combinations of treatments.

Most of these options are more invasive and destructive than home whitening. The preparation for crowns (particularly the new all-porcelain crowns) requires removal of at least 1 to 1.5 mm of tooth tissue (even 2 mm).

THE PROTOCOL

Once a patient has expressed an interest in having his or her teeth lightened, several aspects need to be discussed, before the first whitening visit. After assessing the patient's medical history, it may be useful to ask the patient to complete a tooth discoloration questionnaire to ascertain which foods or drinks are causing the staining (see Figure 5.1). Patients should reduce the intake of foods that are causing the staining of the teeth before whitening treatments are begun. Patients should be warned of the possibility of experiencing caffeine withdrawal symptoms if they stop drinking coffee or tea immediately.

The dentist needs to assess whether the patient is taking any medication that can affect whitening treatment, such as antihistamines, which make the mouth dry (see Chapter 4). Any allergies to components of the whitening product, such as glycerin, flavoring agents, or preservatives, or the whitening tray components need to be checked (see Figure 5.3). Patients who smoke should be counseled to stop smoking before any whitening treatments are begun. Patients are advised that they should not whiten their teeth if they are smoking.

Initial consultation

The initial discussion with the patient should address the following:

- The advantages and disadvantages of tooth whitening.
- Alternatives to whitening treatments.
- Any side effects that may be experienced (such as sensitivity, gingival irritation; see Figure 5.15).
- The risks and benefits of the procedures; the patient's informed consent should be obtained (see Figure 5.15).
- All treatment options, including the possibility that more than one whitening treatment may need to be undertaken.
- The duration of treatment.
- Further esthetic treatment that may be needed.
- Further dental treatment such as replacement of stained and leaking composites.

It is essential to set whitening goals before treatment. Use the appropriate procedures for diagnosis, treatment planning, and evaluation of the teeth, which were discussed in Chapter 4.

Clinical examination of all teeth

A comprehensive examination should be performed to assess the oral environment (Fischer 2000b), soft tissues, mucosae, teeth, gingivae, and oral health status of the patient. Check the integrity of the existing restorations. Check recent radiographs for dental disease and periapical radiolucencies (Haywood 1997b). The size and vitality of the pulps of the teeth can be assessed on radiographs to predict sensitivity levels. The vitality of the teeth should be tested, particularly single discolored teeth. Teeth that are nonvital should be root-treated with a good apical seal before whitening treatment. Cervical recession, periodontal health, and any cracking of the anterior teeth should be assessed. Translucency should be measured because highly translucent teeth do not whiten as well; they sometimes appear grayer rather than whiter. Patients should be informed that translucent teeth do not whiten as well.

Preexisting shade evaluation

Before treatment is begun, discuss with the patient the possible shade lightening that can be achieved. This is normally two shades lighter on a normal porcelain shade guide (Vita Classic shade guide) or 1–3 shades lighter on a value-oriented shade guide (Vita 3D master). Shade taking can be done via the normal methods—that is, using the porcelain shade guide or the shade guide supplied with the whitening kit (see Figure 5.5 and Table 5.1). The patient should be fully involved in the shade-taking process, should acknowledge the preoperative shade that was taken, and may sign the notes for verification.

Planning the treatment

It is normally advisable to whiten only one arch at a time so that the patient has the opportunity for a comparison. Often the patient forgets how dark the teeth were to begin with and wants to carry on with the treatment, perhaps unwisely. Both arches can be whitened when time is short, such as for a forthcoming wedding celebration.

It is also essential to discuss with patients that their existing composite restorations may not match after whitening and that it may be necessary to replace these composites with lighter ones after the whitening procedures. Photographs with the shade tab that currently matches the teeth are taken (see Figure 5.7). Intraoral photographs can also be taken. These images can be enhanced so that the patient can see the possible outcome before treatment, but no guarantees are given if the images are enhanced. Other factors to take into account are listed in Table 5.2.

Table 5.2 Factors that have a guarded prognosis for home whitening success

- A history or presence of sensitive teeth
- Extremely dark gingival third of tooth visible during smiling
- Extensive white spots that are very visible
- Presence of temporomandibular joint dysfunction or bruxism
- Translucent teeth
- Excessive gingival recession and exposed root surfaces

Impression taking

Excellent impressions reproducing the surfaces of the upper and lower teeth should be taken so that whitening trays can be made. Alginate or another accurate material can be used. In mixing the materials, attempts should be made to eliminate as many air bubbles as possible (see Figure 5.6). Alginate mixing machines can be used to reduce air bubbles. A small amount of alginate can be rubbed onto the occlusal surface of the teeth to achieve good detail. Closed-mouth techniques are used to eliminate the possibility of distortion of the mandible. Alginate impressions should be poured and cast very soon to prevent distortion of the casts. Whitening trays are made from these impressions (see Chapter 6).

Selecting the appropriate whitening material

A vast array of whitening materials is available. It is important to select the appropriate material for each particular patient. The greater the concentration of carbamide peroxide, and the thicker the material, the more quickly the whitening will take place and the less the trays will need to be worn. Some systems have graded concentrations of active agent, such as 5%, 10%, 15%, and 20%, or even 35%, to enable the patient to get used to whitening without experiencing tooth sensitivity. Studies comparing whitening agents have shown that they all work and there is minimal difference among them (Lyons and Ng 1998). There is an inverse relationship: if the concentration of the whitening agent is decreased, the treatment time must be increased. The concentration of whitening gel is restricted to 6% hydrogen peroxide in Europe according to the European directive that was introduced in 2012.

The choice of which whitening agent to use depends on the following information (Table 5.1):

Table 5.1 The Vita value-oriented shade guide with 16 shades ranked from lightest color on left to darkest color on the right

B1/A1/B2/D2/A2/C1/C2/D4/A3/D3/B3/A3,5/B4/C3/A4/C4
1- 2- 3- 4- 5- 6- 7- 8- 9- 10- 11- 12- 13- 14- 15- 16-
Lightest.. Darkest

- **The discoloration**
  - The source of the discoloration (see Figures 5.16A and 5.16B)
  - The form, shape, depth (whether superficial or deep), and extent of the discoloration
  - The existing color (darker teeth will take longer to whiten)
  - The location of the staining (i.e., within the enamel or dentin) (Touati et al. 1999)
- **The whitening material**
  - The cost of the material (is the cost of the tray fabrication included?)
  - CE Mark (type and classification)/American Dental Association (ADA) Seal of Approval
  - Chemical constituents of the base material (hydrogen peroxide, carbamide peroxide or perborate)
  - Mode of action: pH values?
  - Dispensing method
  - Tissue tolerance
  - Safety studies: have the products been evaluated by the Food and Drug Administration?
  - Suggested wearing times
  - Patient-friendly, clear instruction sheets
  - Ease of use, application
  - The flavor
- **Patient factors**
  - Existing tooth sensitivity
  - Lifestyle
  - Personal schedule
  - Patient dexterity
  - Goals for whitening

Whitening introduction

It is customary to perform an oral prophylaxis before any whitening procedure. This may be done by the hygienist or the dentist. However, a study (Knight et al. 1997) showed that patients who experience sensitivity after an oral prophylaxis are more prone to experience sensitivity and other side effects during whitening. Leonard (1998) advised that patients should wait 2 weeks after an oral prophylaxis before beginning the whitening procedure. Written home whitening instructions are explained to the patient. The whitening record sheet (see Figure 5.1) is completed and the patient signs the consent form. A power whitening session can be done to initiate the whitening at the chairside or to motivate the patient to continue whitening at home, but there would be increased cost for this additional procedure.

Seating the tray

For a full arch

The whitening trays are checked for correct fit, retention, and overextension on the gingival area. If they are overextended, the trays can be trimmed back with small sharp scissors. The rough edge is then polished with a rubber wheel or flame smoothed. The aim is for the tray to fit well, to keep the whitening material in contact with the teeth but not to impinge on the gingivae (see Figure 5.10). The amount of whitening material to be used can be demonstrated to the patient, and the patient is helped to insert and remove the trays (see Figure 5.9). The patient is instructed to place enough material to fill the tray with minimal excess (Leonard et al. 1999) (see Figure 5.11). A demonstration of how to remove the excess whitening material from the soft tissue can be undertaken. Instruct the patient not to swallow the excess but to remove it first using a cotton wool roll, finger, or toothbrush. Patients are instructed to brush and floss their teeth and then to apply the tray with the whitening material in their mouth. They can choose either to whiten their teeth while they sleep or to apply the tray during the day, depending on their schedule.

Supply the whitening material, a few cotton rolls, cotton buds, and the whitening toothpaste (not mandatory) in a home kit. Document the amount of whitening material given to the patient as well as the name of the whitening agent used on the whitening record sheet (Fasanaro 1992) (Figure 5.1). A patient whitening log (see Figure 5.2) is supplied for the patient to document the use of the materials, sensitivity levels, and the amount of time the trays are worn. The patient is instructed to telephone the practice if any adverse reactions are experienced, particularly sensitivity to hot and cold. Normally it is best to start with the whitening of the maxillary teeth because these whiten more quickly. This is thought to be a result of better retention of the upper tray, the effects of gravity, and the reduced effects of salivary flow compared with the mandibular arch.

For single teeth

Full-arch trays are constructed, but patients are instructed to place the whitening material only in the location of the dark tooth. Normally two trays are made. One full arch tray and a second full arch tray with a window cut on either side of the dark tooth so that the patient whitens only the dark tooth in the beginning. Then, the second full arch tray is used to whiten the whole arch. To help patients identify where to place the whitening material, a small notch can be cut into the tray above the tooth (Small 1998). After the teeth are all the same value, the entire arch can be whitened. This could be achieved the other way, by whitening all the teeth first and then titrating the shade by whitening only the single dark tooth.

Discussion of treatment regimen

The decision about when and how long to keep the trays in the mouth depends on the patient's lifestyle, preferences, and schedule (see Figure 5.8). Whitening times will vary according to the patient's schedule. It is useful for the patient to document wearing times so that they can be modified if necessary. Some patients titrate and/or adjust the amount of whitening agent used for certain teeth because they notice some teeth lightening more than

Patient Whitening Record Sheet

Name

Date bleaching started	Age	
Patient's main complaint		
Discoloration type	Preoperative shade	Shade guide used
Patient's desired color		

Informed consent: The patient is informed that there are no guarantees as to the amount of lightening that can be achieved with whitening treatment. Further dental treatment may be required to whiten the teeth. These options may include microabrasion, bonding, porcelain laminate veneers, crowns, or combinations of the above. The patient is instructed to discontinue the whitening treatment should any problems occur.

Patient's Signature: **Date:**

Whitening method			
Nonvital tooth: tooth number		Root canal treatment present	
Patency of apical seal		Radiograph checked	
Bleaching method: walking bleach		Inside/outside technique	
Bleaching material used		Concentration	
Power bleach	Upper teeth		Lower teeth
Bleaching material		Concentration	
Radiographs checked			
Home bleach	Upper teeth		Lower teeth
Presence of anterior composites		Patient informed they may need to be replaced	
Bleaching material used		Concentration	

Whitening Audit

	Appointment date	Arch	Bleach used	Amt dispensed	Problems
1					
2					
3					
4					
5					
6					
7					
8					
9					
10					

Postoperative assessment	
Shade preoperative	Shade postoperative
Recommended rebleaching	Problems encountered
Maintenance	Further aesthetic treatment

Figure 5.1

Patient whitening record sheet (adapted from Fasanaro 1992).

Patient Log for Home Whitening Teeth

Linda H. Greenwall Dental Practice

Patient's name: ______________________________

Date: ______________________

Present shade of teeth:	Desired shade:
Date bleaching started:	To bleach upper/lower/both

Day	Date	No. of hours the trays were worn	Upper/lower/both	Sensitivity

Please complete this log while you are bleaching your teeth at home so that we can see the amount of progress you are making. Store it together with your kit for ease of access. If you have any untoward problems, please call the practice. Please bring this log sheet to each appointment. You will be asked to return the trays once bleaching is completed.

Figure 5.2

Whitening log sheet, which the patient completes during whitening at home so that the dentist can monitor the patient's progress and make any recommendations for timing of treatment. The patient should fill in the log sheet every day. The log sheet should be brought to every appointment so that treatment times can be modified if necessary. Patient compliance can also be assessed.

Home Whitening Instructions and Consent Form

Patient's name: ______________________________

Date: ______________________________

We are planning to whiten your teeth using carbamide peroxide solution. Please read the following instructions carefully.

The active ingredient is carbamide peroxide in a glycerine base. If you know of any allergy or are aware of an adverse reaction to this ingredient, please do not proceed with this treatment.

As with any treatment there are benefits and risks. The benefi tis that teeth can be whitened fairly quickly in a simple manner. The risk involves the continued use of the peroxide solution for an extended period of time such as a few years. Research indicates that using peroxide to bleach teeth is safe. There is new research indicating the safety for use on the soft tissues (gingivae, cheek, tongue, throat). The long-term effects are as yet unknown. Although the extent of the risk is unknown, acceptance of treatment means acceptance of risk.

This type of whitening treatment has been done for some patients for over 40 years. During that time, nobody needed a root canal or damaged a tooth following home bleaching treatment.

The amount of whitening varies with the individual. Most patients achieve a change within 2–5 weeks. Try to reduce the amount of tea, coffee, and red wine and refrain from eating berries or curries during or after treatment for at least 1 month. You may use the toothpaste supplied with the kit to clean your teeth during treatment.

It is advisable not to smoke during the course of bleaching treatment for at least 5–8 weeks.

Sensitivity may result after a few days. This is usually slight and temporary. If this should occur refrain from using the bleaching treatment for 1day or apply the soothing gel into the tray that you will be given.

Do not use the bleaching treatment if you are pregnant. There have been no reports of adverse reactions, but long-term clinical effects are unknown.

Wear the tray overnight or for a minimum of two hours per day.

Some teeth do not bleach evenly particularly around gum recession on the lower premolar teeth. The enamel bleaches well but the exposed dentine does not bleach as well.

When the treatment is completed, please keep the trays so that they can be used for a top-up maintenance treatment. It may be necessary to do a top-up treatment in 18–24 months depending on the amount of staining.

**

I have read the above information and agree to return for examination after the treatment begins and at any recommended time afterwards. I have read and received a copy of this information sheet. I consent to the treatment and accept the risks described above.

I consent to photographs being taken. I understand that they may be used for documentation and for illustration of my treatment.

Signed ______________________ ***Patient*** ______________________ ***Date:*** ______________

Figure 5.3

Whitening instruction and consent form.

How to Manage Sensitivity during Whitening Treatment

Sensitivity of teeth is the most common side effect of whitening treatment. This usually occurs around the necks of the teeth. Patients can experience some degree of sensitivity, which ranges from mild awareness to a throb on a specific tooth. Up to 50% of patients suffer with some sensitivity.

If you are experiencing sensitivity during your whitening treatment these are the different treatments that you should follow.

1. We will provide you with a desensitizing material called Soothe to place in your bleaching trays. This should be placed in the trays in exactly the same way that the bleaching material is placed. You should alternate each night, one night with the Soothe and the following night with the bleaching material, or you can apply it onto the tray for one hour per night. This should be continued until the sensitivity disappears.
2. We will provide you with some preformed trays which are called Ultra-eze trays. You should wear these trays for one night only. These should relieve your sensitivity.
3. We will provide you with GC Tooth Mouse. Either this can be put in your bleaching trays, or you can rub it into an individual tooth where it is sensitive.
4. You can also use a desensitizing toothpaste such as Sensodyne. You can also brush with the desensitizing toothpaste during the whitening treatment. Place a small amount of the toothpaste on your finger and rub it into the sensitive area. You should repeat this each night until the sensitivity disappears.
5. You can stop the whitening for one night if the sensitivity is too severe. Do not stop for more than two nights; otherwise, the effect of the whitening will slow down. Sometimes the gums may also feel a little sensitive. If you notice the gums are feeling sore, you need to refrain from bleaching for one day or reduce the concentration of the whitening gel.

**

Dr Linda Greenwall
BDS MGDS MSC MRD RCS FFGDP BDBS

Figure 5.4

How to manage sensitivity form.

What to Expect during Your Whitening Treatment

Your dentist has given you a bleaching kit to take home with you together with your bleaching trays. It is essential that you follow the instructions given by your dentist and the manufacturer's instructions in wearing the trays and applying the bleaching agent. Below are answers to the most frequent questions.

How long should I wear the trays?

This depends on the amount of lightening that you desire and the original shade of the teeth. If your teeth are quite dark or very yellow/gray/tetracycline-stained, it will take longer to bleach the teeth. If you are not experiencing any sensitivity you may wear the trays for at least 1–2 hours and even sleep with the trays in your mouth. It is very important to remove all the excess material around the gums or the palate prior to sleeping with the trays.

The darker your teeth, the longer your teeth will take to get lighter. Tetracycline-stained teeth can take 6 months to one year to bleach the teeth. Some teeth can whiten after one month.

If you cannot wear the trays for a few days because of your hectic schedule, it does not matter. Bleach your teeth according to your own schedule. Some people put the trays in after dinner and wear them for the first hour while watching TV or doing the dishes. Then if everything is fine they replenish the trays and sleep with them in the mouth.

What do I do if I have any sensitivity?

Sensitivity of teeth is the most common side effect of home bleaching. In fact many patients suffer from sensitive teeth anyway. This occurs usually around the necks of the teeth where the gums have receded. If you are experiencing any sensitivity you should stop bleaching your teeth for a few days. You can resume after about 3–4 days. If the teeth become ultrasensitive you can place sensitive toothpaste into the bleaching trays for an hour a day. That will usually stop the sensitivity. Alternatively you can rub the desensitizing toothpaste into the gum margins with your finger 5 times per day for a few days.
If you are at all concerned, please call your dentist.

Figure 5.5

(A) Commonly asked questions about whitening treatment.

continued on the next page

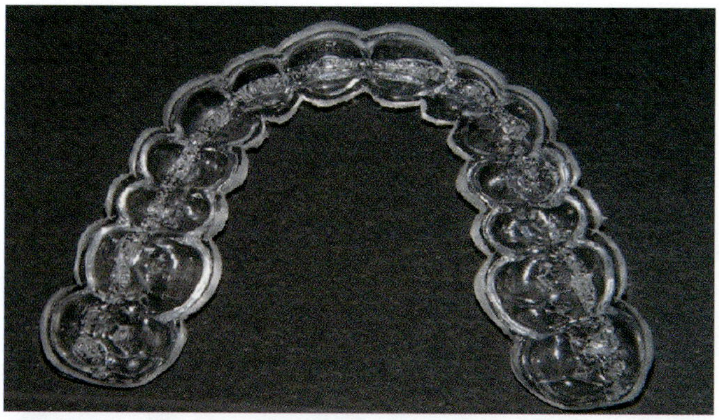

(A)

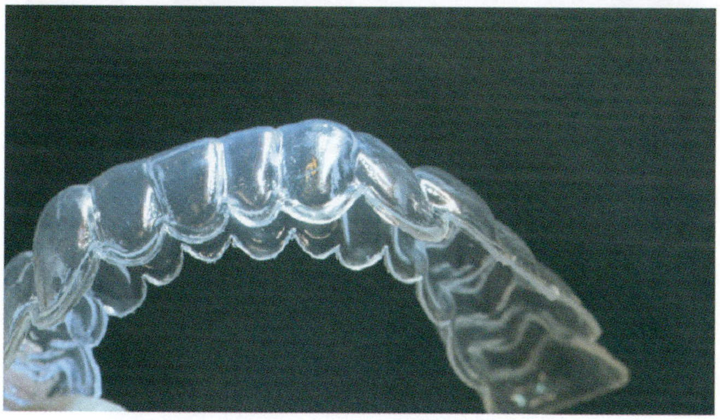

(B)

Figure 5.11

(A) The exact shape of the whitening tray once it is finished in the laboratory. (B) The tray should be trimmed around the gingival area to prevent any irritation.

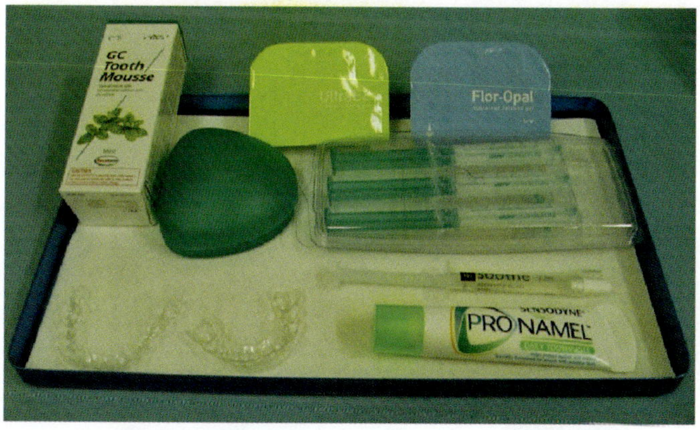

Figure 5.12

The tray is set up to discuss sensitivity that might occur during the first home whitening session. Normally two different soothing products are dispensed to patients so they can self-manage the sensitivity according to their symptoms.

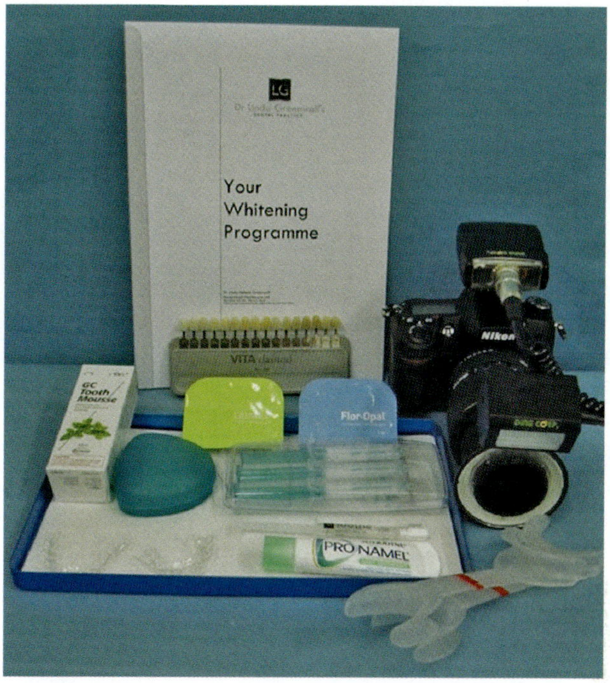

(A)

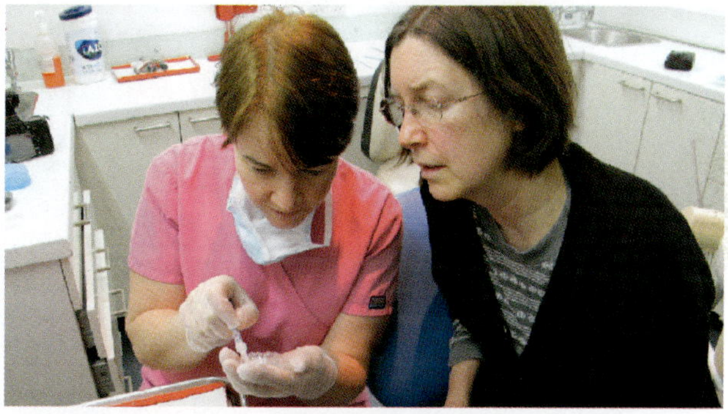

(B)

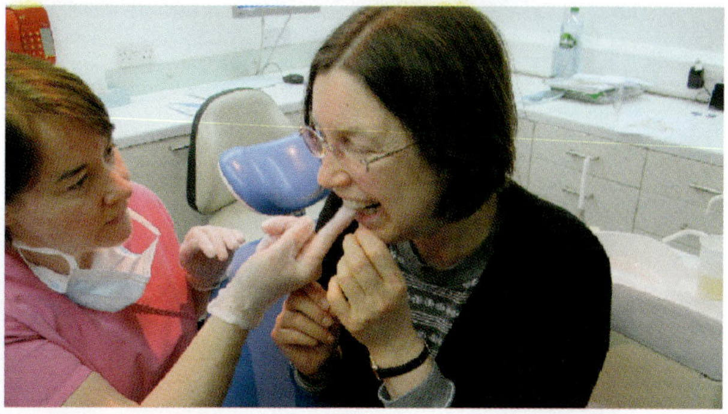

(C)

Figure 5.13

(A) The tray setup for home whitening stage 1. This should be included in any procedure manual for dental assistants so they know exactly how to set up the trays for the home whitening procedure. (B) The patient is shown exactly where and how to place the whitening gel by running a line into the middle of the tray. (C) The patient is then shown how to seat the aligner with the tooth whitening gel inside. *continued on the next page*

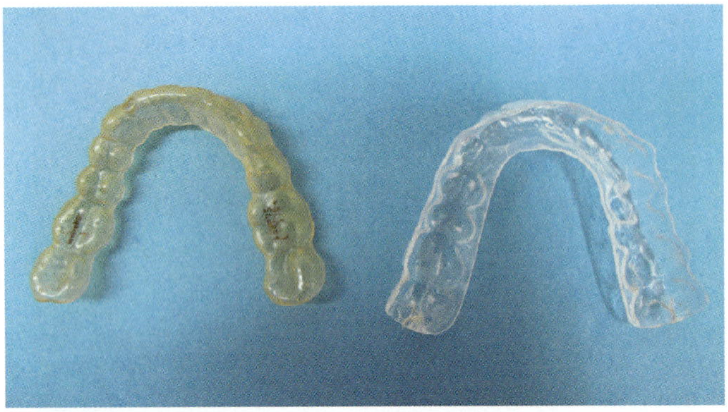

(D)

Figure 5.13 continued

(D) The appearance of the patient's aligner, which has discolored slightly from tea drinking before bed. The patient's whitening tray has not discolored.

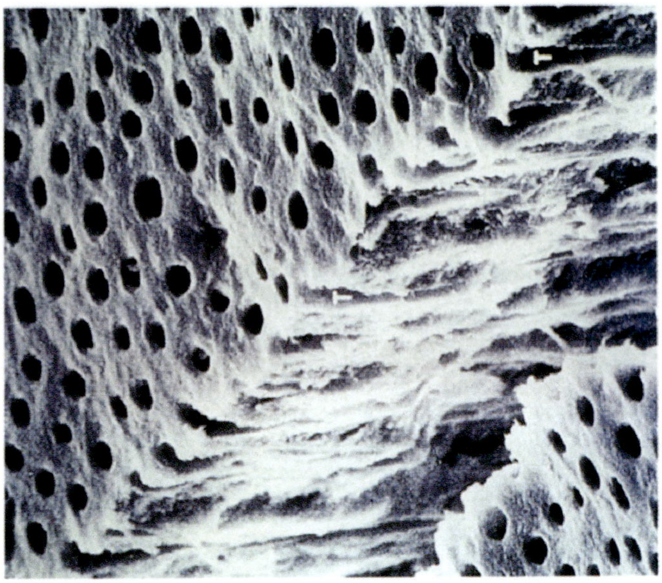

Figure 5.14

The structure of dentin, as revealed on a scanning electron micrograph. (Courtesy of Dr. Ilan Rotstein.)

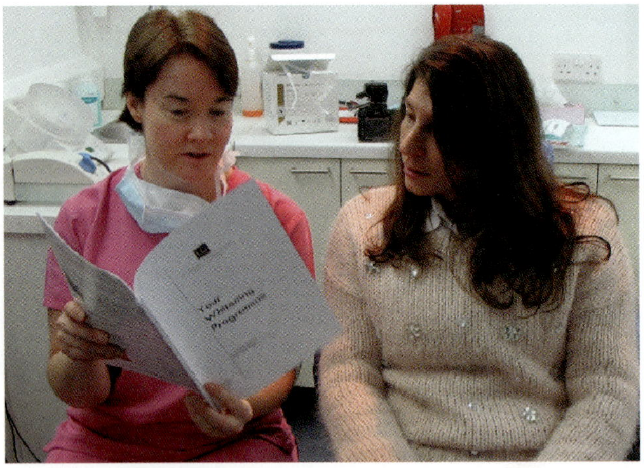

(A)

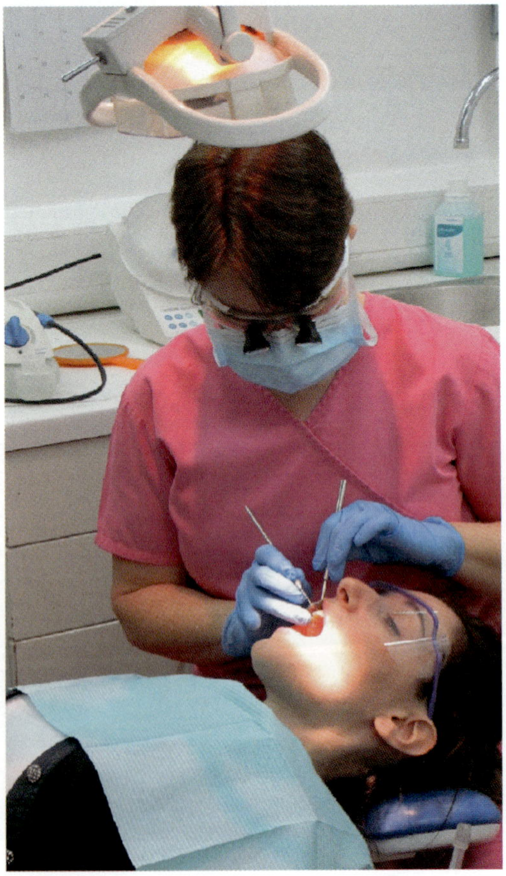

(B)

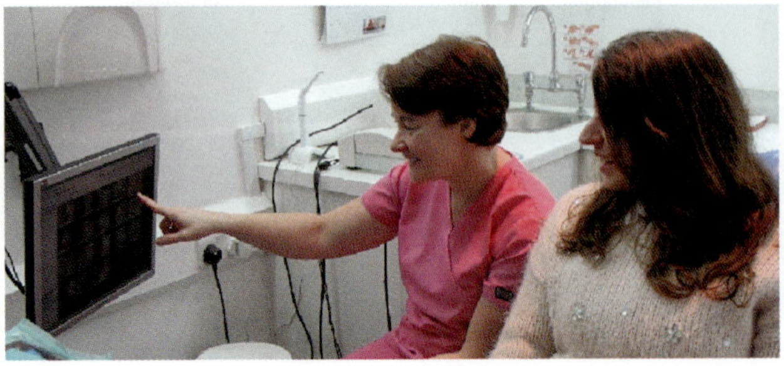

(C)

Figure 5.15

(A) The patient is given a whitening booklet containing all the information that he or she needs to know to undertake the whitening treatment at home. This booklet contains the consent forms, information on how to manage sensitivity at home, and the whitening log to complete. (B) When the patient returns for the second visit the gingivae are checked for any gingival irritation or ulceration. (C) An intraoral camera photograph can be taken of the area of gingival irritation to show the patient and to assess whether the tray should be cut back if it is overextended.

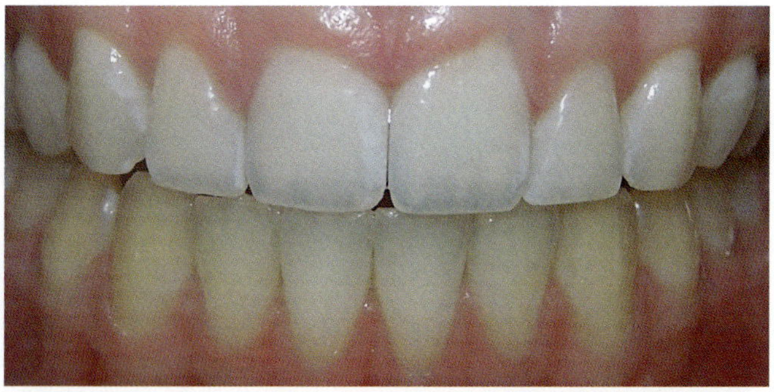

(A)

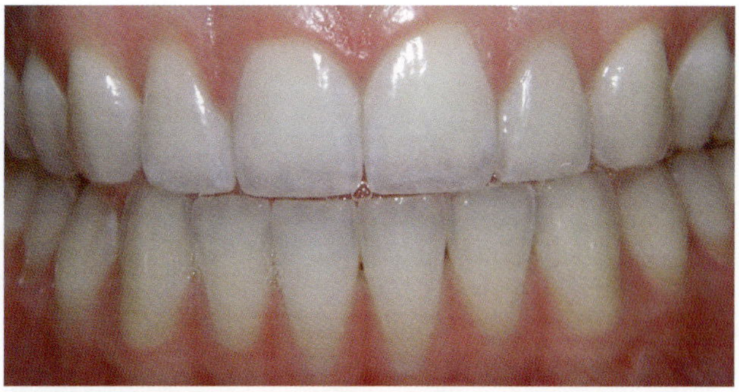

(B)

Figure 5.16

(A) This patient had yellow staining on her teeth from tea and coffee drinking and had noticed that her teeth had recently become more yellow. This picture shows the contrast that occurs halfway through the whitening treatment when the whitening of the upper teeth is completed and the lower teeth whitening can commence. Normally it is just a matter of lightening the lower teeth to match the upper teeth. The treatments are separated to make it easier for the patient to manage and so that the lower teeth remain as a color control throughout the upper whitening. (B) Appearance of the teeth after completion of the whitening treatment, showing that the upper and lower teeth are the same shade of white.

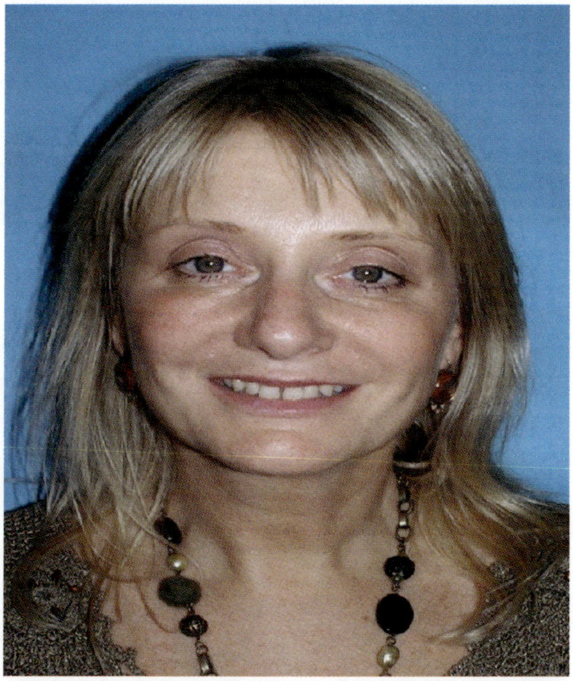

(A)

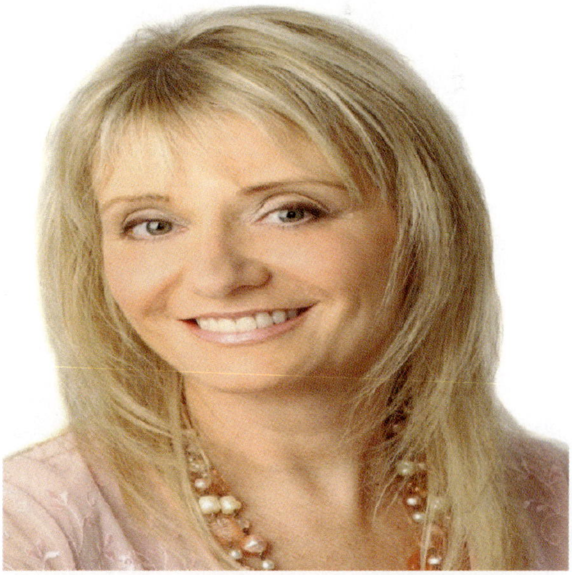

(B)

Figure 5.17

(A) Portrait view of the patient before esthetic treatment. The upper teeth were not whitened because these teeth were prepared for veneers. The lower teeth were whitened first to establish the whiter shade and then the shade of the upper teeth was measured against the new whiter lower teeth. (B) The portrait view of the patient after completion of six upper porcelain laminate veneers and lower whitening treatment using the home whitening technique.

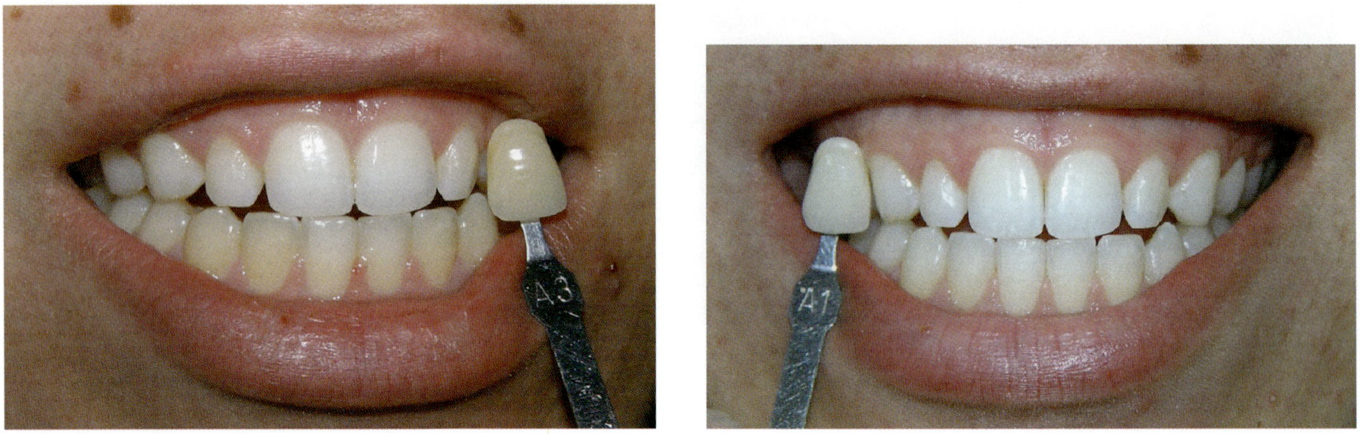

(A) (B)

Figure 5.18

(A) The appearance of the teeth before whitening. The upper teeth are lighter than the Vita A3 shade tab. The lower teeth are darker in this case, and it is important to explain this observation to the patient. In this case it may be more appropriate to whiten the lower teeth first; the whitening will take longer because the existing shade of the lower teeth is darker. (B) The appearance of the teeth after completion of upper and lower whitening.

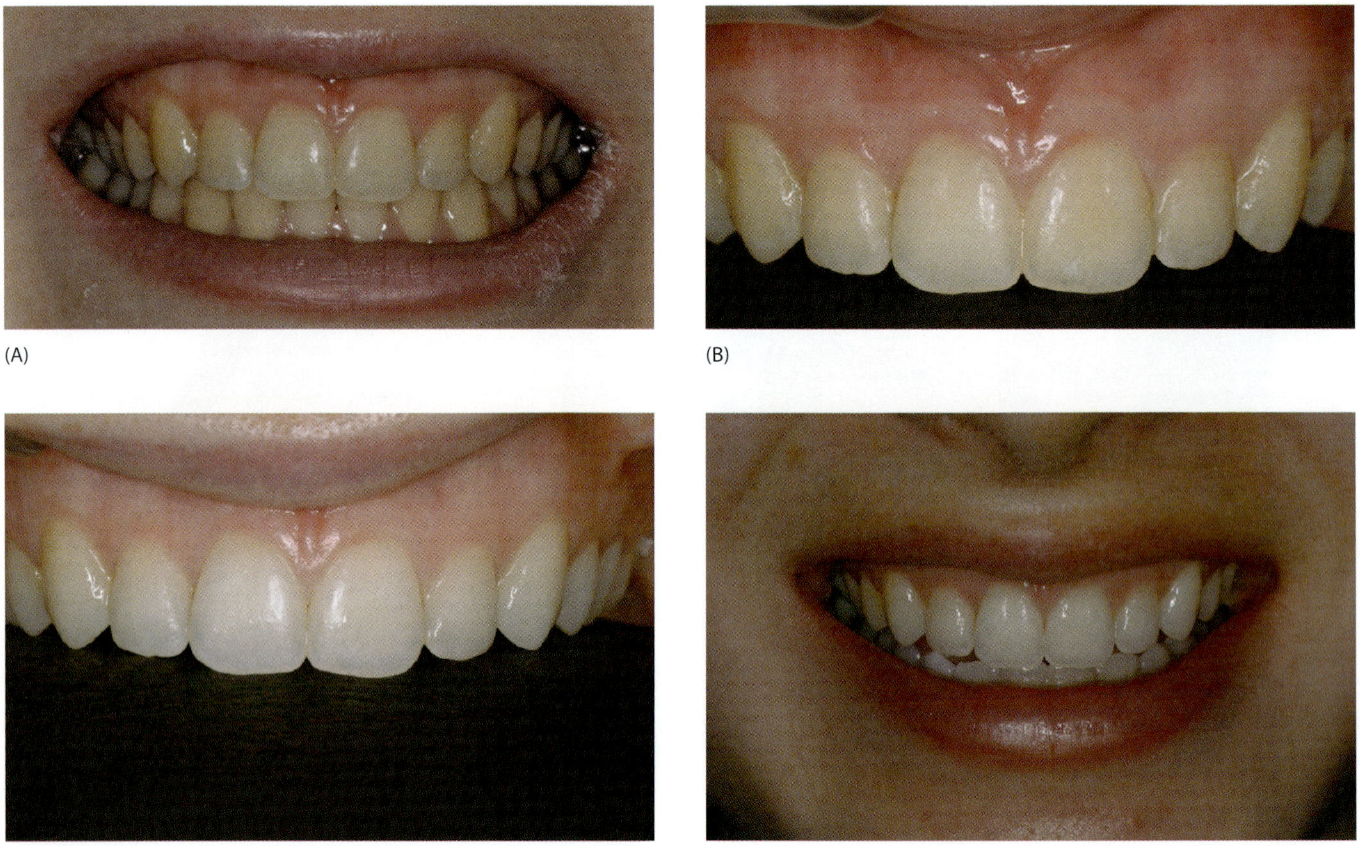

(A) (B) (C) (D)

Figure 5.19

(A) The appearance of the smile of the patient before whitening. The teeth have a yellow hue to them. (B) The appearance of the upper teeth during the whitening treatment. This shows that the tips are white but the rest of the teeth remains yellow. Further whitening treatment is necessary to obtain an even white shade throughout the whole tooth. (C) The appearance of the upper teeth after completion of the upper whitening treatment. (D) The patient's smile at the end of whitening treatment.

continued on the next page

6 HOME WHITENING TRAYS
How to Make Them

Linda Greenwall

INTRODUCTION

The appropriate design, construction, and fit of the whitening tray is essential for successful whitening treatment and patient compliance. It is essential that the patient wear a well-fitting whitening tray, and although much has been written about designs of different whitening trays, this chapter will enumerate the important features that such trays should have. Excess tray material will impinge on the soft tissues and irritate the gingivae if the tray is overextended. This could cause discomfort to the patient, and if the tray is uncomfortable the patient may fail to comply with the home whitening regimen and thus discontinue treatment. This chapter will discuss different tray design features and fabrication options and demonstrate the step-by-step procedure of how to make the whitening trays.

PROPERTIES OF THE IDEAL WHITENING TRAY

The ideal whitening trays (see Figure 6.20) should:

- Be strong enough to avoid damage by the patient during wear.
- Not distort during use.
- Not wear during use.
- Be easy to fit and easy to remove after a treatment session.
- Be made from a material that is bioinert (Greenwall 1999).
- Not cause irritation to the soft tissues, gingivae, mucosa, tongue, or teeth.
- Not impinge too far on the papillae.
- Be thin enough to be well tolerated in the mouth.
- Be smooth and well polished so that there are no rough edges.
- Fit comfortably and passively and not feel too tight in places.
- Not extend into deep undercuts.
- Be correctly trimmed with freedom of movement for the frenum attachments if the full vestibule design is used.
- Have good retention.
- Be easy to clean and rinse.
- Not distort during storage.

Several designs can be used depending on the nature and location of the discoloration and the specific case (Haywood 1991). For example, if the front teeth are particularly dark and discolored but the color of the rest of the teeth is satisfactory, a tray can be designed with cut-out sections to lighten the central incisors only. Conversely, windows can be cut into the trays to exclude certain teeth (see Figure 6.26).

TRAY DESIGN FEATURES

Several types of trays can be used for at-home whitening (Table 6.1).

- Full vestibule upper or lower trays.
- Trays with reservoirs (some whitening manufacturers insist on reservoirs, but new research has demonstrated that this may not be necessary).
- Trays with no reservoirs.
- Trays with a foam liner (Haywood et al. [1993] do not recommend this design because its use does not shorten the whitening time and may impinge on the occlusion).
- Trays with or without windows.
- Trays with scalloping or anatomic cutout (the tray follows the tooth-gingiva interface).
- Nonscalloped: straight-line trays.
- Tray with shortened borders.

Reservoirs

A reservoir (see Figure 6.25) is a void or space that has been created in the whitening tray. The reservoir can also be called a spacer. The reservoir in the tray acts as a receptacle for the whitening material and is supposed to retain the whitening material in the tray, thus allowing it to contact the teeth for a longer period of time. The reservoir is made by placing light-cured composite resin on the buccal surfaces of the teeth on the plaster model. Some manufacturers recommend a reservoir made of plaster so that it will not distort the tray during tray manufacture.

Trays with no reservoirs

Research has shown that it is not necessary to have a reservoir placed and that trays used for tooth whitening do not need to have reservoirs any more. The advantages of this are that the trays are better retained and that less material is used for each application. A better fitting tray allows for the material to compress against the tooth surface and allows for better, quicker penetration of the whitening material into the tooth.

Table 6.1 Tray design options

Design	*Indication*	*Comments*
Full vestibule	This type of tray is not commonly used.	Would provide excellent retention, but the impingement on the gingivae would cause irritation.
Scalloped on the buccal and lingual areas plus reservoir	This type of tray is used where minimal tissue contact is desired. It is useful for highly viscous materials that supply retention. It is used for the maxillary arch to conserve material use.	Saliva ingress is a problem unless insoluble material is used (thick and viscous). Special trimming scissors facilitate fabrication.
Nonscalloped, nonreservoir	This design provides maximum retention of the whitening tray. It provides maximum retention of the material at the cervical area of the tooth. It is useful for fluid and honey-like whitening materials. It is indicated for the mandibular arch where the occlusion contacts the buccal and facial aspects of the tooth.	It allows tissue contact, which may cause gingival irritation. It cannot extend into undercuts. It should not terminate on soft tissue peaks such as rugae or impinge on frenum movement or the canine eminence.
Facial and lingual scalloped reservoir	This type of design is used when taste is a problem for the patient. It can also be used when there has been a problem with tongue irritation from the edges of the tray.	It avoids spill over the material onto the tongue from the lingual side. It provides a smooth edge for tongue contact.
Scalloped reservoir, buccal and lingual surfaces, no occlusal surface	This type of tray can be used for temporomandibular joint dysfunction (TMD) patients who cannot tolerate fine changes to the occlusal surfaces.	Using a viscous whitening gel will allow excellent whitening of the teeth. There should be no difference in whitening rates with the occlusal surfaces removed.
Scalloped, no reservoir (my choice for tray design)	This type of tray is used for gel materials, when tissue avoidance is desired, but allowing for maximum retention of the tray. Orthodontic clear aligners fall into the category and can be used for whitening.	There is no apparent difference in the whitening rate with or without reservoirs. Because there is no apparent difference between whitening rates, Miller (2000) has suggested that the reservoirs are not necessary anymore.
Nonscalloped, no reservoir	This design is used when seating a tray with viscous material and when a better seal is desired. This can be an orthodontic aligner, which can be used for whitening during or after orthodontic treatment.	The mandibular arch is best with the nonscalloped design for retention of the material and tissue comfort.

Adapted from Haywood 1997.

Function of the tray reservoir

It has been determined that the reservoir or spacer performs many important functions.

Advantages

- It retains and contains the whitening material better, particularly the more viscous whitening materials such as Opalescence (Ultradent Products, South Jordan, UT; supplied by Optident, UK) and prevents it from leaking around the gingivae.
- It allows the whitening material to stay in contact with the tooth for longer.
- It may help to keep the whitening material active for longer (Matis et al. 1999).
- It allows gel in areas with a higher concentration of carbamide peroxide to be transferred to areas with a lower concentration (Matis et al. 1999).
- It holds more whitening material (Miller 1999).
- It prevents washout of the whitening agent.
- It aids in seating highly viscous materials (Oliver and Haywood 1999).
- It prevents the occurrence of pinching pressure.

Disadvantages

- It causes the tray to become less retentive (Haywood 1995).
- More whitening material is required to fill the tray.
- It makes the tray more bulbous and slightly thicker.
- There may be the potential for occlusal interference on the mandibular arch.
- It requires additional time and products to be made.

Reservoirs are normally placed on the facial surfaces of the tooth. There is no apparent difference in whitening rate with or without reservoirs (Haywood 1997). Reservoirs can be used depending on the following:

- *The viscosity of the whitening material used.* Some materials (e.g., Opalescence) are very viscous. The material is retained in place better if there is a reservoir that allows for easier seating. If the whitening agent has a thin viscosity, a reservoir is not needed (Heymann and Haywood 1995).

- *Tooth anatomy.* If a tooth is more bulbous than the rest it may not be necessary to place a reservoir. Teeth with lower esthetic demands (e.g., second molar teeth) do not require placement of reservoirs.
- *Tooth darkness.* A darker tooth can have a reservoir (see Figure 6.25).
- *A dark cervical margin.* These cases should have the tray designed to extend 1 mm over the gingivae and could have a reservoir because more whitening material is required to go into the dark cervical margin.

Where should the reservoir be placed?

The reservoir should be placed on the buccal surfaces of the model of the teeth at least 1 mm away from the gingivae. This will seal the tray at the gingivae. The block-out resin can be placed to the incisal edge.

Scalloped trays

Scalloped trays allow for minimal soft tissue contact. They cause minimal gingival irritation and use a minimal amount of whitening material. The tray follows the tooth-gingiva interface. The tray should be cut back 1 mm so that it does not impinge on the gingivae in patients with a high lip line. Scalloping prevents soft tissue contact and reduces gingival irritation. However, saliva may ingress at the neck of the tooth and may remove material from the tray. Furthermore, the tongue or lip can become irritated from the scalloped edges of the tray. Additional time is required to make this type of tray.

Nonscalloped straight-line trays

These trays are cut out 2 mm over the labial incisors. Touati et al. (1999) recommend using this type of tray. They state that this design is easier to use, is simpler to carry out, is less traumatic to the rest of the mouth, and provides a better border seal than the anatomic tray design. This design has the interproximal spaces filled in and a central thin reservoir in the middle of each tooth.

Trays with shortened borders

Although this tray design is not ideal, it can be made in certain circumstances such as for a patient with excessive gingival recession or preexisting sensitivity or one who gags easily. Capillary action will transmit the whitening material to the cervical part of the tooth. This is not often recommended because the trays could theoretically act as an orthodontic retainer or anterior bite splint if the tray is worn for a long period. Intrusion and uncontrolled orthodontic movement of the teeth could result from prolonged wearing of a shortened whitening tray. It is usually better to have full occlusal coverage of all the teeth. The cervical 1 mm can be cut back from the tray if this is found to be irritating the gingivae. This cut-back has been shown to make no difference to the efficacy of the whitening treatment.

Trays with windows

Use of trays with windows depends on the location of the discoloration and can allow for a single or group of teeth to be whitened. Windows can be used to exclude certain teeth from the whitening process. This is usually for a single dark vital or nonvital tooth. Windows can be cut to block out the adjacent lighter teeth (see Figure 6.26). Through placement of a window or cut-back, the darker tooth is able to lighten first. Otherwise the lighter tooth will get too light before the dark tooth has lightened sufficiently. Windows can also be used when further restorative dentistry may be contemplated after whitening treatment.

Thickness of the tray

There are many varying thicknesses of plastic used for trays, and the choice depends on the patient. If the patient has a bruxing habit, it is advisable to use a thicker tray material because the patient may wear through a thin tray in a matter of days. The thicker tray should be 0.05 inches thick. If the patient gags easily, it would be advisable to use a very thin tray that is scalloped well so that it is easily tolerated. It is possible to make trays with no occlusal coverage for those patients who have temporomandibular joint dysfunction (TMD) syndrome. In this case the tray material would cover the labial and lingual surfaces and be cut away from the occlusal surfaces. The standard thickness is the Sof-Tray size 0.035 inch (Ultradent Products). Rigid orthodontic trays can also be used as whitening trays after orthodontic treatment.

PREPARING THE PLASTER MODELS

There is much debate as to whether the plaster models should be specially prepared to receive the whitening trays (see Figures 6.1–6.4). The plaster models should be properly poured to avoid air bubbles on the occlusal surface. There should be no bubbles at the cervical margins because these would interfere with the tray fit. There are recommendations that the plaster model be specially scored with a plaster knife to create deeper indentations at the cervical area. This is to allow for a closer fit of the trays. The dental technician should check the model, remove air bubbles, and tidy the gingival margins on the plaster model. Deeper scoring with a plaster knife has been recommended by some whitening companies.

MAKING THE TRAY

Equipment needed

- Plaster cast of the teeth.
- Block-out resin and applicator (not used much these days).
- Curing light box or light-cure hand-held machine (if block-out resins used).
- Cold mold seal (see Figures 6.2–6.5) and applicator.
- Sheet material (i.e., plastic sheets ready cut to the appropriate shape [Sof-Tray, Ultradent; see Figure 6.6]).

- Heat/vacuum tray-forming machine (see Figure 6.7).
- Pair of scissors for trimming the gross excess.
- Scalpel handle (Bard Parker) and blade (No. 12) with access to a flame.
- A polishing trimmer, cotton wheel (see Figure 6.18).
- Straight/laboratory slow handpiece.
- Stone, spatula, and mixing machine (if available) (Greenwall 1999).

Step-by-step guide

1. Take a good alginate impression

Spatulate the alginate well. Alginator machines can be used to reduce the occurrence of air bubbles in the alginate mix. (See Chapter 5 on home whitening for further detail on impression taking.) Alginate can be wiped on the occlusal surface with a finger to avoid air entrapment (Haywood and Powe 1998). Load the tray and seat it gently. Leave the alginate to set for 1 minute. Once the alginate has set, remove the impression from the mouth. Ensure that there are no air bubbles on the occlusal, facial, or lingual surfaces of the impression. Disinfect the impression and rinse away the disinfectant to ensure that the impression is not distorted. Wrap the models in a damp paper towel and send to the laboratory.

2. Cast a model

Pour stone into the impression and ensure that there is no air entrapment in the stone. Suggestions for stone include Microstone (Whip Mix, Louisville, KY) and a fast-setting stone, Snapstone (Whip Mix), which can set in 8 minutes. Follow the manufacturer's instructions on the setting times carefully. The cast should be free from bubbles, voids, or excess plaster. Any minor voids can be blocked out. Any excess plaster bubbles should be removed from the occlusal and cervical areas (see Figure 6.1).

3. Trim the model

The model should be carefully trimmed so that the base of the model is flat and parallel to the occlusal plane (see Figure 6.1). The cast can be trimmed further around the base into a horseshoe shape so that removal of the heated plastic from the cast is easier. However, the model should not be overtrimmed because this could make it too weak and thin (Miller 1999), potentially causing it to fracture. It is best to allow the model to dry for 24 hours to allow the stone to set fully and to stop further expansion of the stone. This will prevent distortion of the tray. However, the fast-setting stone models can be trimmed after 10 minutes.

4. Place the block-out resin

(This step is no longer mandatory and is not often used.)

Gently place the block-out composite material in the middle of each tooth. Start in the midline and work your way back. The block-out kit comes with an applicator, which has a brush tip on the end to enable ease of placement.

5. Cure the resin on the reservoir

(This step may be excluded because reservoirs are not mandatory.)

Once the desired amount of block-out resin has been added around the teeth, it can be placed in a light box (the one used in our laboratory is the Triad 2000 light box from Dentsply/York Division). The cast is placed in the center of the stand to ensure an even cure.

6. Apply separator/cold mold seal

Once the curing is complete, place a thin layer of cold mold seal over the model. This will facilitate ease of removal of the plastic press-down from the model at a later stage. Remove the excess seal by air drying with compressed air.

7. Choose the tray sheet material

Several types of plastic can be used to make the trays. Some manufacturers supply the tray material inside the whitening kits. The most common tray material is ethyl vinyl acetate (EVA). EVA is a flexible material of the type used for sports guards but is much thinner (Newman and Bottone 1995). The size 0.035 inch is the most common thickness used, but there are thinner ones at 0.02 inch and thicker ones for patients with a bruxing habit at size 0.05 inch. For the purpose of demonstration we have used the Sof-Tray size 0.035 inch made by Ultradent Products. The sheets come in squares with a protective backing.

Some press-down machines take only round sheets, not square ones (see Figures 6.5–6.9). These can be cut down by using a specific template and scalpel. It is also possible to buy precut round sheets. The machine should be preheated for 10 minutes before the procedure is started. It is essential to remove the protective backing before placing the plastic sheet in the machine (see Figure 6.6). Ensure that the sheet is placed into the correct location and in the center of the holder. It is kept in place with three lugs.

8. Cast the plastic in the vacuum tray-forming machine

Place the cast with the teeth face-up in the center of the machine, making sure that the plastic sheet is directly above it. Wait until the plastic has melted and is hanging down and just touching the cast before pulling the machine down over the cast (see Figure 6.9). The machine should be pulled down slowly to avoid generating any creases in the plastic. Sufficient time should be allowed for the vacuum to be properly adapted to the cast (see Figure 6.10). The resultant effect will be the heated plastic sheet vacuum-suctioned over the cast. To avoid tray distortion, the plastic should cool down sufficiently before the trays are trimmed. Remove the plastic sheet from the case; the gross excess can be removed using a small pair of scissors.

9. Trim the tray

Continue trimming the tray with scissors to about 1 cm above the gingival margin (see Figures 6.13 and 6.17.) Put the whitening tray back on the model, and with a heated scalpel carefully trim the palatal margins close to the clinical crown margin of the teeth (see Figure 6.15). Remove the excess flash (see Figure 6.16). The buccal and facial parts of the tray can be scalloped first (see Figure 6.18). Once the buccal part has been completed, start trimming the palatal margins by using the same technique—that is, with the heated scalpel—and polish with a polishing brush (see Figure 6.19). This time, scallop the edge 1–2 mm above the clinical crown margin.

Where should the tray be finished? (See Figures 6.20–6.24.)

- At the gingival margin. This is the most favored design.
- 1 mm above the gingival margin. This is for sensitive teeth.
- 1 mm over the gingival margin. This is for darker gingival margins.

If there is an abrasion or wear lesion at the gingival margin, it may be best to place a glass ionomer restoration on the cervical margins before making an impression of the mouth. Otherwise these defective areas can be temporarily filled in with plaster; if the lesion creates too much of an undercut, this may make tray fabrication difficult.

If the patient has particularly sensitive teeth before starting the whitening procedure, the tray should be cut back to 1 mm below the clinical crown height. This design of tray is good for patients who have particularly dark cervical margins.

10. Polish the tray

Remove the tray from the model again and start polishing and finishing the edges with a soft cotton wheel so that there are no rough parts (see Figure 6.18). To ensure that the frenum attachments have freedom of movement (see Figure 6.24), the tray may need to be further relieved in certain areas. Place the tray back on the model for the final polishing because at this stage it can easily distort. Some techniques advise flame polishing of the edges if it distorts.

THE FINISHED TRAY

The finished tray is shown in Figure 6.24. Once the trays are completed they are returned to the dentist and put back on the plaster models. It is useful to demonstrate how to wear the trays on the model. The dentist will check the tray for correct fit and make any necessary adjustments.

REFERENCES

Greenwall LH. (1999) How to make home bleaching trays. *Indep Dent* **4**(7):71–5.

Haywood VB. (1991) Overview and status of mouthguard bleaching. *J Esthet Dent* **3**(2):157–61.

Haywood VB. (1997) Nightguard Vital Bleaching: current concepts and research. *J Am Dent Assoc Suppl* **128:**19S–25S.

Haywood VB, Leonard RH, Nelson CF. (1993) Efficacy of foam liner in 10% carbamide peroxide bleaching technique. *Quintessence Int* **24:**663–6.

Haywood VB, Powe A. (1998) Using double poured alginate impressions to fabricate bleaching trays. *Oper Dent* **23:**128–31.

Heymann HO, Haywood VB. (1995) In: Goldstein RE, Garber DA, editors. *Complete dental bleaching.* Quintessence Publishing: Chicago, 71–100.

Matis BA, Gaiao U, Blackman D, Schultz FA. (1999) In-vivo degradation of bleaching gel used in whitening teeth. *J Am Dent Assoc* **130**(2):227–35.

Miller MB, editor. (1999) *Reality: The information source for esthetic dentistry,* Vol 13. Reality Publishing: Houston, Texas.

Miller MB, editor. (2000) *Reality: The information source for esthetic dentistry,* Vol 14. Reality Publishing: Houston, Texas.

Newman SM, Bottone PM. (1995) Tray forming technique for dentist supervised home bleaching. *Quintessence Int* **26**(7):447–53.

Oliver TL, Haywood VB. (1999) Efficacy of Nightguard Vital Bleaching technique. Beyond the borders: a shortened tray. *J Esthet Dent* **11**(2):95–101.

Touati B, Miara P, Nathanson D. (1999) *Esthetic dentistry and ceramic restorations.* Martin Dunitz: London.

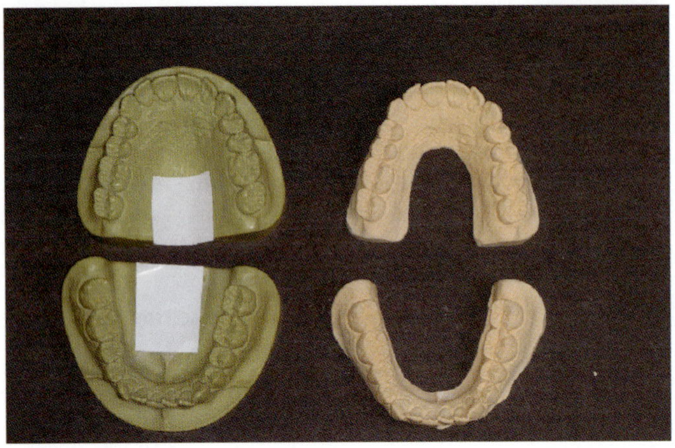

Figure 6.1

The plaster models are prepared for whitening tray models. A horseshoe shape is cut on the model trimmer so that it is easy to prepare the whitening tray models and remove the trays from the model afterward. Check that the model is free from surface blebs or air bubbles that can interfere with the exact fit of the tray at the cervical edges and thus interfere with the correct seating of the tray.

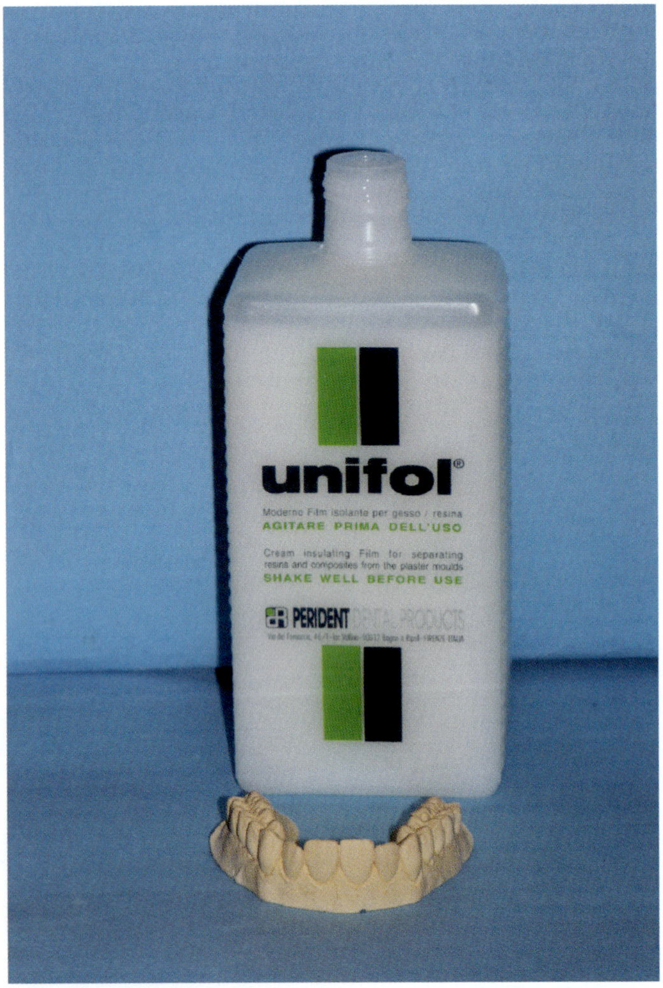

Figure 6.2

A separator can be placed directly onto the plaster teeth to help with ease of removal of the tray after use of the vacuum machine. The tray is always extended onto all the teeth.

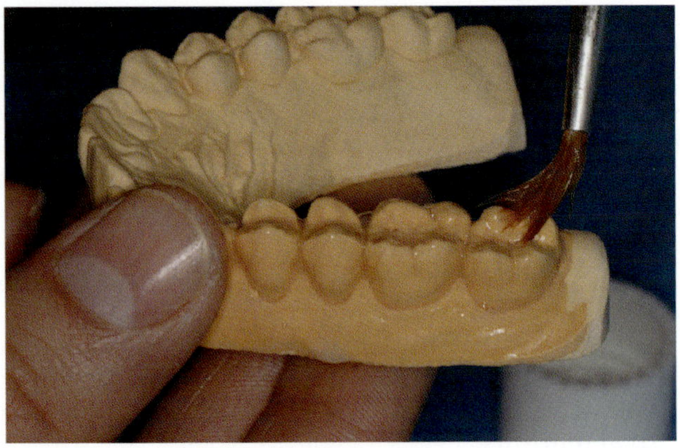

Figure 6.3

The separator is placed directly onto plaster teeth.

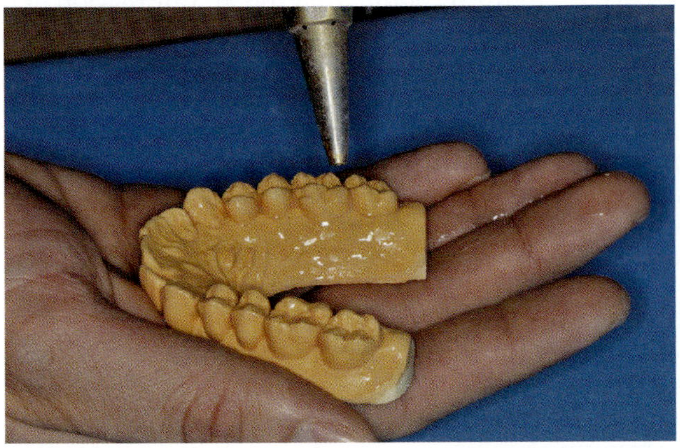

Figure 6.4

The separator is air dried onto the plaster teeth.

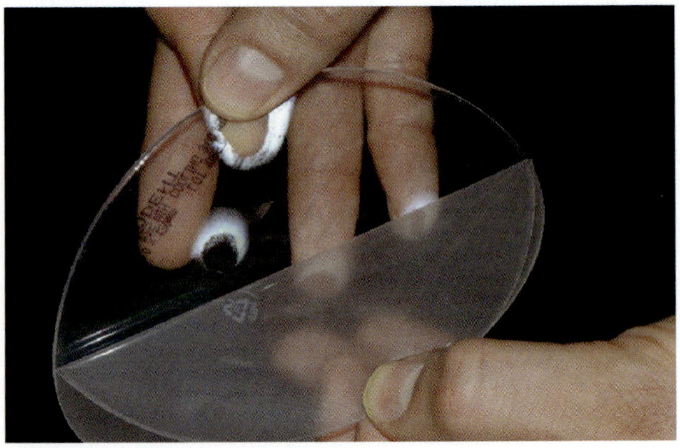

Figure 6.5

The plastic tray material. Some machines have circular devices for the tray material, which can be cut into circles; some machines cut squares. The tray material is separated from its protective backing. The sheets come in varying sizes, shapes, and thicknesses. The 0.035-inch thickness is the standard size; these sheets come in 25-sheet boxes. Because the machine takes only round sheets, these are cut into the correct shape using a template and scalpel. It is essential to remove the backing from the round plastic sheet; otherwise it will not melt properly. Ensure that the plastic sheet is placed into the holder correctly. The machine has three holding lugs to keep the plastic in place. Place the model on the base section of the vacuum tray-forming machine. Ensure that the plastic sheet is properly placed over the model.

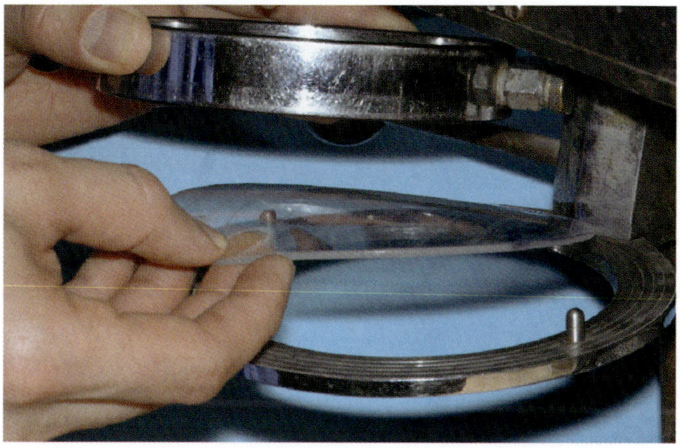

Figure 6.6

The round tray material is placed into the vacuum tray-forming machine.

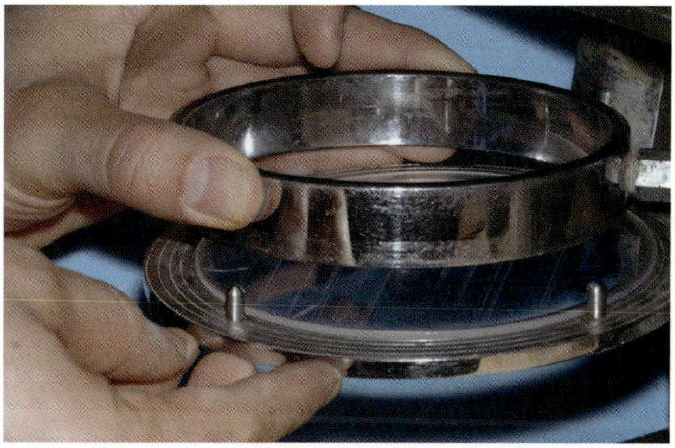

Figure 6.7

The tray material is secured tightly onto the vacuum tray-forming machine. The machine is closed.

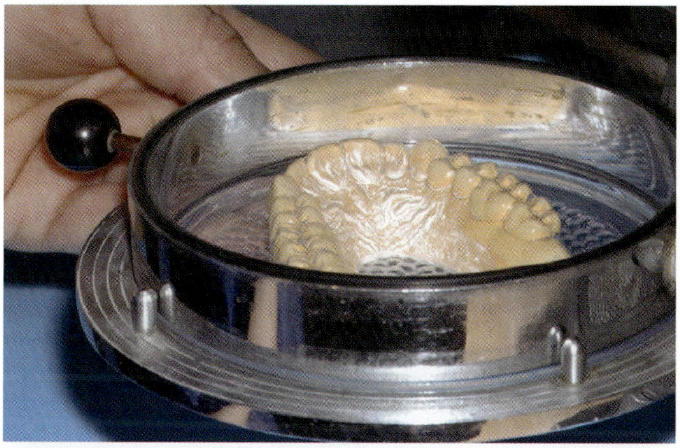

Figure 6.8

The model is placed into the vacuum tray-forming machine.

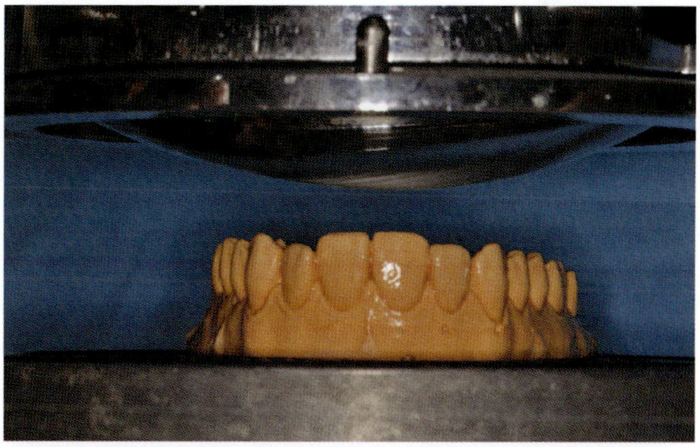

Figure 6.9

The plaster model is positioned in the center of the vacuum machine. The plastic tray material is heated so that it forms a deep crescent shape. It is essential to wait sufficient time for this to happen before pulling the machine down over the teeth.

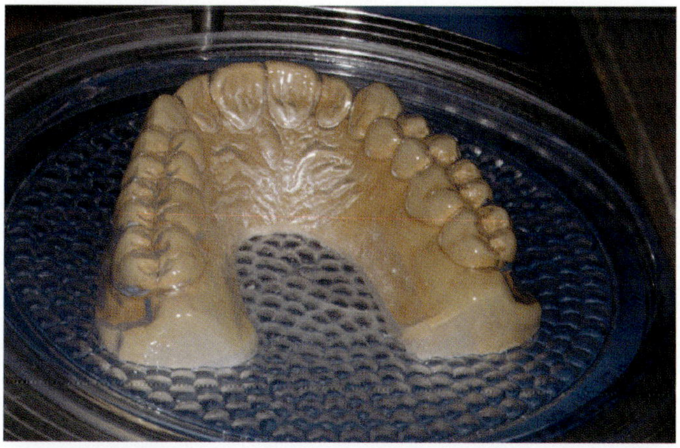

Figure 6.10

The vacuum machine is opened. Sufficient time should be allowed for the heated material to cool down. If the material is removed too quickly, the tray will distort.

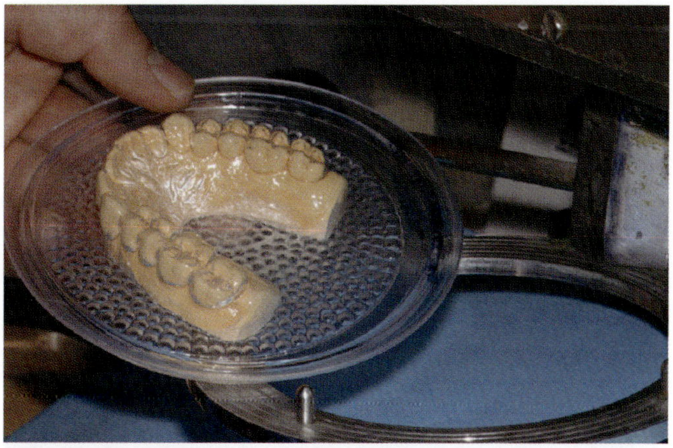

Figure 6.11

The vacuum-formed plastic with the model is removed from the machine. It is important not to remove the tray from the model at this stage. If the tray is removed too early, the tray can distort. Raise the model to the heating element at the correct height. When the plastic has sufficiently melted it will hang over and just touch the model. At this stage it is ready for starting the press-down procedure.

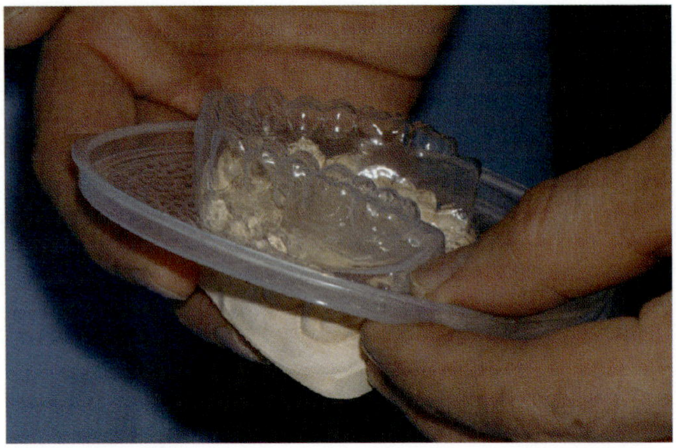

Figure 6.12

Sufficient time should be allowed for the heated tray material to cool down before removal of the tray from the plaster model. The plaster model should be at room temperature before removal. The plastic sheet is now more easily removed from the press. The application of the cold mold seal underneath the plastic leaves a white residue.

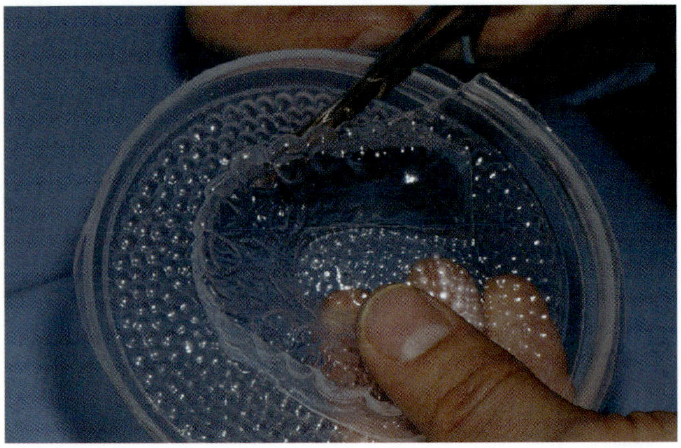

FIGURE 6.13

Cut the plastic with a large pair of scissors to remove the excess material.

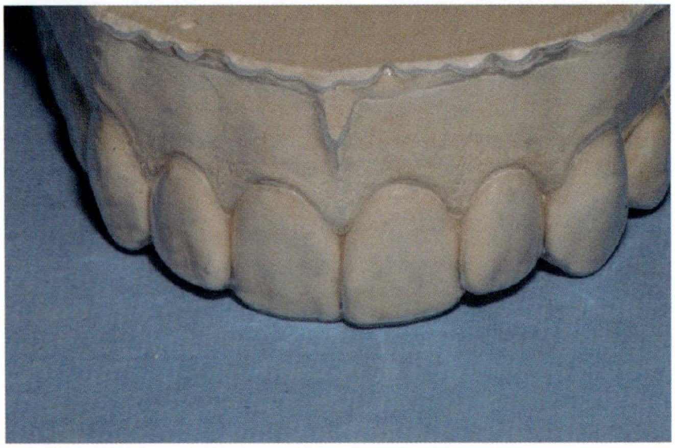

FIGURE 6.14

The excess is removed and the plaster model remains firmly in place over the plastic.

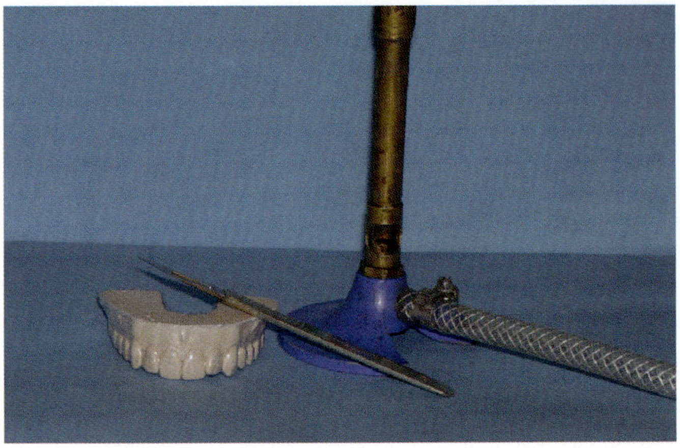

Figure 6.15

The fine trimming and the scalloping can be undertaken using a heated scalpel or a specially designed pair of scissors. The scalpel with a No. 11 blade gives accurate and neat trimming.

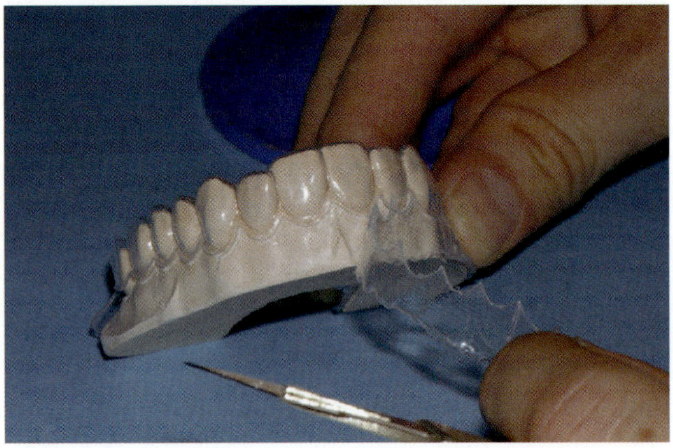

Figure 6.16

The excess is peeled back.

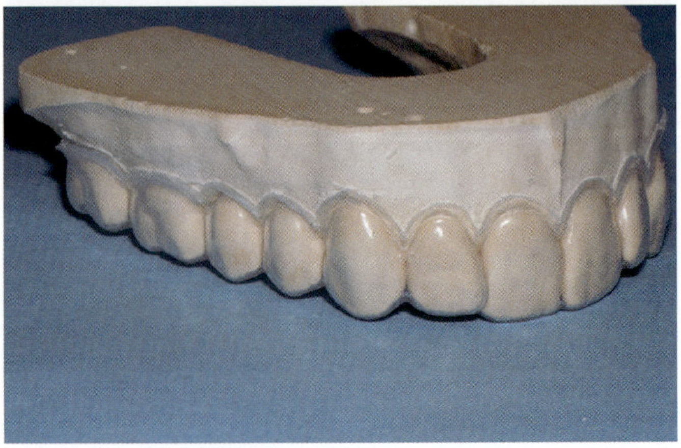

Figure 6.17

Final trimming of the tray on the model.

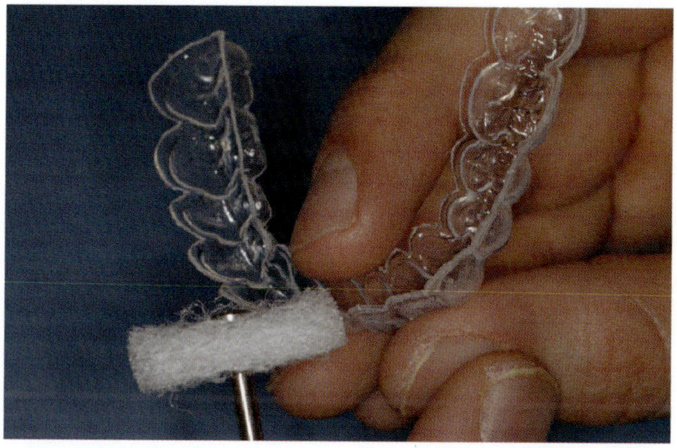

Figure 6.18

The tray is smoothed with a polishing wheel from the buccal aspect.

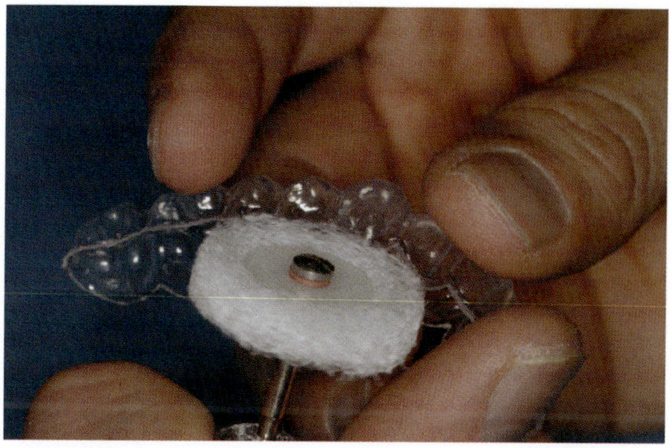

Figure 6.19

The tray is trimmed from the lingual and palatal aspect.

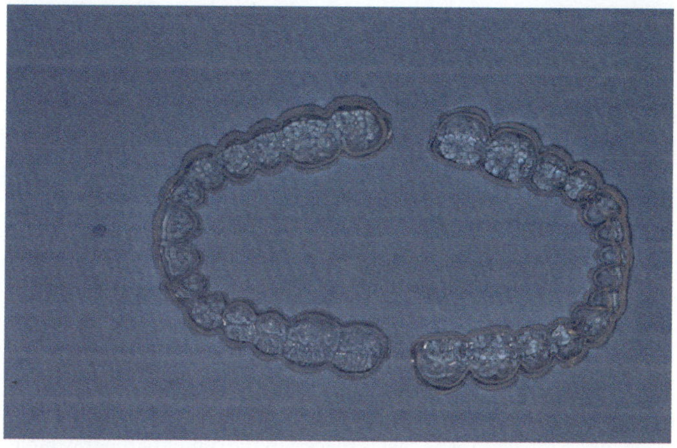

Figure 6.20

The scalloped design of upper and lower trays completed. The trays are scalloped lingually and buccally.

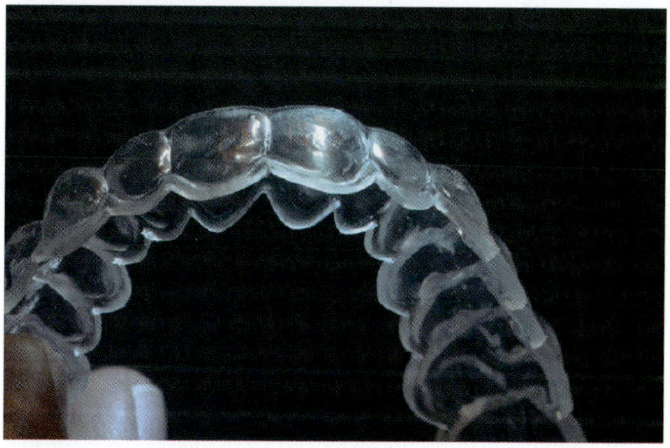

Figure 6.21

Completed tray from the buccal aspect.

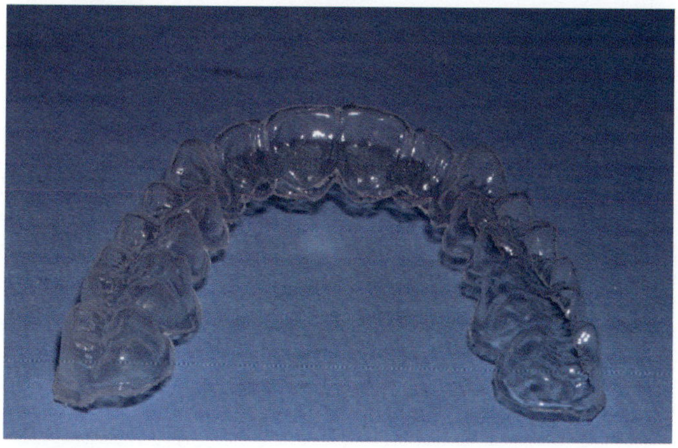

Figure 6.22

Completed upper scalloped tray.

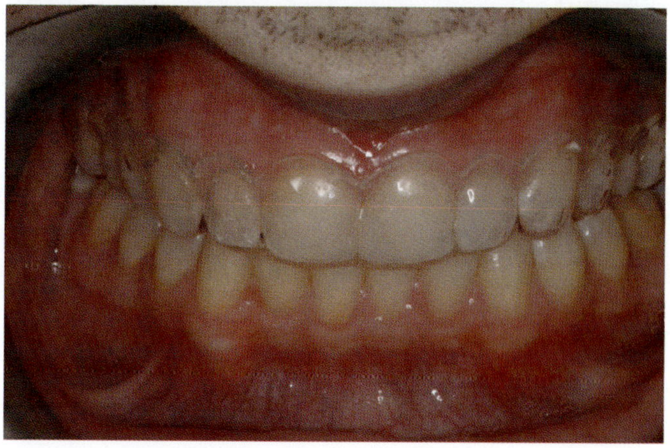

Figure 6.23

Completed tray positioned in the mouth.

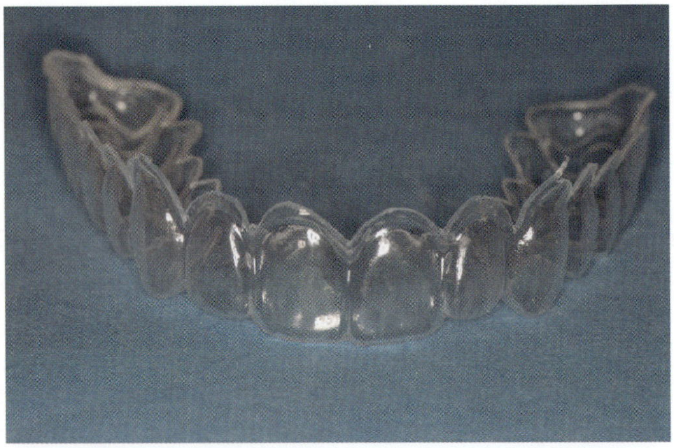

Figure 6.24

Completed tray before final polishing from the labial aspect.

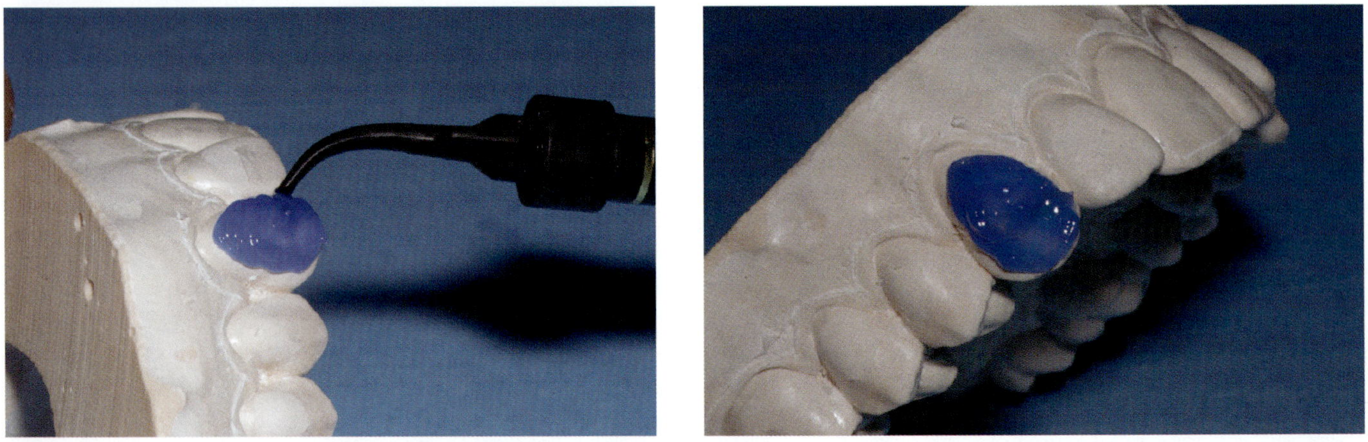

(A) (B)

Figure 6.25

(A) It is rare to use reservoirs, but if the canine teeth are much darker the reservoirs can be placed on these upper canine teeth. The light box is set for 4 minutes to fully cure all the resin if the decision is made to use a reservoir on the teeth. The cast is placed in the center of the tray table. The tray table rotates around the light source for 4 minutes to ensure an even cure. Once the blue resin has set, it is firm and has a slightly oily feel to it. It is advisable to place a thin layer of cold mold seal separating medium over the teeth and the model. This will facilitate easy removal of the tray material from the model after it has been vacuum formed. The cold mold seal is applied to the buccal and lingual surfaces of the model. The excess is blown from the cold mold seal using the compressed air hose. (B) Final reservoir on single canine.

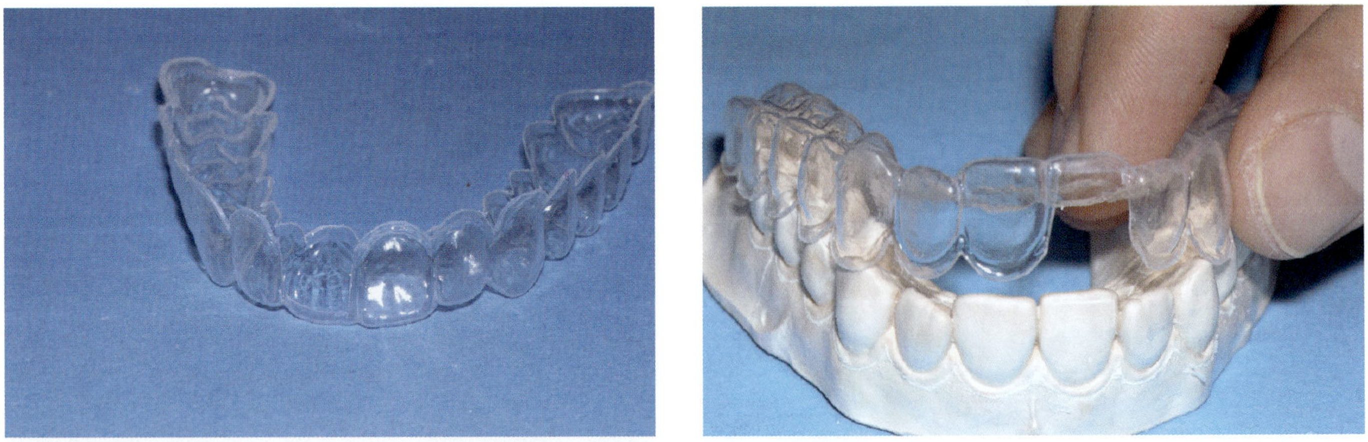

(A) (B)

Figure 6.26

(A) A tray with a window cut on each side. The tooth to be lightened is the upper left central incisor. The teeth adjacent to this tooth are cut back from the labial aspect. This is to prevent the adjacent teeth from becoming lighter while the darker tooth takes longer to whiten because of the complex anatomy of the root canal structure or the tertiary dentin that has been laid down in response to trauma. (B) Another window tray is seated back on the model to prevent distortion of the tray.

7 IN-OFFICE POWER BLEACHING

Joe C. Ontiveros and Rade D. Paravina

Power bleaching or *professional in-office bleaching* is a term used to describe the treatment of discolored dentition with high-concentration oxidizing agents by the dentist chairside. Different techniques, devices, and material choices have been used in dentistry for treating discoloration with varying success. Some situations are better suited for extended treatment outside the dental office with lower concentrations of peroxide delivered in custom trays, whereas the appearance of a severely discolored nonvital tooth may best be treated using a classic "walking bleach" technique. The primary focus of this chapter will be on the power bleaching technique used to achieve more immediate results on *multiple* vital teeth, with special consideration given to treatment of the *single* vital tooth and when combined techniques may be employed.

HISTORICAL BACKGROUND

In 1864, Dr. James Truman of the Pennsylvania College of Dental Surgery published *Discolored and Necrosed Teeth,* in which he described the technique for bleaching nonvital teeth. He is credited with the first successful method for bleaching teeth. His method included treating the patient every day for 1 to 4 weeks with chloride of lime combined with a weak acetic acid (Truman 1864). Techniques were refined throughout the decades using direct or indirect heat in attempts to accelerate the oxidation process (Harlan 1884, Nutting and Poe 1963, Cohen 1968, Chandra and Chawla 1974, Hanosh and Hanosh 1992). Direct heat techniques eventually became less prevalent because of the risk associated with cervical resorption. Chemical techniques using sodium perborate and/or superoxyl in the absence of heat continued with some success on nonvital teeth, but efficient techniques for multiple vital teeth were still lacking. Improvement in bleaching products in the mid-1990s including photosensitive formulas, and delivery systems such as light-cured barrier materials, increased use of in-office bleaching for multiple vital teeth (Barghi 1998). Combined with the introduction of at-home bleaching trays using carbamide peroxide, bleaching emerged as one of the most sought-after procedures in dentistry (Haywood and Heymann 1989).

TREATMENT PLANNING

Clinical and radiographic examination

As with all dental bleaching, a comprehensive oral examination should be performed before power bleaching. A thorough clinical and radiographic examination of the hard and soft tissues should rule out the presence of any oral pathology or dental disease and determine the cause of the stain. The clinician should make special note of any existing dental restorations, formulating a plan with the patient to replace any restorations because of postbleaching color mismatch (see Figure 7.1), and note with the patient any clinical white spot lesions that may appear accentuated immediately after bleaching (see Figure 7.2). A history of tooth sensitivity should be discussed by asking the patient if the teeth are generally sensitive to thermal changes such as when drinking hot or cold beverages.

Case selection for in-office technique

During the treatment planning process, observing the character and depth of discoloration can help discriminate whether the patient is a suitable candidate for in-office power bleaching.

Class I: Good candidate for in-office bleaching

Mild to moderate extrinsic stain (standard patient)

These are the standard patients with all forms of mild to moderate extrinsic staining. Superficial yellow to light-brown discolorations are typically from external sources such as dietary chromogens (tea, wine, coffee), poor dental hygiene, tobacco use, or staining mouth rinse (chlorhexidine); combined with aging, all of these can contribute to extrinsic staining (see Figures 7.3A and 7.3B).

Class II: Moderate candidate for in-office bleaching

Severe extrinsic to mild intrinsic stain

When the cause of the discoloration is intrinsic in nature, including hemorrhagic sources resulting from trauma, the outcome becomes less predictable. Vital teeth with mild intrinsic discoloration may respond well to in-office power bleaching after one appointment if the pulp chambers are not calcified (see Figures 7.4A–D). If the tooth is nonvital and pulpless, then it can be bleached both internally and externally simultaneously, improving the chances for a good outcome as compared with a vital tooth with no access to the pulp chamber (see Figure 7.5A–F). Although the procedure can be successful after one treatment, the patient's expectations should be prepared for the possibility of multiple treatments for severe extrinsic to mild intrinsic stains, especially if a calcified pulp chamber is observed on the radiograph.

Class III: Poor candidate for in-office bleaching

Moderate to severe intrinsic stain

Teeth that may not be suitable for in-office power bleaching include those with moderate to severe intrinsic discoloration. The single nonvital tooth with severe intrinsic stain typically will require multiple treatments such as with the "walking bleach" technique. Improved bleaching can still be expected for the severely discolored tooth; however, patients must be motivated to continue with weekly appointments for multiple sessions. In some cases the patient may tire of repeated office visits and elect to discontinue treatment before reaching maximum expected outcome (see Figures 7.6A–E).

Dense vital tooth

A single vital tooth that has a calcified or reduced pulp chamber may not respond well to in-office bleaching. When a calcified pulp chamber is noted on the radiograph, the presumption is an increased tooth density in which the peroxide will not readily diffuse. In this case, long-term at-home bleaching may improve the color, but the patient ultimately should be prepared for restorative coverage with a laminate veneer if bleaching is unsuccessful (see Figures 7.7A–D).

Setting expectations

As part of the initial patient interview, the advantages and disadvantages of in-office professional bleaching should be discussed relative to at-home bleaching and expected outcomes. The relatively higher cost and increased risk of sensitivity will be important disadvantages to note. By far the most appealing advantage for most is the prospect of "instant" results. The total time savings is material and tooth dependent. Clinical studies have shown that 7 days of at-home bleaching with 10% carbamide peroxide equals 45 minutes with 38% hydrogen peroxide (Auschill et al. 2005), or a 1-hour treatment with 28% hydrogen peroxide using supplemental light (da Costa et al. 2010). Patients should understand that results may vary.

Some patients have unrealistic expectations based on a distorted perception of their existing tooth color. The patient with extremely white teeth from habitual bleaching may in fact believe that his or her teeth appear yellow. These patients may have an obsession with or addiction to bleaching, colloquially known as "bleachorexia," and should be advised against continual bleaching. Time should be taken to educate the patient regarding the extreme light color relative to the color of the lightest natural tooth shades. This can be accomplished by demonstrating to the patient his or her extreme white teeth next to, for example, the B1 tab from the VitaPan classical shade guide (Vita Zahnfabrik, Bad Säckingen, Germany) (see Figure 7.8).

MATERIAL SELECTION

One- and two-component systems

Some bleach formulas will combine all the component materials into one syringe, or products may package activators and additives as separate components that require mixing.

One-component systems are typically bleach formulas that do not require mixing for activation. They consist primarily of highly concentrated hydrogen peroxide as the active ingredient in a gel form matrix such as glycerin or propylene glycol, along with stabilizers or photosensitizers (see Figure 7.9).

Two-component systems may require mixing of the active ingredient with a catalyst. Some systems require hand mixing of the components (see Figure 7.10), others may use syringe-to-syringe mixing (see Figures 7.11A and 7.11B), and still others may combine the components through an automix tip of a dual-barrel syringe (see Figure 7.12).

Active agents

Carbamide peroxide has been shown to be effective for at-home bleaching (Hasson et al. 2006) when used in concentrations ranging from 10% to 22%. Higher concentrations ranging from 35% to 44% have been applied by dentists using an assisted bleaching technique. The carbamide peroxide, in this case, may be warmed and applied with a custom tray or directly to the teeth, avoiding the gingiva, and monitored in the office (Miller 1999). In-office bleaching with carbamide peroxide has generally been replaced with techniques using higher concentrations of hydrogen peroxide. Carbamide peroxide is considered less effective for in-office bleaching because of its slower rate of decomposition to form active oxygen and peroxide radicals.

Chlorine dioxide has also been used chairside by nondental providers, especially in the United Kingdom. However, because of its acidic pH, reported damage to enamel, and lack of investigation for dental use in the scientific literature to date, the dental professional has not adopted the use of chlorine dioxide for in-office power bleaching (Greenwall 2008).

Hydrogen peroxide (H_2O_2) in high concentrations ranging from 15% to 40% has been used most effectively by the dental professional as the active ingredient for in-office power bleaching. As concentration increases, fewer applications of hydrogen peroxide are usually required (Sulieman et al. 2004).

Activators and pH

pH of bleach formula

The common recommendation for professional bleaching formulas is to have a neutral pH to avoid damage to enamel (American Dental Association Council of Scientific Affairs 2009). The optimum pH for hydrogen peroxide decomposition is considered to be around 9.5 to 10.8 (Goldstein and Garber 1995). Some bleach formulas may still contain acidic components to keep the active ingredient stable. A recent study showed the bleaching effect of *acidic* 30% hydrogen peroxide versus *neutral* 30% hydrogen peroxide to be equivalent (Sun et al. 2011).

The pH becomes an important issue if it falls below the critical point of 5.2, at which enamel demineralization is expected to occur (Driessens et al. 1986, Shannon et al. 1993, Joiner 2007). However, an abundance of mineral ions found in human saliva and the formation of a natural salivary pellicle in vivo should have a protective effect against enamel demineralization (Hannig and Balz 1999, Hannig et al. 2004).

Activators and additives

In addition to hydrogen peroxide, power bleach formulas may contain proprietary activators, which may include a combination of alkaline pH adjusters, metal ions, or photosensitive catalysts to absorb and transfer energy to the peroxide and accelerate decomposition. Other added ingredients may include stabilizers for extended shelf life or materials to improve viscosity.

BLEACHING LIGHT DEVICES

The use of light to supplement the bleaching process in dentistry was reported as early as 1918 (Abbot 1918). Not until recently has the use of bleaching lights begun to become widespread. Although there are several light sources with different spectral distributions and efficiencies currently on the market, they all purport to accelerate or enhance the bleaching process. Initially, bleaching lights relied more on heat or thermal decomposition of the bleaching agent, whereas contemporary bleaching lamps aim to achieve photolysis of the bleaching agent at specific wavelengths.

Heat lamps (19th century–1980). Early bleaching lamps made use of an incandescent or photographic floodlight (see Figure 7.13). This type of light source produced a continuous spectrum with high infrared emission, which supplied a source of indirect heat. For vital teeth, temperatures were recommended in a range of 46°C to 60°C (115°F to 140°F). For nonvital teeth temperatures as high as 71°C (160°F) were recommended (Goldstein and Garber 1995). The risk of increasing the pulpal temperature beyond the critical threshold of 5.5°C, at which irreversible pulpal damage can occur, is a concern with any system that raises the temperature of vital teeth (Zach and Cohen 1965, Baik et al. 2001). The use of heating lamps has fallen out of favor for vital teeth and may be considered obsolete by today's standards.

Halogen lamps (1980s–2000). These lights are a refinement of the incandescent light source with halogen gas added. The halogen gas causes evaporated tungsten to redeposit on the filament, improving the filament life and allowing a higher color temperature than the standard incandescent lamp. The higher color temperature supplies a cooler (more blue-green) continuous spectrum of light from near ultraviolet to deep infrared filtered to the usable region for the bleaching agent (see Figure 7.14).

High-intensity discharge (HID) lamps (1990s–current). These are high-powered lamps that produce light by ionizing noble gases (xenon, krypton) or metal halides between two electrodes. Depending on the conducting elements added to the arc stream, HID lamps may properly be referred to as *metal halide lights* and are often referred to as "plasma arc lights" in dentistry. These lamps are typically wide-spectrum lamps using bandpass filters to narrow the emission primarily to the short ultraviolet to blue light (380–500 nm) (see Figure 7.15).

Light-emitting diode (LED) lamps (2000–current). These are solid-state, semiconducting energy sources that supply near-monochromatic light. LED lamps are currently one of the most energy-efficient and rapidly developing light technologies. Because LEDs produce a discrete or narrow spectrum of light, the light source requires no additional filtration of extraneous energy and produces very little heat. As a result, an LED bleaching light system is dependent less on heat and more on the wavelength-specific photochemistry of the bleaching formula and possible energy absorption of the natural tooth chromogens contributing to bleaching effect (Figure 7.16).

Lasers. The popular consumer term for in-office bleaching with any type of light is often referred to as *laser bleaching*. However, a laser by definition is a device that produces a nearly parallel, monochromatic, and coherent beam of light by exciting atoms and causing them to radiate their energy in phase (coherent). Lasers have been slow to gain wide acceptance for dental bleaching because of a lack of scientific clinical trials and the high cost compared with alternative light devices. Deleterious effects associated with increased pulpal temperature of teeth are also a concern with the use of lasers (Luk et al. 2004, Baik et al. 2001).

The role of bleaching lights in dentistry is a topic for which there has been controversy and a lack of agreement. This lack of agreement can be attributed to variability associated with methods used to measure color, different light sources, and bleaching formula interactions (Ontiveros 2011). Some clinical studies have reported significant effects with bleaching lights (Tavares et al. 2003, Ziemba et al. 2005), whereas others have shown no effectiveness (Papathanasiou et al. 2002, Hein et al. 2003). Still others have found mixed results depending on tooth inclusion (Calatayud et al. 2010) or method of color measurement (Gurgan et al. 2009, Kugel et al. 2009, Ontiveros and Paravina 2009). The trend for future lamps may rely more on specialized light sources such as LEDs or lasers rather than filtered light to illuminate the teeth. As refinements in material photochemistry and improvements in spectral properties of bleaching lamps continue, the use of supplemental light devices in dentistry is expected to remain popular and continue to grow in the foreseeable future.

MONITORING OF BLEACHING

Bleaching can be monitored using visual and/or instrumental methods. Both methods can provide credible results if used appropriately.

VISUAL MONITORING

Visual monitoring is by far the predominant method for evaluation of bleaching efficacy. The most important aspects of this method are observer and patient recruitment, shade-matching conditions, method, and tools.

Observers

It is not justified to recruit experienced practitioners or female observers for visual monitoring of tooth bleaching because there is insufficient evidence that experience and gender influence shade-matching performance for observers with normal color vision. However, significant evidence shows that differences exist among individuals of the same gender or people with similar experience. These differences can be quantified through various professional (nondental) tests such as Ishihara charts or the Farnsworth–Munsell 100-hue test. In the latter test, color discrimination ability of color-normal individuals ranges from low (16%), through average (68%), to superior (16%). There is also evidence that education and training can improve one's color-matching skills.

A simple nonprofessional test for color discrimination competency in dentistry has been suggested as mandatory according to the International Standards Organization (ISO) (International Organization for Standardization 2011). Test subjects should match pairs of tabs from two identical shade guides under controlled conditions, ideally in a viewing booth. One set of tabs should have original markings on tab holders, and the markings on the other set of tabs should be masked with custom letters, numbers or symbols. Tabs should be removed from joint tab holders, and scattered on the floor of the viewing booth. After a period of adaptation by observing the gray surface (walls of the viewing booth), the observers should begin matching pairs of tabs. One point should be assigned for each correctly matched pair. An observer who correctly matches at least 60%, 75%, or 85% of pairs corresponds to poor, average, and superior color discrimination competency, respectively. At least three observers with superior or average color discrimination competency should participate in monitoring of bleaching.

Conditions and method

Similarly to the conditions described for testing color discrimination competency, color-corrected light (such as D65) with a color rendering index (CRI) of 90 or greater should be used for visual shade matching in the dental office or laboratory. Light should be neither too intense nor too dimmed; 1000 lux is considered optimal for visual color matching.

Shade matching should be performed at the beginning of the appointment, at a distance of 25–35 cm (10–14 inches). Tabs should be either illuminated at 45° (or 2 × 45°) and observed perpendicularly (at 0°), or vice versa. A single shade-matching trial should last no more than 5–7 seconds, and a light-gray card should be observed during the breaks between two color-matching trials.

Tools and patient recruitment

The so-called value scale of the Vita classical A1–D4 (VC) shade guide is the accepted standard for bleaching monitoring. The value scale is supposed to represent a light-to-dark arrangement from B1 (shade 1) to C4 (shade 16). A visual method based on this scale depends on calculating the difference in shade guide units (SGUs) before and after bleaching. However, the VC value scale has numerous shortcomings, including the following:

- A narrow color range.
- A lack of very light shades. This results in the exclusion of a large percentage of the population from bleaching research (adding group 0 from 3D-Master is not appropriate or logical).
- An inconsistent color distribution. This is most emphasized in the range of primary interest (3–6 SGUs).
- A poor correlation with the increase in chroma from B1 to C4.

The aforementioned inconsistencies in value scale can be misleading and compromise findings to a certain extent. The lack of very light tabs (lighter than B1) excludes more than 52% of the population—for example, in studies that recruit patients with an initial shade of A3 or darker (probably the most frequent design in bleaching studies) (Paravina and Majkic 2007). The addition of group 0 (0M1, 0M2, and 0M3) from the 3D-Master shade guide to the VC value scale does not solve this problem, and it is neither logical nor appropriate: the color difference between 0M3 and B1 is too great ($\Delta E^* = 8.0$). The same is true for the difference in lightness ($\Delta L^* = 7.1$). The difference is less pronounced for the blue-yellow coordinate ($\Delta b^* = 3.7$) and the least pronounced for the green-red coordinate ($\Delta a^* = 1.0$). However, the problem with the Δa^* is that this difference is in the opposite direction: 0M3 has higher a^* than B1 (redder).

The inconsistent color distribution (lack of uniformity of color differences among the adjacent tabs) is another major concern with the classical shade guide. The average color differences (ΔE^*) among adjacent VC tabs and 2, 3, 4, 5, and 6 tabs apart are 5.4, 4.8, 6.6, 6.4, 7.8, and 7.1, respectively ($R^2 = 0.72$). Therefore, the ΔE^* between mean differences 1 and 6 tabs apart is only 1.7, whereas the difference between mean differences 3 and 6 tabs apart (majority of bleaching-dependent color differences are within this range) is only 0.5.

The Vita Bleachedguide (BG) 3D-Master is the first shade guide developed specifically for visual evaluation of tooth bleaching. The current BG has additional numeric markings as shown in Figure 7.17 (see also Figure 4.13). The existing tabs are marked with odd numbers 1 to 29, representing 29 original 3D-Master tabs, from 0M1 to 5M3. Interpolated SGUs are marked with even numbers to comply with the current ADA recommendation that 1 ccu = 1 SGU = 1 ΔE* (American Dental Association Council of Scientific Affairs 2006) and to increase precision (when a tooth shade is between two shade tabs) and sensitivity of the BG. This is justified by the finding that 1 SGU_{BG} = 2 SGU_{VC} (Paravina et al. 2007).

The manufacturer-suggested light-to-dark tab arrangement of the BG is consistent with visual observation. The BG arrangement was found to be identical to tab arrangement independently determined by a panel of observers, which was not the case with VC and some other products. The same is true for changes in chroma from the lightest to the darkest tabs (Paravina 2008).

Inclusion of very light shades into the BG complements contemporary esthetic dentistry and enables the capturing of tooth shades for patients in bleaching studies and practice that are lighter than B1. Indeed, the safe way to obtain comprehensive and credible information on bleaching efficacy of a certain agent would be documentation of tooth shade using visual shade guides designed for monitoring bleaching that overcome the shortcomings of the classic tools and are used under the correct conditions and methods for accurate shade matching.

Instrumental monitoring

The instrumental method is based on the calculation of color difference (ΔE*) before and after bleaching. Frequently used devices for instrumental color assessment in dentistry are spectrophotometers, spectroradiometers, colorimeters, imaging systems for traditional digital imaging, and spectral imaging. It is of essential importance to ensure repeated measurements of the same area through accurate repositioning of the measuring device and/or use of other methods.

IN-OFFICE VITAL TEETH TECHNIQUE

Precautionary statements and management of side effects

No anesthesia and patient monitoring

Anesthesia should *not* be used with this procedure. The doctor is monitoring for sensitivity at all times. The patient can be instructed to raise a hand to signal if any burning, tingling, or discomfort is experienced. The procedure may need to be abandoned if patient sensitivity cannot be overcome.

Sensitivity

Sensitivity should be minimized by proper screening of the patient during the initial interview and dental examination. Some of the risk factors for tooth sensitivity include existing decay, gingival recession, cervical abrasions, or a history of tooth sensitivity. Greater tooth sensitivity has been reported for in-office bleaching with adjunct light compared with no light (Ontiveros and Paravina 2009). Patients reporting a history of tooth sensitivity may prebrush for 2 weeks with a potassium nitrate–containing toothpaste to alleviate or minimize discomfort (Haywood 2005, Haywood et al. 2005). The identified high-risk patient may be provided with 600 mg of ibuprofen 30 minutes before treatment to reduce the incidence of tooth sensitivity (Charakorn et al. 2009). This may allow the patient to complete the procedure with minimal discomfort and to get the greatest benefit out of the appointment. Another strategy may be to provide a 3–6% potassium nitrate gel to the lingual surface of the teeth if the patient experiences sensitivity during the appointment.

Tissue burn or swollen lip

The ideal method to avoid chemical burn is through meticulous application of the gingival barrier. If the bleach penetrates beneath the barrier or accidental soft tissue contact is made, immediately flush the site with copious water spray and apply mineral oil, such as vitamin E. The oil should provide relief from the stinging sensation within a few minutes, and the white oxidation appearance will normally resolve within a few hours (see Figure 7.18). The patient may be provided with additional oil or topical anesthetic for home use. The need for antihistamine administration should be considered for allergic skin reactions.

White spots

Any white spot lesions or striations should be identified before the appointment if possible because they may become accentuated during the bleaching process (see Figure 7.2). As the teeth begin to rehydrate over the next 24 hours these white spots may blend, or subsequent microabrasion techniques may be planned. If the blemishes are suspected to be recent lesions, successful treatment has been demonstrated using fluoride-containing casein phosphopeptides and amorphous calcium phosphate (CPP-ACP) (Robertson et al. 2011). High concentrations of fluoride (≥5000 ppm) should be avoided because rapid remineralization of superficial enamel may impede remineralization of the deeper layer of the lesions, resulting in white enamel opacities that will not allow return to the normal opalescence of sound enamel. This is based on the rapid remineralization of the surface layer with high concentrations of fluoride and lack of remineralization with the deeper demineralized areas of clinically evident white spot lesions (Hicks 2010, personal communication).

Photosensitivity

The dentist should be aware of any patient taking phototoxic drugs or those with certain skin conditions associated with photosensitivity before using a light device for bleaching. There have been reports of patients experiencing negative skin reactions after light exposure, especially ultraviolet light, manifesting as swelling of the lips and surrounding tissues (see Figure 7.19).

Pregnant or lactating women and young children

It is most prudent to postpone treatment for pregnant or lactating women and young children as a precautionary matter. We generally advise postponement of in-office bleaching of vital teeth of young children until beyond the mixed dentition stage.

Step 1: Tray impressions

If models were not poured at a prior appointment, then impressions of the patient's teeth should be taken at the start of the in-office power bleach appointment for the fabrication of custom bleach trays. The trays allow the patient to supplement the in-office procedure with at-home bleaching to minimize any rebound effect or continue to lighten the teeth for more stubborn stains or future maintenance. The trays also can be used post-treatment for delivering desensitizing gel.

Step 2: Prophy

In preparation for bleach application, tooth plaque or superficial stain is removed using prophy paste or pumice of flour paste in a rubber polishing cup (see Figure 7.20).

Step 3: Initial shade

Document the prebleaching shade using visual and/or instrumental methods (see section on monitoring of bleaching). Patients often have a vague recollection of pretreatment color and desire to see the immediate outcome. The initial shade will be an aid in demonstrating to the patient the color change along with the post-treatment shade (step 10).

Step 4: Light-protective glasses and light guides

When using a supplemental light device, it is essential to provide the patient with light-protective eyewear to filter harmful radiation. It has been shown that many lamps exceed standards set for eye exposure to direct blue light (Bruzell et al. 2009). Protective light guides surrounding the exit window of bleaching lamps are also recommended to minimize scattered optical radiation (see Figure 7.21).

Step 5: Lip protection and cheek retraction

A barrier cream or oil is applied to the lips before insertion of the cheek and lip retractors (see Figure 7.22). Vitamin E oil (α-tocopherol), a fat-soluble antioxidant, may neutralize accidental soft tissue contact with the peroxide. If the lips are exposed to potential ultraviolet emission, then a sunblock cream may be used on the lips. Various types of cheek and lip retractors are available and suitable for in-office bleaching. Retractors that shield the lips, especially when a lamp is used, and guard the tongue from contacting the bleaching agent are preferred (see Figures 7.23A and 7.23B). The protective bib or isolation napkin is slipped over the retractors to further shield the perioral skin (see Figure 7.24).

Step 6: Gingival isolation

After retractors are in place, long cotton rolls are placed in the vestibules. A light-cure resin barrier material is carefully applied using a small-tipped syringe at the gingival crest to protect the gingiva from chemical burn. When a bleaching light device is used, additional resin barrier material is extended apically 5–10 mm and sealed against the cotton rolls to protect the gingiva from light radiation. The barrier is completely cured by waving the light tip back and forth for 1–2 minutes (approximately 10 seconds per tooth). Unfolded gauze squares can be placed to cover the remaining soft tissue exposed in vestibules. The material is initially cured for 2–3 seconds, two teeth at a time. Care should be taken to seal the gingival crest from one papilla tip to the next without overlapping too much onto the tooth yet ensuring that no gingival tissue is exposed. The curing light tip should remain moving because some materials are exothermic and high-powered lights can cause soft tissue discomfort for the patient (see Figures 7.25A–G).

Step 7: Activation of bleach, if required

A syringe-to-syringe mixing product will require the user to attach the syringe with the bleaching agent to a second syringe with the activator. The contents of one syringe are then pushed into the other, going back and forth about a dozen times until completely mixed and finally pushing all contents back into one syringe before applying the applicator tip (see Figures 7.11A and 7.11B). Bleach materials that have been refrigerated should be brought to room temperature or slightly warmer by placing them in a water bath, or should be warmed in running water (see Figure 7.26).

Step 8: Application and reapplication of bleach

The bleach material is applied to the teeth in a layer 1–2 mm thick, generally for 15–20 minutes per application with three or four applications per session (see Figures 7.27A and 7.27B). To avoid bleach splatter and dislodgement of the barrier material, surgical suction is used to remove the bleach between repeat applications of fresh material. If patient experiences any burning, immediately suction off the bleach and thoroughly rinse. To avoid dislodgement of the barrier material, surgical suction is preferred over high-volume suction (see Figure 7.28). If the gauze gets wet, it can be replaced with dry gauze between applications. The cotton rolls attached to the gingival barrier should remain in place between applications so as not to disturb the barrier.

Step 9: Removal of barrier

At the end of the bleaching session the resin barrier is ready for removal and typically can be lifted in one piece by grabbing hold of the attached cotton rolls or dislodged using an explorer instrument (see Figures 7.29A and 7.29B).

Step 10: Postbleaching shade

The post-treatment shade is taken to document the color change for the patient record and to demonstrate to the patient the immediate outcome (see Figure 7.30 and section on monitoring of bleaching).

Step 11: Postbleaching instructions

Postbleaching instructions may include a recommendation to wait a minimum of 6 hours after in-office bleaching before drinking any chromogenic drinks such as coffee or grape juice (Ontiveros et al. 2008). Patients requiring pretreatment ibuprofen for sensitivity may benefit from an additional dose immediately after the appointment (Charakorn et al. 2009). To maintain the bleaching results, the patient can be provided a custom at-home bleach tray for periodic maintenance or for continued bleaching using the combination technique.

IN-OFFICE/AT-HOME COMBINATION EXAMPLES

An in-office/at-home combination bleaching technique can be offered as an alternative. The combination technique has been shown to be more effective than in-office bleaching alone (Matis et al. 2009). This technique allows patients to use a custom tray at home after the in-office procedure to accentuate the bleaching effects, or for longer term treatment as in cases of moderate intrinsic staining (see Figures 7.31A and 7.31B). The custom bleach trays are delivered at the completion of the in-office procedure, instructing the patient to start bleaching after 24 hours if further bleaching is desired. If immediate results are satisfactory, the patient may reserve the trays for touch-up bleaching at-home. Patients who reject or cannot wear a bleaching tray at home for one reason or another should be prepared for the possibility of multiple in-office treatments to achieve an optimal result.

REFERENCES

Abbot CH. (1918) Bleaching discolored teeth by means of 30% perhydrol and the electric light rays. *J Allied Dent Soc* **13**:259.

American Dental Association (ADA) Council of Scientific Affairs. (2006) *Acceptance program guidelines: professional in-office tooth bleaching products.* Chicago: ADA.

American Dental Association (ADA) Council of Scientific Affairs. (2009) *Tooth whitening/bleaching: treatment considerations for dentists and their patients.* ADA: Chicago, IL.

Auschill TM, Hellwig E, Schmidale S, Sculean A. (2005) Efficacy, side-effects and patients' acceptance of different bleaching techniques (OTC, in-office, at-home). *Oper Dent* **30**(2):156–63.

Baik JW, Rueggeberg FA, Liewehr FR. (2001) Effect of light-enhanced bleaching on in vitro surface and intrapulpal temperature rise. *J Esthet Restor Dent* **13**(6):370–8.

Barghi N. (1998) Making a clinical decision for vital tooth bleaching: at-home or in-office? *Compend Contin Educ Dent* **19**(8):831–8; quiz 40.

Bruzell EM, Johnsen B, Aalerud TN, Dahl JE. (2009) In vitro efficacy and risk for adverse effects of light-assisted tooth bleaching. *Photochem Photobiol Sci* **8**(3):377–85.

Calatayud JO, Calatayud CO, Zaccagnini AO, Box MJ. (2010) Clinical efficacy of a bleaching system based on hydrogen peroxide with or without light activation. *Eur J Esthet Dent* **5**(2):216–24.

Chandra S, Chawla TN. (1974) Clinical evaluation of heat method for bleaching of discoloured mottled teeth. *J Indian Dent Assoc* **46**(8):313–8.

Charakorn P, Cabanilla LL, Wagner WC, Foong WC. (2009) The effect of preoperative ibuprofen on tooth sensitivity caused by in-office bleaching. *Oper Dent* **34**(2):131–5.

Cohen S. (1968) A simplified method for bleaching discolored teeth. *Dent Dig* **74**(7):301–3.

da Costa JB, McPharlin R, Paravina RD, Ferracane JL. (2010) Comparison of at-home and in-office tooth whitening using a novel shade guide. *Oper Dent* **35**(4):381–8.

Driessens FC, Theuns HM, Borggreven JM, van Dijk JW. (1986) Solubility behaviour of whole human enamel. *Caries Res* **20**(2):103–10.

Goldstein RE, Garber DA. (1995) *Complete dental bleaching.* Quintessence Publishing: Chicago, 26.

Greenwall L. (2008) The dangers of chlorine dioxide tooth bleaching. *Asth Den Today* **2**(2):20–2.

Gurgan S, Cakir FY, Yazici E. (2009) Different light-activated in-office bleaching systems: a clinical evaluation. *Lasers Med Sci* **25**(6):817–22.

Hannig M, Balz M. (1999) Influence of in vivo formed salivary pellicle on enamel erosion. *Caries Res* **33**(5):372–9.

Hannig M, Fiebiger M, Guntzer M, Dobert A. (2004) Protective effect of the in situ formed short-term salivary pellicle. *Arch Oral Biol* **49**(11):903–10.

Hanosh FN, Hanosh GS. (1992) Vital bleaching: a new light-activated hydrogen peroxide system. *J Esthet Dent* **4**(3):90–5.

Harlan AW. (1884) The removal of stains from the teeth caused by the administration of medicinal agents and bleaching of pulpless teeth. *Am J Dent Sci* **18**:521–24.

Hasson H, Ismail AI, Neiva G. (2006) Home-based chemically-induced whitening of teeth in adults. *Cochrane Database Syst Rev* **4**:CD006202.

Haywood VB. (2005) Treating sensitivity during tooth whitening. *Compend Contin Educ Dent* **26**(9 Suppl 3):11–20.

Haywood VB, Cordero R, Wright K, Gendreau L. (2005) Brushing with a potassium nitrate dentifrice to reduce bleaching sensitivity. *J Clin Dent* **16**(1):17–22.

Haywood VB, Heymann HO. (1989) Nightguard Vital Bleaching. *Quintessence Int* **20**(3):173–6.

Hein DK, Ploeger BJ, Hartup JK, Wagstaff RS. (2003) In-office vital tooth bleaching—what do lights add? *Compend Contin Educ Dent* **24**(4A):340–52.

International Organization for Standardization. (2011) *ISO/TR 28642 dentistry—guidance on color measurement.* International Organization for Standardization: Geneva.

Joiner A. (2007) Review of the effects of peroxide on enamel and dentine properties. *J Dent* **35**(12):889–96.

Kugel G, Ferreira S, Sharma S, Barker ML. (2009) Clinical trial assessing light enhancement of in-office tooth whitening. *J Esthet Restor Dent* **21**(5):336–47.

Luk K, Tam L, Hubert M. (2004) Effect of light energy on peroxide tooth bleaching. *J Am Dent Assoc* **135**(2):194–201, 228–9.

Matis BA, Cochran MA, Wang G, Eckert GJ. (2009) A clinical evaluation of two in-office bleaching regimens with and without tray bleaching. *Oper Dent* **34**(2):142–9.

Miller MB, editor. (1999) Bleaching materials. In *Reality: the information source for esthetic dentistry*. Reality Publishing: Houston, Texas.

Nutting EB, Poe GS. (1963) A new combination for bleaching teeth. *J South Calif Dent Assoc* **31**(9):289–91.

Ontiveros JC, Eldiwany MS, Benson B. (2008) Time dependent influence of stain exposure following power bleaching. *J Dent Res* **87**(Spec Iss B): 1083.

Ontiveros JC, Paravina RD. (2009) Color change of vital teeth exposed to bleaching performed with and without supplementary light. *J Dent* **37**(11): 840–7.

Ontiveros JC. (2011) In-office vital bleaching with adjunct light. *Dent Clin North Am* **55**(2):241–53, viii.

Papathanasiou A, Kastali S, Perry RD, Kugel G. (2002) Clinical evaluation of a 35% hydrogen peroxide in-office whitening system. *Compend Contin Educ Dent* **23**(4):335–8, 40, 43-4 passim; quiz 48.

Paravina RD, Johnston WM, Powers JM. (2007) New shade guide for evaluation of tooth whitening—colorimetric study. *J Esthet Restor Dent* **19**(5):276–83; discussion 83.

Paravina RD, Majkic G, Imai FH, Powers JM. (2007) Optimization of tooth color and shade guide design. *J Prosthodont* **16**(4):269–76.

Paravina RD. (2008) New shade guide for tooth whitening monitoring: visual assessment. *J Prosthet Dent* **9**(3):178–84.

Robertson MA, Kau CH, English JD, Lee RP. MI (2011) Paste Plus to prevent demineralization in orthodontic patients: a prospective randomized controlled trial. *Am J Orthod Dentofacial Orthop* **140**(5):660–8.

Shannon H, Spencer P, Gross K, Tira D. (1993) Characterization of enamel exposed to 10% carbamide peroxide bleaching agents. *Quintessence Int* **24**(1):39–44.

Sulieman M, Addy M, Macdonald E, Rees JS. (2004) A safety study in vitro for the effects of an in-office bleaching system on the integrity of enamel and dentine. *J Dent* **32**(7):581–90.

Sun L, Liang S, Sa Y, Wang Z. (2011) Surface alteration of human tooth enamel subjected to acidic and neutral 30% hydrogen peroxide. *J Dent* **39**(10):686–92.

Tavares M, Stultz J, Newman M, Smith V. (2003) Light augments tooth whitening with peroxide. *J Am Dent Assoc* **134**(2):167–75.

Truman J. (1864) Discolored and necrosed teeth. *Dent Times* **2**(2):69–72.

Zach L, Cohen G. (1965) Pulp response to externally applied heat. *Oral Surg Oral Med Oral Pathol* **19:**515–30.

Ziemba SL, Felix H, MacDonald J, Ward M. (2005) Clinical evaluation of a novel dental whitening lamp and light-catalyzed peroxide gel. *J Clin Dent* **16**(4):123–7.

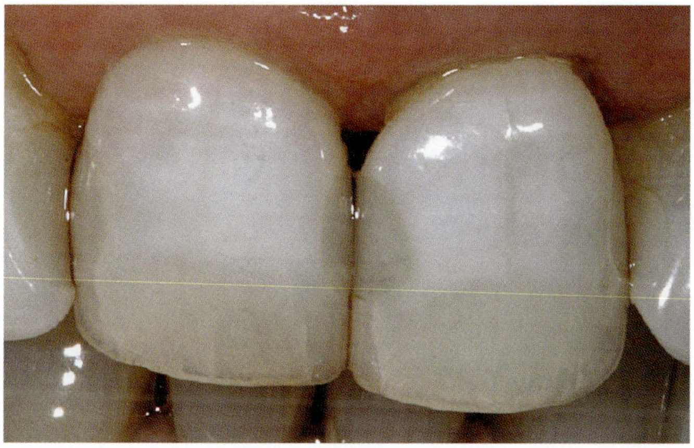

Figure 7.1

Postbleaching color mismatch.

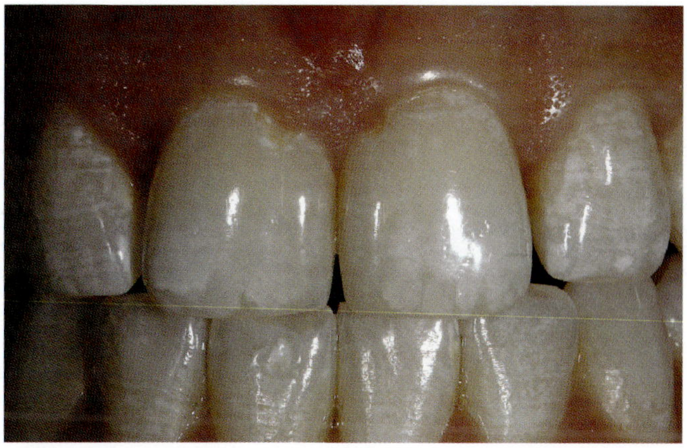

Figure 7.2

White spot lesions after bleaching.

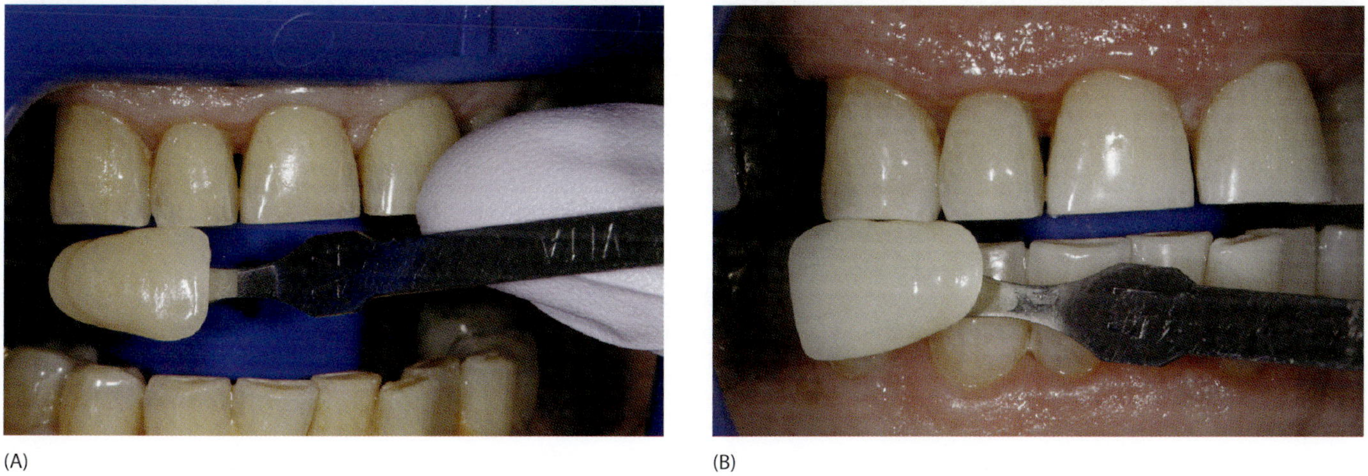

Figure 7.3

Class I, moderate discoloration; vital case. (A) Pretreatment shade A4 from extrinsic stain and aging. (B) Post-treatment shade A1 after three 15-minute cycles with 28% hydrogen peroxide using supplemental light (high-intensity discharge [HID] lamp).

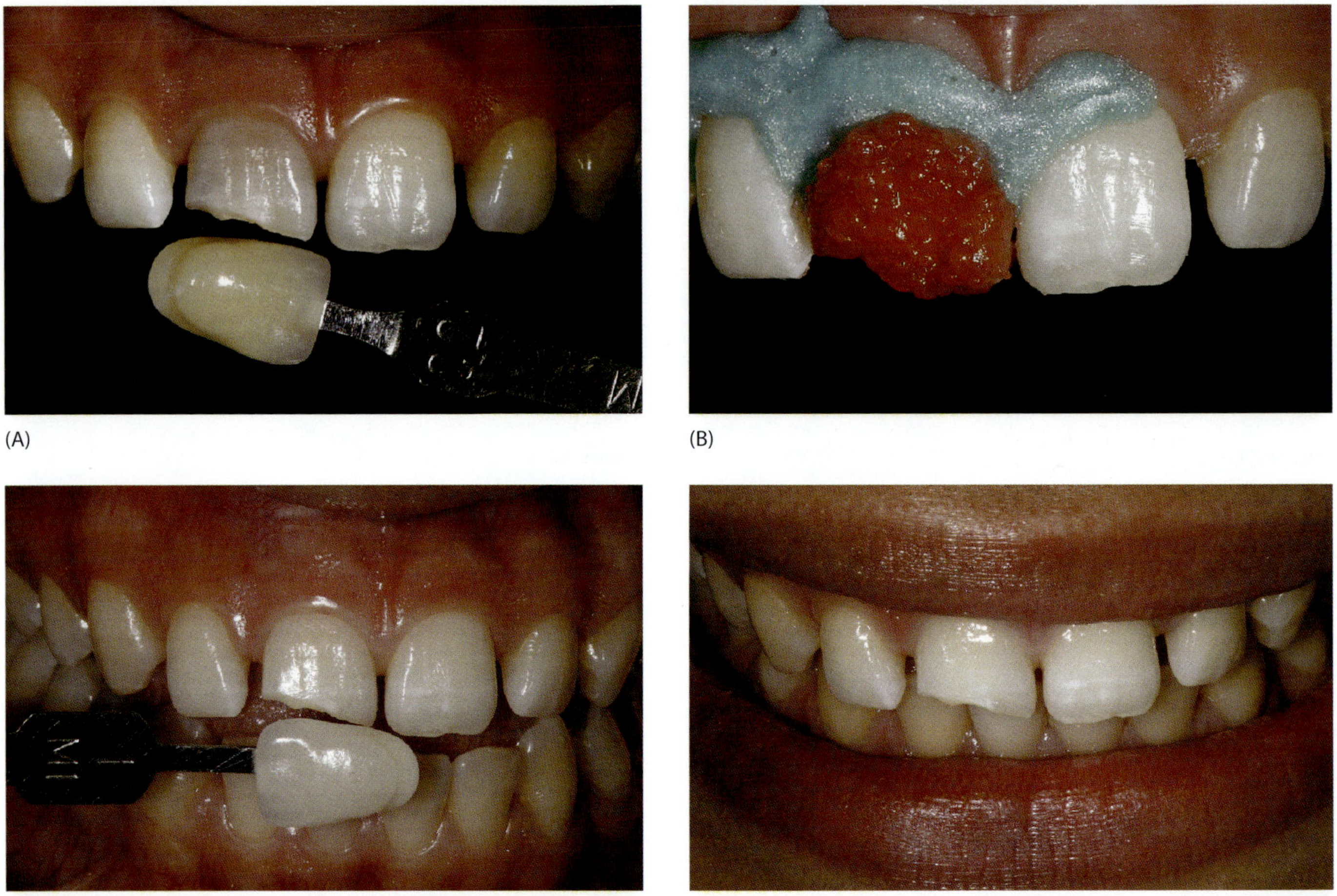

(A) (B) (C) (D)

Figure 7.4

Class II, mild intrinsic stain; vital case. (A) Vital single central incisor before treatment. (B) In-office treatment with 38% hydrogen peroxide, three 20-minute applications, external application only. (C and D) Good response to treatment after a single in-office visit shown 6 days after treatment.

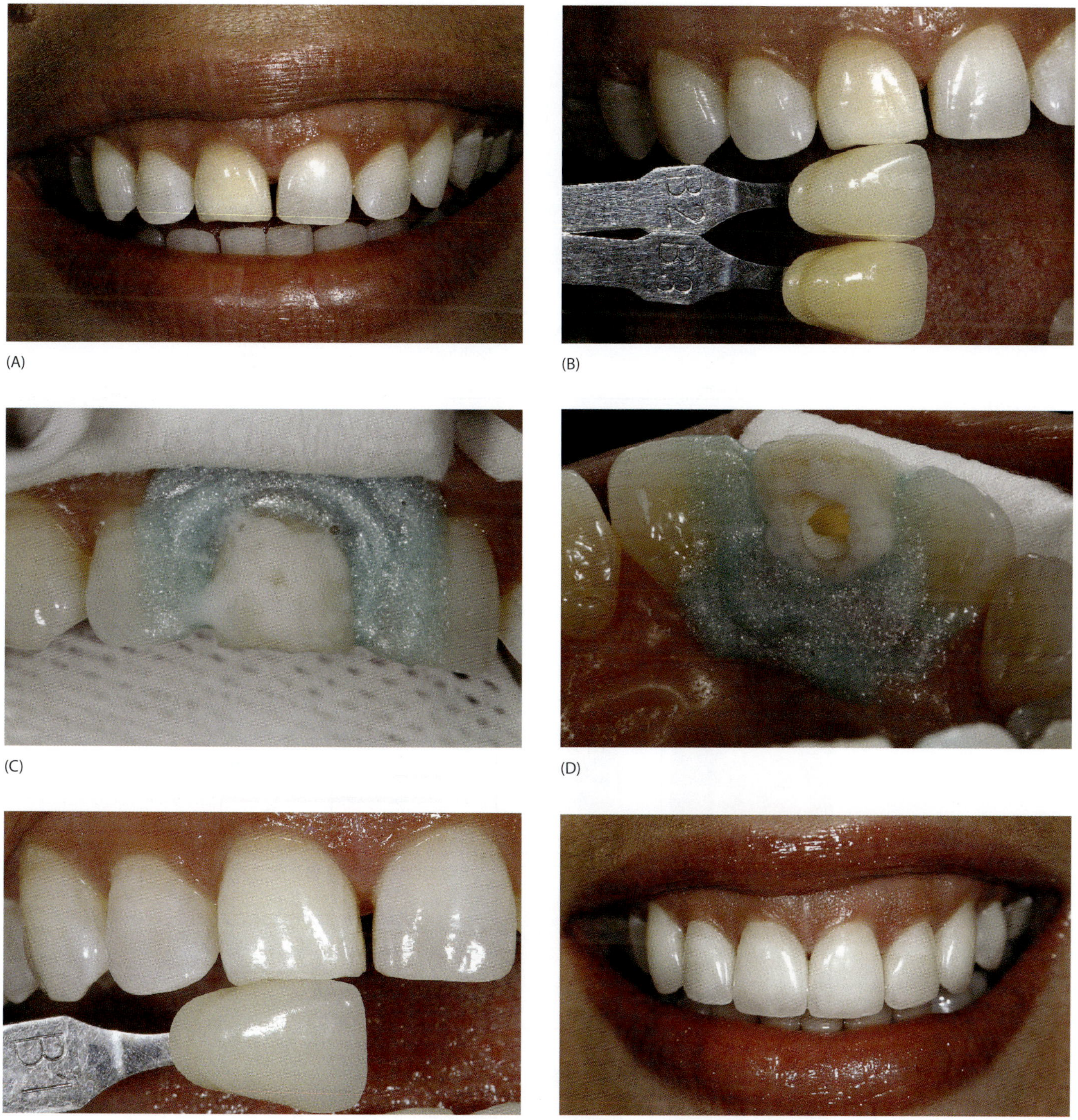

(A) (B) (C) (D) (E) (F)

Figure 7.5

Class II, mild intrinsic stain; nonvital case. (A) Nonvital single central incisor before treatment. (B) Pretreatment shade is documented. (C) In-office treatment with 35% hydrogen peroxide applied on the labial tooth surface and (D) on the lingual surface applied both externally and internally within the pulp chamber after sealing the gutta percha 2 mm below the cementoenamel junction with resin ionomer. (E) Successful bleaching outcome after 1-hour treatment. (F) Patient elected to close spaces with translucent porcelain veneers.

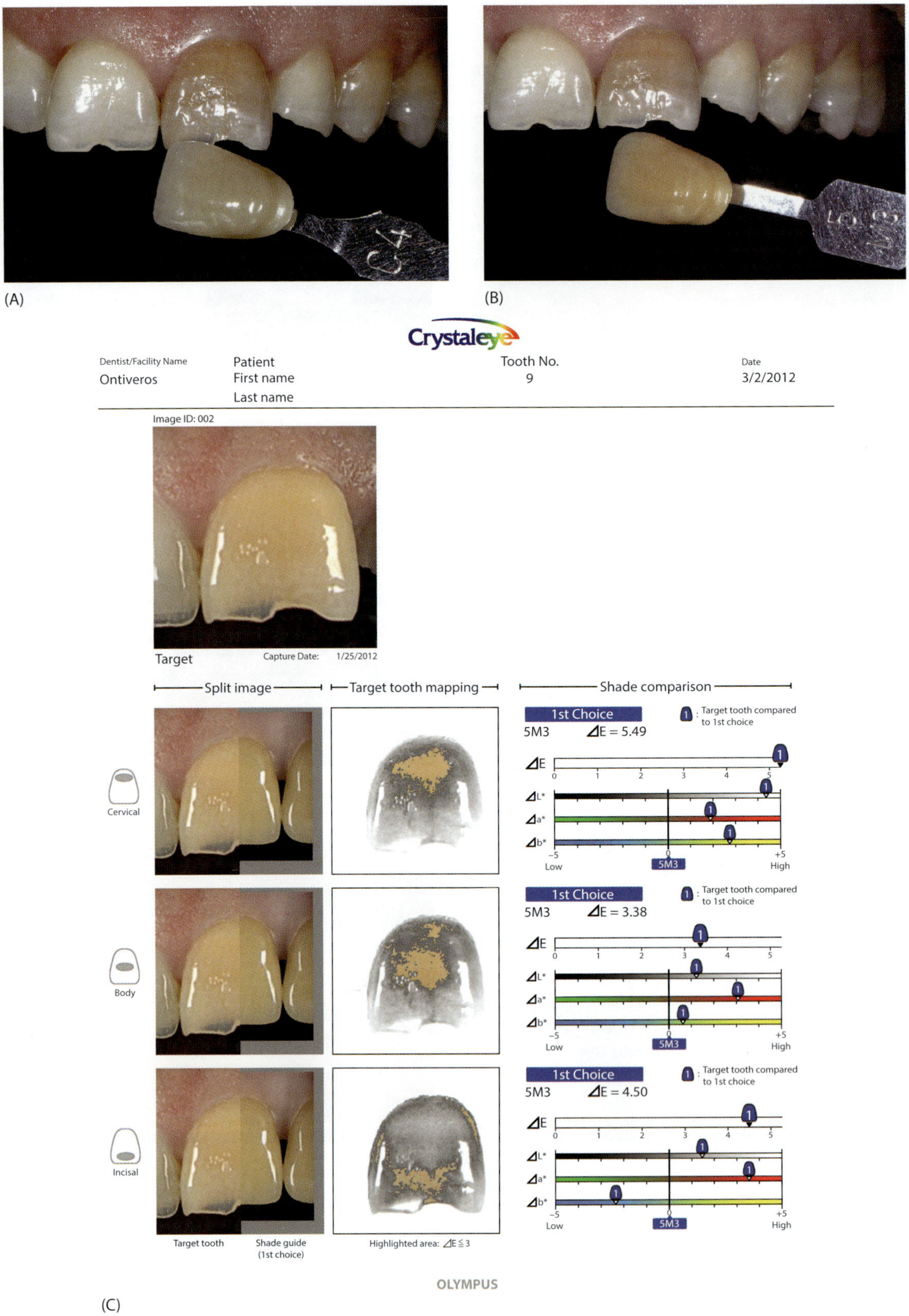

Figure 7.6

Class III, severe intrinsic stain; nonvital case. (A) Severe discoloration of nonvital tooth, which appears darker than the last shade of the Vita classical shade guide (C4). (B and C) Tooth matches more closely to the last shade of the Vita Bleachedguide (5M3), yet is more reddish as verified instrumentally.

continued on the next page

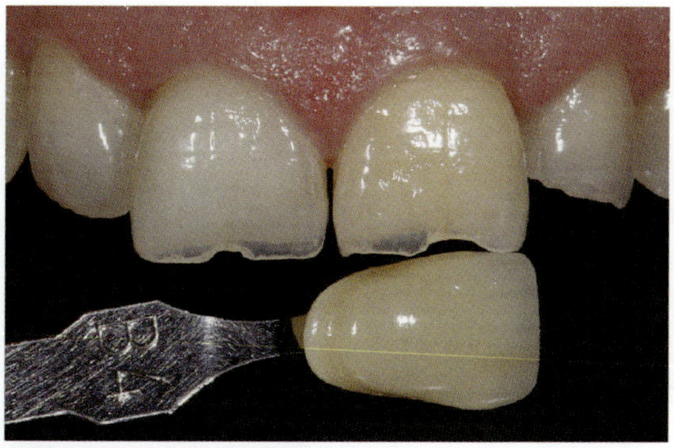

(D)

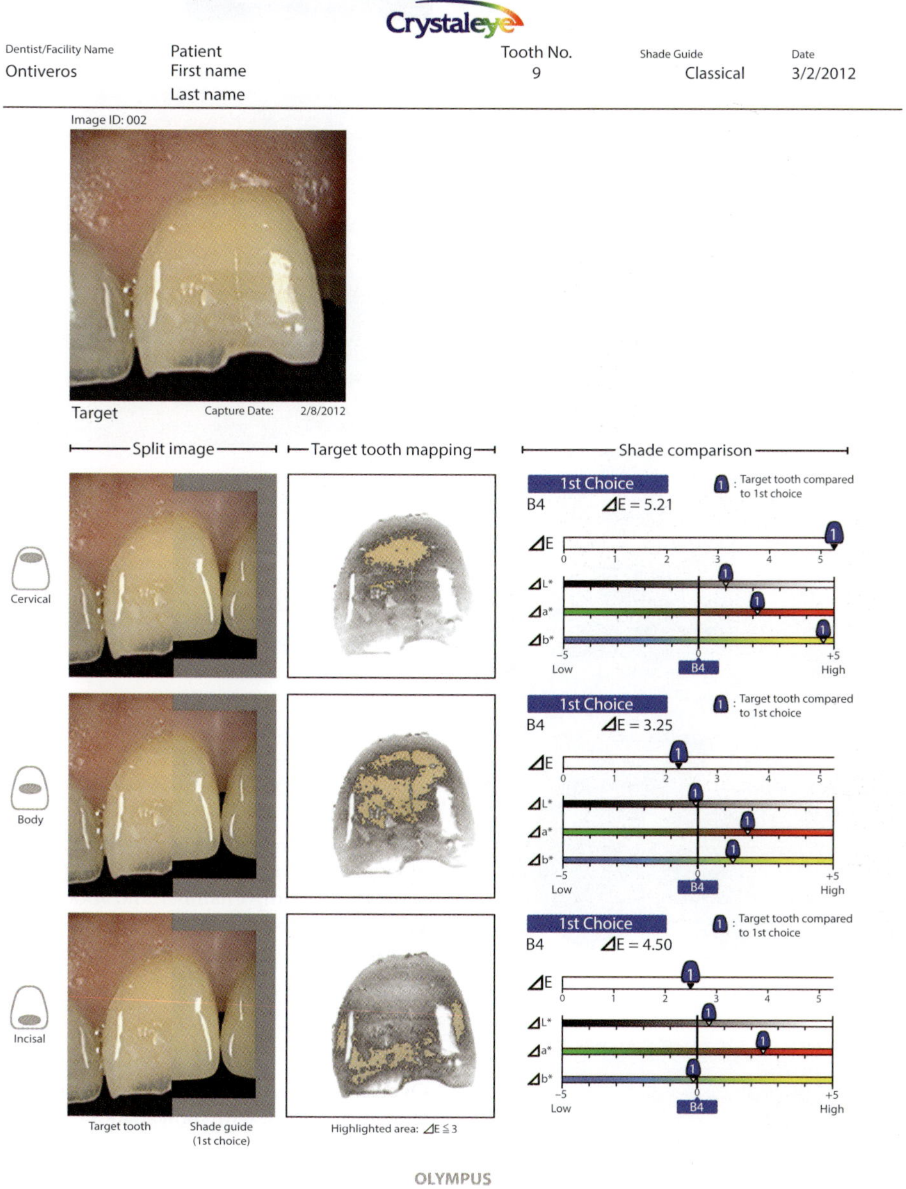

(E)

Figure 7.6 continued

Class III, severe intrinsic stain; nonvital case. (D and E) Color change after three weekly applications of sodium perborate with 3% hydrogen peroxide using the "walking bleach technique" matches closely to shade B4. Although a color mismatch still exists, the patient was pleased with the improved outcome and elected to discontinue treatment.

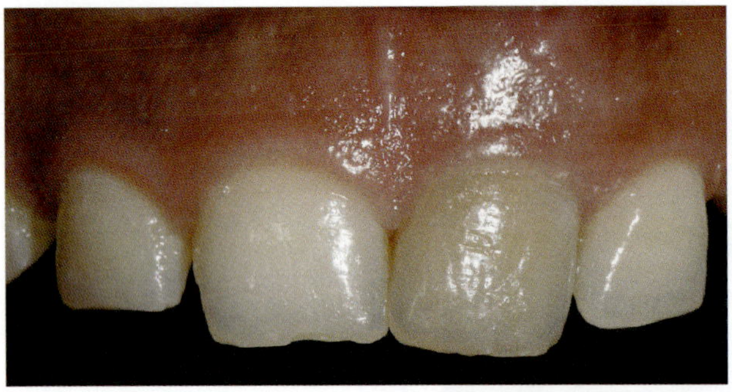

(A)

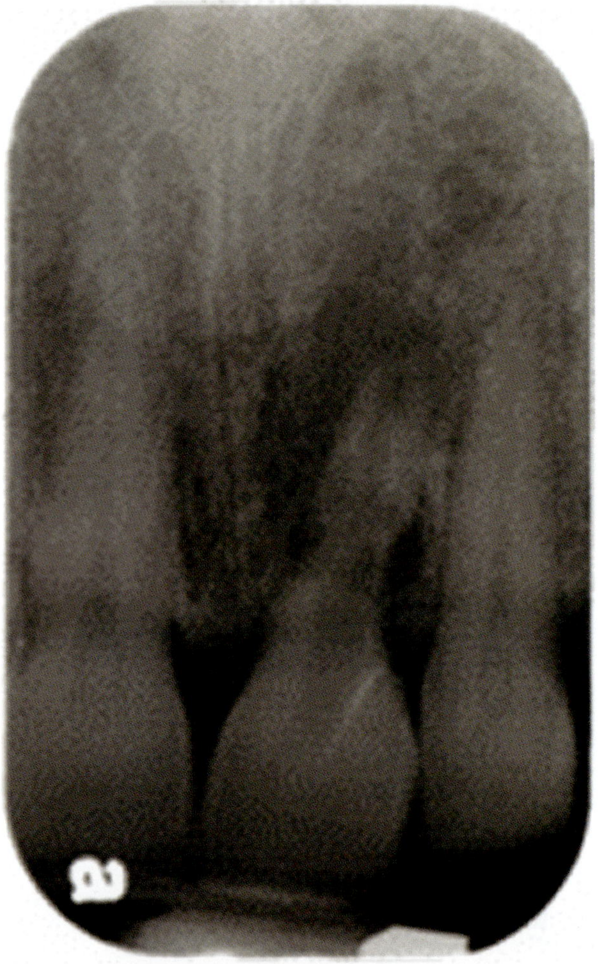

(B)

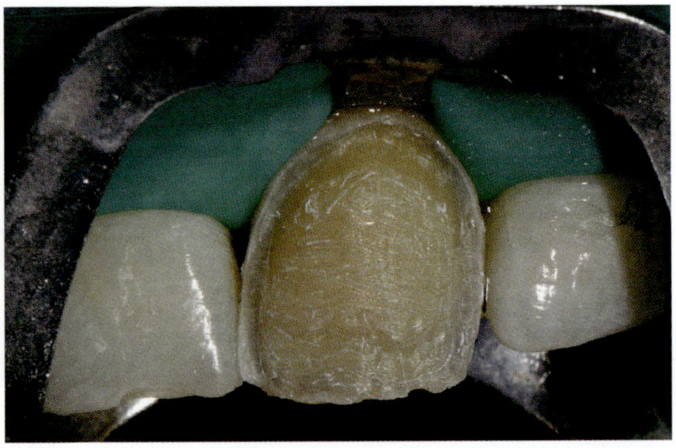

(C)

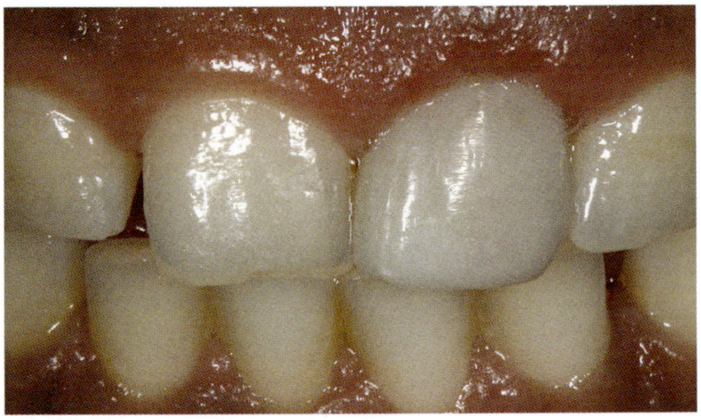

(D)

Figure 7.7

Class III, moderate intrinsic stain; vital case. (A) Intrinsic discoloration of vital tooth as a result of trauma. (B) Radiograph of central incisor shows dense pulp chamber and root resorption present for several years; not a good candidate for in-office bleaching. (C and D) Patient elected restorative coverage with opaque composite resin.

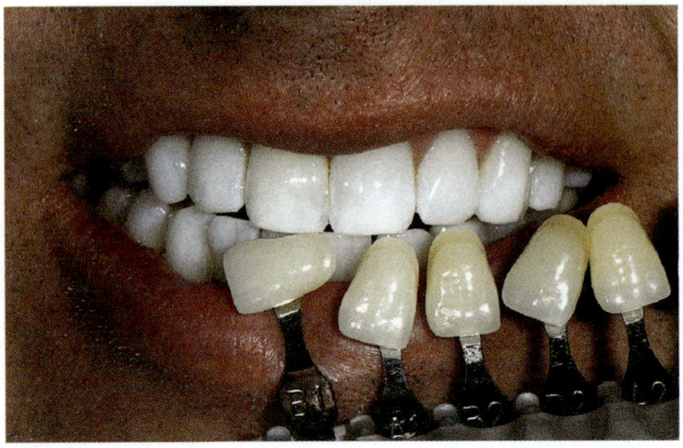

Figure 7.8

Overbleached teeth. Educate patient with extremely white teeth by showing contrast with light shades of the Vita classical shade guide.

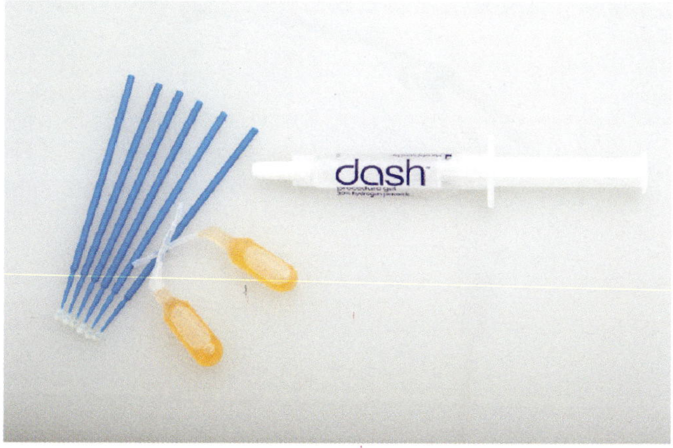

Figure 7.9

One-component system; no-mix formula. Examples of 25% hydrogen peroxide supplied in ampules (PowerBrite) and 30% hydrogen peroxide supplied in syringe (Dash).

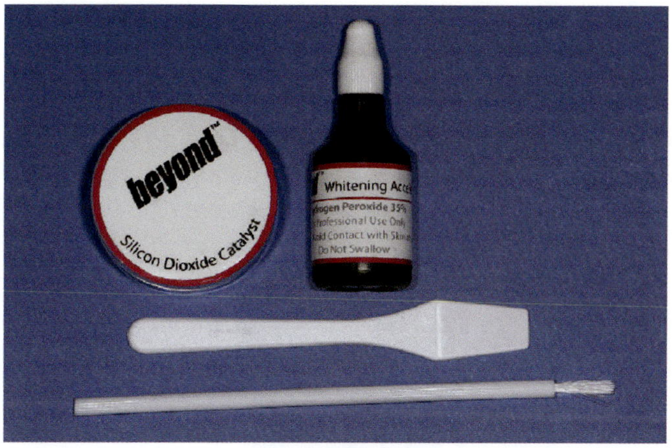

Figure 7.10

Two-component system (Beyond, Stafford, TX) that requires hand mixing 35% hydrogen peroxide with a silicon dioxide catalyst.

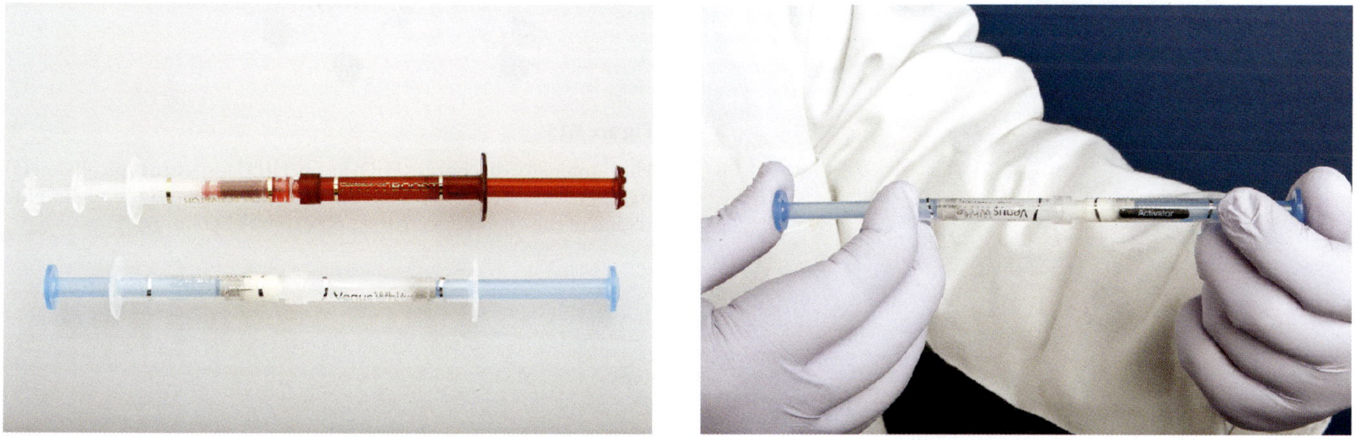

(A) (B)

Figure 7.11

Two-component systems that use syringe-to-syringe activation. (A) Forty percent hydrogen peroxide (Opalescence Boost, Ultradent Products, South Jordan, UT) and 38% hydrogen peroxide (Venus White Max, Heraeus Kulzer, South Bend, IN) ready for mixing. (B) For mixing, the syringe of hydrogen peroxide is connected to a separate catalyst syringe and is pushed to and from the catalyst syringe until completely mixed.

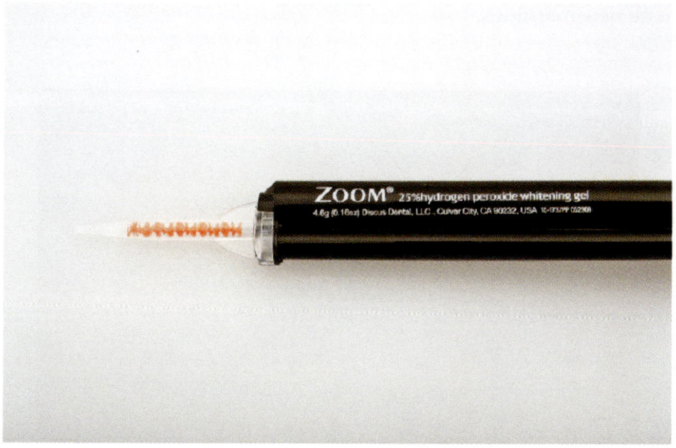

Figure 7.12

Two-component system that combines 25% hydrogen peroxide (Zoom, Philips Oral Healthcare, Stamford, CT) with catalyst using an automix tip from a dual-barrel syringe.

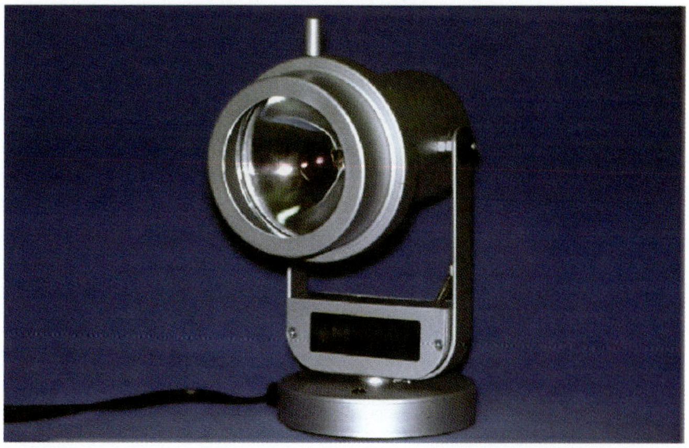

Figure 7.13

Heat lamp. Early bleaching lamp from New Image. This lamp could be used on a bracket table for bleaching multiple vital teeth. (Courtesy of Edward J. Swift, Jr, University of North Carolina at Chapel Hill School of Dentistry.)

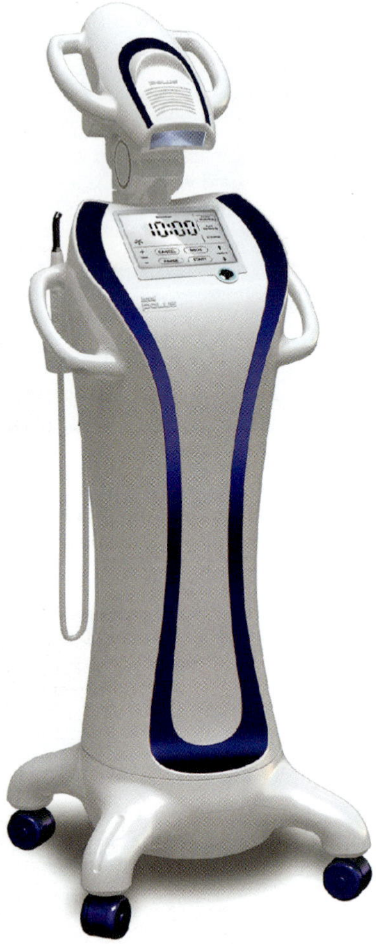

Figure 7.14

Modern halogen lamp. Polus Bleach Light by Beyond is marketed as a multifunctional-system halogen-powered bleaching light, light-emitting diode (LED) curing light, and low-level laser therapy (LLLT) light.

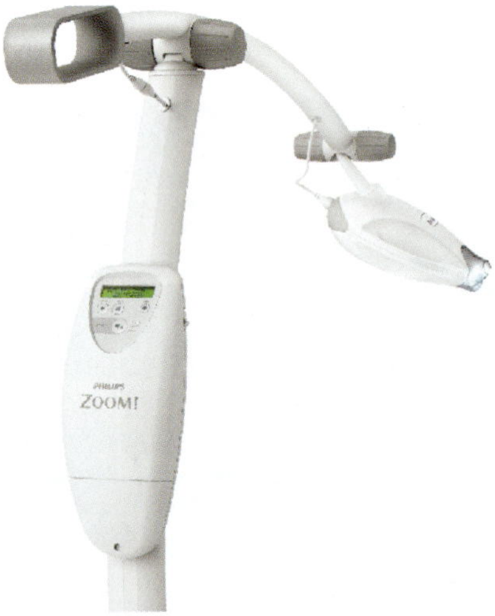

Figure 7.16

Light-emitting diode (LED) bleaching lamp. LED lamps produce near-monochromatic light using LED arrays as a light source—for example, Zoom WhiteSpeed.

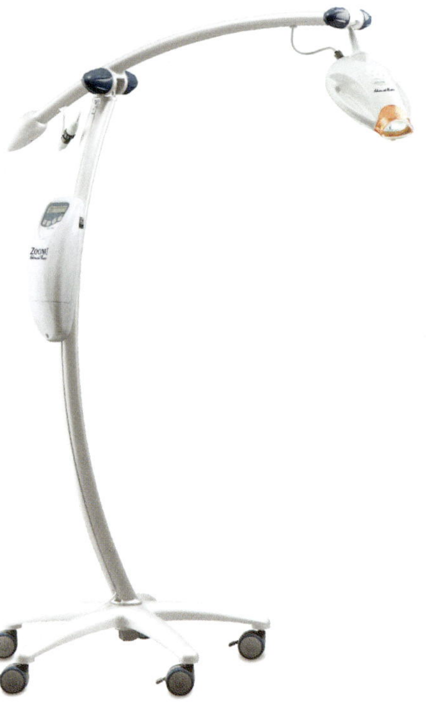

Figure 7.15

High-intensity discharge (HID) lamp. HID lamps are typically metal halide lamps with light sources that filter down to the violet-blue region of the visible spectrum—for example, Zoom AP.

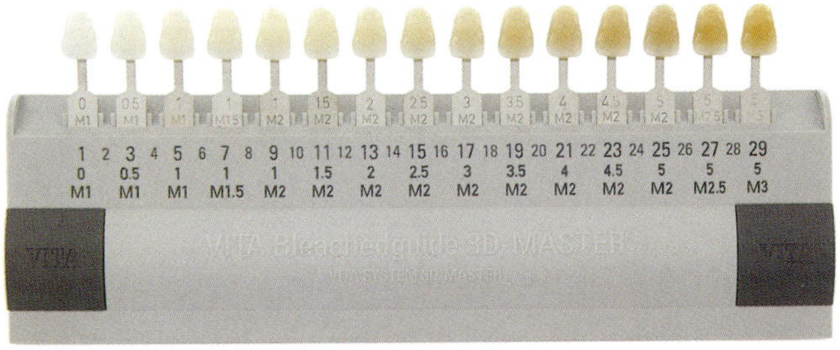

Figure 7.17

Shade guide designed for bleaching monitoring: Vita Bleachedguide with new markings.

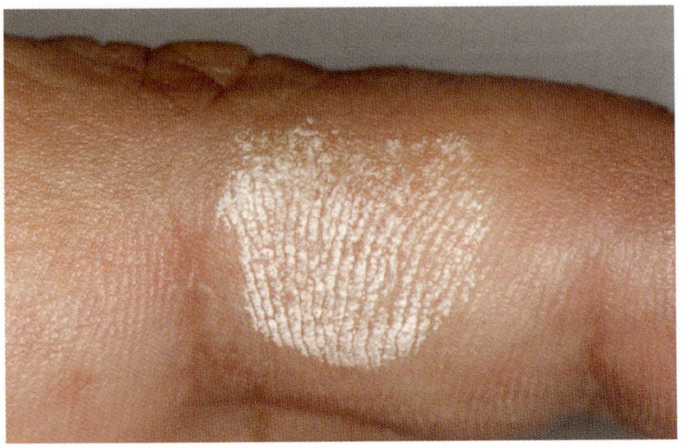

Figure 7.18

Chemical skin burn from 30% hydrogen peroxide.

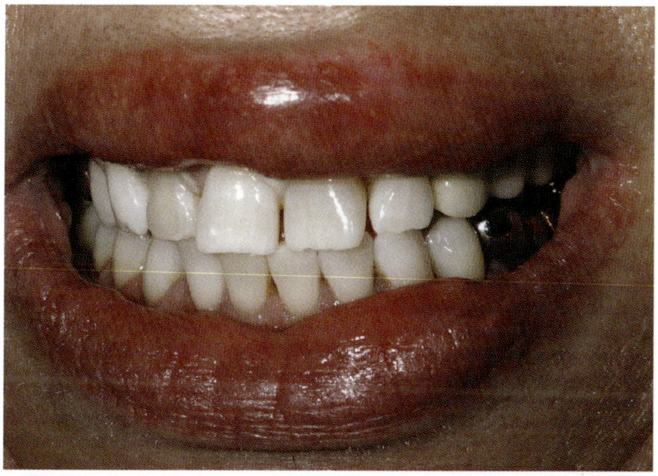

Figure 7.19

Swollen lips.

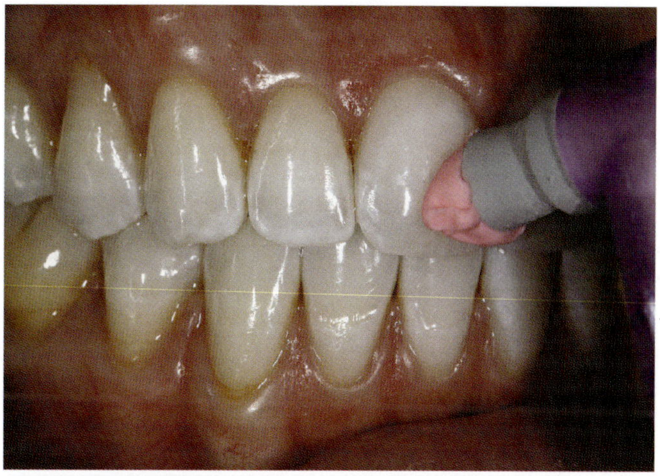

Figure 7.20

Re-treatment prophy to remove plaque and superficial stain.

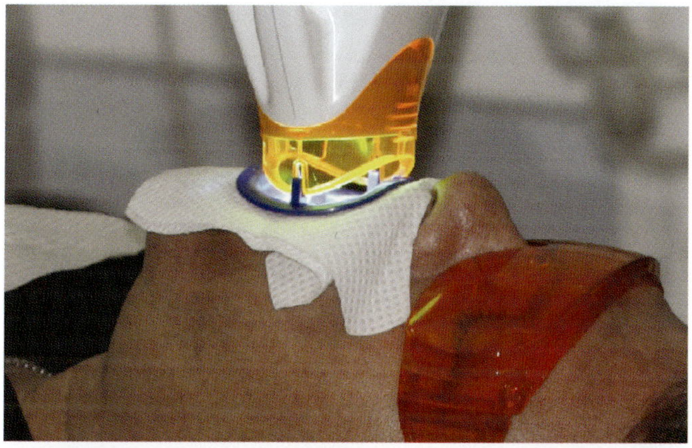

Figure 7.21

Light-protective glasses provided to patient and light guide or shield around the exit window of the lamp are used to control direct and scattered radiation.

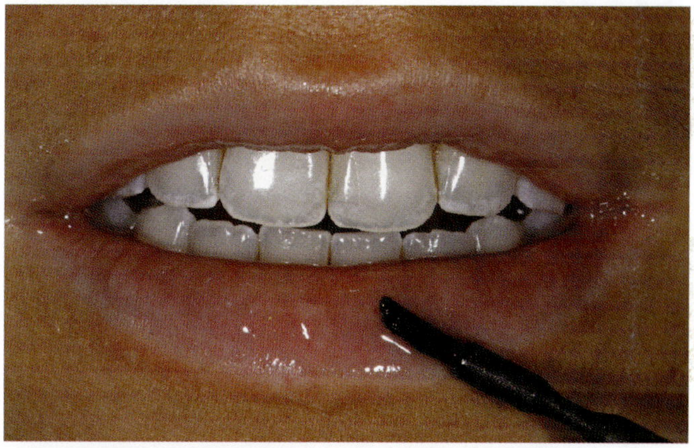

Figure 7.22

Vitamin E oil being applied to lips.

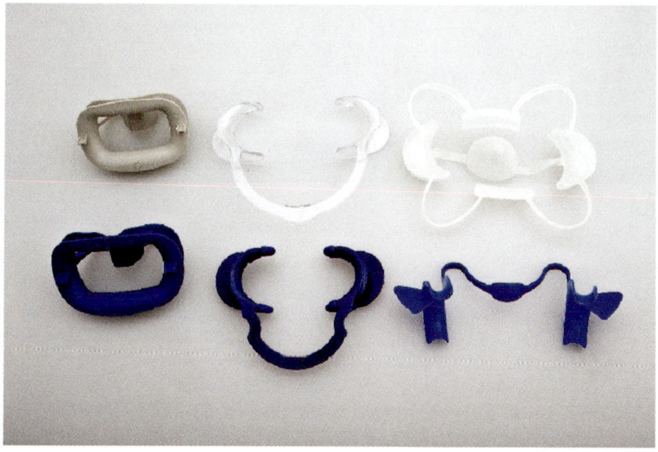

(A)

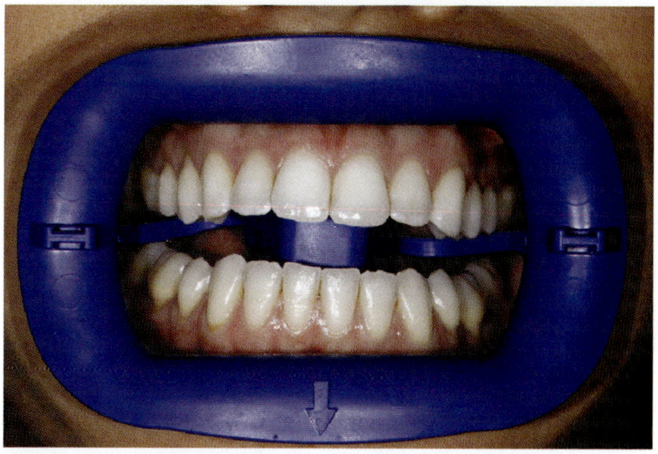

(B)

Figure 7.23

(A) Cheek retractors of various sizes and levels of protection are available. (B) Lip coverage with retractors is preferred when a bleaching lamp is used.

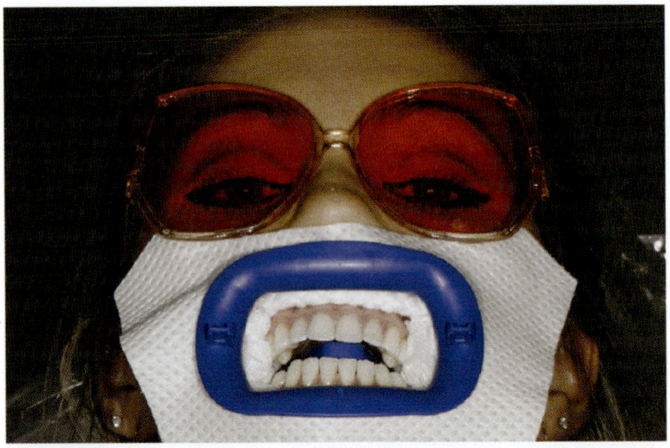

Figure 7.24

A protective bib or isolation napkin is slipped over the retractors.

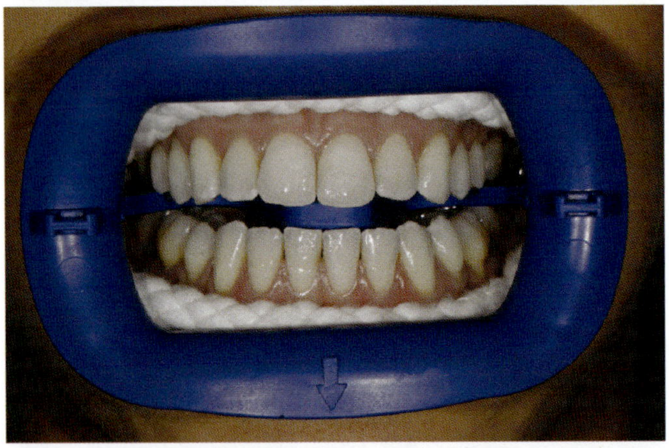

(A)

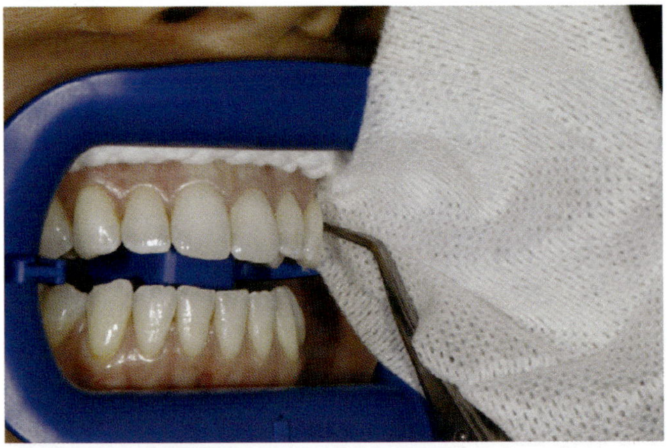

(B)

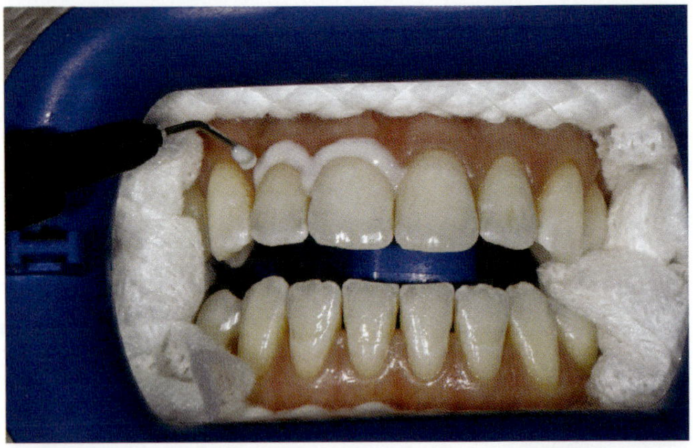

(C)

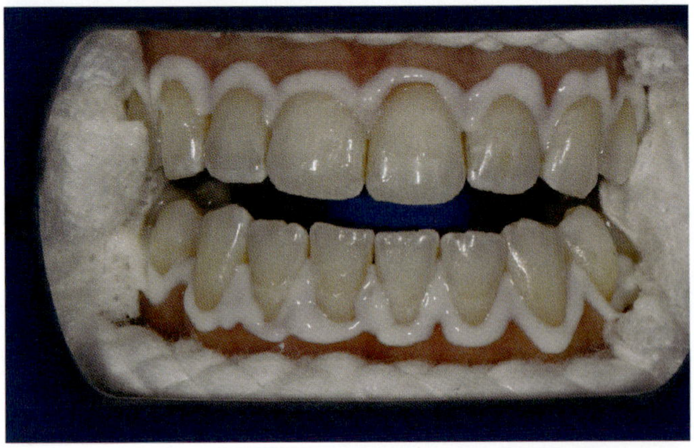

(D)

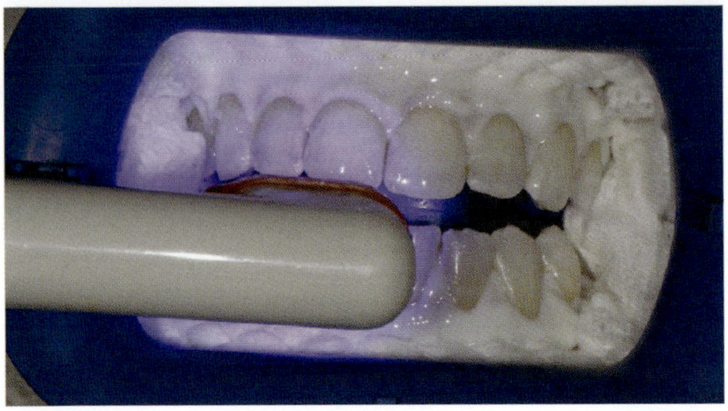

(E)

Figure 7.25

(A) Long cotton rolls are placed in vestibules. (B) Folded gauze may be placed to further protect soft tissue. (C) Resin barrier material being placed two teeth at a time and tacked in place. (D) Resin barrier material is scalloped from papilla to papilla. Tooth 9 shows an inadequate seal at the gingival crest that was corrected before application of bleach material. (E) Additional resin barrier material is extended apically 5–10 mm and cured while slowly moving the curing light to avoid overheating. *continued on the next page* the gel and then place glass ionomer as an interim restoration.

13. Remove the dental dam and inform the patient that the bleaching agent works slowly and that significant lightening may not be evident for several days.
14. Evaluate the patient approximately 2 weeks later; if necessary, repeat the procedure several times. Repeat treatments are similar to the first one.
15. As an optional procedure, if initial bleaching is not satisfactory, strengthen the walking bleach paste by mixing the sodium perborate with gradually increasing concentrations of hydrogen peroxide (3% to 30%) instead of water. The more potent oxidizers may have an enhanced bleaching effect but are not used routinely because of the possibility of permeation into the tubules and damage to the cervical periodontium by these more caustic agents. In such cases, a protective cream, such as Orabase, Vaseline, or cocoa butter must be applied to the surrounding gingival tissues before dental dam placement.
16. In most cases, discoloration will improve after one or two treatments. If after three attempts there is no significant improvement, reassess the case for correct diagnosis of the cause of discoloration and treatment plan.

SODIUM PERBORATE BLEACHING MATERIAL

Sodium perborate ($NaBO_3$) is an oxidizing agent available in a powdered form or as various commercial preparations. When fresh, it contains about 95% perborate, releasing about 9.9% available oxygen. Sodium perborate is stable when dry but, in the presence of acid, warm air, or water, decomposes to form sodium metaborate, hydrogen peroxide, and nascent oxygen. It can act synergistically with hydrogen peroxide (Nutting and Poe 1963).

Various types of sodium perborate preparations are available: monohydrate, trihydrate, and tetrahydrate. They differ in oxygen content, which determines their bleaching efficiency (Weiger et al. 1994). Commonly used sodium perborate preparations are alkaline, and their pH depends on the amount of hydrogen peroxide released and the residual sodium metaborate (Rotstein and Friedman 1991).

Sodium perborate is more easily controlled and safer than high concentrations of hydrogen peroxide solutions. However, sodium perborate has been banned by the European directive. It is not permissible to use any sodium perborate materials in dentistry in Europe.

THERMO/PHOTO BLEACHING PROCEDURES

Thermo/photo bleaching involves placement of the oxidizing agent, usually 30–35% hydrogen peroxide, in the pulp chamber followed by heat application from electric heating devices, light application from specially designed lamps, or both (Buchalla and Attin 2007) (see Figure 8.3). Care must be taken when using these heating devices to avoid overheating the teeth and surrounding tissues. Intermittent treatment with cooling breaks is preferred over one long continuous session. In addition, the surrounding soft tissues should be protected with Vaseline, Orabase, or cocoa butter during treatment to avoid heat damage.

Potential damage from the thermo/photo bleaching approach is external root resorption caused by irritation to the cementum and periodontal ligament. This is possibly attributed to hydrogen peroxide combined with heat (Madison and Walton 1990, Rotstein et al. 1991a). Therefore, application of highly concentrated H_2O_2 and heat during intracoronal bleaching should not be carried out routinely. This technique is now not used much owing to the high heat generated.

In general, the technique involves the following steps:

1. Familiarize the patient with the probable causes of discoloration, the procedure to be followed, the expected outcome, and the possibility of future rediscoloration.
2. Assess the status of periapical tissues and the quality of endodontic obturation (see Figure 8.4D). Endodontic failure or questionable obturation should be re-treated before bleaching (see Figures 8.4 and 8.10).
3. Evaluate tooth color with a shade guide and take clinical photographs before and throughout the procedure. Assess the quality and shade of any restoration present and replace if defective.
4. Apply a protective cream to the surrounding gingival tissues and isolate the teeth with rubber dam and waxed dental floss ligatures. If a heat lamp is used, avoid placing rubber dam metal clamps; they are subjected to heating and may also be painful to the patient.
5. Do not use anesthesia.
6. Position protective sunglasses over the patient's and operator's eyes.
7. Apply a sufficiently thick layer, at least 2 mm, of protective white cement barrier, such as polycarboxylate cement, zinc phosphate cement, glass ionomer, or IRM on top of the endodontic obturation. The coronal height of the barrier should protect the dentin tubules and conform to the external epithelial attachment (Steiner and West 1994). It is best to use glass ionomer as a barrier because it does not interfere with the hydrogen peroxide in the gel.
8. Soak a small amount of 30–35% hydrogen peroxide solution on a small cotton pellet or a piece of gauze and place it in the pulp chamber. A bleaching gel containing hydrogen peroxide may be used instead of the aqueous solution.
9. Apply heat with a heating device or a light source. The temperature should be less than the patient can comfortably tolerate, usually between 50°C and 60°C. Re-wet the cotton pellet and pulp chamber with hydrogen peroxide as necessary. If the tooth becomes too sensitive, discontinue the bleaching procedure immediately. Preferably, bleaching should be limited to separate 5-minute periods rather than being

performed during a long continuous period (Rotstein et al. 1991b).

10. Remove the heat or light source and allow the teeth to cool down for at least 5 minutes. Then wash with warm water for 1 minute and remove the dental dam.
11. Dry the tooth and place walking bleach paste of sodium perborate mixed with water in the pulp chamber.
12. Recall the patient approximately 2 weeks later and evaluate the effectiveness of bleaching. Take clinical photographs with the same shade guide used in the preoperative photographs for comparison purposes. If necessary, repeat the bleaching procedure.

INTENTIONAL ENDODONTICS AND INTRACORONAL BLEACHING

The technique involves standard endodontic therapy of a vital pulp followed by intracoronal bleaching. It should not be done routinely and should be offered to patients only in limited clinical situations. This technique was mainly advocated for treating severe intrinsic tetracycline discolorations. Such discolorations and other similar stains are incorporated into tooth structure during tooth formation, mostly into the dentin, and therefore are very difficult to treat from the external enamel surface. Intracoronal bleaching of tetracycline-discolored teeth has been shown to be predictable and to improve tooth shade without significant clinical complications (Abou-Rass 1982). These days it is not necessary to intentionally devitalize a tooth merely for the sake of bleaching the tooth because the home bleaching technique can bleach the most severe discoloration over a period of time. Normal home bleaching techniques using higher carbamide peroxide are used instead.

COMPLICATIONS AND ADVERSE EFFECTS

External root resorption

Clinical reports (Harrington and Natkin 1979, Lado et al. 1983, Montgomery 1984, Shearer 1984, Cvek and Lindvall 1985, Goon et al. 1986, Latcham 1986, Friedman et al. 1988, Gimlin and Schindler 1990, Al-Nazhan 1991, Heithersay et al. 1994) and histologic studies (Madison and Walton 1990, Rotstein et al. 1991a, Heller et al. 1992) have shown that intracoronal bleaching may induce external root resorption mainly when 30–35% hydrogen peroxide is being used. The mechanism of bleaching-induced damage to the periodontium or cementum has not been fully elucidated. Presumably, the irritating chemical diffuses via unprotected dentinal tubules and cementum defects (Rotstein et al. 1991c, Koulaouzidou et al. 1996) and causes necrosis of the cementum, inflammation of the periodontal ligament, and finally root resorption. The process may be enhanced if heat is applied (Rotstein et al. 1991b) or in the presence of bacteria (Cvek and Lindvall 1985, Heling et al. 1995). Previous traumatic injury (see Figure 8.7) and age may act as predisposing factors (Harrington and Natkin 1979, Tredwin et al. 2006).

Chemical burns

Hydrogen peroxide (30–35%) is highly caustic and can cause chemical burns and sloughing of the gingiva. When such solutions are used, the soft tissues should always be protected with Vaseline, Orabase, or cocoa butter.

High-strength hydrogen peroxide may not be used in Europe. No more than 6% hydrogen peroxide may be used for bleaching in Europe. In this case, 16% carbamide peroxide is sealed into access cavities of teeth. The lower strength has the advantages of causing less chemical burning and less soft tissue discomfort.

Damage to restorations

Bleaching with hydrogen peroxide may affect bonding of composite resins to dental hard tissues (Titley et al. 1993). Scanning electron microscopy observations suggest a possible interaction between composite resin and residual peroxide causing inhibition of polymerization and increase in resin porosity (Titley et al. 1991). This presents a clinical problem when immediate esthetic restoration of the bleached tooth is required. It is therefore recommended that residual hydrogen peroxide be totally eliminated from the pulp chamber before composite placement. This may be done by treating the dentin surface with catalase before bonding (Rotstein 1993). Catalase removes the residual oxygen from the dentin. A glass ionomer restoration can be placed immediately and the rest cut back 2 weeks later for the composite restoration.

It has also been suggested that immersion of peroxide-treated dental tissues in water at 37°C for 7 days prevents the reduction in bond strength (Torneck et al. 1991).

SUGGESTIONS FOR SAFER NONVITAL BLEACHING

See Table **8.5**.

- *Isolate tooth effectively.* Intracoronal bleaching should always be carried out with dental dam isolation. Interproximal wedges and ligatures may also be used for better protection.
- *Protect oral mucosa.* Protective cream, such as Orabase, Vaseline, or cocoa butter, must be applied to the surrounding oral mucosa to prevent damage associated with chemical burns by caustic oxidizers. Animal studies suggest that catalase applied to oral tissues

Table 8.5 Suggestions for safer intracoronal nonvital bleaching

- Isolate tooth effectively
- Protect oral mucosa
- Verify adequate endodontic obturation
- Use protective barriers
- Avoid acid etching
- Avoid strong oxidizers
- Avoid heat
- Recall periodically

before hydrogen peroxide treatment totally prevents the associated tissue damage (Rotstein et al. 1993b).

- *Verify adequate endodontic obturation* (see Figure 8.4). The quality of root canal obturation should always be assessed clinically and radiographically before bleaching. Adequate obturation ensures a better overall prognosis of the treated tooth. It also provides an additional barrier against damage by oxidizers to the periodontal ligament and periapical tissues.
- *Use protective barriers.* This is essential to prevent leakage of bleaching agents (see Figure 8.4D), which may infiltrate between the gutta-percha and root canal walls, reaching the periodontal ligament via dentinal tubules, lateral canals, or the root apex. In none of the clinical reports of postbleaching root resorption was a protective barrier used. Various materials can be used for this purpose (Rotstein and Walton 2015). Barrier thickness and its relationship to the cementoenamel junction are most important (Rotstein et al. 1992, Steiner and West 1994). The ideal barrier should protect the dentinal tubules and conform to the external epithelial attachment (see Figure 8.5).
- *Avoid acid etching.* It has been suggested that acid etching of dentin in the pulp chamber to remove smear layer and open the tubules would allow better penetration of oxidizer. This procedure has not proven beneficial (Casey et al. 1989) and therefore usually is unnecessary. The use of caustic chemicals in the pulp chamber is undesirable because periodontal ligament irritation may result.
- *Avoid strong oxidizers.* Procedures and techniques applying strong oxidizers should be avoided if they are not essential for bleaching. Solutions of 30–35% hydrogen peroxide, either alone or in combination with other agents, should not be used routinely for intracoronal bleaching. Sodium perborate is mild and quite safe, and usually no additional protection of the soft tissues is required. In general, however, oxidizing agents should not be exposed to more of the pulp space and dentin than absolutely necessary to obtain a satisfactory clinical result.
- *Avoid heat.* Excessive heat may damage the cementum and periodontal ligament as well as dentin and enamel, especially when combined with strong oxidizers (Madison and Walton 1990, Rotstein et al. 1991a). Although no direct correlation was found between heat applications alone and external cervical root resorption, it should be limited during bleaching procedures.
- *Recall patients periodically* (see Figure 8.6). Bleached teeth should be frequently examined both clinically and radiographically. Root resorption may occasionally be detected as early as 6 months after bleaching. Early detection improves the prognosis because corrective therapy may still be applied.

REFERENCES

Abou-Rass M. (1982) The elimination of tetracycline discoloration by intentional endodontics and internal bleaching. *J Endod* **8**:101.

Al-Nazhan S. (1991) External root resorption after bleaching: a case report. *Oral Surg* **72**:607.

American Association of Endodontists (AAE). (2010) *Guide to clinical endodontics*, AAE: Chicago, 39.

Attin T, Paqué F, Ajam F, Lennon AM. (2003) Review of the current status of tooth whitening with the walking bleach technique. *Int Endod J* **36**:313.

Buchalla W, Attin T. (2007) External bleaching therapy with activation by heat, light or laser—a systematic review. *Dent Mater* **23**:586.

Casey LJ, Schindler WG, Murata SM, Burgess JO. (1989) The use of dentinal etching with endodontic bleaching procedures. *J Endod* **15**:535.

Cvek M, Lindvall AM. (1985) External root resorption following bleaching of pulpless teeth with hydrogen peroxide. *Endod Dent Traumatol* **1**:56.

Friedman S, Rotstein I, Libfeld H, Stabholz A. (1988) Incidence of external root resorption and esthetic results in 58 bleached pulpless teeth. *Endod Dent Traumatol* **4**:23.

Gimlin DR, Schindler WG. (1990) The management of postbleaching cervical resorption. *J Endod* **16**:292.

Goon WW, Cohen S, Borer RF. (1986) External cervical root resorption following bleaching. *J Endod* **12**:414.

Harrington GW, Natkin E. (1979) External resorption associated with bleaching of pulpless teeth. *J Endod* **5**:344.

Heithersay GS, Dahlstrom SW, Marin PD. (1994) Incidence of invasive cervical resorption in bleached root-filled teeth. *Aust Dent J* **39**:82.

Heling I, Parson A, Rotstein I. (1995) Effect of bleaching agents on dentin permeability to *Streptococcus faecalis*. *J Endod* **21**:540.

Heller D, Skriber J, Lin LM. (1992) Effect of intracoronal bleaching on external cervical root resorption. *J Endod* **18**:145.

Holmstrup G, Palm AM, Lambjerg-Hansen H. (1988) Bleaching of discoloured root-filled teeth. *Endod Dent Traumatol* **4**:197.

Koulaouzidou E, Lambrianidis T, Beltes P, Lyroudia K. (1996) Role of cementoenamel junction on the radicular penetration of 30% hydrogen peroxide during intracoronal bleaching in vitro. *Endod Dent Traumatol* **12**:146.

Lado EA, Stanley HR, Weisman MI. (1983) Cervical resorption in bleached teeth. *Oral Surg* **55**:78.

Latcham NL. (1986) Postbleaching cervical resorption. *J Endod* **12**:262.

Madison S, Walton RE. (1990) Cervical root resorption following bleaching of endodontically treated teeth. *J Endod* **16**:570.

Montgomery S. (1984) External cervical resorption after bleaching a pulpless tooth. *Oral Surg* **57**:203.

Nutting EB, Poe GS. (1963) A new combination for bleaching teeth. *J South Calif Dent Assoc* **31**:289.

Rotstein I. (1993) Role of catalase in the elimination of residual hydrogen peroxide following tooth bleaching. *J Endod* **19**:567.

Rotstein I, Friedman S. (1991) pH variation among materials used for intracoronal bleaching. *J Endod* **17**:376.

Rotstein I, Friedman S, Mor C, Katznelson J. (1991a) Histological characterization of bleaching-induced external root resorption in dogs. *J Endod* **17**:436.

Rotstein I, Mor C, Friedman S. (1993a) Prognosis of intracoronal bleaching with sodium perborate preparations in vitro: 1 year study. *J Endod* **19**:10.

Rotstein I, Torek Y, Lewinstein I. (1991b) Effect of bleaching time and temperature on the radicular penetration of hydrogen peroxide. *Endod Dent Traumatol* **7**:196.

Rotstein I, Torek Y, Misgav R. (1991c) Effect of cementum defects on radicular penetration of 30% H_2O_2 during intracoronal bleaching. *J. Endod* **17**:230.

Rotstein I, Walton RE. (2015) Bleaching discoloured teeth. In Torabinejad M, Walton RE, editors. *Endodontics: principles and practice*, 5th edn. Elsevier: St Louis, 428.

Rotstein I, Wesselink PR, Bab I. (1993b) Catalase protection against hydrogen peroxide-induced injury in rat oral mucosa. *Oral Surg* **75**:744.

Rotstein I, Zalkind M, Mor C, Tarabeah A. (1991d) In vitro efficacy of sodium perborate preparations used for intracoronal bleaching of discolored non-vital teeth. *Endod Dent Traumatol* **7**:177.

Rotstein I, Zyskind D, Lewinstein I, Bamberger N. (1992) Effect of different protective base materials on hydrogen peroxide leakage during intracoronal bleaching in vitro. *J Endod* **18**:114.

Shearer GJ. (1984) External resorption associated with bleaching of a non-vital tooth. *Aust Endod Newsl* **10**:16.

Spasser HF. (1961) A simple bleaching technique using sodium perborate. *N Y State Dent J* **27**:332.

Steiner DR, West JD. (1994) A method to determine the location and shape of an intracoronal bleach barrier. *J Endod* **20**:304.

Titley KC, Torneck CD, Ruse ND, Krmec D. (1993) Adhesion of a resin composite to bleached and unbleached human enamel. *J Endod* **19**:112.

Titley KC, Torneck CD, Smith DC, Chernecky R. (1991) Scanning electron microscopy observations on the penetration and structure of resin tags in bleached and unbleached bovine enamel. *J Endod* **17**:71.

Torneck CD, Titley KC, Smith DC, Adibfar A. (1991) Effect of water leaching on the adhesion of composite resin to bleached and unbleached bovine enamel. *J Endod* **17**:156.

Tredwin CJ, Naik S, Lewis NJ, Scully C. (2006) Hydrogen peroxide tooth-whitening (bleaching) products: review of adverse effects and safety issues. *Br Dent J* **200**:371.

Weiger R, Kuhn A, Löst C. (1994) In vitro comparison of various types of sodium perborate used for intracoronal bleaching. *J Endod* **20**:338.

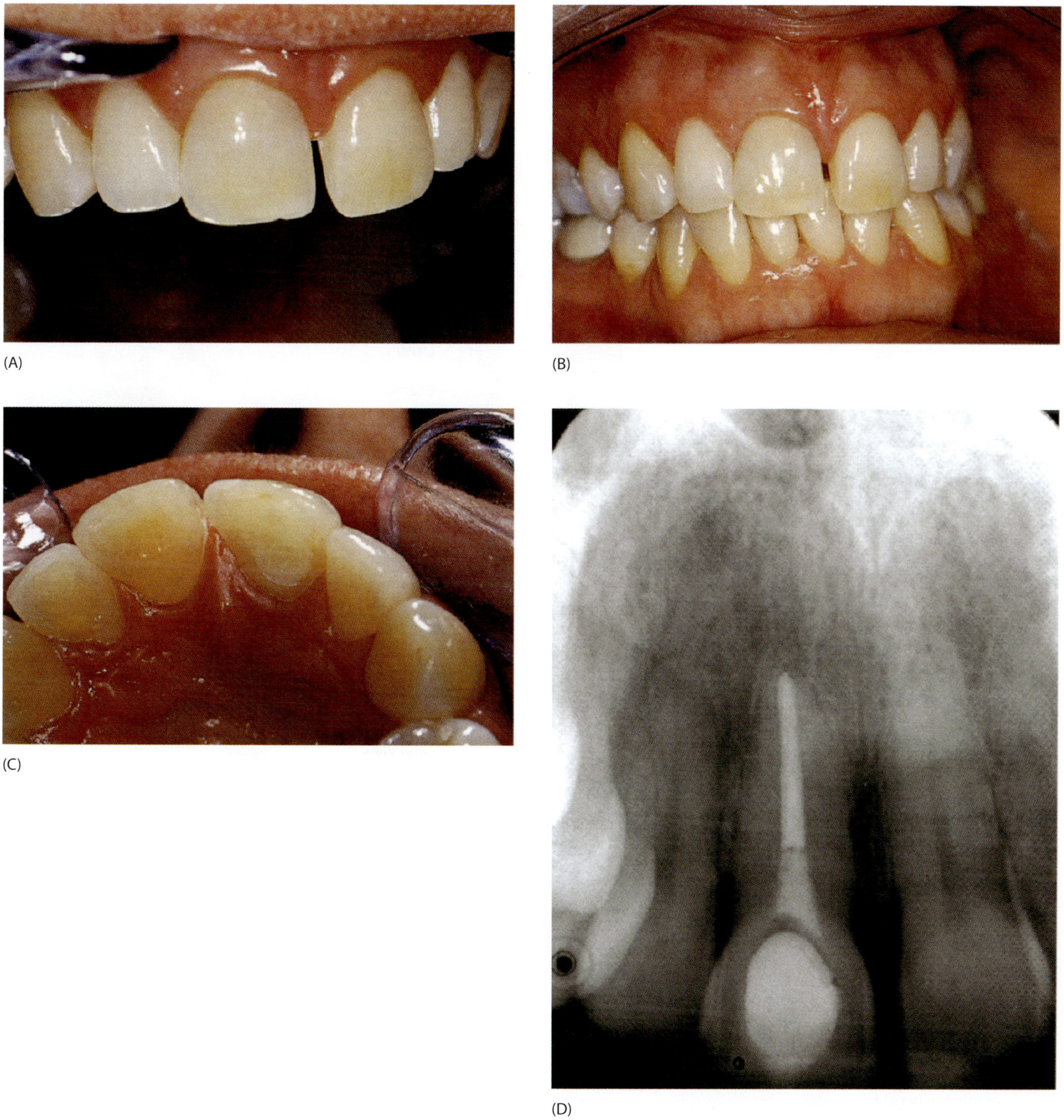

Figure 8.1

Long-term success with intracoronal bleaching. (A) This patient reported that her tooth changed color following pulp damage and a root canal treatment 25 years ago. She had intracoronal bleaching on the maxillary left central incisor 20 years ago. The shade of the tooth has remained stable. The composite restoration in the palatal part has been replaced once since then. (B) The tooth in occlusion. The color match is excellent and the nonvital tooth cannot be differentiated from the adjacent central incisor. (C) The palatal view of the tooth shows a well-sealed palatal composite restoration, which has contributed to the success of the treatment. (D) Periapical radiograph of the tooth that was bleached. The barrier was placed at the cementoenamel junction. A well-condensed root canal is in place. *continued on the next page*

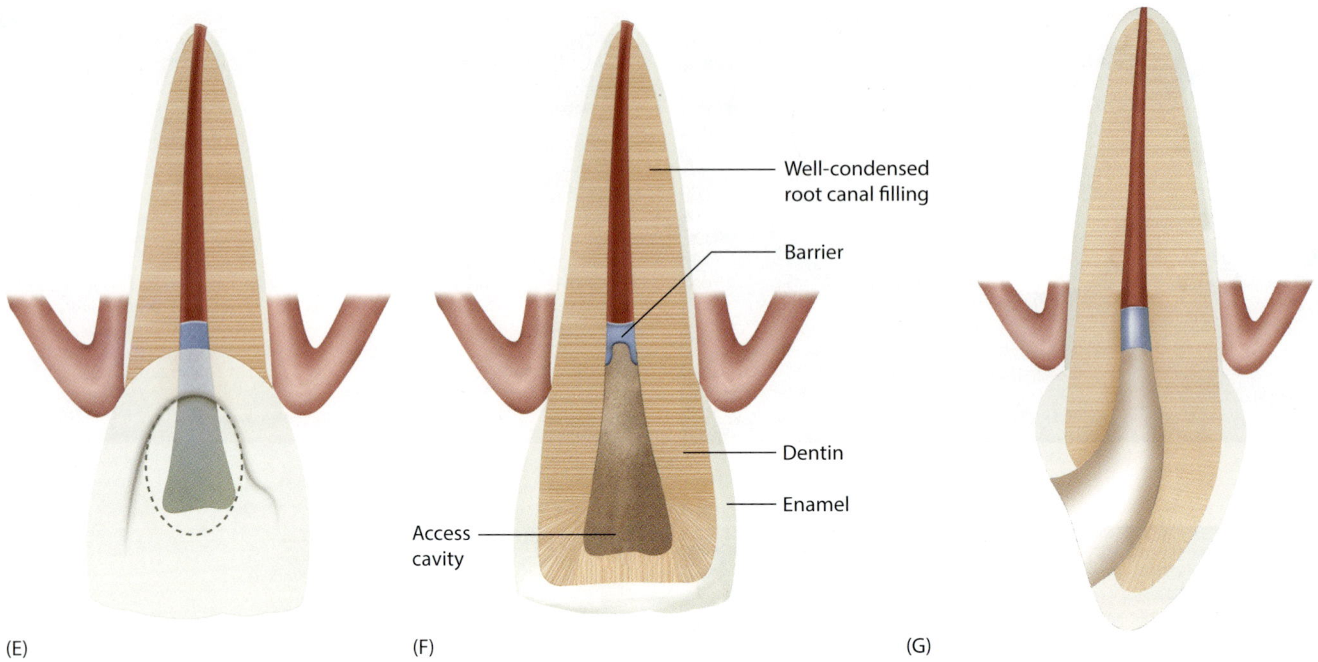

Figure 8.1 continued

Long-term success with intracoronal bleaching. (E) All existing restorative material is removed. Root filling is removed to 2 mm apical to cementoenamel junction. A small quantity of glass ionomer is packed to form a 1.5–2.00 mm sealing plug. (F) The design of the barrier from the facial view (E) or the palatal view (F) and from the proximal view (G).

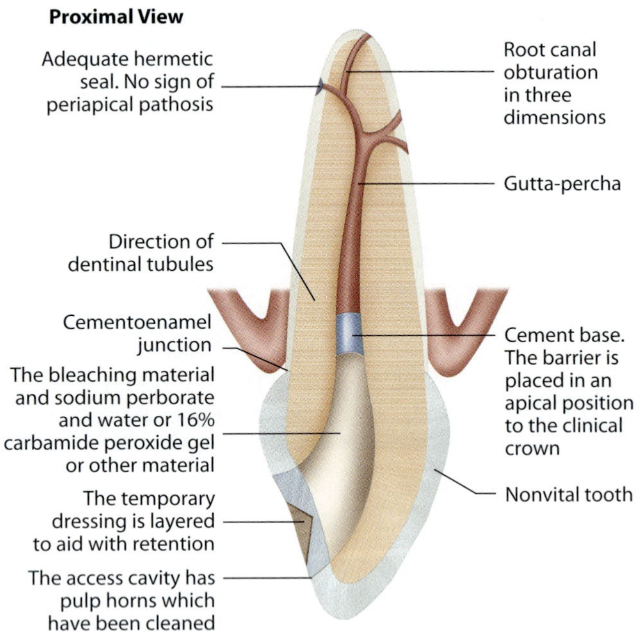

Figure 8.2

The walking bleach technique.

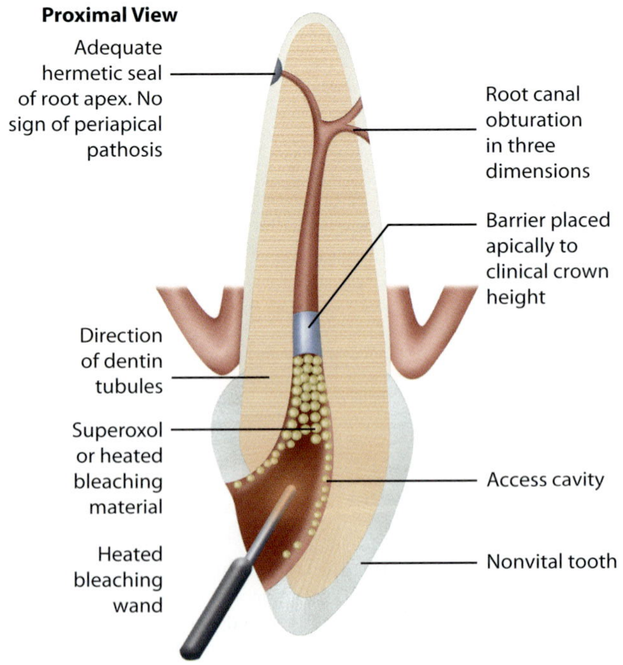

Figure 8.3

The thermocatalytic technique. This technique using heat, a heated instrument, and high concentration is no longer recommended because the possible heat generated could cause damage to the surrounding tissues and lead to possible cervical resorption.

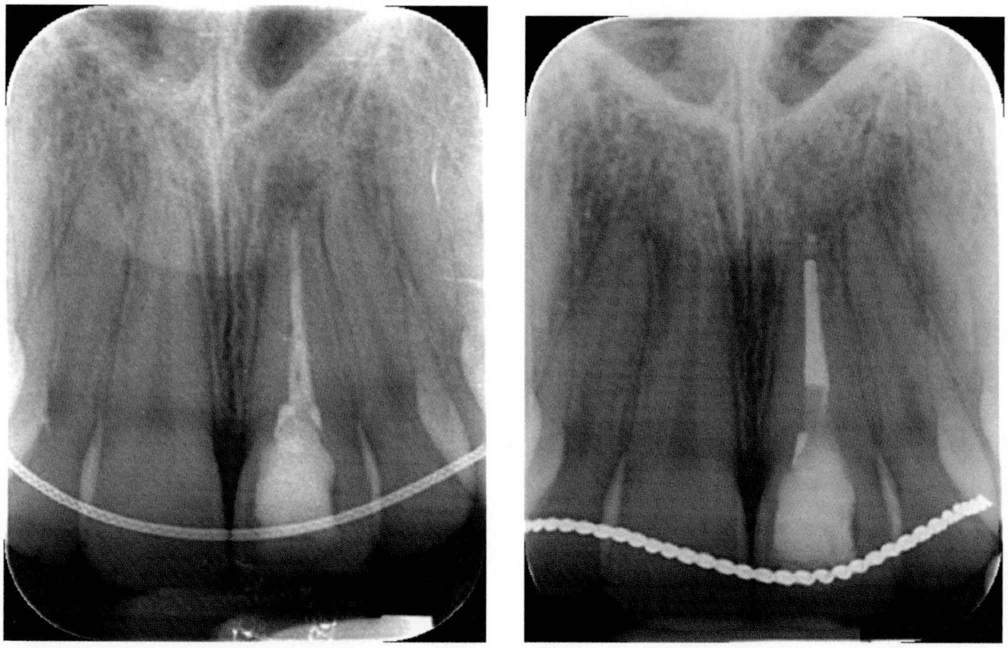

(A) (B)

Figure 8.4

(A) This patient's maxillary left central incisor tooth (tooth 9) became nonvital during her orthodontic treatment at the age of 13. Radiograph before assessment for undertaking internal bleaching. This tooth is unsuitable to be bleached at present because it shows a periapical radiolucency and a poorly condensed root canal filling. The endodontic treatment should be re-treated, allowing for healing for 1 month and no further symptoms before proceeding to the bleaching treatment. (B) Results after the treatment and preparation of the barrier. The barrier should be 2–3 mm below the cementoenamel junction and at least 2 mm in thickness to protect the surrounding dentin. Once the tooth had been successfully lightened, a new fixed retainer was placed onto the tooth. The periapical radiolucency has resolved.

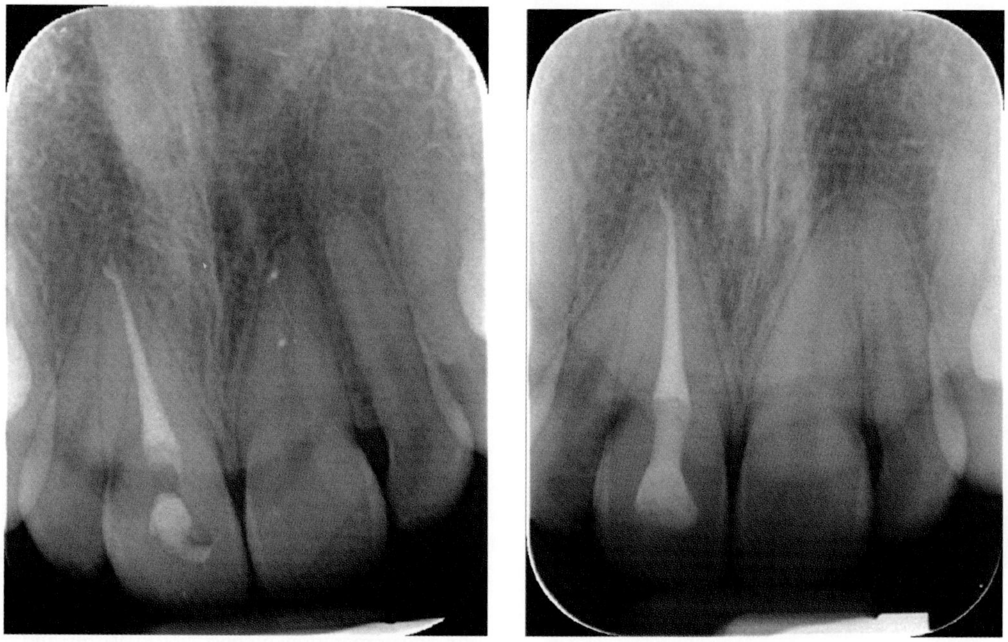

(A) (B)

Figure 8.5

(A) Radiograph taken after completion of the root canal treatment. Patient had traumatized the maxillary right central incisor during a sporting injury. The tooth needed to be endodontically treated and had become discolored as a result of the trauma. Treatment involved preparing the barrier of the root canal first, using a glass ionomer light-cured material shaped into a bobsled design to follow the shape of the cementoenamel junction. The barrier was 2 mm in thickness and placed 2 mm below the cementoenamel junction. Enough space was given for the bleaching material, which was sealed into the tooth and a glass ionomer restoration was placed as a temporary cover. (B) Periapical radiograph taken a year later as a follow-up shows the barrier preparation.

continued on the next page

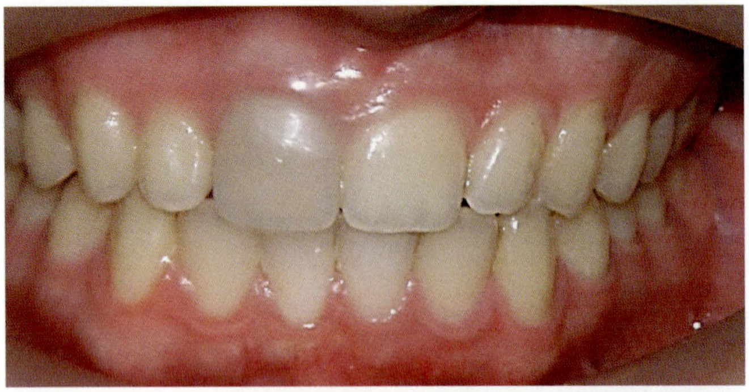

(C)

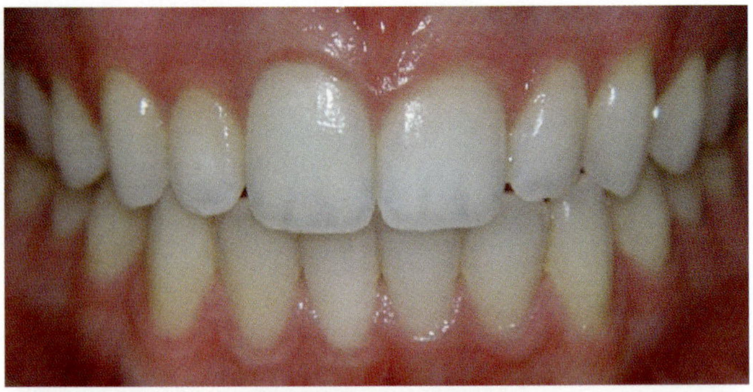

(D)

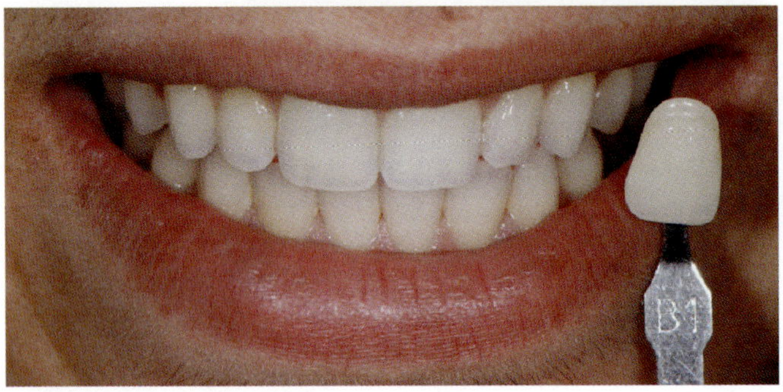

(E)

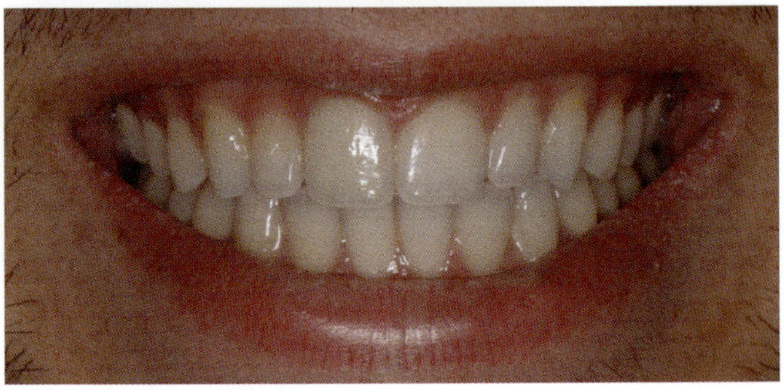

(F)

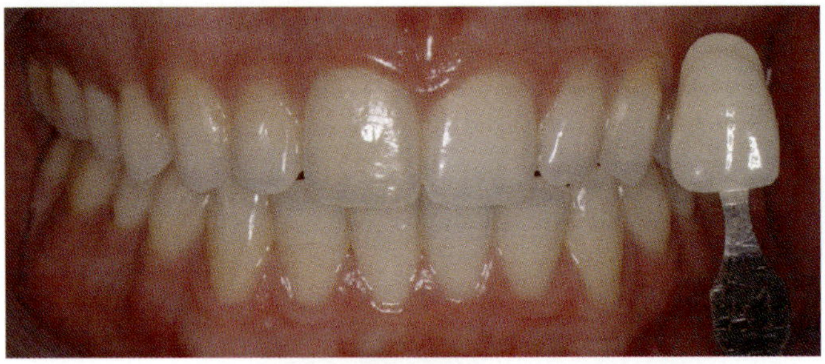

(G)

Figure 8.5 continued

(C) Appearance of all the teeth before bleaching. Nonvital bleaching was administered using 16% carbamide peroxide sealed into the access cavity. This was followed by home bleaching using 10% carbamide peroxide in trays for a period of 2 weeks on the upper and 3 weeks on the lower teeth. (D) Appearance of the teeth after nonvital bleaching and home bleaching of upper and lower teeth. (E) Appearance of the smile at the end of treatment showing the final shade at B1. (F) Appearance of the smile 5 years later. No further bleaching had been undertaken. (G) Appearance of the teeth 5 years later showing the final shade at A1. No further bleaching had been undertaken.

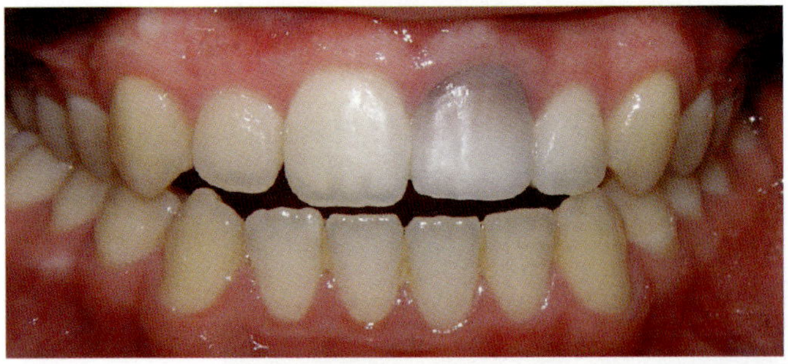

(A)

Figure 8.6

(A) An attempt had been made to undertake a nonvital bleaching on the maxillary left central incisor. The gray area at the cervical neck area shows that the glass ionomer barrier had not been placed deep enough below the cementoenamel junction (CEJ). There are problems associated with undertaking nonvital bleaching for a single tooth only. It is difficult to match the single tooth to the other teeth. It is more realistic to undertake bleaching for the upper and lower teeth. That way there is better control of the shade of the teeth and all the teeth can match the new lighter shade. In this case the barrier was prepared below the CEJ by 2 mm. It is difficult to re-prepare the barrier because the barrier needs to be prepared with either a long bur in a fast handpiece similar to a crown preparation bur or a gooseneck slow-speed bur. The preparation method should be stop and start because visibility and access are difficult. An endodontic probe can be used to check the internal surface of the access cavity and prevent potential perforation of the tooth structure.

continued on the next page

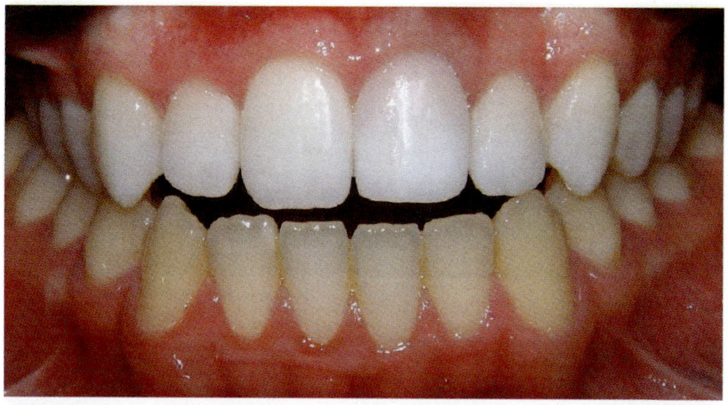

(B)

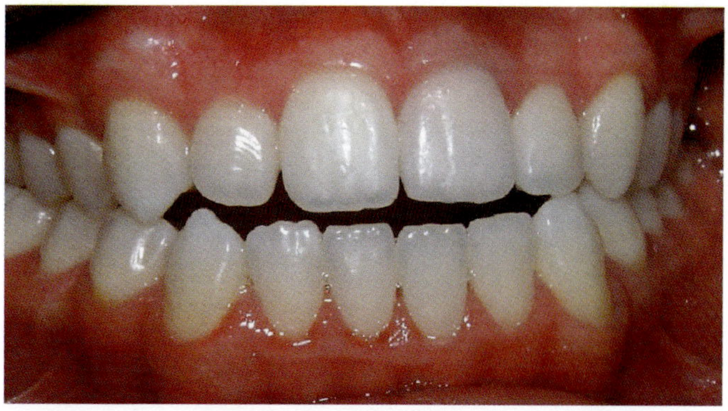

(C)

Figure 8.6 continued

(B) The barrier was re-prepared and the tooth was bleached using the seal-in technique. Sixteen percent carbamide peroxide was sealed into the access cavity. Upper and lower bleaching trays were made. The maxillary teeth were bleached first. The picture shows the result of the nonvital bleaching, which was undertaken for the second time. In addition, the upper bleaching was performed using 10% carbamide peroxide in the bleaching tray. (C) The result of the upper and lower bleaching completed using 10% carbamide peroxide as the home bleaching agent.

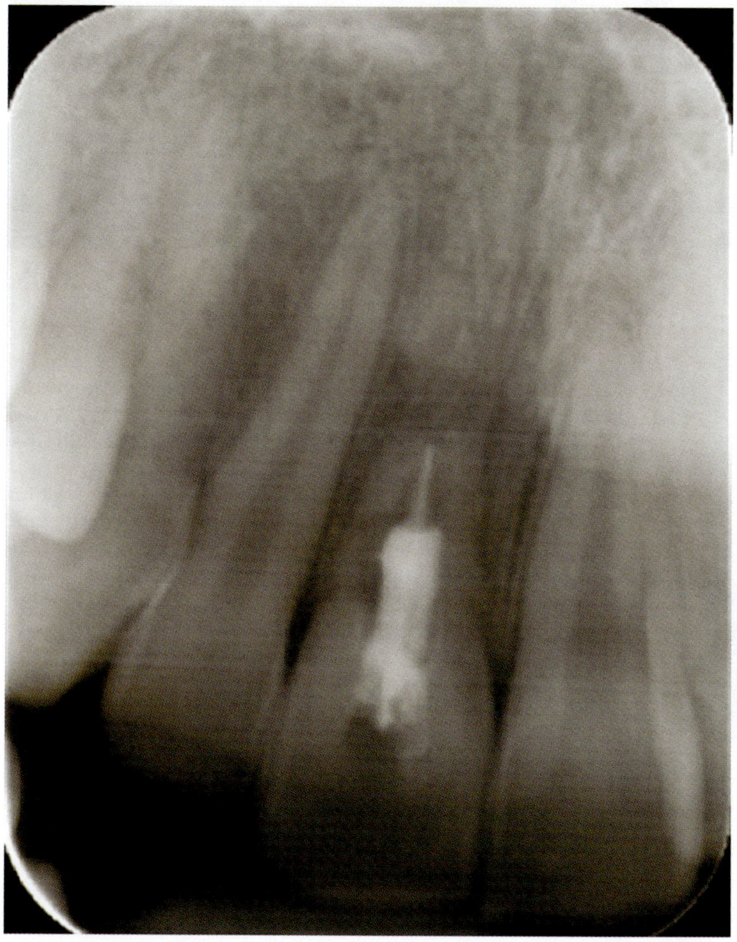

(A)

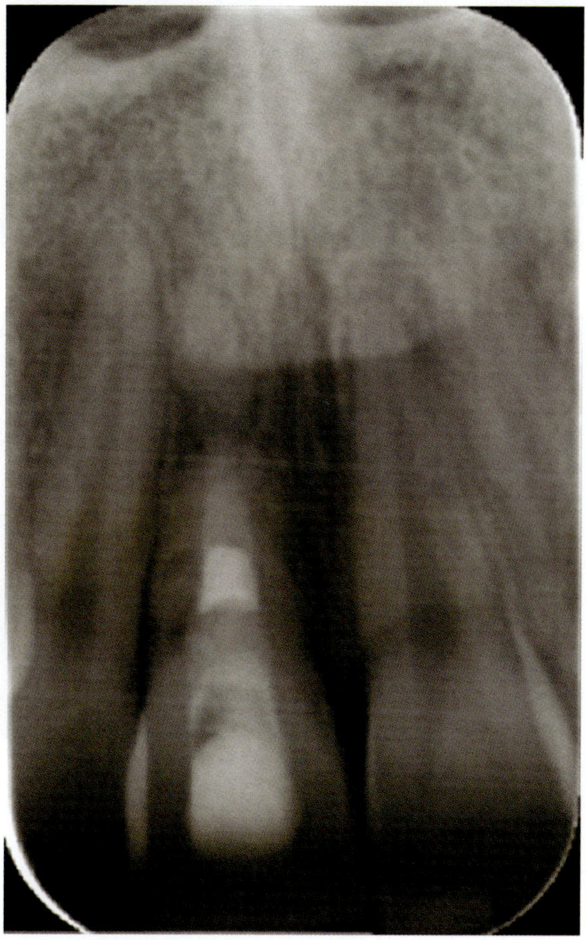

(B)

Figure 8.7

(A) Periapical radiograph shows the appearance of the tooth at presentation. A 14-year-old patient had experienced trauma to the tooth at age 10. The trauma was so severe that the root separated. An attempt at endodontic treatment was made; the radiograph shows that the endodontic treatment is incomplete. Because the presenting tooth was very dark and the child was teased at school it was decided to attempt to improve the endodontic therapy first. (B) The existing root canal material was removed and the tooth was dressed with calcium hydroxide for a period of 3 months in an attempt to heal the area of resorption.

continued on the next page

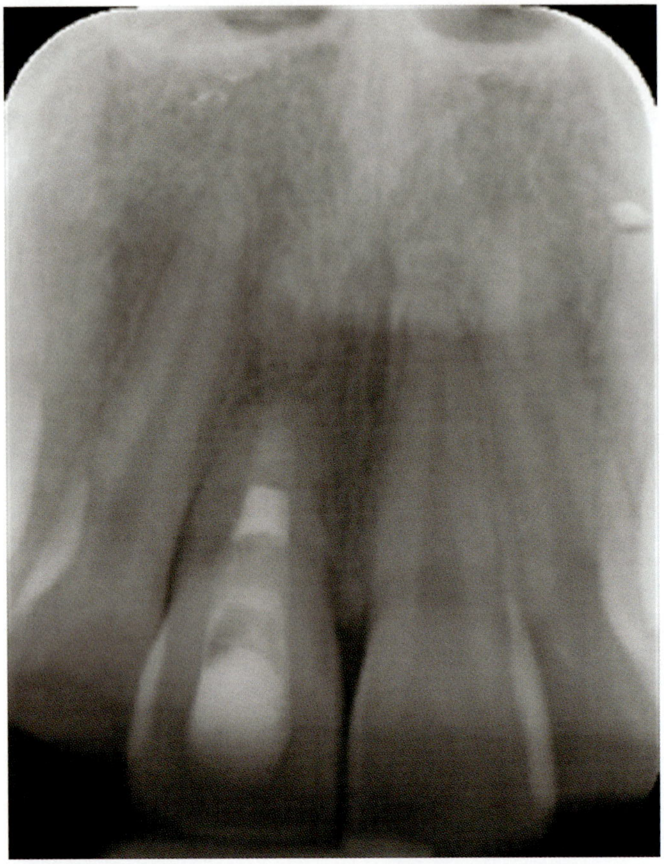
(C)

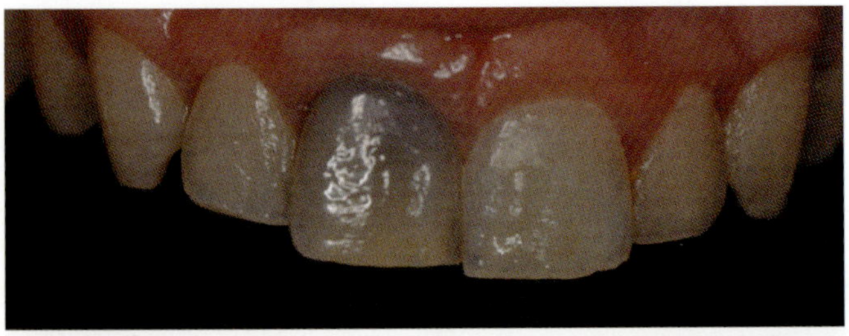
(D)

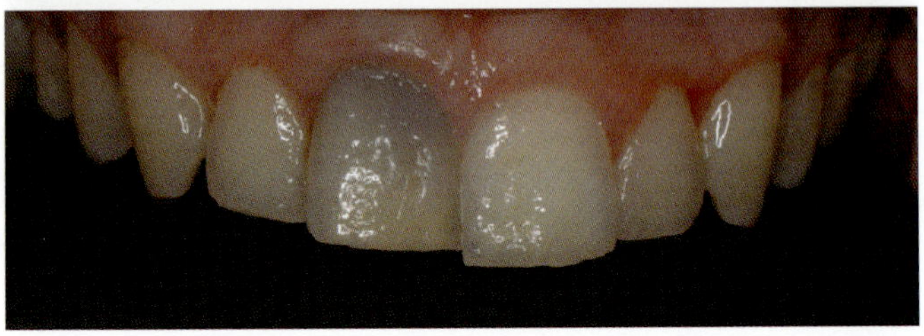
(E)

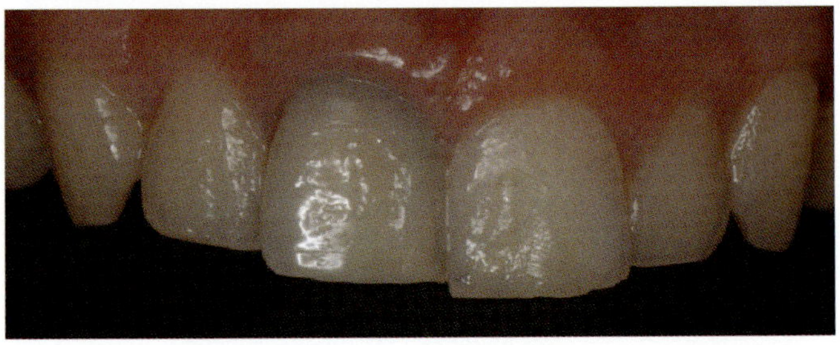
(F)

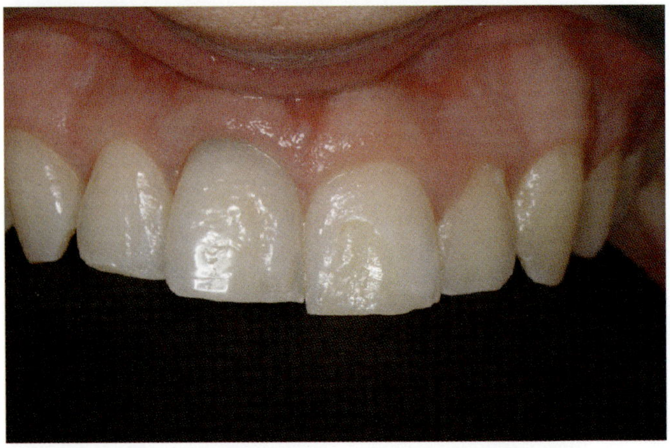
(G)

Figure 8.7 continued

(C) Once healing had taken place it was decided to do a conventional root canal treatment. Even though the tooth had a guarded prognosis, it was better to attempt to save the tooth because the child was very young and the tooth needed to remain in place at least until the age of 22 years, when an implant could be placed. A thick barrier was placed and the tooth was filled with calcium hydroxide to wait for further healing. After another 6 months, the tooth was asymptomatic and external bleaching only was undertaken. (D) Appearance of the teeth at presentation. (E) After 6 months the tooth was bleached using a bleaching tray with no internal bleaching. This shows a slight improvement of the shade of the tooth. The patient bleached his tooth for 1 week only using 10% carbamide peroxide. (F) After another 6 months and further healing, it was decided to undertake nonvital bleaching. The access cavity was cleaned and 16% carbamide peroxide was placed in the access cavity for a period of 1 week. (G) The final improvement in the shade of the tooth. Although the result was not perfect, this was an acceptable improvement for the patient. The tooth will need to be monitored every 6 months, and follow-up radiographs will be taken annually for 5 years.

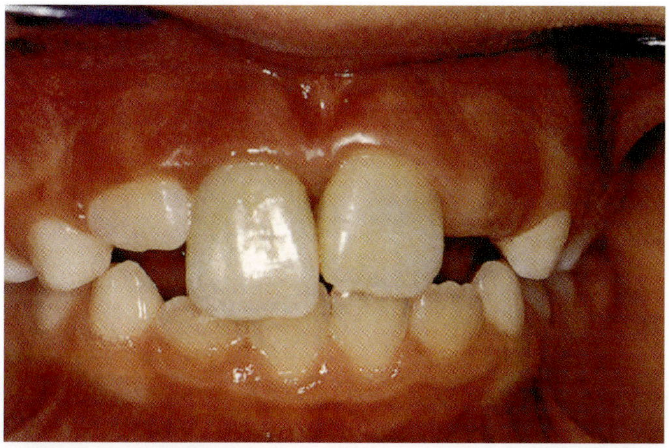

(A)

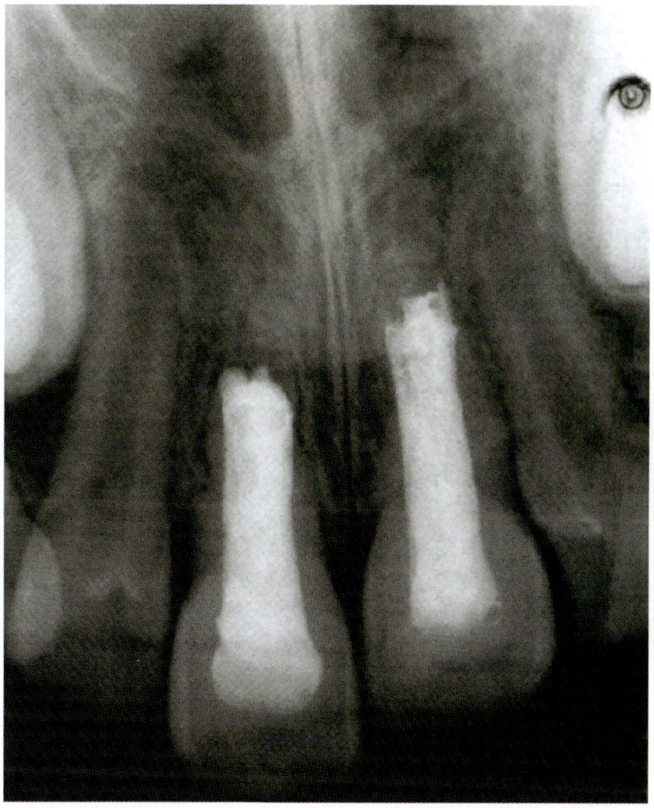

(B)

Figure 8.8

Contraindications to bleaching. (A) This young patient fell onto her two front teeth. The trauma caused the teeth to become devitalized. Because the roots were still immature and apexogenesis had not occurred, the roots remained short and were not yet fully closed. With such a severe traumatic impact and short roots, it is probably best not to attempt intracoronal bleaching. (B) Periapical radiograph of the root-treated teeth.

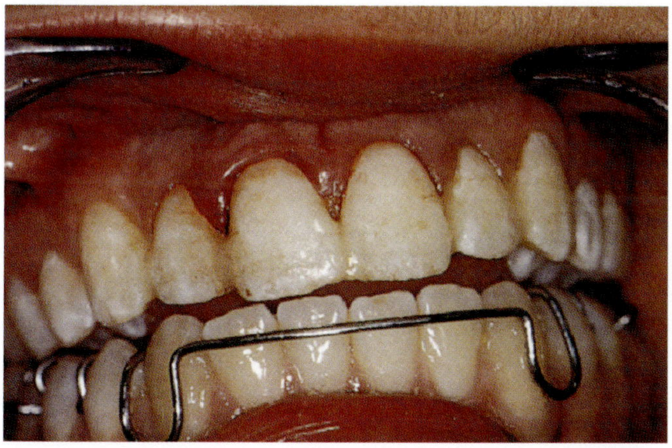

Figure 8.9

This patient tripped and fell onto a hard surface. The upper right central incisor was avulsed completely and the upper left incisor pushed forward out of occlusion. The teeth are shown immediately after the right central was reinserted and the left central was repositioned. The teeth were splinted lightly with composite material. Because the patient had completed orthodontic treatment recently, she was still wearing a retainer. The upper retainer acted as a splint for several weeks. Because of the unpredictable prognosis of these teeth, it is probably best not to attempt intracoronal bleaching.

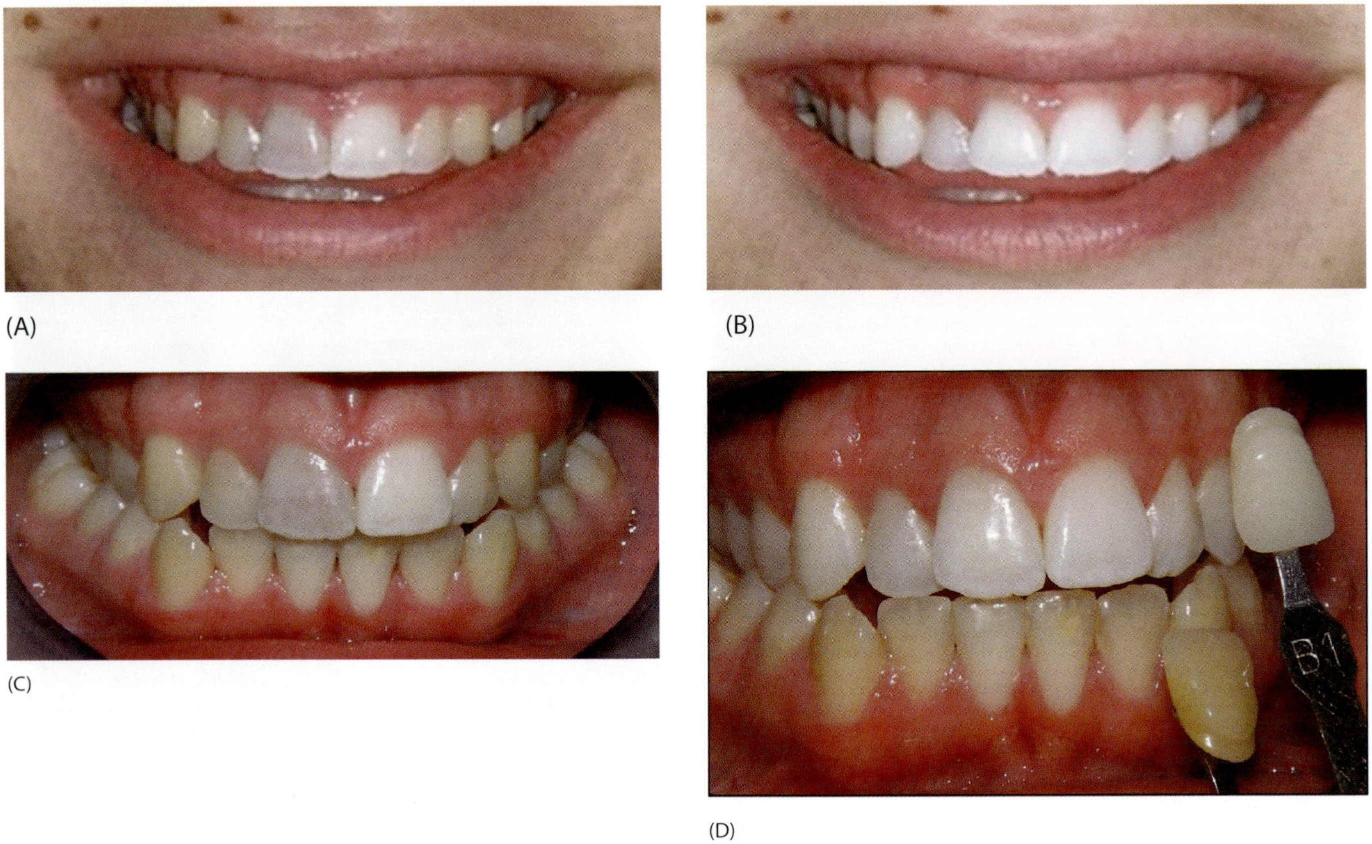

Figure 8.10

(A) The patient after trauma to the maxillary right central incisor sustained in a sporting injury. (B) The portrait view showing the smile at the end of treatment—the results after the root canal treatment to the maxillary right central incisor and the nonvital bleaching treatment that was undertaken. (C) Appearance of the teeth after the completion of the root canal treatment to the maxillary right central incisor. (D) Results of the nonvital bleaching to the maxillary central incisor and the rest of the maxillary teeth. No bleaching was undertaken on the lower teeth.

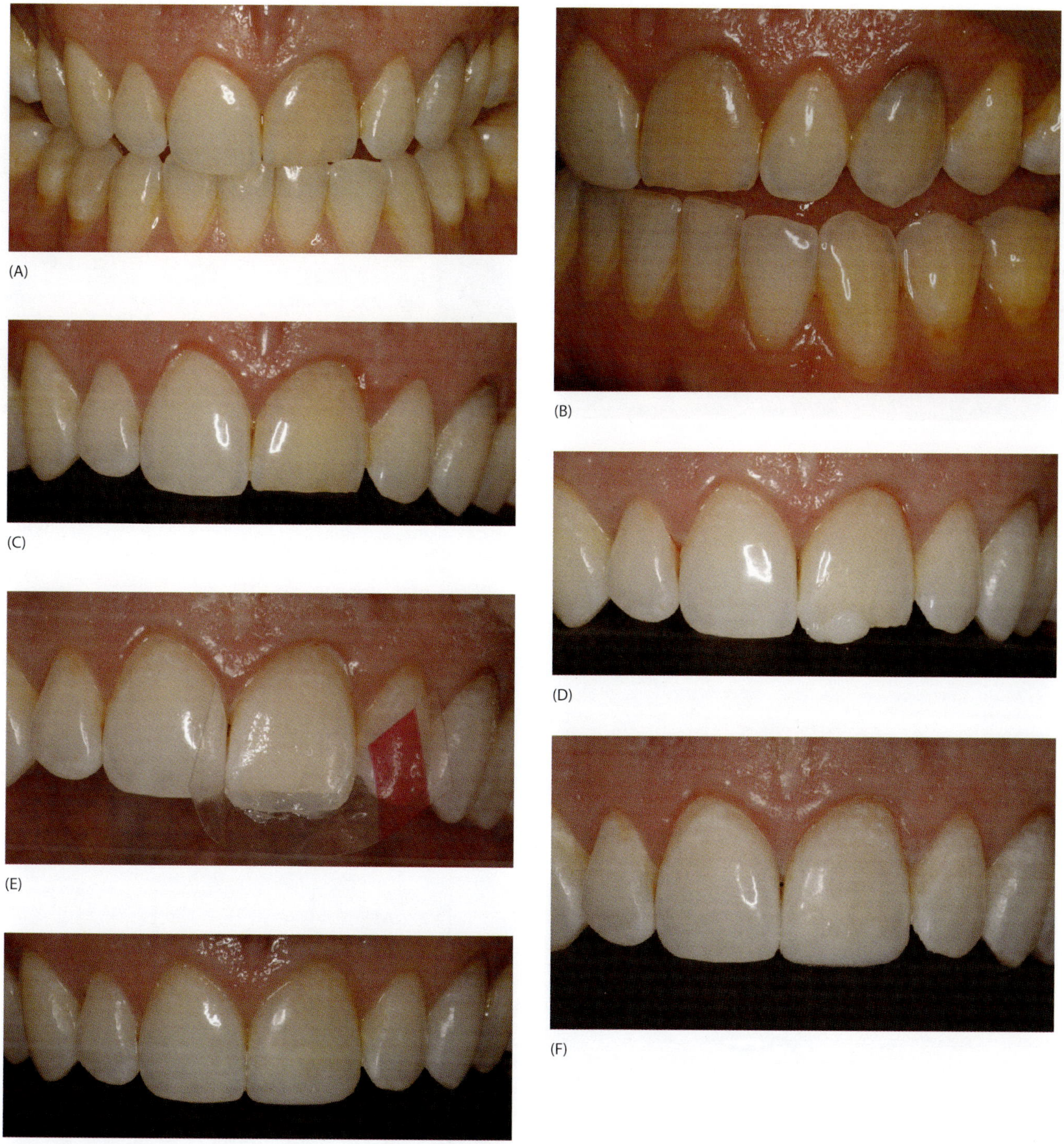

Figure 8.11

(A and B) This patient was unhappy with the appearance of the maxillary left central incisor and canine teeth. Both teeth had previously experienced trauma and had needed endodontic treatment. An assessment was made of the quality of the endodontic treatment; it was decided that the central incisor endodontic treatment was satisfactory but that the maxillary left canine needed to be re-treated. (C) Completion of endodontic treatment before the bleaching treatment. Nonvital bleaching was undertaken on both the central and maxillary left canine teeth. Nonvital bleaching was undertaken by sealing 16% carbamide peroxide into the pulp chamber and making a specially prepared bleaching tray with windows so that only the dark teeth were bleached first. Thereafter, when the two single teeth had bleached sufficiently, the rest of the upper and lower teeth were bleached using normal scalloped bleaching trays. (D) At the end of the bleaching treatment and after allowing sufficient time for the oxygen to dissipate from the tooth, the maxillary central incisor was repaired with a composite bonding. This was followed by making the patient an upper Michigan bite splint to protect the patient from further grinding. (E) The first layer of composite was placed from the palatal section using a clear matrix strip. Thereafter, a dentin layer was placed but mamelons were built into the the incisal structure because the incisal tip showed translucency. (F) Completion of the bleaching and completion of the composite bond on the maxillary left central incisor. (G) Appearance of the teeth 1 year later.

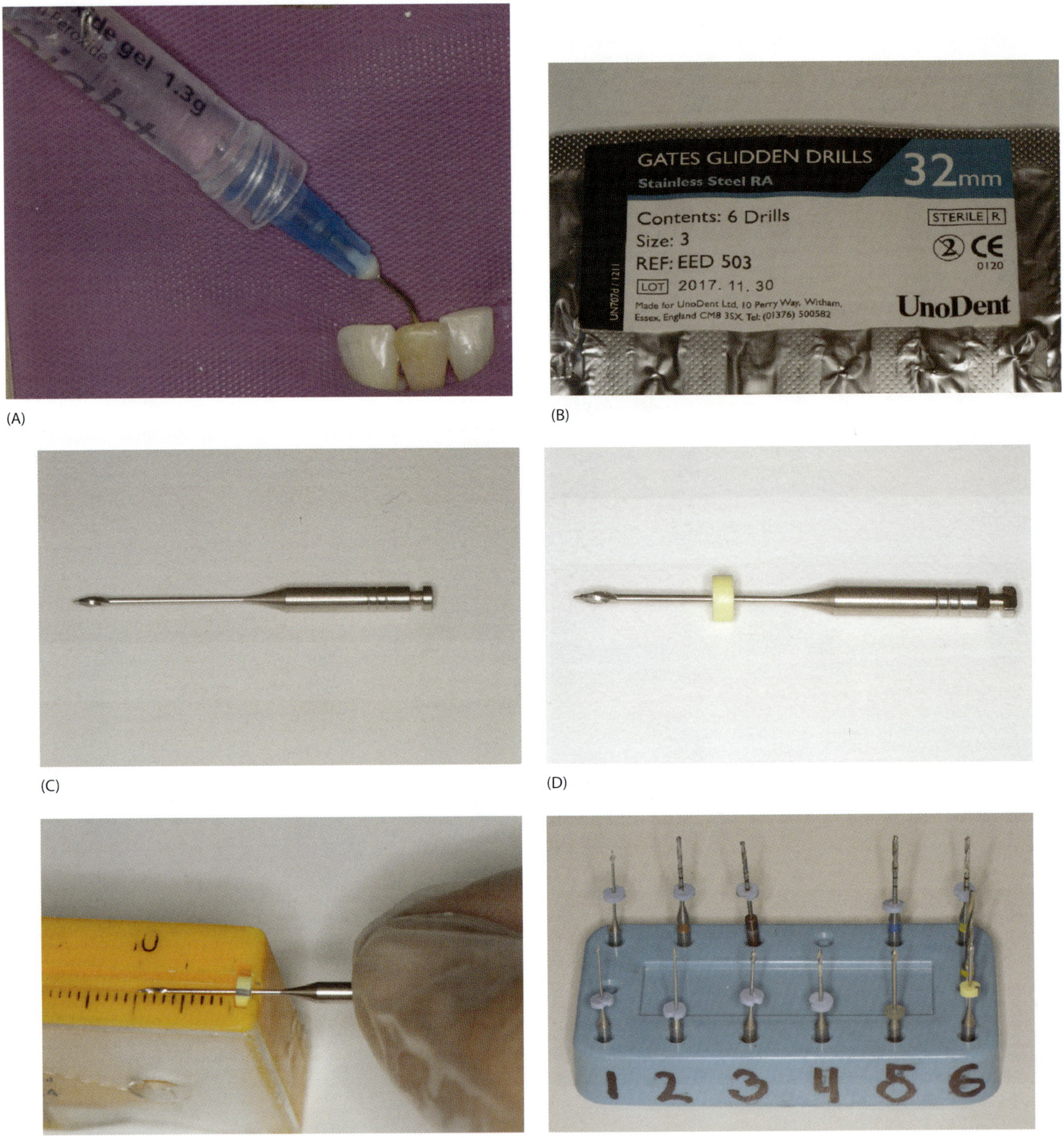

Figure 8.12

(A) Prior to placing any bleaching gel into the tooth, it is important to prepare a barrier. This figure shows a bleaching gel syringe with a smaller diameter syringe tip that has been placed in order to insert the material more effectively into the access cavity of the tooth. (B) Gates Glidden burs can be used for preparation of the barrier to be placed directly over the gutta-percha root canal material. (C) Size 3 Gates Glidden bur without stopper. (D) Rubber stopper placed at 10 mm on the size 3 Gates Glidden bur. (E) The rubber stopper is used to measure the length of the barrier in the specially designated holder for measuring. This measuring device is also used for measuring the length of posts for preparation. (F) Armamentarium used in the walking bleach procedure. A magnetized autoclavable bur stand places all instruments together for efficient use: Gates Glidden burs in ascending order, labeled in black marker pen on the holder. Each size has a stripe near the end for easy identification. The end tip has a safe cutting edge that will not destroy excess dentin. ParaPost burs can be used (shown in the row farther back). The first used is the smallest ParaPost bur, which is the brown bur (size 4), then the yellow bur (size 5), then the blue bur (size 6), just for the initial removal of the gutta-percha. *continued on the next page*

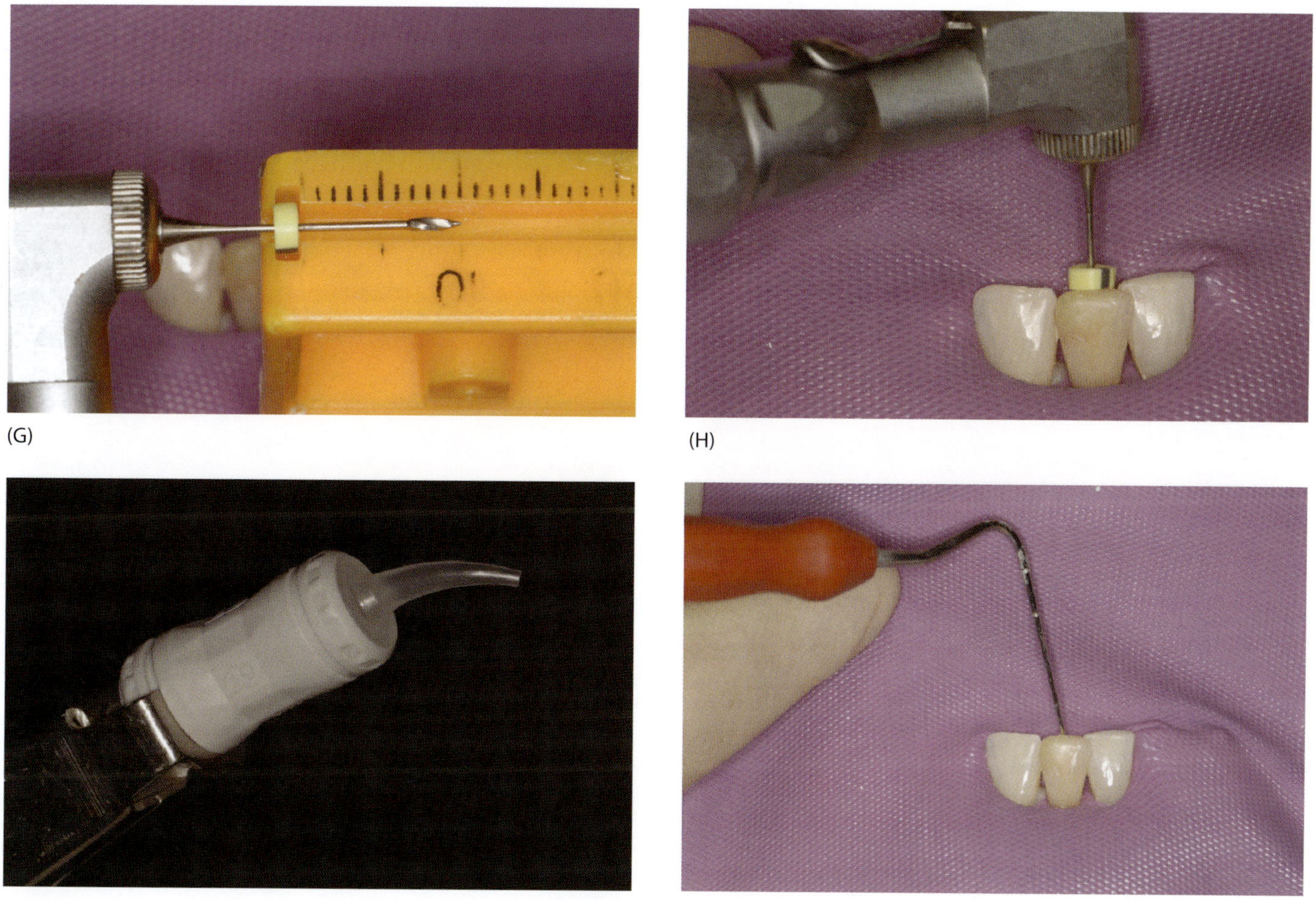

(G) (H) (I) (J)

Figure 8.12 continued

(G) Normally after satisfactory completion of the root canal procedure the size 3 Gates Glidden bur is used first to the correct size. Before the procedure is started, the length of the clinical crown is measured without the dental dam in place. The clinical crown is normally approximately 10–12 mm in length. Because the barrier needs to be 2–3 mm in thickness and the barrier needs to be 3 mm below the cementoenamel junction, the actual length is calculated as 10 + 3 + 3 = 16 mm, where 10 mm = clinical crown, 3 mm = area below the cementoenamel junction for placement of the clinical crown, and 3 mm = thickness of the barrier. Therefore, preparation of the barrier in length is similar to preparation of a post for the tooth. This figure shows the ruler device used to measure the length of the Gates Glidden bur for barrier placement. The size 3 Gates Glidden bur is placed into the holder, and 10 mm is measured first. (H) Preparation for intracoronal bleaching technique. The dental dam is placed on the teeth and they are well isolated. Care is taken that the dam fits tightly at the cervical margin. Rubber wedges can be used to keep the dam in place. The coronal access cavity and restoration are removed. The gutta-percha is situated just underneath the restoration. All restorative material is removed from the access cavity. The dentin should be exposed and the access cavity refined. The gutta-percha can be removed in several ways: by using a heated instrument (electric or manual) directly onto the gutta-percha, or by using Gates Glidden burs measured to the exact barrier depth (about 3 mm below the cementoenamel junction). This figure shows the Gates Glidden bur being inserted. A rubber stopper is placed onto the bur to reach the correct length. Orange solvent, chloroform, or xylene can be used to dissolve the sealer remnants. The pulp remnants can be removed with an excavator as shown here or with an ultrasonic cleaning device. It has been suggested that a small calcium hydroxide layer be placed directly over the gutta-percha before the barrier is placed, but this is empirical. (I) Encapsulated chemically cured glass ionomer material is used for the barrier placement in this case. (J) The material is placed at the correct depth snugly, using a flat plastic or an endodontic plugger. The endodontic plugger (with the red handle) is also shown. This one has a finer diameter.

continued on the next page

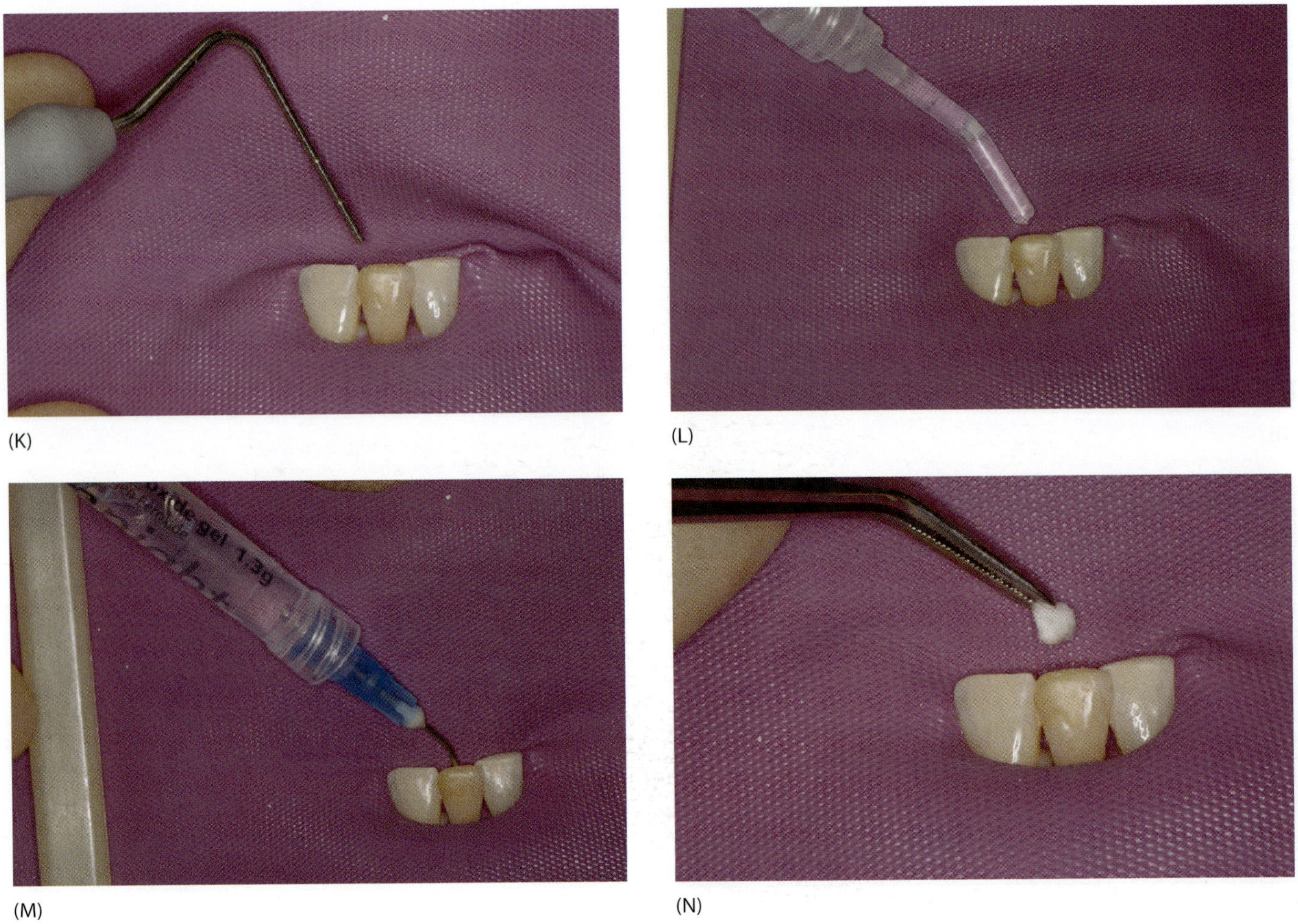

(K) (L) (M) (N)

Figure 8.12 continued

(K) Endodontic plugger with a thicker base is used to plug the glass ionomer barrier down into place; the thinner plugger is then used to ensure that there is no excess on the access cavity walls and that the barrier has a bobsled shape to follow the dentinal odontoblasts at the cervical edge. (L) Once the material is set and the excess scraped away, the intracoronal bleaching material can be placed directly from the bleaching syringe. (M) The bleaching material is placed directly into the access cavity with the bleaching syringe, which has been modified by using a finer tip for easier placement directly into the access cavity. This way fewer voids are placed. (N) Excess gel is removed by tamping with a cotton pellet. This also compresses the gel into all areas of the pulp chamber. Excess bleaching material is removed from the pulp horn and gingival area.

continued on the next page

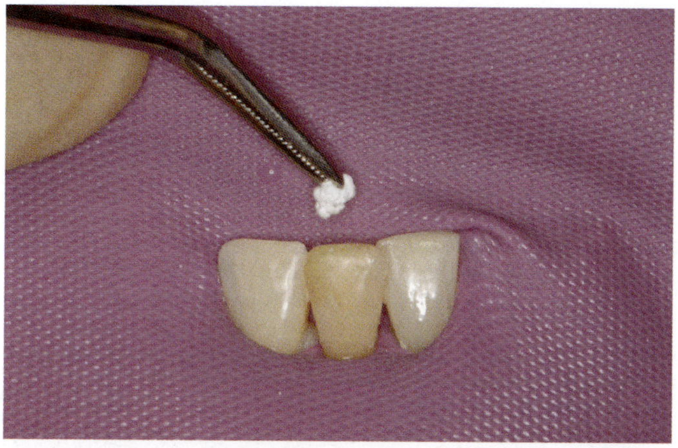

(O)

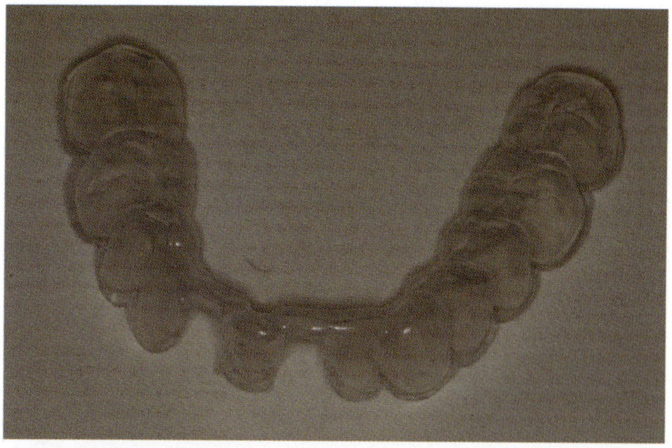

(P)

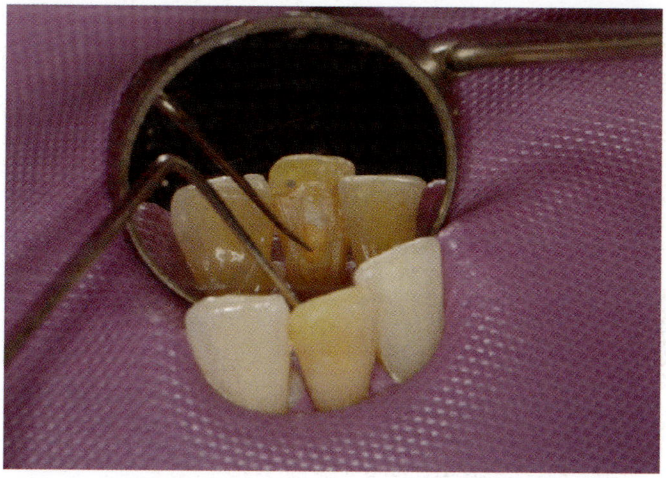

(Q)

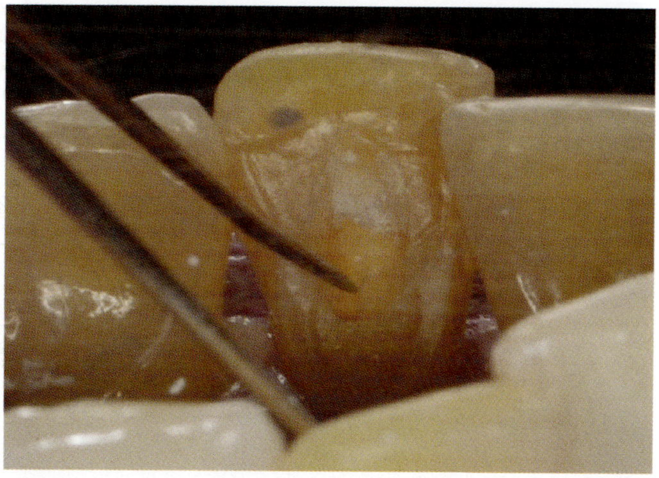

(R)

Figure 8.12 continued

(O) Alternatively, excess material can be plugged down with polytetrafluoroethylene (PTFE) tape rolled into a ball. This is also used directly over the gel before the glass ionomer dressing is placed for ease of placement for the temporary dressing. The glass ionomer is then placed into the access cavity directly with the capsule tip, then this is smoothed with a flat plastic and the material is light cured. A temporary dressing is placed over this to seal the access cavity. This can be sealed with a bonding agent to prevent oxygen escaping; a chemically cured material is used to protect it while it sets. (P) The patient is given a specially constructed bleaching tray that has windows in the design on either side of the dark tooth so that only the dark, nonvital tooth will be bleached with the bleaching tray. This is a lot of coverage from the buccal and the lingual surface. The patient can use 16% carbamide peroxide or 6% hydrogen peroxide in the bleaching tray to speed up the bleaching process from the labial aspect. (Q) When the patient returns after 2 weeks, there are small defects in the restoration where the oxygen has escaped despite placement of bonding agent over the palatal surface. The rubber dam is applied onto the teeth again and the temporary dressing removed. The bleaching material can be changed, or if satisfactory lightening has occurred, the bleaching material is removed. The pulp chamber is rinsed out with water or sodium hypochlorite, and a restoration can be placed into the coronal access cavity. Glass ionomer can be used as a base over the barrier into the full access cavity. (R) An endodontic probe is used to remove the excess temporary material and clean the excess gel from the tooth before the dressing is changed. The access cavity should be clean and free from residual gel.

continued on the next page

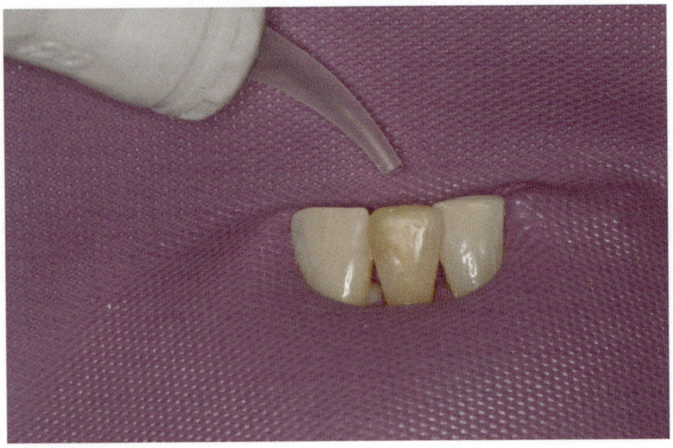

(S)

Figure 8.12 continued

(S) Glass ionomer is used to close the access cavity after completion of the nonvital bleaching because it seals the tooth better. Because after nonvital bleaching there is excess oxygen in the access cavity and clinical crown, it is not advisable to place a composite restoration immediately after completing the nonvital bleaching. This is because with the excess oxygen the enamel bond strength is weakened by 20% and so the coronal restoration will start leaking immediately, causing shade regression almost immediately. Beverages and food will enter the coronal restoration almost immediately, and the coronal seal will be compromised. At a later stage, at least 1 month, composite material can be placed into the access cavity of the tooth. A segmental buildup technique should be employed. The glass ionomer is left at the base of the cavity and the material is then cut back and the enamel and cavosurface margin are etched. A bonding agent is then applied with a fine brush. Composite material is packed into the tooth using a segmental buildup.

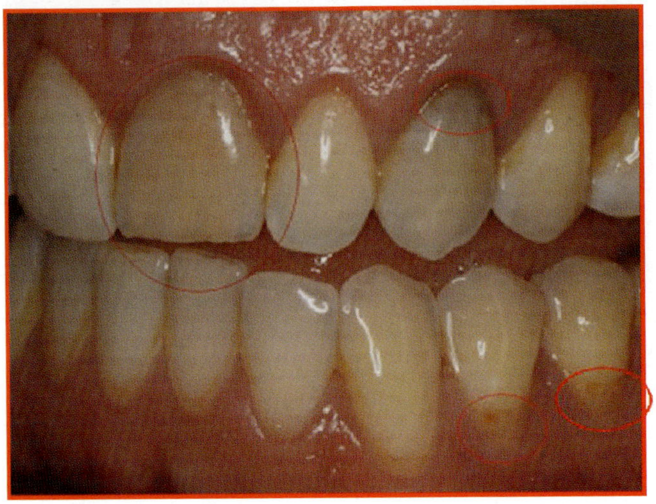

Figure 8.13

Two nonvital teeth 21 and 23. The treatment options are internal bleaching using a bleaching tray; sealed-in bleaching; external bleaching only; combined bleaching; and direct bonding, Componeer (Coltene), or porcelain veneer instead of bleaching. There is no guarantee of the amount of bleaching that can be achieved.

9 SINGLE TOOTH WHITENING OF VITAL TEETH

Linda Greenwall

Many vital teeth experience some degree of mild trauma at some stage. This trauma, which is normally an impact, causes bleeding into the pulp and dentin of the tooth, causing the single tooth to become slightly discolored. It is this slight difference in shade of two adjacent teeth that indicates that there has been some degree of trauma to the tooth. This chapter will explain the trauma process and will outline the process taken to whiten a single vital tooth.

There is a place for whitening single vital and nonvital teeth, but often this treatment needs to be integrated with full whitening of the upper and lower teeth. A specially designed whitening tray can be made to whiten just the single tooth, and the sequencing and timing of the treatment are essential if an excellent result is to be achieved. The aim of treatment is to obtain an even shade of whiteness so that adjacent teeth are a similar matching shade.

HISTORY AND DIAGNOSIS

The tooth normally has sustained some type of mild trauma previously; typically, a single tooth has been knocked. The patient may not necessarily remember the initial trauma but may recall it by the second appointment. The pathologic process is known as calcific metamorphosis (CM).

PROCESS OF DISCOLORATION

The tooth experiences trauma. Bleeding occurs within the tooth. The tooth tries to protect itself by laying down protective dentin. This is laid down in the form of secondary and tertiary dentin. The dentin also coats the pulp chamber, and often the pulp chamber appears almost obliterated (see Figure 9.10E). The blood within the tooth breaks down and the hemolysis releases iron, which reacts with hydrogen sulfide, which breaks down to iron sulfide. If the tooth survives the injury, there is rapid deposition of tertiary dentin near the root canal to protect it from the injury and to encourage healing. This is the reason the tooth becomes gray; as the tooth reorganizes, the color can change from black to brown to yellow. The patient is left with a single tooth that has a slightly different color from that of its neighbor. This color difference often is subtle.

VITALITY TESTING

These teeth are normally vital, but because of the trauma the pulp chamber may be calcified or reduced in size. As a result there will be a slower response from the electric pulp tester.

Normally the dial is turned up to the end reading before the patient reports that he or she can feel the electric current vaguely. It is important to take time in testing the response of the patient because the patient will need time to register the reading. The same is true for the cold or ice test, when a cold cotton pellet which has been soaked in ethyl chloride is placed on the tooth. It will eventually respond and the patient will report that he or she can feel the cold.

RADIOGRAPHIC ASSESSMENT

A periapical radiograph will normally demonstrate canal calcification or obliteration. The whole tooth should be present on the radiograph and there should be no evidence of any type of fracture in the tooth, either in the crown or in the root (see Figure 9.7B). There is normally no periapical area present. The root of the tooth is intact and there is no evidence of external or internal root resorption. Often the pulp chamber appears almost completely obliterated, but a very faint line in the middle can be discerned. Other times a dentin bridge may occur across the margin between the crown and the root.

THE PATHOLOGIC PROCESS

The usual process is that a minor trauma causes some type of bleeding within the tooth (see Figure 9.1). This bleeding causes secondary and tertiary dentin to be laid down within the pulp canal (see Figures 9.1 and 9.2). The secondary dentin is laid down regularly along the dentinal walls as a response to the trauma to protect the sensitive pulp tissue from further damage. This causes the pulp chamber and canal to gradually diminish in size until only a narrow root canal remains. It becomes calcified or sometimes even obliterated.

Histologically, the pulps have an increase in the amount of collagen and varying cell sizes (Lundberg and Cvek 1980). There seems to be no justification for root canal treatment of these teeth (Cvek 2007). Periapical radiolucencies have been reported in only 13–16% of teeth with traumatically induced pulp canal obliteration during observation periods of up to 20 years according to Jacobsen and Kerekes (1977). According to Cvek (2007), the periapical radiolucency that occurs later is associated with caries, inadequate crown restoration, or new trauma.

CM can also be known as dystrophic calcification. It is seen commonly in the dental pulp after traumatic tooth injuries and can be recognized clinically as early as 3 months after injury (Amir et al. 2001). CM is characterized by deposition of hard tissue within the root canal space and yellow discoloration of the clinical crown (see Figure 9.9).

According to Amir et al. (2001), opinion differs among practitioners as to whether to treat these cases on early detection of CM or to observe them until symptoms or radiographic signs of pulpal necrosis are detected.

INCIDENCE OF CALCIFIC METAMORPHOSIS

Approximately 3.8% to 24% of traumatized teeth develop varying degrees of CM (Amir et al. 2001). Studies indicate that of these, approximately 1–16% will develop pulpal necrosis. Pulpal necrosis can be assessed through a radiograph and clinical symptoms.

It is normally not necessary to do root canal treatment for these teeth. Most of the literature does not support endodontic intervention unless periradicular pathosis is detected or the involved tooth becomes symptomatic (Amir et al. 2001). It may be advisable to manage cases conservatively by demonstrating CM through observation and periodic examination and radiographs as necessary.

However, the discoloration in teeth with obliterated pulp chambers is not always caused by pigments from the blood degradation products but may be caused by the presence of secondary and tertiary dentin that has been laid down after the trauma (Dahl and Pallesen 2007). It may be that the light being transmitted through such a tooth gives it a darker appearance.

RESEARCH AND INCIDENCE OF THE OCCURRENCE

The response to minor trauma many years previously can result in the development of dystrophic calcification in 3.8–27% of traumatized teeth (Amir et al. 2001). Up to 16% of cases can develop pulp necrosis (Amir et al. 2001). Robertson and colleagues found that 51% responded to normal electric pulp testing and 40% were clinically and radiographically sound (Robertson et 1996), with tertiary dentin formation occurring (Torneck 1990).

TREATMENT

Table 9.1 shows the options for treatment. It is important to decide whether only the single dark tooth is to be whitened or whether the entire arch is to be whitened. It is more difficult to whiten the single dark tooth to get it to match and is easier to try to whiten the entire arch using a special protocol. If it is decided that only the single tooth should be whitened, then a specially designed whitening tray needs to be made. A full-arch tray is first made and then a window is cut adjacent to the dark tooth on either side of the tooth to be whitened. If this is not done, then the adjacent teeth will lighten more quickly.

Table 9.1 Treatment options for single vital teeth

1. Home whitening
2. Home whitening with a sectional tray
3. Sectional whitening of only dark teeth first, then a full-arch tray to whiten all the teeth to match the same light shade
4. Start with a lower concentration and then ramp up the concentration from 10% to 15–16% carbamide peroxide
5. Use 6% hydrogen peroxide on the teeth

Although some authors have suggested removing the coronal sclerotic dentin and using internal and external whitening as necessary (Pedorella et al. 2000), such extreme methods are not deemed to be necessary.

PROTOCOL FOR WHITENING THE SINGLE TOOTH AND THE FULL ARCH

There are three ways to undertake single tooth whitening.

1. Whiten the dark tooth first using the specially constructed tray, which blocks out the adjacent teeth (see Figures 9.7 and 9.10). That way the lightening potential of the tooth can be assessed. It is essential that the adjacent teeth are not lightened at the same time because the darker tooth will look worse as the lighter adjacent teeth whiten more quickly, and the problem will look worse or more exaggerated. Once a reasonable level of whitening has been achieved on the single tooth, then the whitening can be continued with a full-arch tray to whiten all the teeth at the same time. Thus a good overall color can be achieved.
2. Whiten the dark tooth only.
   - *Whitening a single tooth discolored because of CM:* It is unrealistic to expect to be able to determine to which shade the tooth affected by CM will lighten. Whitening can be unpredictable, and the darker tooth may not necessarily match the adjacent teeth. It is easier to have more control of the lightness by whitening the entire arch. The whitening process will be slower because of the anatomy of the tooth after the trauma (see Figure 9.9).
   - *Whitening a single tooth that is slightly darker than adjacent teeth because of restorations:* This may also be unpredictable with regard to achieving an exact match between the discolored tooth and the adjacent teeth.
3. Whiten the whole arch and then focus on titrating the dose of whitening gel by increasing the concentration of the whitening gel. Normally a full-arch scalloped whitening tray is made. The upper teeth are whitened

for 2 weeks using 10% carbamide peroxide to evaluate the speed and progress of the whitening of the whole arch. Thereafter 16–20% carbamide peroxide gel is placed in the tray adjacent to the single tooth for a period of 4–6 weeks or until the single tooth is matching all the upper teeth and they are all the same shade. Sometimes it may be necessary to continue whitening for a further 2 weeks after this. The progress of whitening the single tooth can be slow because of the nature of the dentin, which had been packed very densely from the secondary and tertiary dentin depositions. However, there is little or no sensitivity experienced by this vital tooth during the whitening treatment.

FOLLOW-UP AND MONITORING

It is important to undertake the appropriate monitoring at intervals that are deemed necessary to follow the progress of the whitening treatment. Because the dentin is compacted tightly together, it will take time for the whitening to reach the same level as in the adjacent teeth. The whitening process is normally assessed by reviewing the patient at 2-weekly intervals. However, if the patient is older, the intervals may be every 3 weeks because the lightening will take place at a slower pace.

Monitoring continues until the patient and dentist are satisfied with the result. Normally the shade of the single whitened tooth will retain well and color regression occurs at a slower rate. It may be necessary to do a touch-up or maintenance treatment for the whole arch about 3 years later.

REFERENCES

Amir FA, Gutmann JL, Witherspoon DE. (2001) Calcific metamorphosis: a challenge in endodontic diagnosis and treatment. *Quintessence Int* **32**(6):447–55.

Barber A, King P. (2014) Management of the single discoloured tooth. Part 1: aetiology, prevention and minimally invasive restorative options. *Dent Update* **41**(2):98–100, 102–4, 106–8.

Cvek M. (2007) Endodontic management and the use of calcium hydroxide. In Andreasen JO, Andreasen FM, Anderssen L, editors. *Traumatic injuries to the teeth,* 4th edn. Blackwell: London.

Dahl JE, Pallesen U. (2007) Bleaching of the discoloured traumatised tooth. In Andreasen JO, Andreasen FM, Anderssen L, editors: *Textbook and colour atlas of traumatic injuries to the teeth,* 4th edn. Blackwell: London.

Denehy GE, Swift EJ Jr. (1992) Single tooth whitening. *Quintessence Int* **23**(9):595–8.

Greenwall LH. (2007) Single tooth whitening. *Aesthet Dent Today* **1**:4, 42–4.

Jacobsen I, Kerekes K. (1977) Long-term prognosis of traumatized permanent anterior teeth showing calcifying process in the pulp cavity. *Scand J Dent Res* **85:** 588–98.

Lundberg M, Cvek M. (1980) A light microscopy study of pulps from traumatized permanent incisors with reduced pulp lumen. *Acta Odontol Scand* **38:**89–94.

Malhotra N, Mala K. (2013) Calcific metamorphosis. Literature review and clinical strategies. *Dent Update* **40**(1):48–50, 53–4, 57–8.

McCabe PS, Dummer PM. (2012) Pulp canal obliteration: an endodontic diagnosis and treatment challenge. *Int Endod J* **45**(2):177–97.

Pedorella CA, Meyer RD, Woollard GW. (2000) Whitening of endodontically untreated calcified anterior teeth. *Gen Dent* **48**(3):252–5.

Torneck CD (1990) The clinical significance and management of calcific pulp obliteration. *Alpha Omegan* **83**(4):50–4.

West JD. (1997) The aesthetic and endodontic dilemmas of calcific metamorphosis. *Pract Periodont Aesthet Dent* **9**(3):289–93.

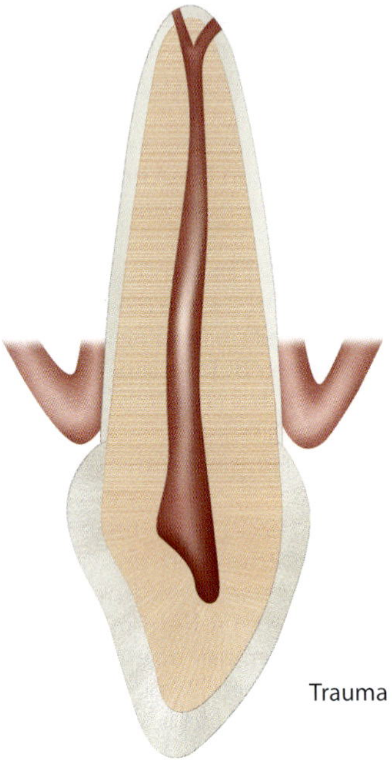

Figure 9.1

The process of trauma and how the trauma affects the tooth.

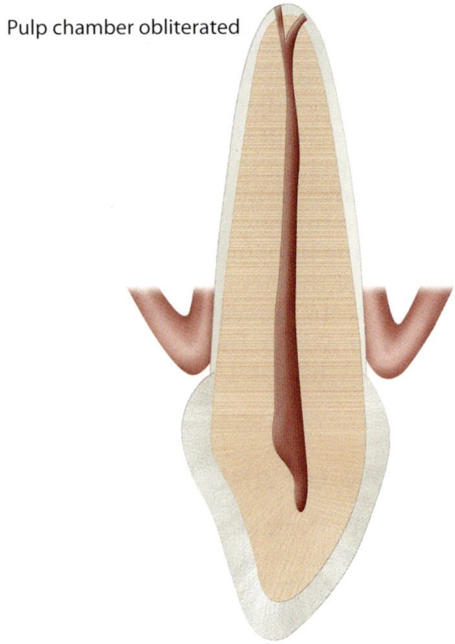

Figure 9.2

After the trauma, bleeding occurs in the tooth, and the pulp canal and pulp chamber start to shrink. Secondary and tertiary dentin is laid down and the pulp canal starts to give the appearance that it is becoming obliterated.

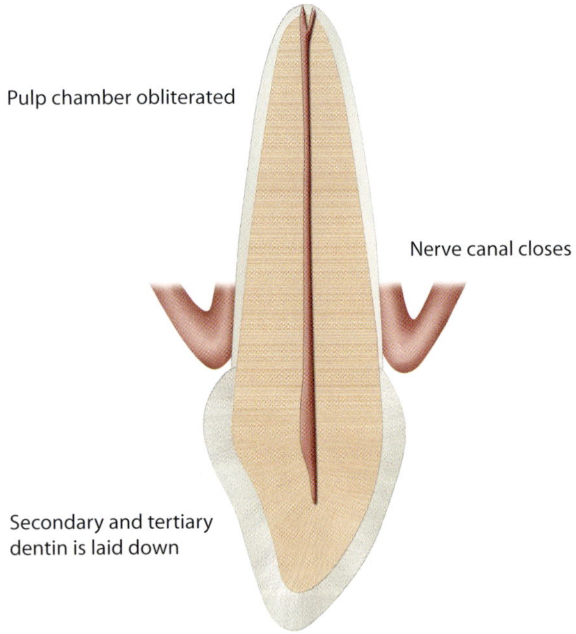

Figure 9.3

Single dark tooth pathologic process. Tertiary dentin is being laid down.

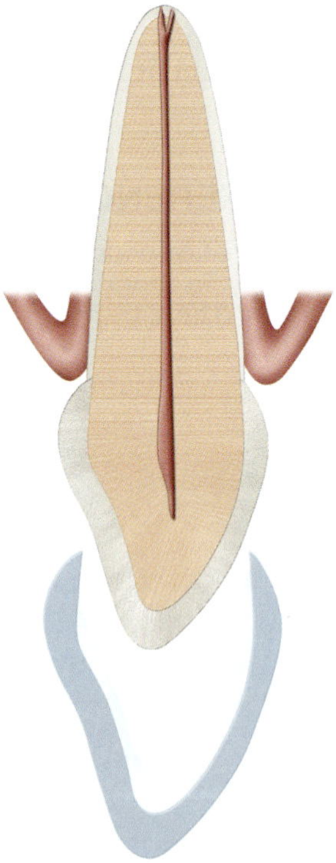

Figure 9.4

Placing the whitening gel into the whitening tray. A higher concentration of gel is placed in the single-arch tray because the tooth is less likely to be sensitive. More gel can be placed into the whitening tray to initiate the whitening process. Whitening will be slower because of the anatomy of the traumatized tooth. This process whereby the pulp chamber is almost obliterated is called calcific metamorphosis.

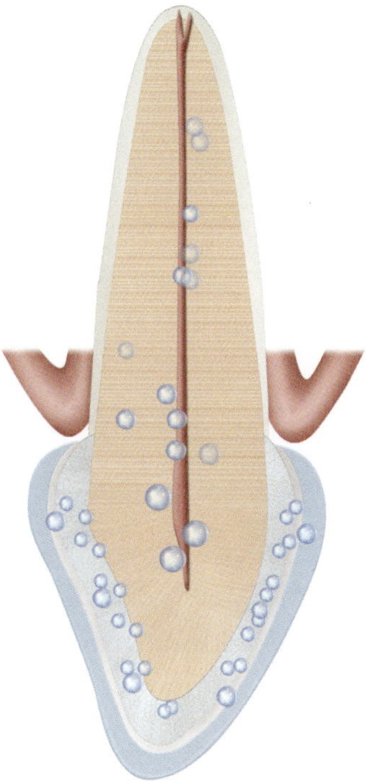

Figure 9.5

The process of whitening as the oxygen moves through the tooth and through the pulp canal, which has been narrowed by the formation of secondary and tertiary dentin. After a period of about 6 weeks, the tooth starts to lighten. It may be that the light being transmitted through such a tooth gives it a darker appearance, so the whitening treatment may take a little longer to achieve the same level of whiteness as in the adjacent teeth.

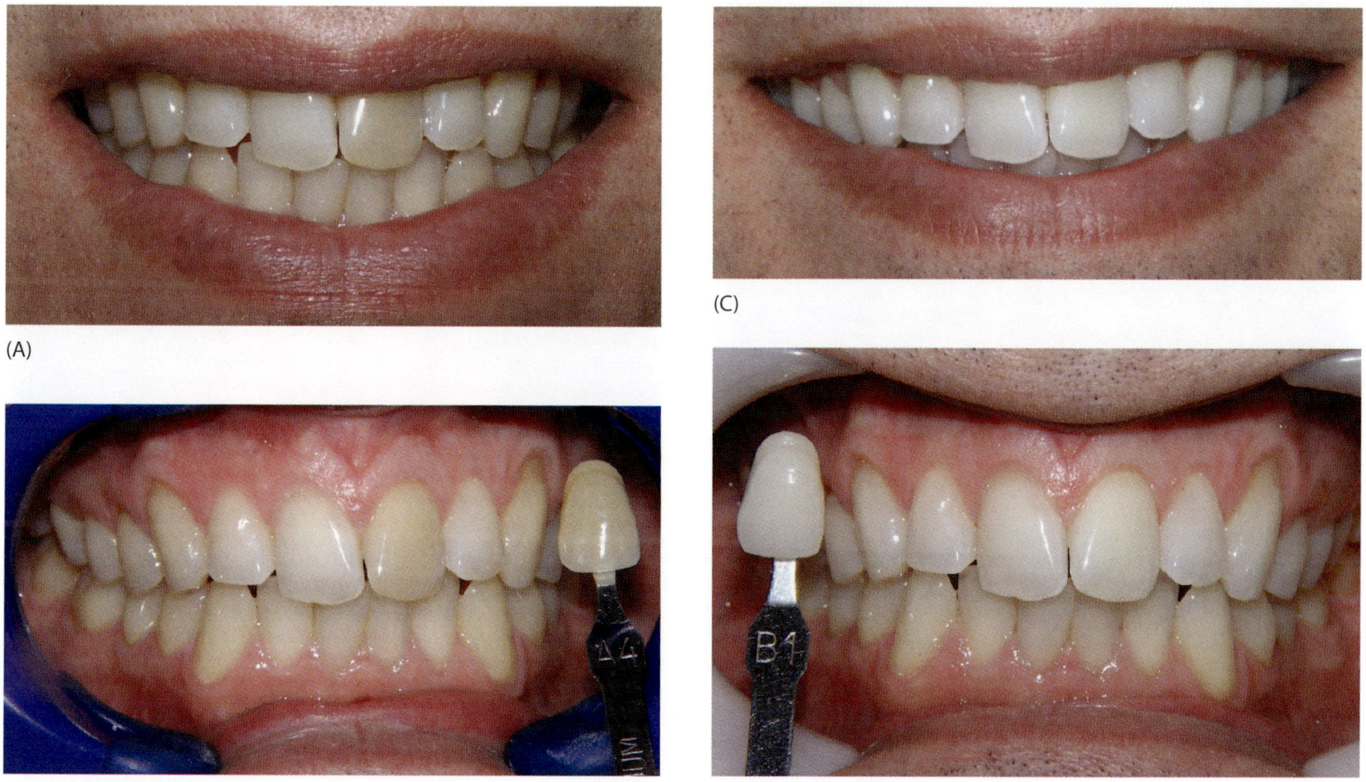

(A) (B) (C) (D)

Figure 9.6

(A–D) Because of the anatomy of the previously traumatized tooth, the whitening gel takes time to penetrate through the layers of secondary and tertiary dentin. The whitening process for the single vital tooth that has undergone calcific metamorphosis takes longer to complete. It is expected that it may take approximately 6 weeks for the tooth to closely match the shade of the adjacent teeth.

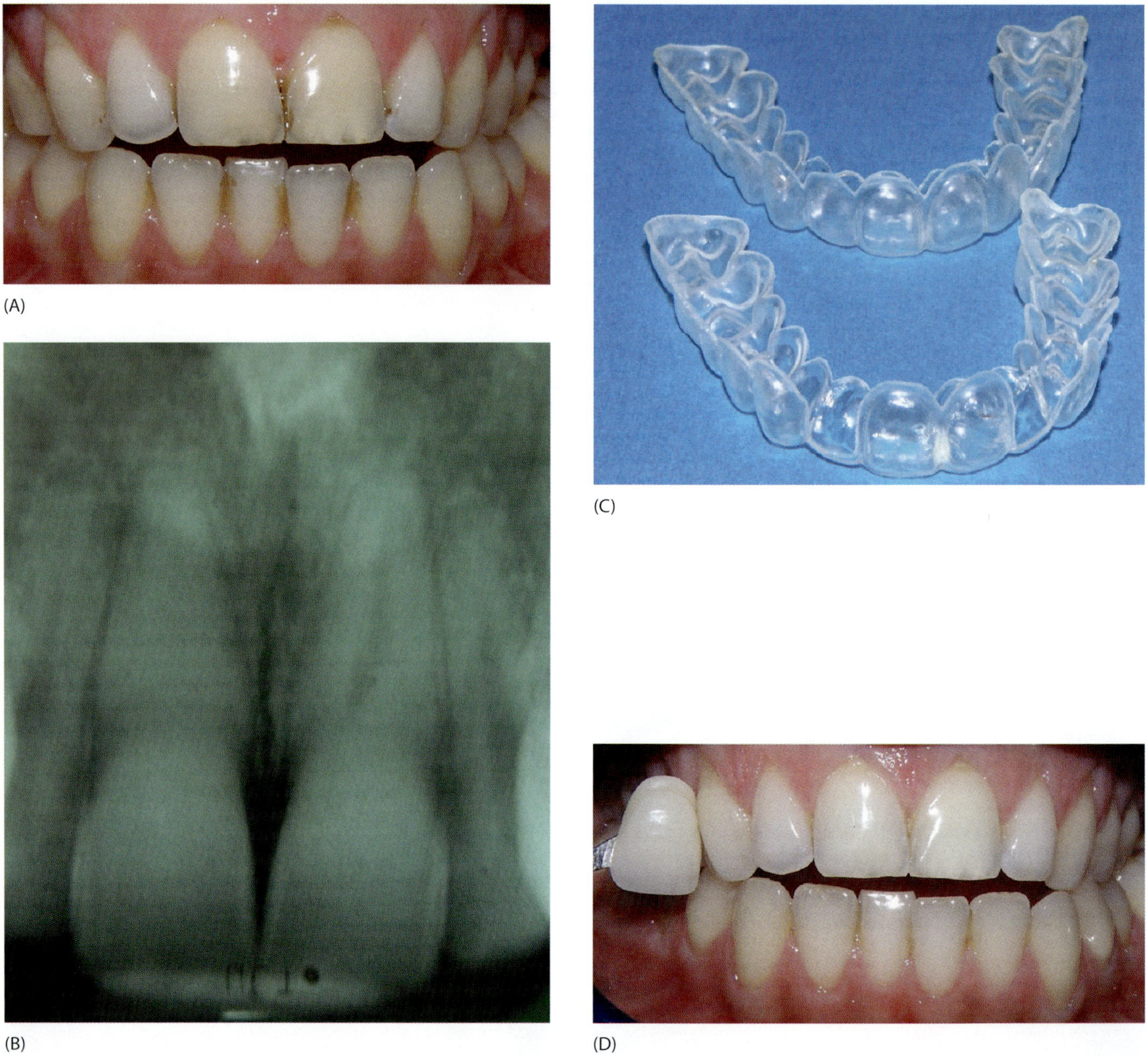

Figure 9.7

(A) Two upper central incisors that were damaged in a minor bicycle accident when the front teeth hit the handlebars. The patient reported that the teeth had darkened within a period of 1 month after the trauma. (B) Periapical radiograph showing the trauma that was sustained by the two upper central incisor teeth. The upper right central incisor shows a completely obliterated pulp canal and chamber, and the upper left central incisor shows the formation of a dentin bridge in the center of the neck of the tooth. The pulp canal can be seen on the latter section toward the apex of the tooth but it is completely impenetrable owing to the thickness of the dentin bridge. (C) A sectional whitening tray and a full-arch tray. The central incisors are darker than the lateral teeth owing to the trauma from the bicycle accident. Two whitening trays were made. One tray is a full upper arch and the second one is a window tray in which the teeth on either side of the dark teeth are cut away. The sectional whitening tray is used first so that the darker teeth can whiten first. Once the shade starts to lighten, the full-arch tray is used to whiten all the teeth so that an even white shade can be achieved. (D) The whitening of the upper central incisors to match the adjacent teeth. The central incisors were first whitened using the specially created sectional whitening tray. Once these teeth had lightened sufficiently, a full-arch whitening tray was used to whiten all the upper teeth.

10 TOOTH WHITENING, THE MICROABRASION TECHNIQUE, AND WHITE SPOT ERADICATION

Linda Greenwall

INTRODUCTION

It has now been 25 years since the introduction of the microabrasion technique. There are many published studies on its 20-year effectiveness as a technique that eradicates and fades white spots, white marks, and white lesions. Microabrasion techniques are used in combination with whitening techniques, and microabrasion is an effective minimally invasive treatment option. It is the intention in this chapter to elaborate on the whitening techniques used for teeth with existing white, brown, and orange spots. The chapter will discuss current whitening techniques, microabrasion, and resin infiltration for the eradication of the white spots.

The small white, brown, or mottled lesions that appear on front teeth can be unsightly, and patients are often concerned about this type of discoloration (see Figure 10.1). Some enamel discolorations, although intrinsic, are confined to the outermost layers of the enamel.

TREATMENT OPTIONS FOR WHITE SPOTS, WHITE MARKS, AND WHITE LESIONS

White spots, marks, and lesions have many possible causes and treatments (Tables 10.1–10.4). There are several treatment options for treating white spots on the labial surfaces of teeth, including the following:

- Tooth whitening
- Application of amorphous calcium phosphate directly to the lesion or in a whitening tray (Abreu et al. 2011)
- Microabrasion using 6.6% hydrochloric acid (Greenwall 2006; Opalustre, Optident, United Kingdom) and 10% hydrochloric acid (Premier Dental Products, Plymouth Meeting, PA)
- Resin infiltration using 15% hydrochloric acid (Icon, DMG, Germany)
- Combination therapy using whitening and increasing concentrations of hydrochloric acid
- Composite bonding directly over the lesion
- Removing the white mark with a fast handpiece and restoring with composite resin, dentin, enamel, and opaque shades
- Direct and translucent resin veneer
- Indirect resin veneer (Edelweiss, Optident)
- Porcelain laminate over the whole labial surface

WHAT IS MICROABRASION?

Enamel microabrasion is a procedure in which a microscopic layer of enamel is simultaneously eroded and abraded with a special compound, leaving a perfectly intact enamel surface behind (Croll 1991b). It is used to treat enamel discolorations that may be the result of hypermineralization, hypomineralization, or staining. Croll (1991b) called the process "enamel dysmineralization," which describes the superficial enamel coloration defects resulting from some disturbance of the normal mineralization process. There are advantages in using a combination of chemical and mechanical surface microreduction. In successful cases enamel loss is insignificant and unrecognizable and the patient is left with tooth surfaces that appear normal (Greenwall 2009). This technique can be used before, after, or during the whitening treatment.

The difference between whitening and microabrasion

Microabrasion improves tooth color by eliminating the superficial discolored enamel. Once the discoloration has been removed, the result is permanent. Microabrasion is preferred when general tooth color changes are not needed, but a defined isolated surface discoloration is present (Haywood 1995).

Whitening treatment improves tooth color by lightening, whitening, and brightening the teeth. Unlike microabrasion, whitening preserves the intact fluoride-rich layer of enamel and the tooth shape. The shade of the teeth over many years may darken slightly, but the teeth never return to their original dark color. Whitening will lighten and whiten the actual tooth color, thus rendering the white spot less noticeable because the background shade is whiter.

The two techniques can be used in conjunction with each other depending on the specific case (see Figure 10.4). Sometimes after microabrasion the tooth appears more yellow or darker. Whitening can thus follow microabrasion to improve tooth color. The best results and improvements are achieved with a combination of both treatments (Croll 1997). Normally whitening is undertaken first when a patient has white spots on the teeth. Many small white spots will fade with whitening and so it may not always be necessary to undertake

Table 10.1 Classification of white spots by cause and appearance

Cause
- Hereditary
- Trauma
- Fluorosis
- Decay hypomineralization
- Molar incisor hypoplasia
- Congenital premature birth
- Lesions: orthodontic bands, enamel solubility, diet, saliva, medication
- Childhood illness, medications, e.g., antibiotics, chemicals (bisphenol A)

Appearance
- Based on size: small, medium, large
- Based on depth: deep, shallow, flecks
- Based on appearance: bright, faint, opaque white spot

Table 10. 2 Treatment options for white spots

- Do nothing
- Monitor
- Chemical therapeutics
- Tooth whitening
- Prolonged whitening
- Microabrasion
- Icon infiltration (Ikon, DMG)
- Megabrasion
- Direct bonding
- Preformed veneers
- Porcelain laminate veneers
- Topical application of amorphous calcium phosphate (ACP)
- Crowns, if severe mottling that does not respond to treatment

Table 10.4 Concentrations of hydrochloric acid that can be used for white spot removal

- 18% Hydrochloric acid—Generic hydrochloric acid can be mixed with pumice as a basic treatment (Sheoran et al. 2014).
- 15% HCl—Used for the resin infiltration treatment (Ikon, DMG, Hamburg, Germany; Greenwall 2013) (see Figures 10.4H–J).
- 10% HCl Prema—Used for microabrasion or white spot eradication; Prema kit (Premier Dental Products, Plymouth Meeting, PA; Croll 1986) is 10% hydrochloric acid in a preparation of fine-grit silicon carbide particles in a water-soluble paste that can be applied manually or with a handpiece (see Figure 10.9).
- 6.6% HCl Opalustre—Also used for microabrasion; a proprietary kit including purple syringes, hydrochloric acid, and silicon carbide microparticles in a water-soluble paste (see Figure 10.10) (Opalustre Kit, Ultradent Products, South Jordan, UT).
- Other materials—37% Phosphoric acid and pumice (Sheoran et al. 2014).

microabrasion. Because whitening is noninvasive, it is best to undertake whitening first followed by microabrasion if necessary.

Hydrochloric acid

The use of hydrochloric acid to whiten teeth and remove stains from teeth has been advocated for many years. Hydrochloric acid and pumice are the main ingredients used for the technique. The use of hydrochloric acid depends on the decalcification of enamel, that is, softening and dissolving the enamel to remove the stain. It should be selectively applied and well controlled

Table 10.3 Possible treatments for different causes

Type of white lesion	*Etiology*	*Possible treatment*
Isolated single white spots with diameter <0.5 mm on adult maxillary incisors	Natural occurrence	Whitening only
White speckled lesions: mottled enamel	Fever during development	Whitening then microabrasion at 6.6%
Multiple lesions: brown and white discolorations	Fluorosis	Whitening then microabrasion
White lines or stripes	More severe developmental disturbance	Whitening then microabrasion
White patches	Trauma to the primary dentition	Whitening followed by resin infiltration
White spots covered with yellow layer	Bleeding that occurred during traumatic injury and seeped into the areas of mineralization	Whitening, microabrasion, then resin infiltration
Faint white lesions, some black edges	Demineralization lesions after removal of orthodontic brackets	Resin infiltration or whitening or microabrasion depending on the size of the mark
Enamel defects and white lesions in deciduous incisors and molars	Celiac disease, molar incisor hypoplasia	Whitening, glass ionomers placed onto the defective molar teeth, resin infiltration of the anterior lesions
White spot or enamel hypoplasia	Preterm birth (prevalence 45% normal birth weight to 92% preterm babies [Lai et al. 1997])	Whitening
Natural occurrence		Microabrasion then resin infiltration

Adapted from Greenwall 2009 with permission.

(McEvoy 1998). Normally less than 200 mm of enamel in total is removed, but it may be much less. Use of the correct concentration, procedure, and application can allow careful control of the degree of enamel loss (Touati et al. 1999). The effects of hydrochloric acid are nonselective and superficial. The technique may be enhanced by adding an abrasive (pumice, as advocated by Croll 1986), heat, or chemicals such as hydrogen peroxide and ether (Touati et al. 1999). Which concentration of hydrochloric acid is used first depends on the case. A higher concentration of hydrochloric acid is used in the resin infiltration technique (Greenwall 2013). This technique allows for the placement of 15% hydrochloric acid directly onto the white lesion for 2 minutes. This is followed by an alcohol preparation to assess the likelihood of the white lesion disappearing. This preparation is called Icon-Dry. This is then followed by the Icon resin, which infiltrates the white lesion. The Icon resin is placed onto the tooth for approximately 3 minutes and then the resin is light cured for 40 seconds. This resin is then applied again and allowed to set, followed by further light curing. If the area does not fade, the technique can be repeated again, this time using a microetcher to sandblast (see Figure 10.4G) the white lesion first to obtain deeper penetration (Greenwall 2013). The resin infiltration technique was first used to treat interstitial lesions showing changes in the enamel causing demineralization interstitially.

What is the best age for treatment of the white spots?

Although the white spots can sometimes be treated at the time of eruption of the permanent tooth, it is best to wait until full eruption of the tooth to understand the nature of the white spot or lesion. Teenagers are at an ideal age to undertake this treatment because this is the age at which individuals become aware of their appearance, especially the appearance of their teeth.

Normally it is best to undertake whitening first because home whitening treatment may eradicate the lesion completely. Once the whitening treatment is completed, then microabrasion can be undertaken. Less treatment may be required because the lesion is smaller. Sometimes despite all available treatment options, the white spot is too large to respond to whitening, microabrasion, and resin infiltration treatment; the only option may be to place a composite bond directly over the white spot area. This can result in a satisfactory outcome as well. Normally the tooth is whitened first to lighten the background shade and then the white patch is surveyed for the results, after which a simple mega-abrasion technique may be used whereby a microscopic layer of the surface enamel is removed and a direct composite resin is placed over the white lesion. Before treatment is begun, the area is cleaned with a mixture of pumice and chlorhexidine soap (Hibiscrub soap; see Figure 10.7E). The tooth is prepared and then the restoration is layered segmentally for a beautiful esthetic result (see Figure 10.7G). The tooth can also be prepared by air abrasion with the Aquacut machine using bioglass for cleaning (Aquacut and Sylc bioglass [Velopex International, London]).

Microabrasion of the enamel surface can be undertaken in patients of all ages: adolescents, adults, and the elderly.

In a study using a split-mouth study design (Sheoran et al. 2014) 37% phosphoric acid and 18% hydrochloric acid were used for removal of visually unesthetic developmental enamel opacities of young permanent maxillary anterior teeth from 25 patients (11–13 years old) by two microabrasion techniques for 10 and 5 seconds. This procedure was repeated four to six times during each clinical appointment. The patients were evaluated about their satisfaction with the treatment. Two blinded evaluators appraised both sides of the mouth using a visual analog scale. The records were analyzed using the Wilcoxon test. The results showed that the majority of the patients (approximately 97%) reported satisfaction at the end of the treatment (P = .001). Statistically significant reduction in enamel opacities was observed by evaluators immediately after microabrasion technique in group 1 (81.75%) and in group 2 (81.4%) (P < .002). Reduction was increased to 97.2% in group 1 and 96.7% in group 2 after 1 month.

Indications for microabrasion

Indications for microabrasion include the following:

- Developmental intrinsic stains from hypoplastic marks attributed to premature birth (Lai et al. 1997).
- Developmental lines and discolorations (see Figure 10.7A) (Croll 1997).
- Superficial surface enamel stains and opacities (see Figure 10.8B).
- Yellow-brown areas (see Figure 10.5A).
- Multicolored stains (brown, gray, or yellow).
- Superficial hypoplastic enamel (Croll [1991a] calls this "enamel dysmineralization").
- Areas of enamel fluorosis (see Figure 10.3A).
- White patches, white spots (see Figure 10.4A).
- Superficial decalcification lesions from stasis of plaque and from orthodontic bands
- Some irregular surface textures.

Contraindications

Microabrasion cannot be used for the following conditions:

- Age-related staining.
- Tetracycline staining.
- Deep enamel hypoplastic lesions.
- Some concentric areas of hypocalcification that extend to the dentin.
- Some amelogenesis imperfecta.
- Most dentinogenesis lesions.
- Carious lesions underlying regions of decalcification (Croll 1997).
- Areas of deep enamel and dentin stains.

Ideal requirements of proprietary kits

- They should use water-soluble gels for ease of application.
- The risk of spillage or splashing should be limited; application procedures should be simple.
- Concentration of the gel should be able to be varied for different situations.
- The acid should have a low concentration for safety in the mouth.
- The abrasive agent should have great hardness to remove enamel easily when combined with the acid.
- The abrasive agent should have a small particle size to prevent the enamel from being damaged.
- The application method should be slow to prevent splattering of the compound.

Effects on the enamel and mechanism of action

The rotary application process allows the material to simultaneously abrade and erode the enamel surface and so remove the stain. The enamel surface layer is restructured to form an amorphous prismless layer that clinically appears smooth and lustrous (see Figure 10.9; Croll 1997). A generalized smoothing effect on the enamel has been documented (Berg and Donly 1991, Donly et al. 1992). It consists of an amorphous layer of compacted mineral. This effect has been called the "enamel glaze" or "abrosion" effect.

Advantages of the technique

- It is easily performed (Rosenthaler and Randel 1998).
- It is a conservative treatment.
- It is inexpensive.
- Teeth require minimal subsequent maintenance.
- It is fast acting (McEvoy 1998).
- It removes yellow-brown, white, and multicolored stains.
- It is effective.
- Results are permanent.

Disadvantages of the technique

- It removes enamel.
- Hydrochloric acid compounds are caustic.
- It requires protective apparatus for patient, dentist, and assistant.
- It requires a visit to the dental office.

THE PROCEDURE

Clinical evaluation of the teeth

When microabrasion treatment is being planned, the teeth should be evaluated when they are moist, hydrated, and saturated with saliva. There is a camouflaging effect in the presence of saliva. Although the enamel stain may still be present, the saliva hides it. It is thus not necessary to remove the stain entirely and this phenomenon should be evaluated first, before more is removed. It is best to be conservative when removing enamel because more applications can be undertaken during another appointment. That is why it is best to undertake whitening treatment first.

Tooth whitening normally removes the brown, orange, and yellow stains that are present on the tooth first, then the natural color of the tooth lightens. The effect on the white spot is then evaluated as the last part of the evaluation process, which takes place over several weeks (see Figure 10.3). When whitening treatments are undertaken, patients need to be warned that the white areas may appear whiter at first. Once the color of the teeth changes, the difference becomes less noticeable. Microabrasion can be used to remove or reduce in size the remaining white areas after the whitening process (see Figure 10.4). Again, the camouflaging effect should be carefully evaluated, and only those white areas that are noticeable should be treated.

Equipment needed

- Contra-angle slow handpiece: Alternating speed reduction 10:1 or normal rotary slow handpiece. The alternating handpiece prevents splashing.
- The microabrasion material.
- Polishing or prophylaxis paste (see Figure 10.9 for polishing after microabrasion).
- Patient protection: Gingival protection in some form, such as a rubber dam or paint-on dam, lip retractors, and protective eyewear are normally required (e.g., OptraGate [Ivoclar Vivadent]).
- Protective coverings: for dentist and assistant.

Treatment planning

Case selection is particularly important with this technique. Careful discussion with the patient and his or her parents (if the patient is underage) regarding the consequences, side effects, benefits, and further options for treatment such as whitening, veneers, bonding, and crowns needs to be undertaken. Do not raise the patient's expectations regarding the results. Rather, be conservative with regard to prognosis; that way the patient will not be disappointed with the results. There can be no guarantee that the technique will definitely remove the white lesion. Further treatments, such as resin infiltration or the removal of the superficial layer of the enamel and placement of a composite resin restoration, may be necessary to completely eradicate the white spot.

The enamel should be assessed from the incisal edge with the aid of a mouth mirror. This way the labiolingual enamel thickness of the tooth and enamel lesion can be assessed. The depth of the enamel lesion can also be checked.

Step-by-step guide

1. Clean teeth with rubber cup and prophylaxis paste or pumice and Hibiscrub combination with a microbrush.
2. Isolation of teeth:

- Rubber dam. Floss ligatures can be tied around the rubber dam to secure the gingival margin. It is not always necessary to use clamps. Interdental rubber strips can be used to hold down the dam (see Figure 10.5D).
- Light-cured resin applied to the gingiva.
- Lip retractor. An OptraGate dam isolates the teeth. It is not always necessary to use clamps. Interdental rubber strips can again be used to hold down the dam.

3. Protect the lips with a Vaseline barrier.
4. Protect the soft tissues.
5. Microreduce the lesion to begin the treatment by using a fine-grit diamond or tungsten carbide bur (Croll 1997). This decreases overall treatment time. This step is not always necessary.
6. Apply the microabrasion compound to the areas in 60-second intervals with appropriate rinsing (see Figure 10.3C). Check manufacturer's instructions on specific timing. A timer can be used to ensure the correct amount of time for application of the compound and bristle cup.
7. The applicator head has special fluting to capture as much material as possible and to compress the compound onto the tooth and to keep it in contact with the tooth (see Figure 10.10).
8. Apply the material for short periods of time only. Cautionary note: Damage to soft tissue can occur if the material is left for too long. This may be in the form of blanching or whitening of the gingiva or soft tissues or small ulcerations of the mucosa (see Figure 10.9A).
9. Wipe off with a wet cotton roll first to prevent splashing, and rinse the teeth. The water-soaked cotton rolls help to rehydrate the teeth so that intermittent observation can be undertaken. The teeth are hydrated and re-evaluated and then rehydrated to ensure that the white spot is fully observed when the tooth is wet. When the teeth are dehydrated, more white spots become obvious; it is not necessary to remove all the white spots present on the teeth—only those that are obvious when the tooth is hydrated.
10. Check periodically from the labiolingual aspect that minimal enamel reduction is taking place.
11. Repeat the procedure.
12. Polish the teeth using a fine-grit fluoridated prophylaxis paste or amorphous calcium phosphate (see Figure 10.9C).
13. Rinse the teeth.
14. Re-evaluate the teeth when wet because some white areas disappear when wet. The rubber dam desiccates the teeth and some of the whiter areas become more vivid; thus evaluation needs to be done when the teeth are wet. It may sometimes be difficult to determine how deep the decalcification is. There is nothing to lose by trying the microabrasion technique first and then continuing with further treatment such as whitening or bonding if the former is not successful.
15. Remove the rubber dam.
16. Apply a topical fluoride (neutral sodium fluoride gel) or amorphous calcium phosphate (Abreu et al. 2011) directly onto the teeth for 1 minute (see Figure 10.9C) (e.g., PreviDent, Colgate Oral Pharmaceuticals; Tooth Mousse or MI Paste, GC America).
17. Re-evaluate the result. More than one visit may be necessary.
18. Explain to the patient that immediately after completion of the first microabrasion treatment the appearance of the teeth may look worse because of the dehydration effect and there may be more white spots visible in the dehydrated state. The following day, when the teeth are rehydrated, the enamel surface will appear smooth and lustrous and will not pick up stains.
19. Assess the patient 4–6 weeks later because the result will continue to improve over time. Take post-treatment photographs (e.g., see Figure 10.8C).

MICROABRASION AND HOME WHITENING TREATMENT

It is best to undertake home whitening treatment in trays first (Greenwall 2006). The whitening treatment for white spots is normally prolonged and falls into the advanced whitening category because it can take 6–8 weeks to completely eliminate the brown, orange, and yellow marks from the teeth. The basic color of the tooth is lightened first; this makes it easier to eradicate the remaining white marks.

MICROABRASION AND ADJUNCTIVE TREATMENT

Additional treatment can be undertaken to manage the white spots. The white spots can be treated after whitening with amorphous calcium phosphate in the same whitening trays to reduce the appearance of the white spots. The teeth can be cleaned with air abrasion and bioglass, they can be resin infiltrated, or direct bonding can be undertaken (see Figure 10.7).

Further treatment using resin infiltration technique and protocol for treatment of labial enamel

The resin infiltration technique (Kugel et al. 2009, Paris et al. 2010, Paris and Meyer-Lueckel 2012) is an erosion-infiltration technique that was proposed as a new product (Icon, DMG) designed to halt caries interproximally in the posterior segment (Meyer-Lueckel and Paris 2008, Pharck et al. 2009); it was launched on the market several years ago (Attal et al. 2014). However, it has now been successfully used on labial enamel to treat many white marks, lesions, and hypocalcifications following orthodontic treatment (Kim et al. 2011), either on its own or in combination with whitening treatment (see Figure 10.6).

The technique consists of four components:

1. The preparation phase: the surface of the teeth is cleaned and prepared with 15% hydrochloric acid for 2–5 minutes (see Figure 10.5).
2. Alcohol is placed onto the surface as a drying agent and left for 30 seconds.
3. Triethylene glycol dimethacrylate (TEGMA) resin is applied onto the tooth for 2–5 minutes.
4. The tooth is light cured.

In addition, the protocol includes the following:

1. Application of hydrochloric acid for 2 minutes (see Figure 10.5).
2. Sand blasting of the lesion if it is deep.
3. Alcohol application to see whether the lesion has faded.
4. Second resin infiltration application.

Research

In a study undertaken by Muñoz et al. (2013) in which suitable teeth were infiltrated with resin, the researchers found that the most successful cases were the ones with fluorosis stains. These cases showed visibly perceptible differences. The hypoplasia areas were not completely eradicated. The researchers reported that the patients recovered their self-esteem as a result of the treatment and thus this was considered a success. The effect of the hydrochloric acid on the enamel was evaluated in a study by Paris et al. (2010). These researchers evaluated the etching effect of the hydrochloric acid versus phosphoric acid on deciduous teeth. They evaluated 36 pairs of primary molars with enamel lesions, then etched for 2 minutes with both phosphoric acid and hydrochloric acid. They examined the results using confocal microscopy. They reported that there was a difference between the two acids on the surface of the teeth and that the hydrochloric acid caused higher erosion on the enamel, thus allowing deeper penetration of the resin infiltrant. The erosion depth of the hydrochloric acid was twice the depth of the phosphoric acid. The phosphoric acid at an etching time of 2 minutes cannot erode the surface of the enamel. It seems that the resin infiltration technique can reduce long-term restorative needs and costs, thus complementing the concept of minimal-intervention dentistry (Kielbassa et al. 2009).

Side effects of resin infiltration

The resin infiltration technique may not always fade the white spot lesion entirely (Meyer-Lueckel and Paris 2008). This may improve over time. In a study by Kim et al. (2011) 20 teeth with a developmental defect of enamel and 18 teeth with postorthodontic decalcification were selected to have resin infiltration. Standardized photographs were taken before, immediately after, and 1 week after treatment. The results were classified into three different groups: completely masked, partially masked, and unchanged. The image analysis of the ΔE results showed that 25% (five) of the teeth were classified as completely masked, whereas 35% (seven) were partially masked and 40% (eight) were unchanged.

Of the postorthodontic decalcification group, 11 (61%) of the teeth were completely masked, six teeth (33%) were partially masked, and one tooth (6%) was unchanged. In some teeth the result improved by 1 week after infiltration rather than immediately after the infiltration. The researchers concluded that the masking effect was dramatic in some cases but not in others. Further research on the long-term effects should be continued.

Further research

There is still further research to be undertaken because there are many unanswered questions, such as how it can be determined which lesions will respond with complete eradication of the white spot and which with partial eradication (Kielbassa et al. 2009). However, it appears that some lesions are located deeper within the enamel and require several sessions to reduce the lesion. The resin, once applied, keeps working on the lesion, and it is advisable to assess the patient a month after the first application to review whether the lesion has become smaller. Questions remain as to whether whitening should be undertaken first before resin infiltration and whether this will improve the overall result. However, in very young children, it may be appropriate to treat isolated lesions first with either microabrasion or resin infiltration, followed by whitening treatment when the child is older.

Other questions involve the effect of the TEGMA resin on further bonding techniques (will the bond be as strong or weaker?). At this stage it does not interfere with other resin bonding techniques and additional direct bonding techniques.

Further adjunctive treatment

1. Composite bonding to mask the defect (see Figure 10.7).
2. Direct bonding over the whole tooth.
3. Porcelain laminate veneer.

Deep enamel hypoplastic lesions, once removed, leave a tooth form defect that requires a composite restoration. Sometimes the depth of a lesion cannot be ascertained until the tooth is treated (see Figure 10.7). A composite restoration may need to be placed to mask the discoloration. When this is necessary, the enamel surface of the lesion can be roughened with a coarse diamond bur to expose fresh enamel for the phosphoric acid to etch. The enamel surface of the microabraded area should be etched for 60 seconds instead of the usual 15–30 seconds because the mineral pattern and density of the enamel changes.

After the treatment, the enamel appears smooth and lustrous (see Figure 10.3). In many cases the results may be permanent. Remineralization of the enamel surfaces can occur. It appears that the surfaces do not retain plaque and stain as easily. The treated surfaces resist dissolution more easily. They colonize fewer *Streptococcus mutans* bacteria (Segura et al. 1997).

CONCLUSION

These days there are more options for treatment of white spots, white marks, and white lesions, which give many more ways to eradicate these lesions. Although it is best to try whitening treatment first because it is the least invasive method, microabrasion and resin infiltration are excellent options for reducing, fading, and eradicating white marks and white lesions and have yielded excellent results.

REFERENCES

Abreu DR, Sasaki RS, Amaral FL, Florio FM. (2011) Effect of home-use and in-office bleaching agents containing hydrogen peroxide associated with amorphous calcium phosphate on enamel microhardness and surface roughness. *J Esthet Restor Dent* **23**(3):158–68.

Atia GS, May J. (2013) Dental fluorosis in the paediatric patient. *Dent Update* **40**(10):836–9.

Attal JP, Atlan A, Denis M, Vennat E. (2014) White spots on enamel: treatment protocol by superficial or deep infiltration (part 2). *Int Orthod* **12**(1):1–31.

Berg JH, Donly KJ. (1991) The enamel surface and enamel microabrasion. In Croll TP, editor. *Enamel microabrasion.* Quintessence Publishing: Chicago, 55–60.

Croll TP. (1986) Enamel colour modifications by controlled hydrochloric acid–pumice abrasion. Techniques and examples. *Quintessence Int* **17**:81–7.

Croll TP. (1991a) *Enamel microabrasion.* Quintessence Publishing: Chicago.

Croll TP. (1997) Enamel microabrasion: observations after 10 years. *J Am Dent Assoc Suppl* **128**(4):45S–50S.

Croll TP. (1991b) Enamel microabrasion: the technique. *Quintessence Int* **20**:395–400.

Croll TP. (1998) Esthetic correction with fluorosis and fluorosis-like enamel dysmineralization. *J Esthet Dent* **10**(1):21–9.

Donly KJ, O'Neill M, Croll TP. (1992) Enamel microabrasion: a microscopic evaluation of the "abrosion effect." *Quintessence Int* **23**:175–9.

Greenwall LH. (2006) Combining home bleaching and microabrasion. *Aesthet Implant Dent* **8**(3):34–41.

Greenwall LH. (2009) White lesions and bleaching treatments. *Aesthet Dent Today* **3**(2):15–8.

Greenwall LH. (2013) White lesion eradication using resin infiltration. *Aesthet Dent Today* June 15–18.

Haywood VB. (1995) Bleaching and microabrasion options. *Esthet Dent Update* **6**(4):99–100.

Kielbassa AM, Muller J, Gernhardt CR. (2009) Closing the gap between oral hygiene and minimal invasive dentistry: a review on the resin infiltration technique of incipient (proximal) enamel lesions. *Quintessence Int* **40**(8): 663–81.

Kim S, Kim EY, Jeong TS, Kim JW. (2011) The evaluation of resin infiltration for masking labial enamel white spot lesions. *Int J Paediatr Dent* **21**(4):241–8.

Kugel G, Arsenault P, Papas A. (2009) Treatment modalities for caries management, including a new resin infiltration system. *Compend Contin Educ Dent* **3**:1–10.

Lai PY, Seow WK, Tudehope DI, Rogers Y. (1997) Enamel hypoplasia and dental caries in very-low birthweight children: a case-controlled, longitudinal study. *Pediatr Dent* **19**(1):42–9.

McCloskey R. (1984) A technique for removal of fluorosis stains. *J Am Dent Assoc* **109**:63–4.

McEvoy SA. (1998) Combining chemical agents and techniques to remove intrinsic stains from vital teeth. *Gen Dent* **46**(2):168-72; quiz 173–4.

Meyer-Lueckel H, Paris S. (2008) Improved resin infiltration of natural caries lesions. *J Dent Res* **87**:1112–1126.

Muñoz MA, Arana-Gordillo LA, Gomes GM, Gomes OM. (2013) Alternative esthetic management of fluorosis and hypoplasia stains: blending effect obtained with resin infiltration techniques. *J Esthet Restor Dent* **25**(1):32–9.

Paris S, Dorfer CE, Meyer-Lueckel H. (2010) Surface conditioning of natural enamel caries lesions in deciduous teeth in preparation for resin infiltration. *J Dent* **38**:65–71.

Paris S, Meyer-Lueckel H. (2012) The potential for resin infiltration technique in dental practice. *Dent Update* **39**(9):623–6, 628.

Pharck JH, Duarte S, Meyer-Leuckel H. (2009) Caries infiltration with resins. A novel treatment option for interproximal caries. *Compend Contin Educ Dent* **Spec No 3**:13–7.

Rosenthaler H, Randel H. (1998) Rotary reduction, enamel microabrasion and dental bleaching for tooth colour improvement. *Compend Contin Educ Dent* **19**(1):62–7.

Segura A, Donly KJ, Wefel JS. (1997) The effects of microabrasion on demineralisation inhibition of enamel surfaces. *Quintessence Int* **28**:463–6.

Sheoran N, Garg S, Damle SG, Dhindsa A. (2014) Esthetic management of developmental enamel opacities in young permanent maxillary incisors with two microabrasion techniques—a split mouth study. *J Esthet Restor Dent* **26**(5):345–52.

Tirlet G, Attal JP. (2011) L'erosion/infiltration: une nouvelle therapeutique pour masque les taches blanches. *Inf Dent* **4**:12–6.

Touati B, Miara P, Nathanson D. (1999) Treatment of tooth discolouration. In *Esthetic dentistry and ceramic restorations.* Martin Dunitz: London, 83–116.

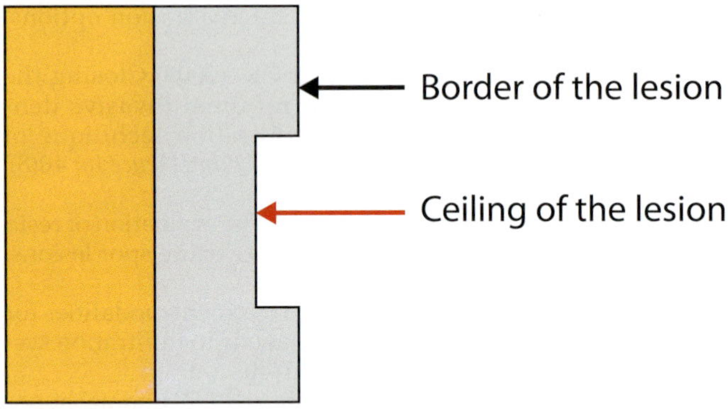

Figure 10.1

Anatomy of a white spot lesion, which extends to the dentinoenamel junction. (Redrawn with permission from Attal et al. 2014).

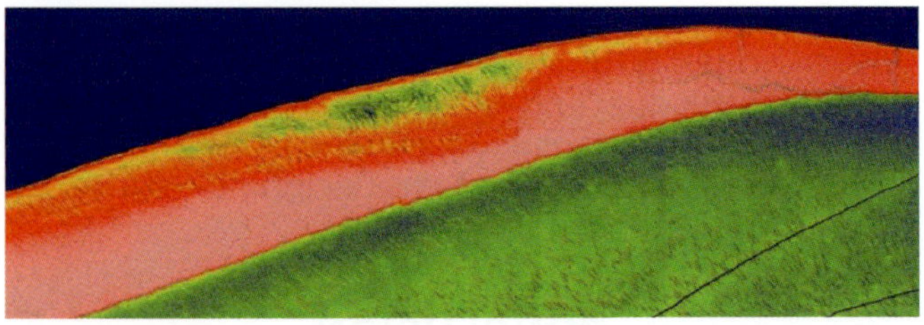

Figure 10.2

Longitudinal section of a deciduous central incisor. Cool colors are at the least dense end of the mineralization density spectrum, and warm colors are at the most dense. (Blue is the embedding resin.) The pink is enamel, which is increasingly demineralized from red, to yellow, to green, to blue; there is a subsurface demineralization in the center of the image. The lower band of green, along with a lower density blue below the dentinoenamel junction, is all normal dentin. (Courtesy of Dr. Timothy Bromage.)

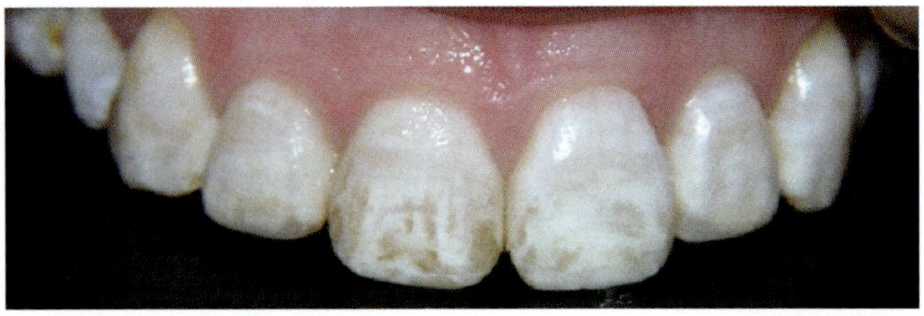

(A)

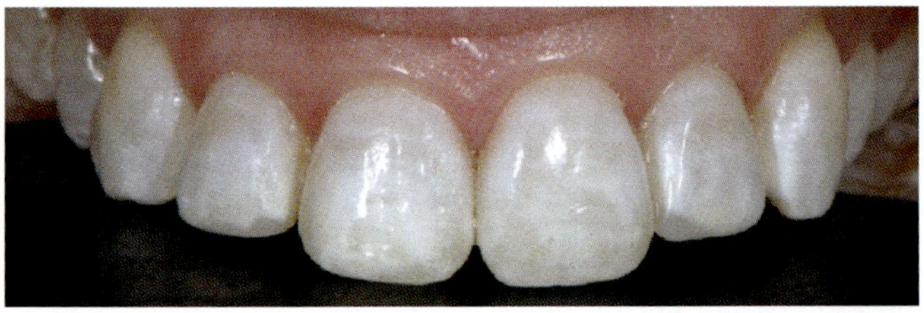

(B)

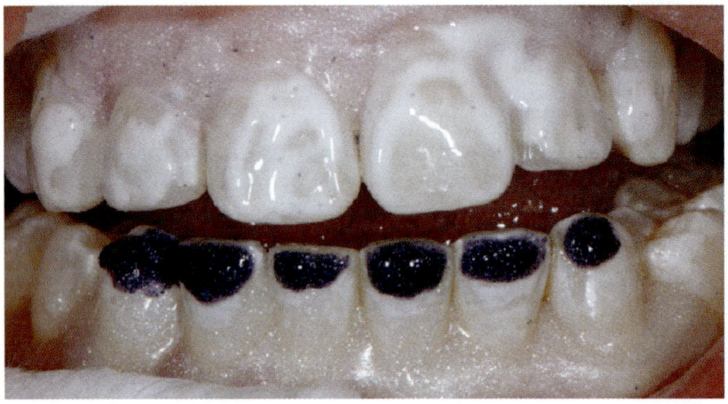

(C)

Figure 10.3

(A) This patient has moderate fluorosis on her anterior teeth. (B) After treatment, which consisted of whitening treatment for 8–10 weeks using carbamide peroxide gel followed by two sessions of microabrasion treatment using 6.6% Opalustre paste. (C) After isolation, the microabrasion material is placed directly onto the buccal surfaces of the teeth. The material is applied and then rinsed off using a wet cotton roll to wipe off the excess. The material is applied at least four to six times during the appointment. After the upper teeth have been treated, a material containing amorphous calcium phosphate is placed directly onto the upper teeth (MI Paste, GC America, Alsip, IL). The lower teeth are then treated.

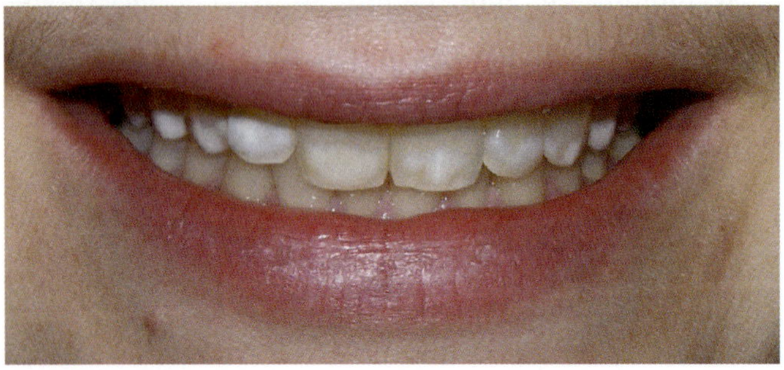

(A)

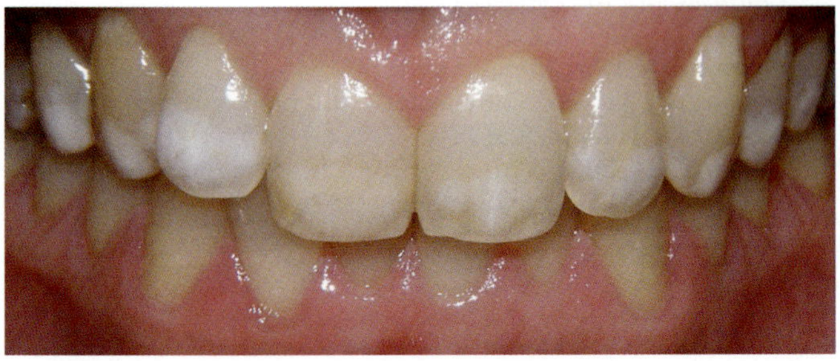

(B)

Figure 10.4

(A) A patient with more extensive white patches on her teeth. The treatment undertaken shows a combined approach wherein whitening, two sessions of microabrasion treatment using 6.6% hydrochloric acid, and two sessions of resin infiltration were undertaken to achieve a good result. The patient wanted to achieve a result using a minimally invasive approach to preserve the enamel as much as possible. (B) Retracted view before treatment showing appearance of white markings.
continued on the next page

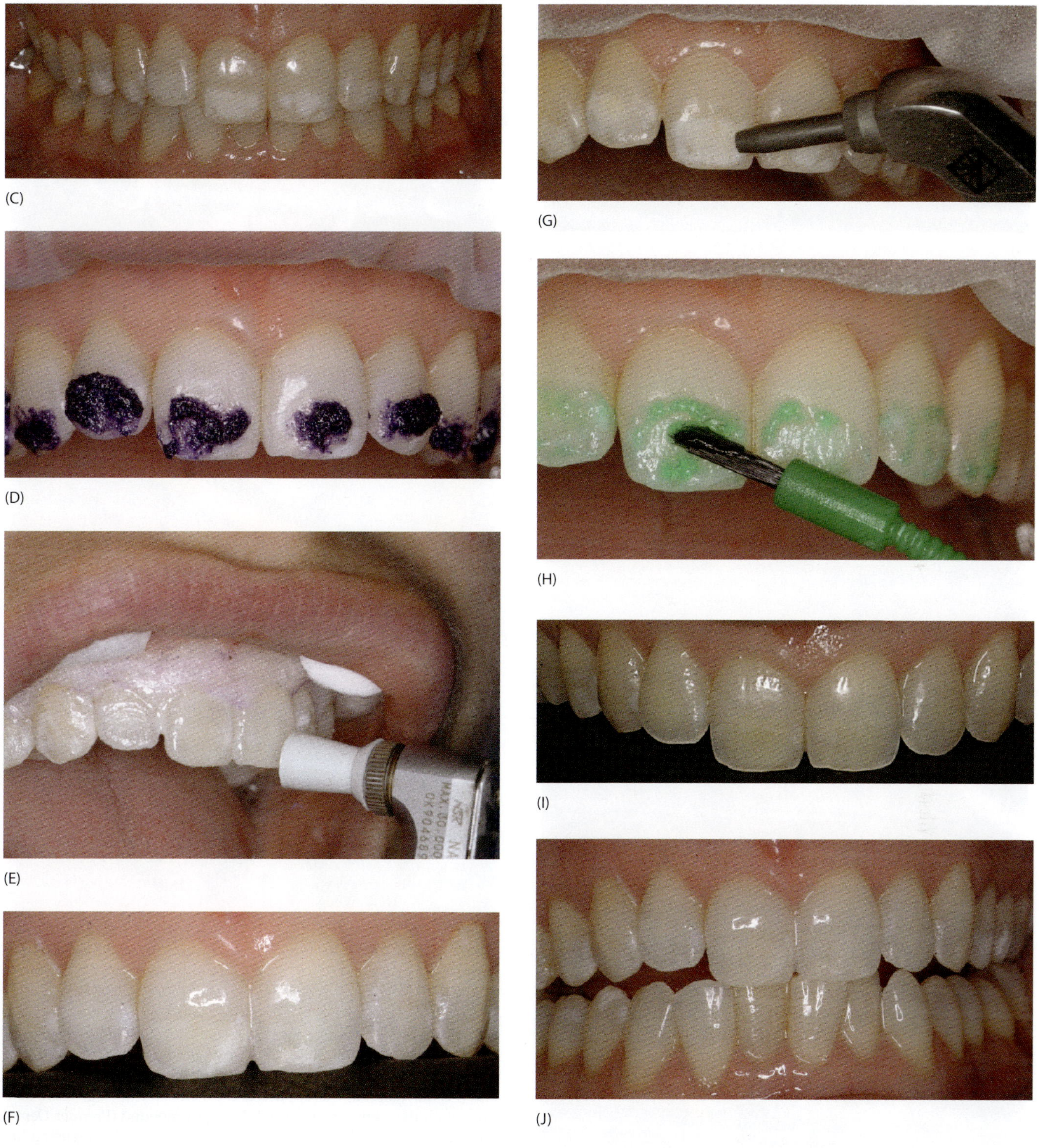

Figure 10.4 continued

(C) Result after 2 weeks of whitening of the upper teeth. (D) First microabrasion treatment. The microabrasion paste Opalustre is placed directly onto the white markings only and the material is polished onto the teeth. (E) After the first stage of treatment, amorphous calcium phosphate is polished directly onto the teeth so that the enamel surface is strengthened. Amorphous calcium phosphate allows calcium and phosphate to be reabsorbed onto the teeth. (F) Results after first stage of microabrasion. (G) Sandblasting to get deeper penetration of the resin. (H) Resin infiltration material icon placed on the teeth directly onto the white patches. (I) Result after one session of resin infiltration treatment. (J) Result after final treatment.

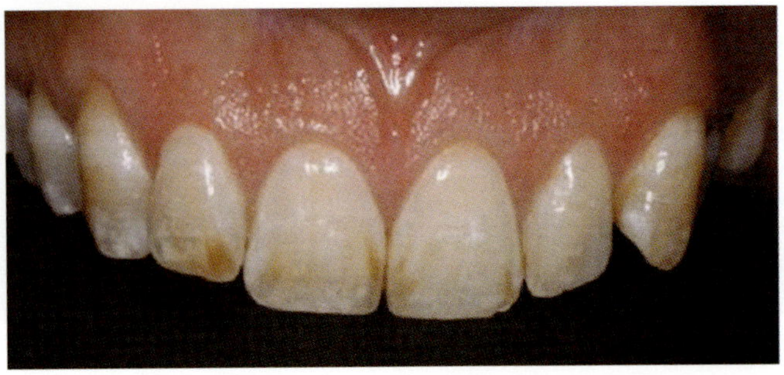

(A)

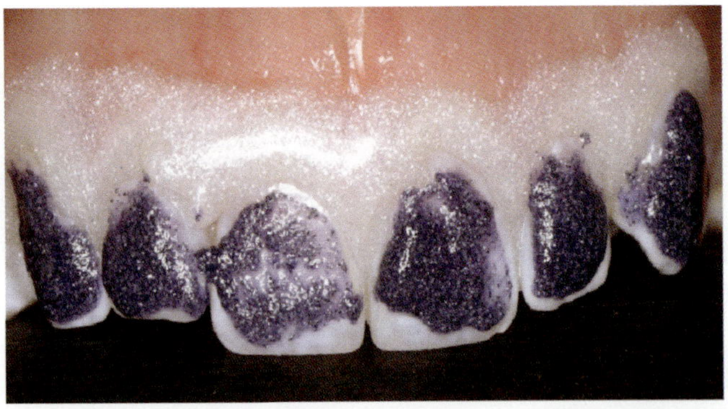

(B)

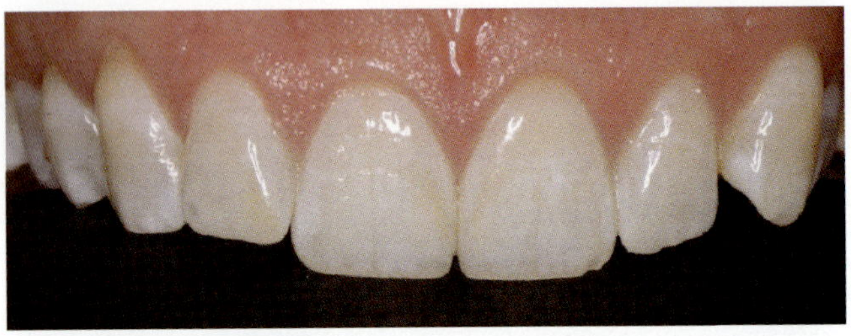

(C)

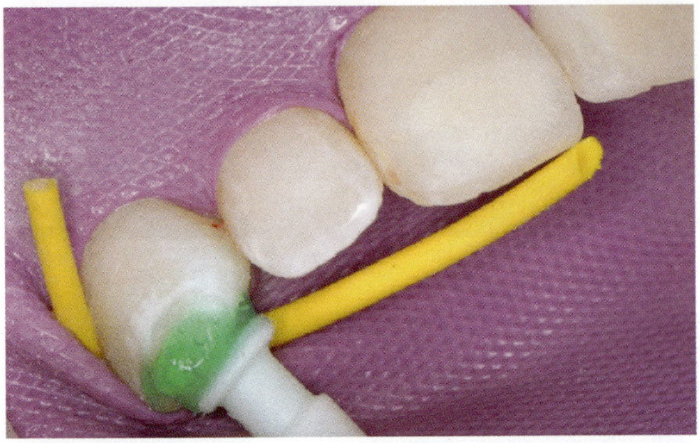

(D)

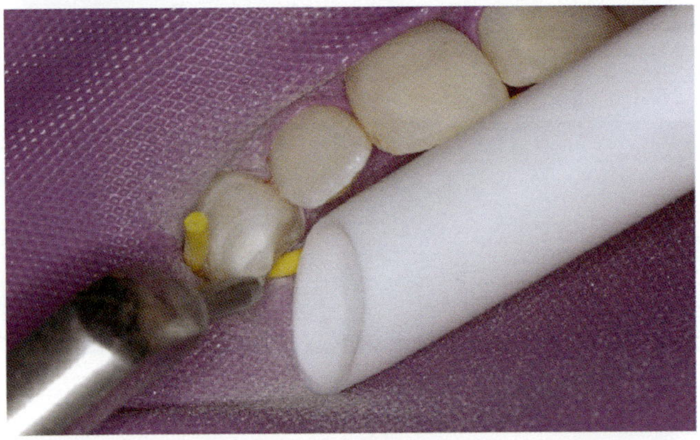

(E)

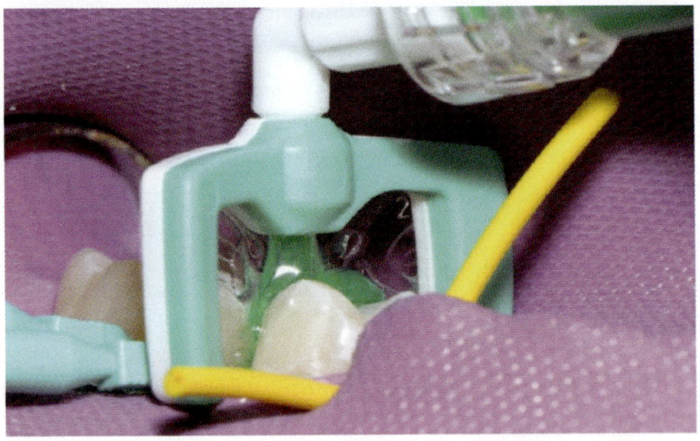

(F)

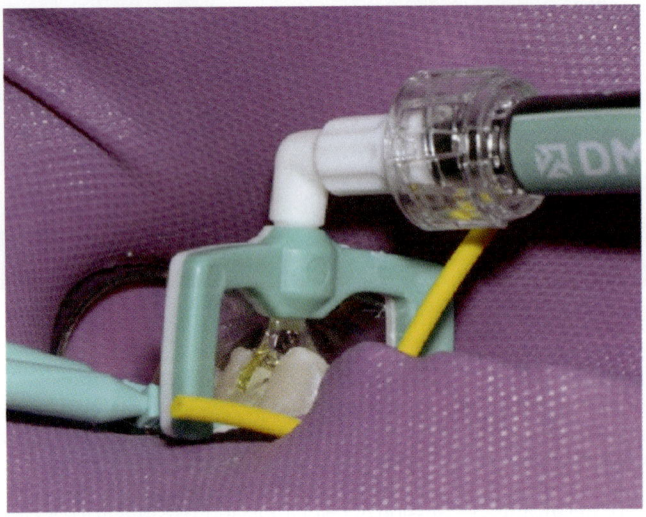

(G)

Figure 10.5

(A) Before whitening and microabrasion. White and brown dysmineralization present on the teeth. (B) After whitening treatment using 10% carbamide peroxide, microabrasion treatment using 10% hydrochloric acid (Prema material) was applied to the teeth. Note the light cure dam present on the teeth. The material Prema Compound (Premier Dental Products, Plymouth Meeting, PA) is applied with a rubber tip using 10:1 gear reduction angle. (C) The result after whitening and Prema microabrasion material. (D) The 15% hydrochloric acid is applied directly onto the tooth with an anterior sponge applicator. (E) Sandblasting the white lesion allows the resin to penetrate deeper. (F) Icon resin infiltration technique was originally designed to arrest interproximal decay. In the picture the 15% hydrochloric acid is place with a special applicator onto the interproximal part of the lesion. The applicator has small apertures, which are placed to face the side of the tooth where the lesion is situated. (G) The resin infiltrating the lesion using the specially created applicator for interproximal spaces.

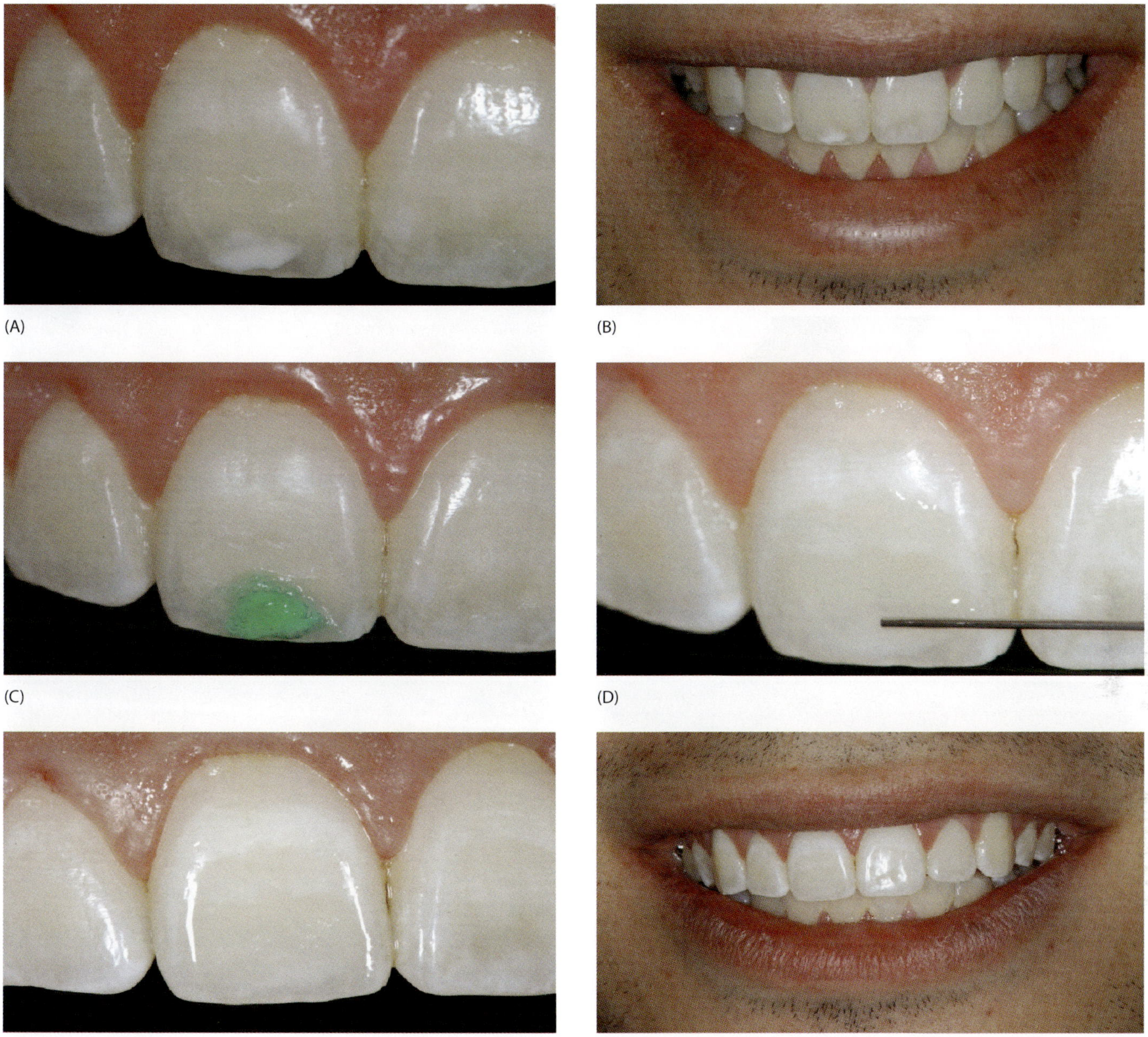

(A) (B) (C) (D) (E) (F)

Figure 10.6

(A) White spot present on the teeth before treatment. (B) Smile view showing the appearance of the white lesion before treatment. (C) Icon-Etch placed onto the white lesion. (D) Alcohol is placed onto the area to assess whether the initial placement of Icon-Etch will resolve the appearance of the white spot. (E) Final result after resin infiltration. (F) Smile view of the lesion after treatment. (With permission from Dr. Jean Pierre Attal, Paris.)

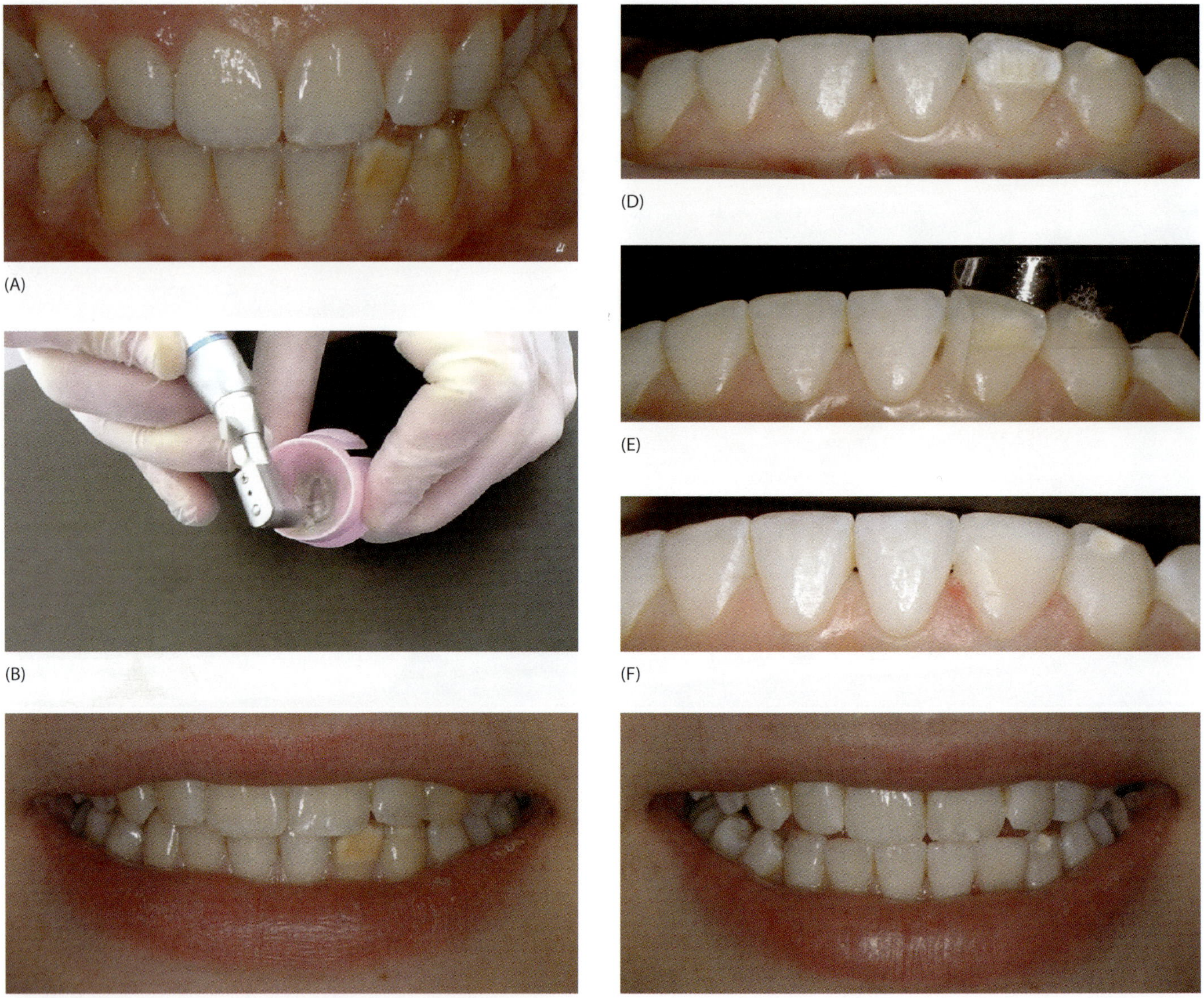

(A) (B) (C) (D) (E) (F) (G)

Figure 10.7

(A) Orange lesion on the lower left second incisor tooth. Treatment involved whitening first then microabrasion and a direct bonding onto the tooth. The patient should be warned that underneath the large orange lesion there is a white lesion that will need to be treated. All options should be discussed with the patient before the start of the whitening treatment. (B) The area is polished and cleaned with a microbrush and a mixture of pumice and chlorhexidine before microabrasion treatment. (C) Smile view before treatment showing the appearance of the orange lesion. (D) The result after whitening showing the large opaque white area remaining. (E) Placement of the clear matrix strip to prevent overhangs of composite material. A segmental layering approach is undertaken to mask the appearance of the white lesion. The tooth is first cleaned with pumice and Hibiscrub chlorhexidine then washed and etched, and the resin bonding material is placed. Then flowable enamel, whitened composite dentin material, and enamel composite are applied. (F) After whitening, microabrasion, resin infiltration of the smaller lesion, and a direct composite bond over the lower left incisor tooth. (G) Result after whitening and composite bonding.

plaque associated with poor oral hygiene or around previous orthodontic braces. On the molar teeth, some severe effects are associated with dental caries. These severely affected teeth are called "cheese molars."

Diagnosis

Early diagnosis is essential for appropriate treatment and to prevent deterioration of the condition in the child. The diagnosis is normally made based on the appearance of the lesions when the permanent teeth erupt (Table 11.1). The differential diagnosis includes enamel hypoplasia, fluorosis, and amelogenesis imperfecta. Rapid breakdown of tooth structure may occur, giving rise to acute symptoms and complicated treatment (Daly and Waldron 2009). There is often rapid breakdown of the first permanent molars from the stage of eruption at around 6 years; thus early detection and treatment are imperative.

Diagnosis can be made using gene evaluation; there are 11 different types of genes involved in enamel matrix formation. Saliva can be collected from the patient and his or her parents. These 11 single-nucleotide polymorphism (SNP) markers can be selected in genes involved in enamel formation and genotyped using predesigned TaqMan genotyping assays (these amplifications were made in a GeneAmp PCR System 9700 [Perkin Elmer Applied Biosystems, Foster City, California]) (Ranade et al. 2001).

For a diagnosis to be made, one to four permanent first molars may be affected as well as the upper central incisors, but the lower central incisors also may be affected (Williams et al. 2006).

Diagnosis can also be made from the color of the permanent molar. Yellow-brown defects have lower Knoop hardness values and greater porosity than white defects and normal enamel and indicate a need for quicker intervention.

Signs and symptoms

Molar teeth with hypocalcification are porous and soft. These affected teeth can be very sensitive to air and cold, warm, and mechanical stimuli. Even tooth brushing may create toothache in these teeth. Children with MIH can have more intense dental sensitivity from temperature variations (Weerheijm et al. 2001), and there is innervation density in the area of the hypoplasia and the subodontoblastic region of hypomineralized teeth compared with sound teeth (Shubna and Hegde 2013).

This is a result of the combination of the chronic pulp inflammation and innervation of the region right under the hypomineralized area (Rodd et al. 2007). Consequently, children with MIH may have hampered anesthetic action, which can affect their behavior (Rodd et al. 2007). The extreme sensitivity that these children experience causes further deterioration of the tooth because the child cannot brush the teeth, which are too sensitive. Older children have more severe manifestations because the tooth continues to deteriorate after eruption (Shubna and Hegde 2013). Bacteria enter these porous areas of the dentin and rapidly break down the enamel (Fagrell et al. 2008). In sections where bacteria were found in the cuspal areas or deeper in the dentin, a zone of reparative dentin was found; and in sections from one tooth, the coronal pulp showed an inflammatory reaction with inflammatory cells. The dentinal tubules with odontoblastic processes were filled with bacteria (Fagrell et al. 2008). The transitional ameloblast is considered most vulnerable, and when these cells do not undergo complete maturation, full-thickness hypomineralization occurs. Enamel maturation involves (1) the removal of acid labile mineral, (2) replacement with more acid-resistant apatite, and (3) an influx of calcium and phosphate ions, increasing the crystal width and thickness (Avery 2002).

Table 11.1 Recommended diagnostic criteria for molar incisor hypoplasia (MIH) from the European Academy of Paediatric Dentistry

Criteria	*Definitions*
Permanent first molars and incisors	One to all four permanent first molars (PFMs) show hypomineralization of the enamel. Simultaneously, the permanent incisors can be affected. To diagnose MIH, at least one PFM has to be affected. The defects can also be seen in second primary molars, incisors, and the tips of canines. The more molars and incisors affected, the more severe the defect.
Demarcated opacities	The affected teeth show clearly demarcated opacities at the occlusal and buccal parts of the crown. The defects vary in color and size. The color can be white, creamy, or yellow to brownish. The defect can be negligible or comprise the major part of the crown. It is recommended that defects less than 1 mm not be reported.
Enamel disintegration	The degree of porosity of the hypomineralized opaque areas varies. Severely affected enamel subjected to masticatory forces soon breaks down, leading to unprotected dentin and rapid caries development.
Atypical restorations	PFMs and incisors with restorations revealing extensions similar to MIH are recommended to be judged as affected.
Tooth sensitivity	The affected teeth may be reported frequently as sensitive, ranging from a mild response to external stimuli to spontaneous hypersensitivity; these teeth are usually difficult to anesthetize.
Extracted teeth	Extracted teeth can be defined as having MIH only in cases where there are notes in the records or demarcated opacities on the other PFMs. Otherwise it is not possible to diagnose MIH.

Adapted from Lygidakis et al. 2010, with permission from Springer.

Treatment options

- Early diagnosis
- Risk assessment—medical and dental history
- Prevention regimens—remineralization

We suggest that these patients receive intensified prevention with fluoride varnish, fissure sealing, and amorphous calcium phosphate varnish placement. A new remineralizing agent based on casein phosphopeptide and amorphous calcium phosphate (CPP-ACP) has been proposed to be effective in hypomineralized enamel, improving also esthetic conditions (Mastroberardino et al. 2012).

Operative options

Mechanical removal of soft material from the tooth is performed first, followed by:

1. Placement of a glass ionomer restoration.
2. Composite restorations.
3. Extracoronal restorations such as stainless steel crowns, composite crowns.
4. Extractions if severely affected, and orthodontic closure of spaces.
5. Implants in extreme cases.

In some cases an interdisciplinary approach with an orthodontist can result in the extraction of the molars in patients aged 8–10 years.

Esthetic options for treating teeth affected by molar incisor hypoplasia

1. Tooth whitening. Tooth whitening has been shown to reduce caries and root caries, and this would be an option in mild to moderate MIH. Otherwise, for the deeper lesions, restorations with glass ionomer would be performed first, followed by whitening treatment.
2. Microabrasion of the labial enamel.
3. Icon treatment on both anterior and posterior mildly affected areas.
4. Direct composite bonding.
5. Preformed veneers over the teeth.
6. Porcelain veneers.

Maintenance and monitoring

- Long-term frequent regular follow-up is necessary for these patients, including regular preventive regimens repeated every 3 months until the mouth is stable.
- Oral health maintenance and health sustainability for the teeth are considerations (see Table 24.3).

CONCLUSION

It is important that the correct diagnosis be made early because multidisciplinary approaches are necessary to treat these children. Options for treatment will range from the least invasive methods to coronal coverage and extraction with orthodontic treatment. A multidisciplinary team may need to be involved to assist with treatment planning to achieve a good long-term outcome.

REFERENCES

Alaluusua S. (2010) Aetiology of molar-incisor hypomineralisation: a systematic review. *Eur Arch Paediatr Dent* **11:**53–8.

Avery J. (2002) *Oral development and histology*, 3rd ed. Thieme: Stuttgart, Germany.

Crombie F, Manton D, Kilpatrick N. (2009) Aetiology of molar-incisor hypomineralization: a critical review. *Int J Paediatr Dent* **19**(2):73–83.

Daly D, Waldron JM. (2009) Molar incisor hypomineralisation: clinical management of the young patient. *J Ir Dent Assoc* **55**(2):83–6.

Edginton AN, Ritter L. (2009) Predicting plasma concentrations of bisphenol A in children younger than 2 years of age after typical feeding schedules, using a physiologically based toxicokinetic model. *Environ Health Perspect* **117:**645–52.

Fagrell TG, Lingström P, Olsson S, Steiniger F. (2008) Bacterial invasion of dentinal tubules beneath apparently intact but hypomineralized enamel in molar teeth with molar incisor hypomineralization. *Int J Paediatr Dent* **18**(5):333–40.

Jälevik B. (2010) Prevalence and diagnosis of molar-incisor-hypomineralisation (MIH): a systematic review. *Eur Arch Paediatr Dent* **11:**59–64.

Jälevik B, Dietz W, Norén JG. (2005) Scanning electron micrograph analysis of hypomineralised enamel in permanent first molars. *Int J Paediatr Dent* **15:**233–40.

Jedeon K, De la Dure-Molla M, Brookes SJ, Loiodice S. (2013) Enamel defects reflect perinatal exposure to bisphenol A. *Am J Pathol* **183**(1):108–18.

Jeremias F, Koruyucu M, Küchler EC, Bayram M. (2013) Genes expressed in dental enamel development are associated with molar-incisor hypomineralization. *Arch Oral Biol* **58**(10):1434–42.

Kellerhoff NM, Lussi A. (2004) ["Molar-incisor hypomineralization"]. *Schweiz Monatsschr Zahnmed* **114**(3):243–53.

Lygidakis NA, Dimou G, Marinou D. (2008) Molar-incisor hypomineralization (MIH). A retrospective clinical study in Greek children. II. Possible medical aetiological factors. *Eur Arch Paediatr Dent* **9**(4):207–17.

Lygidakis NA, Wong F, Jälevik B, Vierrou AM. (2010) Best clinical practice guidance for clinicians dealing with children presenting with molar-incisor hypomineralisation (MIH): an EAPD policy document. *Eur Arch Paediatr Dent* **11**(2):75–81.

Mastroberardino S, Campus G, Strohmenger L, Villa A. (2012) An innovative approach to treat incisors hypomineralization (MIH): a combined use of casein phosphopeptide–amorphous calcium phosphate and hydrogen peroxide—a case report. *Case Rep Dent* **2012:**379593.

Ranade K, Chang MS, Ting CT, Pei D. (2001) High-throughput genotyping with single nucleotide polymorphisms. *Genome Res* **11**(7):1262–8.

Robinson C, Kirkham J, Brookes SJ, Bonass WA. (1995) The chemistry of enamel development. *Int J Dev Biol* **39:** 145–52.

Rodd HD, Morgan CR, Day PF, Boissonade FM. (2007) Pulpal expression of TRPV1 in molar incisor hypomineralization. *Eur Arch Paediatr Dent* **8**(4):184–8.

Sahlstrand P, Lith A, Hakeberg M, Norén JG. (2013) Timing of mineralization of homologues permanent teeth—an evaluation of the dental maturation in panoramic radiographs. *Swed Dent J* **37**(3):111–9.

Shubna AB, Hegde S. (2013) Molar-incisor hypomineralization: review of its prevalence, etiology and clinical appearance and management. *Int J Oral Maxillofac Pathol* **4**:26–33.

Weerheijm KL, Duggal M, Mejàre I, Papagiannoulis L. (2003) Judgement criteria for molar incisor hypomineralisation (MIH) in epidemiologic studies: a summary of the European meeting on MIH held in Athens. *Eur J Paediatr Dent* **4**:110–3.

Weerheijm KL, Jalevik B, Alaluusua S. (2001) Molar-incisor hypomineralization. *Caries Res* **35**(5):390–391.

Weerheijm KL, Merjare I. (2003) Molar incisor hypomineralisation: a questionnaire inventory on its occurrence in member countries of the European Academy of Paediatric Dentistry (EAPD). *Int J Paediatr Dent* **13**:411–6.

Williams V, Messer LB, Burrow MF. (2006) Molar incisor hypomineralization: review and recommendations for clinical management. *Pediatr Dent* **28**(3):224–32.

Willmott NS, Bryan RA, Duggal MS. (2008) Molar-incisor-hypomineralisation: a literature review. *Eur Arch Paediatr Dent* **9**(4):172–9.

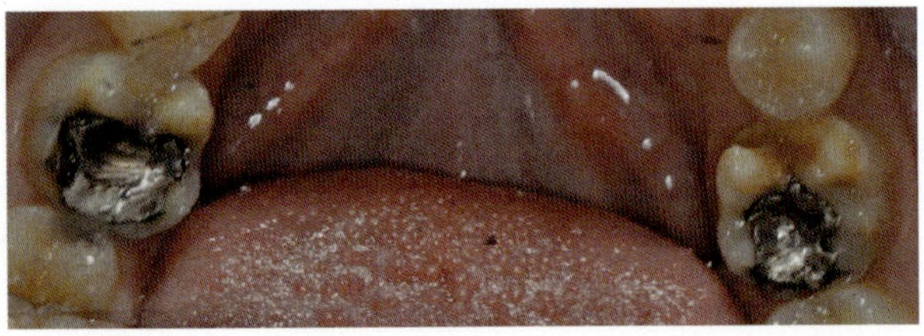

Figure 11.1

This 15-year-old has molar incisor hypoplasia of the lower left and right first molars (36, 46) and of the upper and lower incisors. We carried out whitening, microabrasion, and resin infiltration and replaced the old amalgam filling on the lower left and right first molars with composite.

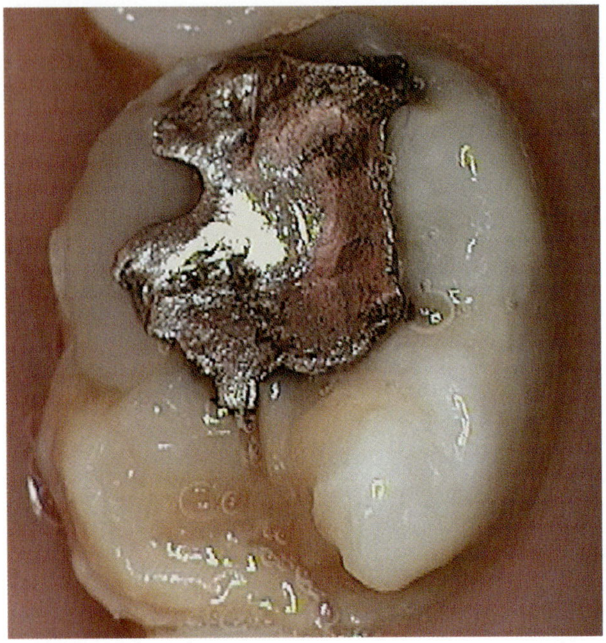

Figure 11.2

The lower first molar (36) was filled with an amalgam filling. The enamel surrounding the filling is very weak and broken down.

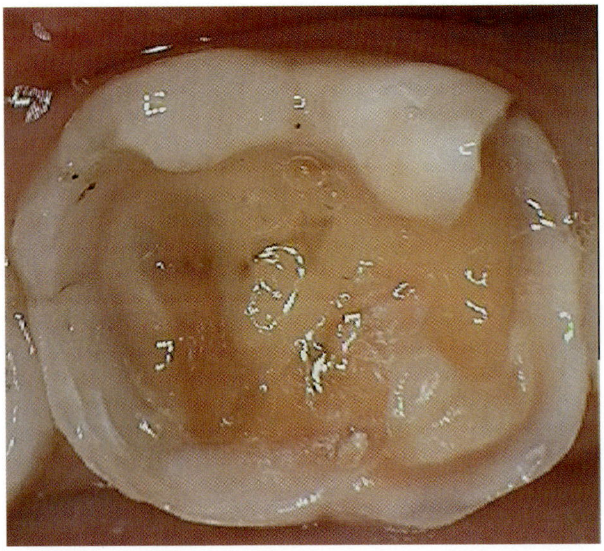

Figure 11.3

The amalgam filling was removed. There is minimal tooth structure left.

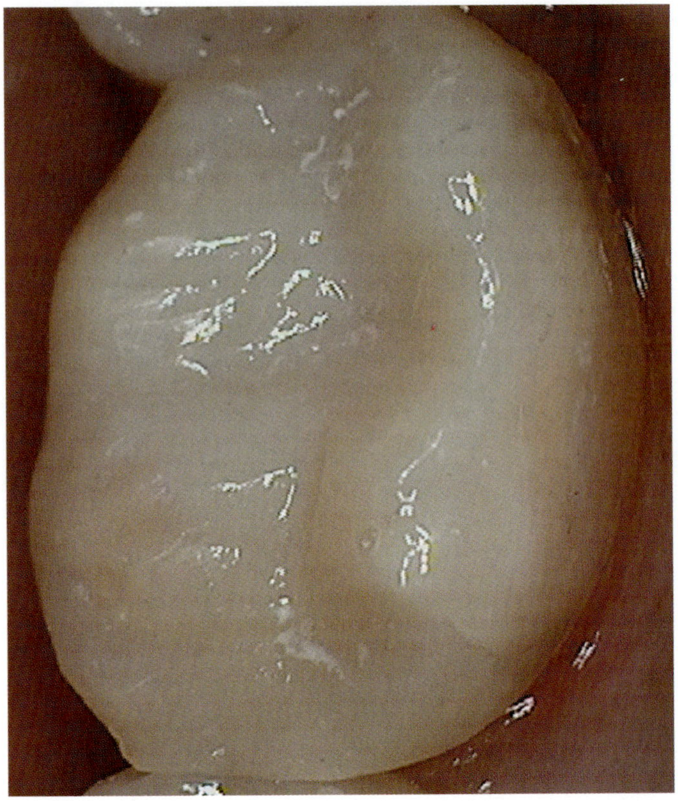

Figure 11.4

The tooth is restored with a composite restoration. In the future this tooth may require an onlay of a crown because of the size of the restoration.

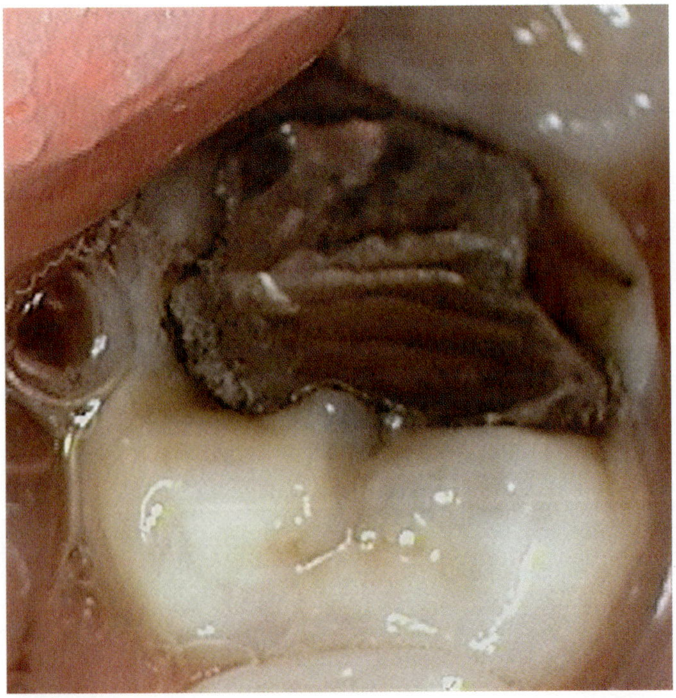

Figure 11.5

The lower right first molar (46) was also restored with an amalgam filling. There is a larger amount of enamel left than on the lower left.

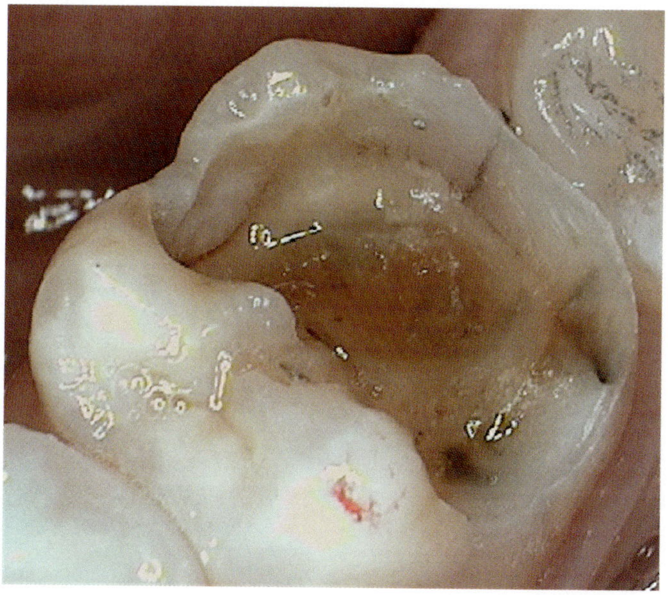

Figure 11.6

Lower right first molar (46) once the amalgam has been removed.

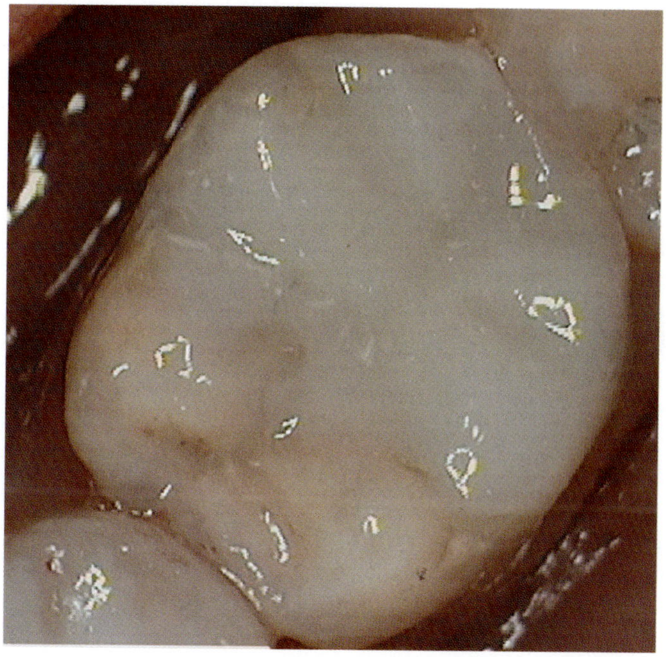

Figure 11.7

The tooth is restored with a composite restoration.

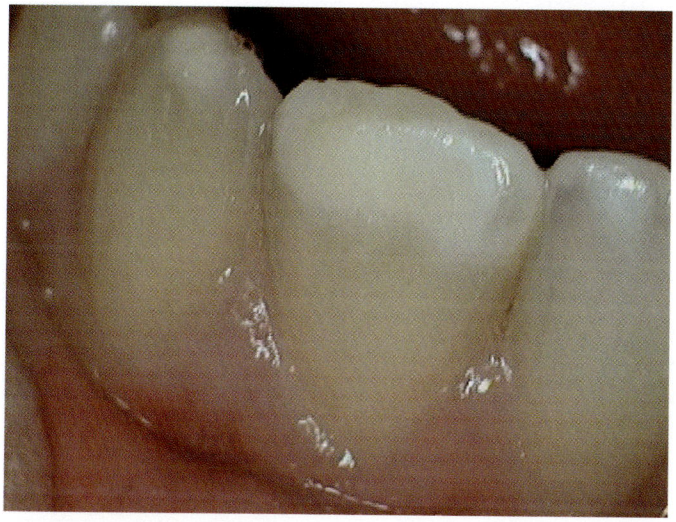

Figure 11.8

Molar incisor hypoplasia on the lower incisor. This tooth has had whitening and microabrasion to help fade the white spot.

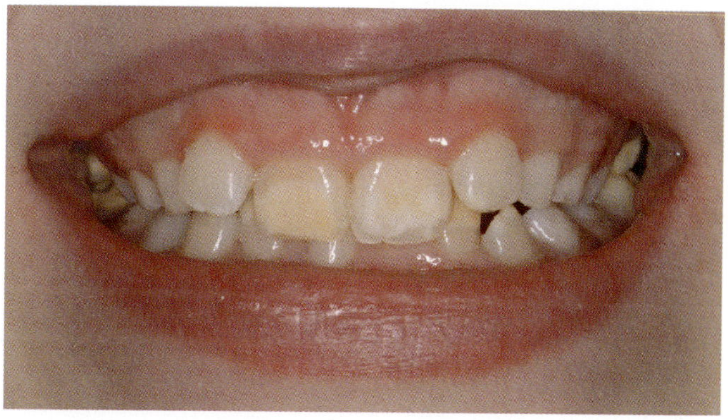

Figure 11.9

This 10-year-old girl has molar incisor hypoplasia on all her first molars and her upper left and right central incisors.

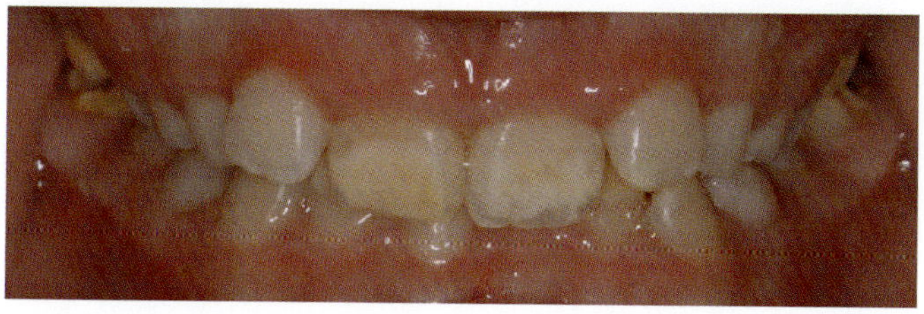

Figure 11.10

Retracted view of the teeth. The first molars have been restored with a glass ionomer because the patient is still young. Long-term treatment would be crowns owing to the enamel destruction. The upper right and left central incisors will receive resin infiltration treatment to help mask the white and yellow spots. In the future whitening, microabrasion and possibly bondings will be performed.

12 MANAGEMENT OF TETRACYCLINE DISCOLORATION

Philip R.H. Newsome

INTRODUCTION

Tetracycline broad-spectrum antibiotics were introduced in 1948 and quickly found favor in the treatment of a multitude of commonly occurring childhood and adult infections. All tetracycline compounds consist of four fused cyclic rings, hence the name *tetracyclines*. More than 60 years later they are still commonly used in the treatment of acne, and in addition there has been a resurgence of interest in them as a result of their beneficial use in combination therapy for bone metastasis (Saikali and Singh 2003) as well as in the treatment and prophylaxis of tuberculosis, anthrax, and malaria. Although they possess undoubted therapeutic benefits, tetracycline compounds have, nevertheless, also been found to exhibit a number of significant systemic side effects. These include hepatic damage in pregnant women (Madison 1963) as well as toxic, damaging effects on the developing fetus as a result their ability to cross the placenta. They are clearly, therefore, contraindicated during pregnancy.

EFFECTS OF TETRACYCLINES ON TEETH

One of the most obvious side effects of tetracycline use (and in particular minocycline [Minocin], which is a semisynthetic tetracycline derivative) is its incorporation as a fluorescent pigment into tissues that are calcifying at the time of administration (Cheek and Heymann 1999). It has the ability to chelate calcium ions and to be incorporated into teeth, cartilage, and bone, to form a tetracycline-calcium orthophosphate complex (Eisenberg and Bernick 1975) resulting in discoloration and enamel hypoplasia of both the primary and permanent dentitions if administered during the period of tooth development. The ability of tetracycline to intrinsically stain teeth during odontogenesis has been well known and documented for almost five decades (Schwachman and Schuster 1956, Davies et al. 1962) and usually causes affected patients considerable distress as well as posing a number of problems for dentists charged with the task of improving the appearance of such teeth.

The severity of the discoloration is considered to be related to dose, frequency, duration of therapy, and, critically, the stage of odontogenesis. The calcification of deciduous teeth begins at approximately the end of the fourth month of gestation and ends at approximately 11–14 months of age. Permanent teeth begin calcifying after birth and are not affected by exposure to tetracycline during the prenatal period. The calcification of permanent teeth is completed at 7–8 years of age with the exception of the third molars (Mello 1967, Jackson 1979). Therefore, in addition to the reasons stated earlier, the administration of tetracycline to pregnant women as well as to children up to 8 years of age must be avoided because it may result in discoloration (see Figure 12.2) and enamel hypoplasia (Conchie et al. 1970). Enamel hypoplasia (see Figure 12.1) can, of course, also be the result of childhood disease, hereditary defects in enamel formation, or prematurity of the child—all of which are known to cause enamel defects. Tetracyclines are excreted in urine and feces, with the urinary route being the most important for the majority of these drugs. The drugs should not be given to nursing mothers because they are also excreted in human milk (van der Bijl and Pitigoi-Aron 1995). Adult-onset tooth discoloration after long-term ingestion of tetracycline has also been reported (Di Benedetto 1985). The prevalence of tetracycline discoloration has ranged from 0.4–6% in various studies (Martin and Barnard 1969, Suckling and Pearce 1984, Berger et al. 1989), the actual figure clearly being a reflection of the prevailing prescribing habits of medical practitioners in any particular region at any given time. For example, King and Wei (1989) reported a prevalence of over 16% in Hong Kong's population.

The ensuing discoloration is permanent and varies from yellow or gray to brown depending on the dose or the type of the drug received in relation to body weight. After tooth eruption and exposure to light, the fluorescent yellow discoloration gradually changes over a period of months and years to a nonfluorescent brown color. The labial surfaces of yellow-stained anterior teeth will darken in time, whereas the palatal surfaces and buccal surfaces of posterior teeth will remain yellow. These changes are thought to be the result of an oxidation product of tetracycline, which is light induced (Bevelander et al. 1961, Atkinson and Hartcourt 1962). A further complication, and one that adds to the stigma associated with tetracycline-discolored teeth, is that tetracycline will fluoresce bright yellow under ultraviolet light in a dark room.

Minocycline hydrochloride, a semisynthetic derivative of tetracycline often used for the treatment of acne, has been shown to cause pigmentation of a variety of tissues including skin, thyroid, nails, sclera, teeth, conjunctiva, and bone (Rosen and Hoffmann 1989). A further side effect of minocycline on the oral cavity is the occurrence of "black bones," "black" or "green roots," and blue-gray to gray darkening of the crowns of permanent teeth. Minocycline differs from other tetracyclines in that it is well absorbed from the gastrointestinal tract and chelates with iron to form insoluble complexes, and this may provoke the tooth staining. It is best to try to avoid the long-term use of minocycline because this discoloration can be the most difficult to bleach. It is also important to discuss this complication with the patient's medical practitioner so that he or she can administer a different medication.

DIAGNOSIS

It is important to recognize other causes of tooth staining to discriminate among tetracycline staining, minocycline staining, and other extrinsic or intrinsic tooth-staining problems (Table 12.1).

TREATMENT

Nowhere does the old adage that "an ounce of prevention is better than a pound of cure" apply better than with the prescription of tetracycline, not only from the patient's point of view but also from that of the clinician, especially when one takes into account possible medico-legal implications. Indeed, a legal precedent was set in 1982 when tetracycline was alleged to have caused discoloration of the teeth of two children with an ensuing, successful, legal action being brought against the prescribing general medical practitioner (Medical Protection Society 1982).

When actual treatment is sought—and this is almost always for esthetic reasons—there are a number of possible treatment options. These are as follows (in increasing degrees of invasiveness):

1. Tooth bleaching only.
2. Tooth bleaching and composite bonding, full or partial, over discolored areas (Figure 12.1).
3. Combination treatment starting with tooth bleaching and continuing to direct veneers (Figure 12.2).
4. Indirect laminate veneers (with or without prior tooth bleaching).
5. Full-coverage restorations.

When considering which of these options one should pursue, Dietschi has wisely observed that "Clinicians should correct restorative challenges by selecting a progressive treatment concept that begins with the most conservative restorative option and progresses to more invasive procedures only as required."

Table 12.1 Causes of tooth staining

Extrinsic factors	*Characteristics*
Chromogenic bacteria stains	Green, black-brown, and orange
Tobacco	Black, brown
Amalgam	Black, gray
Medicaments	Silver nitrate: gray, black
	Stannous fluoride: black, brown
	Chlorhexidine: black, brown
Foods and beverages	Coffee, tea, wine, berries, and others: color of food item
Iron	Black cervical discoloration
Intrinsic factors	*Characteristics*
Dentinogenesis imperfecta	Yellow or gray-brown
Amelogenesis imperfecta	Yellow-brown
Dental fluorosis	Opaque white to yellow-brown patches
Sulphur drugs	Black staining
Tetracyclines:	
Chlortetracycline	Gray-brown hue
Oxytetracycline	Brown-yellow to yellow
Tetracycline hydrochloride	Brown-yellow to yellow
Dimethylchlortetracycline	Brown-yellow to yellow
Minocycline	Blue-gray to gray
Doxycycline	No change
Dental trauma	Transiently red through to black
Hyperbilirubinemia	Yellow-green to blue, brown, and gray
Erythropoietic porphyria	Red or brown
Ochronosis	Brown

TOOTH BLEACHING

The treatment of tetracycline staining with tooth bleaching has been used with varying degrees of success for the last 40 years. Haywood et al. (1997) were the first to show that carbamide peroxide, applied in trays and used overnight, can be effective in the treatment of tetracycline-stained teeth. Since then, other studies have confirmed the beneficial effects of combining in-office bleaching with home use of carbamide peroxide (Fiedler and Reichl 2000) and of hydrogen peroxide within bleaching strips (Kugel et al. 2002). A 90-month follow-up of Haywood's 1997 study has been published and highlights the effectiveness of tray bleaching in reducing discoloration for an extended period of time (Leonard et al. 2003). The success of such treatment largely depends on the depth, severity, and degree of the discoloration; to make a well-informed prediction of likely treatment outcome, it is advisable to grade the degree of discoloration in terms of the following classification as devised by Jordan and Boksman (1984):

1. First degree: mild tetracycline staining. This is yellow to gray with no banding and is uniformly spread throughout the tooth. See Figure 12.1.
2. Second degree: moderate tetracycline staining. This is yellow-brown to dark-gray staining.
3. Third degree: severe tetracycline staining. This is blue-gray or black and is accompanied by significant banding across the tooth. See Figure 12.2.
4. Fourth degree: intractable staining is staining that is so severe that bleaching is ineffective.

5. A fifth degree of severe staining with enamel deficiency (such as white spots and ridges) has also been described (see Chapter 13).

Normally, bleaching can be successful in the first three types—namely, mild, moderate, and severe—and in each the best option is usually to bleach the teeth first and then review the need for further, more invasive, treatment. Types of bleaching treatment for tetracycline staining are as follows:

1. Home bleaching. This is the most predictable option to try.
2. Combination bleaching or deep bleaching (Chapter 15). This may work using both home and chairside treatments.
3. Power bleaching (Chapter 7). This approach will offer limited success for patients with tetracycline staining and may require multiple visits because the bleaching gel is usually unable to penetrate the dentin sufficiently deeply during the 1-hour power bleaching session.
4. Intentional devitalization (Chapter 8) and internal nonvital bleaching. This method has been recommended (Abou-Rass 1982) for severe tetracycline staining and consists of devitalizing the teeth and thereafter undertaking nonvital bleaching using hydrogen peroxide. Clearly, such a radical approach is controversial and it is now very rarely indicated given the success of home bleaching.

The treatment regimen for bleaching tetracycline teeth

Haywood et al. (1997) showed that it takes longer to bleach tetracycline-stained teeth in comparison with teeth yellowed with age and normal wear and tear and it is therefore necessary to set up a well-considered treatment program for these patients. Patients should be seen for an initial assessment during which photographs and radiographs are taken and a full detailed intraoral examination is performed. Tooth discolorations should be classified in terms of severity. All the various options ranging from bleaching and bonding (Haywood and Pohjola 2004) through to more extreme approaches such as porcelain veneers and full-coverage crowns should be discussed, and treatment should be planned to take place in a coordinated, sequential manner. Should bleaching be the preferred option, patients are advised that, according to research, treatment can take up to 3, 6, 9, or 12 months depending on the severity of the condition and its response to treatment. Given this, it is usually a wise precaution to underestimate the likely time taken to achieve a result and even the potential for improvement itself. Once the decision has been made to undertake bleaching, a review is normally set for around 2 to 3 weeks after the start of treatment to assess how much lightening has been achieved in that amount of time. Normally the upper teeth are bleached first using the home bleaching tray. This allows skeptical patients the opportunity to compare directly the treated upper teeth against the untreated lower ones. Patients are instructed about the treatment options for self-managing any possible sensitivity (Chapters 4 and 20). The lower bleaching tray is dispensed at this review appointment and the next review date set. The patient is given a 1-month supply of material, sufficient to treat both upper and lower teeth. Low concentrations of carbamide peroxide (10%) are used initially to prevent the patient from terminating treatment because of sensitivity. If the patient has experienced no sensitivity, the patient may then be given 15% carbamide peroxide gel to use. Matis et al. (2006) described the effects of bleaching using two of three different bleaching concentrations (10%, 15%, and 20% carbamide peroxide used overnight) for a 6-month period and found that bleaching could be accomplished with any of the three concentrations used. They also found that more than 55% of tooth lightening occurred within 1 month and that after 5 years, more than 65% of the maximum tooth bleaching remained for all three concentrations. Finally, the study revealed that cervical staining is the most difficult to correct.

Most of the home gels incorporate desensitizers such as potassium nitrate, fluoride, or amorphous calcium phosphate to reduce the incidence of sensitivity. At the 1-month review appointment the degree of improvement is assessed using the Vita porcelain shade guide and photographs taken. Depending on the result, the patient is then seen 1 month later and thereafter once a month until the bleaching treatment is completed. Often much of the initial lightness can be seen within the first 6 weeks, and thereafter the bleaching process may be a little slower. Further treatment may need to be undertaken; these decisions should be made together with the patient. In most instances patients are delighted with the result.

LAMINATE VENEERS

Indirect laminate veneers (usually ceramic, but occasionally composite) are one of the most commonly used ways of treating tetracycline-discolored teeth by restorative means. Directly applied composite is usually inadequate to mask tetracycline discoloration in all but the most minimally affected teeth.

Ceramic veneers have been around now for three decades and in that time have become a very useful and relatively conservative way of improving esthetics. Their use has grown considerably in recent years in line with developments such as dentin bonding and ultra-thin veneer systems. Not all of these developments have, however, been received entirely favorably, and concerns have been expressed about the widespread proliferation of ceramic veneers (Christensen 2006). When they were first introduced in the early 1980s it was recommended that veneers be restricted to those cases in which a predominantly enamel substrate was available, accompanied by minimal crowding, a favorable occlusion, and relatively little underlying tooth discoloration. Over time, though, these recommendations have increasingly been ignored, with the result that veneers are being used in ever more challenging circumstances. A growing number of "cosmetic" dentists display a worrying willingness to cut veneer preparations deeper than ever before into dentin to (1) mask extreme discolorations; (2) provide a bulk of ceramic capable of withstanding heavier occlusal loading; and (3) correct crowding, so-called "instant orthodontics." The consequences of this are that first, the veneer suddenly ceases to be a particularly conservative treatment option, and second, retention of the restoration becomes almost entirely dependent on the strength and integrity of the bond between the luting cement and the dentin substrate. However, as Swift and Friedman (2006) observed, "Recent reports of 50% failure at 6 years and 34% fracture are disturbing when compared with 93% to 100% success rates of 15 years observation in the 1980s, i.e., at a time when veneers were universally bonded almost entirely to enamel." This view is reinforced by recent data from the United Kingdom indicating a success rate for veneers placed within the General Dental Services in England and Wales of just over 50% at 10 years (Burke and Lucarotti 2009): "These results give a strong message to all clinicians who raise a rotating bur to a tooth, namely that, despite their intended minimal invasiveness, the tooth prepared for a veneer becomes compromised and may be replaced by a more invasive restoration which, in turn, increases the likelihood of pulpal involvement and/or tooth fracture."

Clinical studies

A number of clinical trials involving ceramic veneers are shown in Table 12.2 (Clyde and Gilmoure 1988, Reid et al. 1988, Calamia 1989, Jordan et al. 1989, Strassler and Nathanson 1989, Rucker et al. 1990, Christensen and Christensen 1991, Karlsson et al. 1992, Dunne and Millar 1993, Nordbo et al. 1994, Jager et al. 1995, Pippin et al. 1995, Strassler and Weiner 1995, Walls 1995, Shaini et al. 1997, Friedman 1998, Kihn and Barnes 1998, Meijering et al. 1998, Peumans et al. 1998, Dumfahrt 1999, Dumfahrt and Schaffer 2000, Magne et al. 2000, Aristidis and Dimitra 2002, Peumans et al. 2004, Smales and Etemadi 2004, Fradeani et al. 2005, Murphy et al. 2005, Layton and Walton 2007, Burke and Lucarotti 2009). It can be seen that failure rates range from 0% at 4 years (Kihn and Barnes 1998) to as high as 50% over 5 years (Shaini et al. 1997). Different studies have considerably different criteria for success and failure, but, in general, failure is seen as a breakdown resulting in total or partial loss of the veneer such that it requires replacement (Newsome and Owen 2008b). In addition to the studies shown in Table 12.2 a meta-analysis conducted in 1998 (Kreulen et al. 1998) combined the results of multiple clinical studies of porcelain veneer outcomes and was able to quote a probable survival of greater than 90% only after 3 years. A review of the literature in 2000 (Peumans et al. 2000) reported rates of 0–5% over 0–5 years.

What comes out of these various studies is that veneers, when used appropriately, offer acceptably high levels of durability and extremely high levels of patient satisfaction. However, as Burke and Lucarotti (2009) have warned, "Despite the more minimally invasive nature of the veneer preparation, as compared with a crown, the tooth that is veneered still enters onto a cycle of restorative dentistry which it cannot get off—a tooth which is restored with a porcelain veneer can never be whole again."

Clinical considerations

It is patently clear that great care must be taken in case selection, treatment planning, and clinical execution and that to get the very best out of the veneer technique a number of basic fundamental principles must be taken into consideration.

1. Bond to an enamel substrate wherever possible

The notion of etching enamel to accept resin luting cement is very well accepted and will be familiar to all dentists. It has taken more time, however, for the idea of dentin bonding to be accepted (Perdigao and Lopes 1999). In principle, for dentin bonding to be effective the dentin surface must be conditioned and then primed to form a hybrid layer onto which an adhesive is placed and which copolymerizes with the composite luting agent. The first bonding agents used a four-step process to etch enamel, etch dentin, and prime dentin, finally followed by the application of adhesive. This evolved into the so-called "total-etch" system in which the dentin and enamel are etched simultaneously but the prime and bond remained separate components. More recently "self-etch bonding" systems have been introduced that combine all the aforementioned steps. These have had a mixed reception (Tay 2005) despite the obvious convenience they represent and their possible role in reducing post-treatment sensitivity.

As far as ceramic veneers are concerned, the advent of dentinal adhesives has created the illusion that veneers bonded to dentin will be as successful as those bonded to enamel, thus encouraging dentists to use the technique in a wider range of clinical situations. Why is it that practitioners increasingly feel the need to extend veneer preparations into dentin and interproximally to the extent of breaking contacts with adjacent teeth? The main reasons would seem to be the ability of a thicker layer of porcelain to hide dark discolorations and to "correct" mild crowding of teeth, as well as greater ease of handling. Technicians also tend to find making thick ceramic veneers less challenging than very thin ones. As a result, tooth reduction into enamel alone can lead to bulky veneers, and so in many cases the dentist will cut further into the tooth to prevent overbuilding of the final restoration. Unfortunately, in spite of the considerable advances made in the field of dentin bonding, the longevity of a veneer continues to be a direct function of the amount of enamel substrate supporting it (Friedman 2001). There is an almost complete lack of clinical evidence to support the technique of bonding veneers to dentin as opposed to enamel, with Calamia and Calamia (2007) observing that "The key concept of preservation of enamel somehow

Table 12.2 Studies of veneer longevity

Author	*No. of veneers*	*No. of patients*	*Observation period (years)*	*Success rate (%)*
Clyde and Gilmoure 1988	200	Not specified	1–2.5	99
Reid et al. 1988	217	50	4	79
Calamia 1989	115	17	2–3	97
Jordan et al. 1989	80	12	4	97
Rucker et al. 1990	44	16	2	100
Christensen and Christensen 1991	163	45	3	87
Karlsson et al. 1992	119	36	0.25–2.5	100
Dunne and Millar 1993	315	96	5.25	89
Nordbo et al. 1994	135	41	3	95
Jager et al. 1995	80	25	1–7	99
Strassler and Nathanson 1989	291	60	1.5–3.5	98
Pippin et al. 1995	120	60	5	100
Strassler and Weiner 1995	115	21	7–10	93
Walls 1995	54	12	5	72
Shaini et al. 1997	372	104	6.5	50
Meijering et al. 1998	56	Not specified	2.5	Not specified
Peumans et al. 1998	87	25	5–6	93
Kihn and Barnes 1998	59	12	4	100
Friedman 1998	3,500	—	—	—
Dumfahrt 1999	—	—	—	—
Dumfahrt and Schaffer 2000	205	72	10.5	1
Magne et al. 2000	48	16	4.5	100
Aristidis and Dimitra 2002	186	61	5	98
Smales and Etemadi 2004	110	50	7	96 and 86*
Peumans M et al. 2004	87	25	10	64
Fradeani et al. 2005	182	46	12	95
Murphy et al. 2005	62	29	5	89
Layton and Walton 2007	304	100	15	81
Burke and Lucarotti 2009	2562	1177	11	53

* This study specifically looked at preparation design; the 96% success rate refers to veneers with incisal coverage, whereas the 86% success rate refers to veneers without incisal coverage.

has gone by the wayside or is considered less important. This may be a huge mistake."

Why is this the case when reported dentin bond strengths appear to match those achieved when bonding to enamel? Most longitudinal studies of dentin adhesives are performed using composite restorations directly bonded onto noncarious Class V lesions where the strength and elastic modulus of the teeth are hardly affected (Peumans et al. 2005). The difficulty of dentin bonding in the context of ceramic veneers is the disparity in flexibility between a rigid veneer and less rigid dentin. As Barghi and Overton (2007) observed, removal of facial enamel or selection of teeth without facial enamel for veneer restorations is an attempt to match up high–elastic modulus porcelain with lower elastic modulus dentin. It is predictable that functional loading of the veneered tooth will transfer this energy to the interface, resulting in debonding or cracking in the porcelain. For this reason, the smaller the amount of enamel available for bonding and the greater the amount of dentin that is exposed during laminate veneer preparation, the greater the likelihood that a full-coverage restoration should be chosen.

2. Avoid tooth wear and heavy occlusal loading cases

Although a veneer gains considerably in strength once it has been bonded to the tooth surface, it is nevertheless a relatively brittle restoration especially vulnerable to heavy occlusal loading. A prospective study carried out by Walls (1995) used a patient population with a high likelihood of parafunctional habits along with a large amount of dentin substrate; unsurprisingly, the combined high-risk factors resulted in a decreased survival rate. In cases where occlusal loading is likely to be high, the decision to use veneers in the first place should be thought through very carefully and consideration perhaps given to the use of stronger, more durable, full-coverage restorations. If veneers are to be used, then clearly a high-strength porcelain would be preferable (e.g., an aluminum oxide ceramic such as Procera

Alumina), and the accompanying higher opacity means that esthetics may have to be compromised.

3. Do not overpromise the ability of a veneer to mask deep discolorations

There is often tremendous temptation to suggest to patients the use of veneers as a relatively conservative means of masking deep discolorations. It has been shown that placement of veneers, in combination with prior tooth bleaching, is an effective treatment for teeth with *mild* discoloration. Veneers, however, become less and less useful the deeper the tooth discoloration becomes. This is because the ceramic needs to be of sufficient thickness to mask the dark color effectively, which usually means cutting a deeper preparation than is normally recommended. This in turn results in the veneer being retained primarily by the luting agent's bond to dentin and for the reasons outlined earlier this is undesirable. In addition, as one cuts deeper and deeper into the tooth its shade usually becomes progressively darker, making it harder for the veneer to provide an effective mask. Whenever veneers are chosen to treat discolored teeth, the use of a more opaque porcelain is desirable, as is the ability to deliver this level of opacity while still maintaining as thin a cross section as possible. Hence the porcelain should also be very strong, and once again an aluminum oxide ceramic such as Procera Alumina would be appropriate.

Attempts have been made to overcome these difficulties by cutting a standard veneer preparation and then either bleaching the tooth before cementation (Sadan and Lemon 1998) or carrying out what is referred to as sub-opaquing—that is, the selective removal of the darkest bands of dentin and replacement with a lighter composite (Nixon 1996). The latter can be done either at the tooth preparation phase or, as has been advocated recently, at the cementation phase, in order to (1) prevent the provisional veneers from adhering to the composite restoration and (b) enhance the bond strength achieved by removing the need to etch and silanate the freshly placed composite (Lowe et al. 2005).

4. Avoid using veneers to provide "instant orthodontics"

Although veneers are, in many ways, ideal restorations for the treatment of spacing, their use for the correction of tooth crowding is somewhat problematic, and the greater the degree of crowding the more likely it is that tooth preparation will involve dentin, something which, as described earlier, is to be avoided if at all possible. The use of a pretreatment diagnostic wax-up and trial preparations will provide a useful indication of the degree of tooth reduction required and whether this is likely to be excessive and even result in pulpal involvement. In most cases it is far preferable to treat the crowding orthodontically first, and only after this has been completed determine whether or not veneers are still required.

5. Replace old restorations before veneer placement

It is now widely recommended that old composite restorations, which may otherwise form part of the veneer preparation, be removed before bonding in order to ensure the best possible bond to the luting agent. This is usually done at the preparation stage itself, although in some cases it can also be performed simultaneously with veneer cementation. This latter approach has the advantage of ensuring the composite substrate is "fresh" and has not been contaminated in any way, although doing things this way can be quite difficult to accomplish and is practical only when the restoration being replaced is relatively small.

6. Pay meticulous attention to clinical technique

Veneers are notoriously technique sensitive and demand an understanding of dental materials, design principles, and, above all, tremendous attention to detail. Through the years there have been various recommendations made regarding veneer preparations. Meijering et al. (1998) followed 263 veneer cases and observed that because of the number of potential variables such as the dentist's skill, materials used, hard tissue substrate, occlusion, degree of tooth discoloration, outcome criteria, and so on, a definitive answer to which veneer design is most effective is very hard to provide. Various basic principles have, nevertheless, emerged.

- Tooth preparation should remain wherever possible in enamel.
- Sufficient thickness of porcelain should be present to allow masking of any underlying tooth discoloration without the need to overbuild tooth contour.
- In treating discolored teeth, margins should be placed slightly subgingivally and interproximally to hide the transition between veneer and dark tooth. In such cases retraction cord is usually necessary unless the veneer margin is being placed supragingivally, and careful impression technique is vital.
- The preparation should result in a smooth transition between tooth and restoration and in the gingival region should maintain the correct emergence profile.
- Restoration margins should not be placed in positions where there is a high degree of occlusal loading.
- If using a material such as Procera, which requires the model to be scanned, make sure that all margins are very clear and that the chamfer does not become a weak "J" margin with unsupported enamel that the scanner cannot register. Similarly, it is usually advisable to break the contact points so that the scanner can detect the margins fully. This also helps to hide the interproximal margins.
- Sharp line angles should be avoided to prevent the propagation of undesirable stress fractures in the bonded ceramic material.
- The shade of the prepared tooth (if possible together with photographs) should be sent to the laboratory to help them achieve the best possible result.
- At the bonding stage it is vital to use a selection of different water-soluble try-in pastes to determine the most appropriate shade of luting cement. The more translucent the veneer, the more critical this step becomes.

- Should bleaching be performed before placement of veneers, it is important to leave a period of at least 2 weeks between the final bleaching and bonding; otherwise the bond strength will likely be compromised as oxygen trapped within the tooth is slowly released (Titely et al. 1988).

A number of studies have looked specifically at the incisal edge preparation. This is a critical area, and variations range from the very conservative window approach, through one in which the margin is sited on the incisal edge itself, to the overlap reduction, which in turn can be finished either as a butt margin or as a palatal chamfer. Of these, incisal coverage preparations appear to be the preferred option. Various studies have been carried out to examine the effect of preparation design on veneer longevity. Smales and Etemadi (2004), for example, investigated long-term survival rates of veneer restorations after a 7-year period and found a 96% cumulative survival rate when incisal coverage preparations were used compared with 86% survival without incisal coverage. Priest (2004) found that incisal butt joints provide the best solution, resulting in not only a relatively simplified tooth preparation but also stronger, longer lasting restorations.

Ceramic selection

Should veneers be the treatment of choice, then the question arises as to which ceramic system is the most appropriate (Newsome and Owen 2008a). Clearly, in most cases, highly translucent ceramics are not recommended, and for this reason moderately filled glass materials such as IPS Empress Esthetic (Ivoclar Vivadent, Liechtenstein) are usually unsuitable because they allow too much of the underlying discoloration to shine through. More opaque systems such as IPS e.max Press (Ivoclar Vivadent) and Procera Alumina (Nobel Biocare, Zurich, Switzerland) are better able to mask out dark underlying hues. Although zirconium-based polycrystalline ceramics are totally opaque, they cannot be etched to provide a micromechanical bond and so are currently not used in laminate veneers.

Bonding

The bonding phase is critical. The operator and, just as important, the chairside assistant must be fully versed in the sequence of events that have to take place for successful veneer placement. Just how taxing this phase of the treatment is should not be underestimated. If necessary, a number of dry-runs can be carried out to ensure that the whole process will be as well practiced and choreographed as possible. Some operators recommend the use of a rubber dam during the bonding phase of the treatment, the main benefit clearly being moisture control, not only of saliva and gingival fluid, but also of the moist air present during exhalation. Such considerations assume even greater significance when bonding veneers in the lower arch, where moisture control is usually a considerable problem. Dunne and Millar (1993), however, found that use of rubber dam was not a significant factor in the long-term performance of porcelain veneers. The downside of using rubber dam is that they can be extremely difficult to apply properly when large numbers of veneers are being placed, especially when veneer preparations are subgingival.

Full-coverage restorations

The inherent difficulties of using laminate veneers to mask tetracycline discoloration as previously outlined have led many to abandon their use in all but the mildest cases and opt for full-coverage restorations. Doing so allows the teeth to be more aggressively prepared so that the covering layer of porcelain is thicker. Full coverage also places less reliance on bonding as a means of retention because a more conventional means of retention is now present. Although under "normal" circumstances there are usually more esthetic alternatives for anterior teeth, zirconia crowns are useful in the treatment of tetracycline-stained teeth, especially if the preparation has a deep enough chamfer to allow a sufficiently thick veneering layer of esthetic porcelain. The need to use porcelain-fused-to-metal crowns would appear to be limited except in the most extreme cases where great strength is an advantage—for example, when parafunctional habits, such as bruxism, are combined with deep tooth discoloration.

CONCLUSION

The management of tetracycline-discolored teeth poses a number of problems. As with treatment of any kind, the most conservative option should be used first. Here this means tooth bleaching, and it is becoming clear that excellent results can be achieved by means of long-term home bleaching. Even if this approach does not yield the desired result, then sufficient improvement in tooth color can usually be achieved to make the task of masking the discoloration by means of ceramic restorations easier. Care must be taken, especially when using veneers, to balance the desire to remove sufficient tooth structure to provide enough thickness of ceramic to mask discoloration with the need to maintain enamel for bonding purposes.

REFERENCES

Abou-Rass M. (1982) The elimination of tetracycline discolouration by intentional endodontics. *J Endod* **8**:101.

Aristidis GA, Dimitra B. (2002) Five-year clinical performance of porcelain laminate veneers. *Quintessence Int* **33**:185–9.

Atkinson HF, Hartcourt JK. (1962) Tetracyclines in human dentine. *Nature* **295**:508–9.

Barghi N, Overton JD. (2007) Preserving principles of successful porcelain veneers. *Contemp Esthet* **11**:48–51.

Berger RS, Mandel EB, Hayes TJ, Grimwood RR. (1989) Minocycline staining of the oral cavity. *J Am Acad Dermatol* **21**:1300–1.

Bevelander G, Rolle GK, Cohlan SG. (1961) The effect of the administration of tetracycline on the development of teeth. *J Dent Res* **40**:1020–4.

Burke FJ, Lucarotti PS. (2009) Ten year outcome of porcelain laminate veneers placed within the General Dental Services in England and Wales. *J Dent* **37**:31–8.

Calamia JR. (1989) Clinical evaluation of etched porcelain veneers. *Am J Dent* **2**:9–15.

Calamia JR, Calamia CS. (2007) Porcelain laminate veneers: reasons for 25 years of success. *Dent Clin North Am* **51**:399–417.

Cheek CC, Heymann HO. (1999) Dental and oral discolorations associated with minocycline and other tetracycline analogs. *J Esthet Dent* **11**:43–8.

Christensen GJ. (2006) Are veneers conservative treatment? *J Am Dent Assoc* **137**:1721–3.

Christensen GJ, Christensen RP. (1991) Clinical observations of porcelain veneers: a three year report. *J Esthet Dent* **3**:174–9.

Clyde JS, Gilmoure A. (1988) Porcelain veneers: a preliminary review. *Br Dent J* **164**:9–14.

Conchie JM, Munroe JD, Anderson DD. (1970) The incidence of staining of permanent teeth by the tetracyclines. *Can Med Assoc J* **103**:351–6.

Davies PA. Little K, Aherne W. (1962) Tetracycline and yellow teeth. *Lancet* **1**:742–3.

Di Benedetto DC. (1985) Tetracycline staining in an adult. *J Mass Dent Soc* **34**:217.

Dumfahrt H. (1999) Porcelain laminate veneers. A retrospective evaluation after 1 to 10 years of service: Part I: clinical procedure. *Int J Prosthodont* **12**:505–13.

Dumfahrt H, Schaffer H. (2000) Porcelain laminate veneers. A retrospective evaluation after 1 to 10 years of service: Part II: clinical results. *Int J Prosthodont* **13**:9–18.

Dunne SM, Millar BJ. (1993) A longitudinal study of the clinical performance of porcelain veneers. *Br Dent J* **175**:317–21.

Eisenberg E, Bernick SM. (1975) Anomalies of the teeth with stains and discolourations. *J Prev Dent* **2**:7–20.

Fiedler RS, Reichl RB. (2000) Combined professional and home care Nightguard bleaching of tetracycline-stained teeth. *Gen Dent* **48**:257–61.

Fradeani M, Redemagni M, Corrado M. (2005) Porcelain laminate veneers: 6- to 12- year clinical evaluation—a retrospective study. *Int J Peridont Restor Dent* **25**:9–17.

Friedman MJ. (1998) A 15-year review of porcelain veneer failure—a clinician's observations. *Compend Contin Educ Dent* **19**:625–32.

Friedman MJ. (2001) Porcelain veneer restorations: a clinician's opinion about a disturbing trend. *J Esthet Restor Dent* **13**:318–27.

Haywood VB, Leonard RH, Dickinson GL. (1997) Efficacy of 6 months of Nightguard Vital Bleaching of tetracycline-stained teeth. *J Esthet Dent* **9**:13–9.

Haywood VB, Pohjola R. (2004) Bleaching and esthetic bonding of tetracycline stained teeth. *Contemp Esthet Restor Pract* **October**:16–20.

Jackson R. (1979) Tetracycline staining of wisdom teeth. *Cutis* **23**:613–6.

Jager K, Stern M, Wirz J. (1995) Laminates—reif fur die Praxis? *Quintessenz* **46**:1221–30.

Jordan RE, Boksman L. (1984) Conservative vital bleaching treatment of discoloured dentition. *Compend Contin Educ Dent* **10**:803–7.

Jordan RE, Suzuki M, Senda A. (1989) Clinical evaluation of porcelain laminate veneers: a four-year recall report. *J Esthet Dent* **1**:126–37.

Karlsson S, Landahl I, Stegersjö G, Milleding P. (1992) A clinical evaluation of ceramic laminate veneers. *Int J Prosthodont* **5**:447–51.

Kihn PW, Barnes DM. (1998) The clinical evaluation of porcelain veneers: a 48-month clinical evaluation. *J Am Dent Assoc* **129**:747–52.

King NM, Wei SH. (1989) Developmental defects of enamel in Chinese girls and boys in Hong Kong. *Adv Dent Res* **3**:120–5.

Kreulen CM, Creugers NH, Meijering AC. (1998) Meta-analysis of anterior veneer restorations in clinical studies. *J Dent* **26**:345–53.

Kugel G, Aboushala A, Zhou X, Gerlach RW. (2002) Daily use of whitening strips on tetracycline-stained teeth: comparative results after 2 months. *Compend Contin Educ Dent* **23**:29–34.

Layton D, Walton T. (2007) An up to 16-year prospective study of 304 porcelain veneers. *Int J Prosthodont* **20**:389–96.

Leonard RH Jr, Van Haywood B, Caplan DJ, Tart ND. (2003) Nightguard Vital Bleaching of tetracycline-stained teeth: 90 months post treatment. *J Esthet Rest* **15**:142–53.

Lowe E, Rego N, Rego J. (1963) A delayed sub-opaquing technique for treatment of stained dentition: clinical protocol. *Pract Proced Aesthet Dent* **17**:A–H.

Madison JF. (1963) Tetracycline pigmentation of teeth. *Arch Dermatol* **88**:58–9.

Magne P, Perroud R, Hodges JS, Belser UC. (2000) Clinical performance of novel-design porcelain veneers for the recovery of coronal volume and length. *Int J Periodont Restor Dent* **20**:441–57.

Martin ND, Barnard PD. (1969) The prevalence of tetracycline staining in erupted teeth. *Med J Aust* **1**:1286–9.

Matis BA, Wang Y, Eckert GJ, Cochran MA. (2006) Extended bleaching of tetracycline-stained teeth: a 5-year study. *Oper Dent* **31**:643–51.

Medical Protection Society. (1982) Annual report and accounts. *Med Prot Soc* **90**:30–1.

Meijering AC, Creugers NH, Roeters FJ, Mulder J. (1998) Survival of three types of veneer restoration in a clinical trial: a 2.5-year interim evaluation. *J Dent* **26**:563–8.

Mello HS. (1967) The mechanism of tetracycline staining in primary and permanent teeth. *J Dent Child* **34**:478–87.

Murphy E, Ziada HM, Allen PF. (2005) Retrospective study on the performance of porcelain laminate veneers delivered by undergraduate dental students. *Eur J Prosthodont Restor Dent* **13**:38–43.

Newsome PR, Owen SA. (2008a) Ceramic veneers in general dental practice. Part two: choice of materials. *Aesthet Dent Today* **2**(1):8–14.

Newsome PR, Owen SA. (2008b) Ceramic veneers in general dental practice. Part five: aftercare and dealing with failure. *Aesthet Dent Today* **2**:10–3.

Nixon RL. (1996) Masking severely tetracycline-stained teeth with ceramic laminate veneers. *Pract Periodont Aesthet Dent* **8**:227–35.

Nordbo H, Rygh-Thoresen N, Henaug T. (1994) Clinical performance of veneers without incisal overlapping: 3-year results. *J Dent* **22**:342–5.

Perdigao J, Lopes M. (1999) Dentine bonding—questions for the new millennium. *J Adhes Dent* **1**:191–209.

Peumans M, De Munck J, Fieuws S, Lambrechts P. (2004) A prospective ten-year clinical trial of porcelain veneers. *J Adhes Dent* **6**:65–76.

Peumans M, Kanumilli P, De Munck J, Van Landuyt K. (2005) Clinical effectiveness of contemporary adhesives: a systematic review of current clinical trials. *Dent Mater* **21**:864–81.

Peumans M, Van Meerbeck B, Lambrechts P, Vanherle G. (2000) Porcelain veneers: a review of the literature. *J Dent* **28**:163–77.

Peumans M, Van Meerbeek B, Lambrechts P, Vuylsteke-Wauters M. (1998) Five-year clinical performance of porcelain veneers. *Quintessence Int* **29:**211–21.

Pippin DJ, Mixson JM, Soldon-Els AP. (1995) Clinical evaluation of restored maxillary incisors: veneers vs PFM crowns. *J Am Dent Assoc* **126:**1523–9.

Priest G. (2004) Proximal margin modifications for all-ceramic veneers. *Pract Proced Aesthet Dent* **16:**265–72.

Reid JS, Murray MC, Power SM. (1988) Porcelain veneers—a four year follow-up. *Restor Dent* **4:**60–6.

Rosen T, Hoffmann TJ. (1989) Minocycline-induced oral discoloration of the permanent teeth. *J Am Acad Dermatol* **21:** 569.

Rucker ML, Richter W, MacEntee, Richardson A. (1990) Porcelain and resin veneers clinically evaluated: 2-year results. *J Am Dent Assoc* **121:**594–6.

Sadan A, Lemon RR. (1998) Combining treatment modalities for tetracycline-discoloured teeth. *Int J Periodont Restor Dent* **18:**565–71.

Saikali Z, Singh G. (2003) Doxycycline and other tetracyclines in the treatment of bone metastasis. *Anticancer Drugs* **14:**773–8.

Schwachman H, Schuster A. (1956) The tetracyclines: applied pharmacology. *Pediatr Clin North Am* **3:**295–303.

Shaini FJ, Shortall AC, Marquis PM. (1997) Clinical performance of porcelain laminate veneers. A retrospective evaluation over a period of 6.5 years. *J Oral Rehabil* **24:**553–9.

Smales RJ, Etemadi S. (2004) Long-term survival of porcelain veneers using two preparation designs. *Int J Prosthodont* **17:**324–6.

Strassler HE, Nathanson D. (1989) Clinical evaluation of etched porcelain veneers over a period of 18 to 42 months. *J Esthet Dent* **1:**21–8.

Strassler HE, Weiner S. (1995) Seven to ten year clinical evaluation of etched porcelain veneers. *J Dent Res* **74:**176 (Abstract 1316).

Suckling GW, Pearce EI. (1984) Developmental defects of enamel in a group of New Zealand children: their prevalence and some associated etiological factors. *Community Dent Oral Epidemiol* **12:**177–84.

Swift EJ Jr, Friedman MJ. (2006) Critical appraisal: porcelain veneer outcomes. Part II. *J Esthet Restor Dent* **18:**110–3.

Tay FR. (2005) Degradation of resin-dentin bonds from above and below. Presented at 83rd General Session AADR; March 2005; Baltimore MD.

Titely KC, Torneck CD, Smith DC, Adifar A. (1988) Adhesion of composite resin to bleached and unbleached bovine enamel. *J Dent Res* **67:**1523–8.

van der Bijl P, Pitigoi-Aron G. (1995) Tetracyclines and calcified tissues. *Ann Dent* **54:**69–72.

Walls AW. (1995) The use of adhesively retained all-porcelain veneers during the management of fractured and worn anterior teeth. Part II: clinical results after 5-years follow-up. *Br Dent J* **178:**337–9.

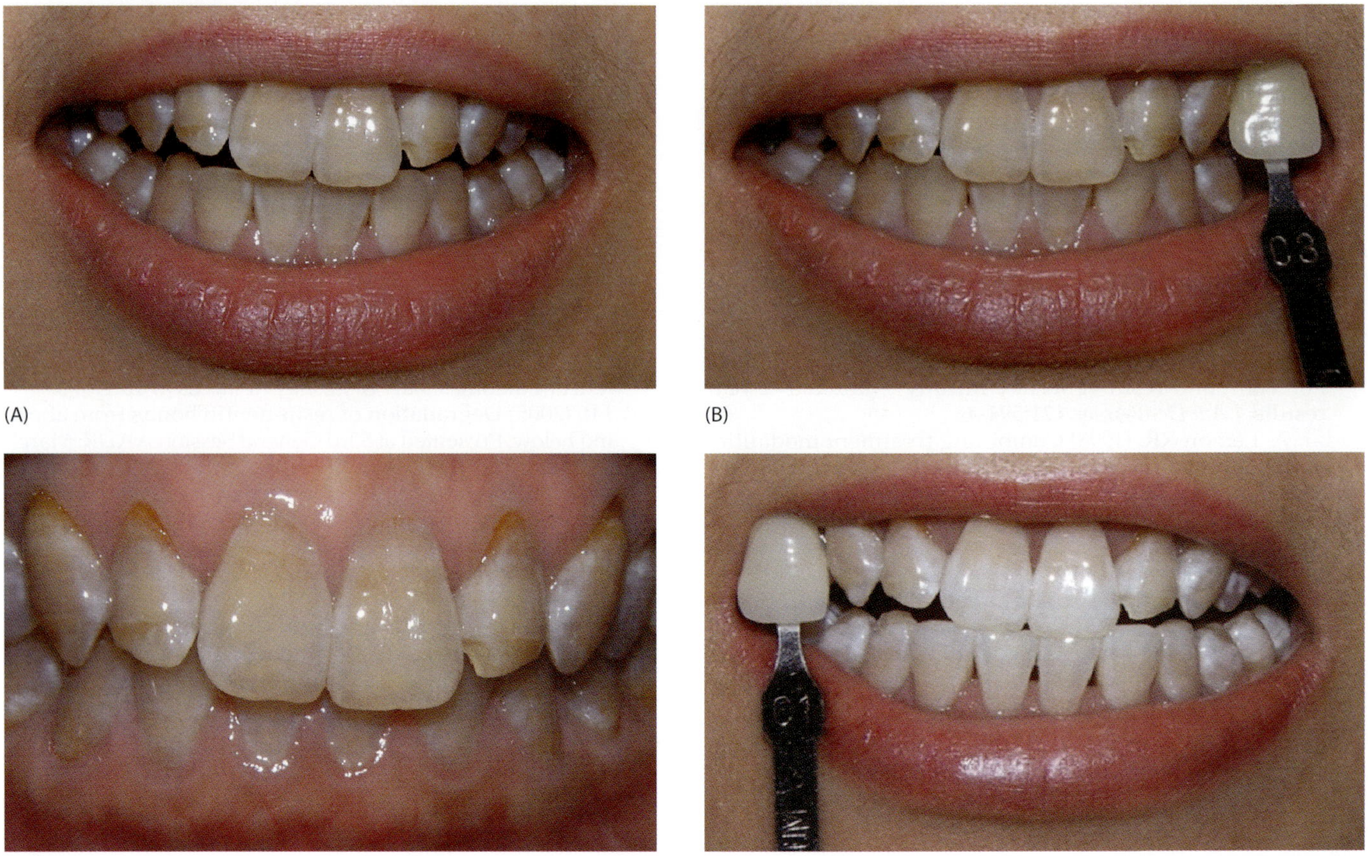

(A) (B)

(C) (D)

Figure 12.1

(A) Tetracycline discoloration in addition to white spots and defective enamel. Treatment options included bleaching, prolonged bleaching, microabrasion, and bonding; all options were discussed with the patient and a sequential approach was taken. Bleaching was the first part of the treatment plan. Because the patient had white markings, the patient was warned that the white spots would get whiter during the initial parts of the bleaching treatment. (B) The baseline shade was recorded. This shade was noted to be C3. This shade is on the gray spectrum, which is indicative of patients with tetracycline discoloration. (C) Retracted view of the appearance of the tetracycline discoloration. There is cervical erosion and gingival recession. The roots appear orange. It is essential to explain to the patient that the necks of the teeth in the cervical erosion will not bleach to the same level as the clinical crown of the teeth. It is important that a thorough treatment plan document that further restorations are needed—Class V restorations on the cervical areas to repair the defects and bleach the restorations to the new shade of the bleached teeth. Further blocking out of the area can be undertaken by placing segmental layering of the composite restorations and by placing an opaquer into the darkest part of the cervical lesion. There is defective enamel on the lateral incisors, and this will need to be built up in composite material. The patient specifically requested that no porcelain laminates be placed to mask the discoloration and the discrepancy of the laterals to the central incisors. (D) Final shade of the bleaching, which was completed within 6–8 weeks. The shade matches the A1 shade, which is a good result. The white opaque marks are more noticeable and will require microabrasion.

continued on the next page

increased the rate of whitening obtained with carbamide in a study by Gimeno et al. (2008).

LONGEVITY OF HOME WHITENING TREATMENT USING 10% CARBAMIDE PEROXIDE FOR TETRACYCLINE-STAINED TEETH

Research studies undertaken by Leonard et al. (1999, 2003) have shown that the whitening that takes place with use of carbamide peroxide in trays can last up to 7.5 years or longer. In their study, 21 patients with moderate to severe tetracycline staining participated. Baseline evaluations and procedures included consent forms, medical and dental history, oral examination, and radiographs of the maxillary incisor teeth. Patients were included in the study if they had upper teeth with no restorations. All participants were at least 18 years of age with no health problems. The darkest portion of the tooth from the middle one third was used for shade determination. The Vita classical shade of some of the teeth was difficult to ascertain owing to the nature of the pattern of tetracycline discoloration. In these cases the shade of the untreated lower teeth was assessed and photographs were used to determine whether the maxillary anterior teeth had a different shade. Participants were instructed to place enough material to fill the tray without excess and to brush and floss their teeth before bed and seat the tray. The tray remained in place during sleep. The patients removed the tray in the morning and applied the gel the following evening again. The untreated mandibular arch served as a control. A log form was given to the patients to log the number of hours the tray was worn each night. Patients were instructed to discontinue if the teeth became too uncomfortable. After 6 months of tray wearing, a single examiner assessed the shade of the maxillary teeth. Photographs and post-treatment impressions were taken to assess the buccal surfaces of the maxillary teeth. Patients were seen at 6, 12, 54, and 90 months.

Results

The extended treatment time of 6 months using 10% carbamide peroxide gel was effective in lightening tetracycline-stained teeth. The mean treatment time was 860 hours (range 150–1440 hours). Fifteen of 21 patients completed the course of treatment. Of those who finished, all had lightening of their teeth. The proportion of patients who reported a shade change was 86%. The mean Vita shade of participants before treatment was C4. Immediately after treatment the mean shade was B1 (range B1–C2). The degree of improvement after treatment was significant ($P < .005$). Side effects were reported. There was no correlation between the age of the patient and the incidence of sensitivity or reported allergy and sensitivity. Six participants did not complete the study for reasons including side effects, taste, time involvement, and job relocation. The results at 90 months showed that no patient's shade had returned to the original shade and that all had a significant degree of lightening with only slight darkening of the post-treatment shade. After 7.5 years, 27% of patients rewhitened their teeth. No patient needed to have a crown or a root canal treatment after prolonged whitening treatment. Of the patients, 93% said they would rewhiten their teeth again if necessary. The texture, contour, and color of the patients' gingivae were assessed and found to be within normal limits. Of the patients who were seen at recall, 88% had teeth at least two shades whiter than the baseline record. It was thought that the tenacious and thick nature of the whitening gel allowed for deeper penetration of the whitening gel into the tooth surface during the extended whitening treatment. The sustained release of the oxygen into the tooth helped to achieve efficient whitening of the tetracycline-stained teeth. The prognosis for the tetracycline whitening depended on the region of discoloration within the tooth. If the discoloration was deeply embedded at the neck of the tooth, it was more difficult to whiten than if the discoloration was situated at the incisal tip of the tooth.

Eighty-three percent of patients participating in the study who reported at 6, 50, and 90 months perceived that there had been no obvious tooth color change after whitening, or only slight darkening.

Side effects

Patients in the study reported that there were no obvious side effects that persisted after the termination of whitening for 6 months. There were initial reports of tooth and gingival sensitivity during the treatment phase.

SUCCESS RATE OF WHITENING TETRACYCLINE-STAINED TEETH

A success rate of 95% has been reported for non–tetracycline-stained teeth (Haywood et al. 1994); there was a 97% success rate reported in the later study by Haywood et al. (1997). Eighty-six percent of tetracycline-stained teeth whitened for 6 months (Leonard et al. 2003).

WHITENING OF TETRACYCLINE STAINING USING PREFORMED STRIPS

In a study to assess the effectiveness of 6.5% hydrogen peroxide whitening strips on teeth with tetracycline stain, use of the treatment under the supervision of a dentist was shown to be effective (Kugel et al. 2002, 2011). A randomized clinical trial compared the efficacy of two at-home vital whitening systems on tetracycline-stained teeth. Daily whitening was conducted for 2 months using 6.5% hydrogen peroxide whitening strips, which were preformed strips coated with the whitening beads. Eligibility was limited to healthy adult volunteers who had 16 or more natural teeth, including at least three gradable maxillary incisors with significant tetracycline staining. Individuals demonstrating tooth sensitivity or an immediate need for dental treatment were excluded from participating in this trial. After informed consent was obtained and baseline measurements were taken, subjects were randomized 3:1 to a strip-based, hydrogen peroxide tooth-whitening system (Crest Professional Whitestrips) or a marketed tray-based, carbamide peroxide whitening system control (Opalescence 10%). Both groups were given a standard dentifrice (Crest Cavity Protection Regular Paste) and an extrasoft toothbrush (Crest Complete) for use throughout the study. The first product application was supervised for instructional purposes, but all other treatment was unsupervised. Only the maxillary arch was treated. Participants in the strip group were instructed to wear a whitening strip for 30 minutes twice daily. Individuals in the tray group had a custom soft, full-arch whitening tray fabricated with gingival scalloping and gel reservoirs using materials supplied by the manufacturer. Subjects in that group were instructed to place half to three quarters of the contents of a whitening syringe into the custom tray and wear the device for 2 hours daily. Shade assessments were made in a neutral-colored dental operatory under color-balanced lighting conditions by a trained and calibrated examiner. Tolerability was assessed by intraoral examination and subject report at each study visit. Individual shade scores were determined by ranking the 16 shade tabs, arranged from dark to light, according to the rank order suggested by the manufacturer. To account for unusually dark colors (often seen with tetracycline staining) or white colors (often seen after whitening), this 16-step guide was supplemented by two additional values (C4+ and B1–) representing shades darker than C4 or lighter than B1. Effectiveness was determined by calculating the change in shade scores from baseline at each post-treatment visit.

The results of the study showed that twice-daily use of the 6.5% hydrogen peroxide whitening strips was well tolerated over the 2-month treatment period. The side effects in this study, which were transient tooth sensitivity and gingival irritation, were similar in nature and severity to those reported in other longitudinal trials using the at-home tray-based whitening systems. In the current study, in which the whitening strips were used for a total of 60 contact hours over a 2-month period, no subject in the strip group discontinued treatment because of an adverse event.

A second study, in 2011, showed that the strips averaged shade reduction in month 1, 2, and 3 visits. Of all the subjects, 65% reached B1 color by month 6. Treatment was generally well tolerated. Mild and transient tooth sensitivity (46.7%) and oral discomfort (43.3%) were the most common adverse events associated with daily whitening, yet neither affected study participation (Kugel et al. 2011).

A new version of 6% whitening strips has been launched for the United Kingdom and Europe (Oral B, Proctor and Gamble, 2015). These strips are available only via dental practices for supervision of patients.

POWER WHITENING FOR TETRACYCLINE-STAINED TEETH

Because more contact time is needed to whiten the tetracycline-stained teeth, one treatment session of power whitening is insufficient.

Use of a potassium titanyl phosphate (KTP) laser for tetracycline-stained teeth has been reported in the literature (Kinoshita et al. 2009). The KTP laser is a type of neodymium:yttrium-aluminum-garnet (Nd:YAG) laser. It seems to be appropriate for whitening of tetracycline-stained teeth because its laser beam at a wavelength of 1064 goes through the solid medium of KTP crystal. Its wavelength then decreases to 532 nm, just half of the original wavelength. This means that KTP has very similar characteristics to Nd:YAG, plus a few unique characteristics. The green visible light of KTP is absorbed well in hemoglobin and melanin but not in hydroxyapatite or water. KTP tends to penetrate into dentin with less damage. The temperature does not increase much during the whitening procedure; the cooler temperature and stronger photon energy make it suitable for whitening without damaging the pulp tissue. Its photons have high energy that facilitates the chemical and photodynamic reactions without damage to both hard and pulp tissues. It has been shown that the KTP laser is capable of producing significantly greater effect than LED or diode laser.

Because of the low molecular weight of hydrogen peroxide, it can penetrate into organic substances among hydroxyapatite crystals. Given the KTP laser's efficient acceleration, hydrogen peroxide cuts the chain and opens the carbon rings, resulting in brightening of the color of collagen.

SUMMARY

Dentists can feel confident about offering long-duration dental whitening to their patients who have tetracycline discoloration (Croll 2003). This helps to postpone further advanced invasive restorative treatment to mask the tetracycline discoloration.

REFERENCES

Abou-Rass M. (1982) The elimination of tetracycline discoloration by intentional endodontics and internal bleaching. *J Endod* **8**:101–6.

Bernier C, Dréno B. (2001) [Minocycline]. *Ann Dermatol Venereol* **128**:627–37.

Boksman L, Jordan RE. (1983) Conservative treatment of the stained dentition: vital bleaching. *Aust Dent J* **28**(2): 67–72.

Bowles WH. (1998) Protection against minocycline pigment formation by ascorbic acid (vitamin C) *J Esthet Dent* **10**: 182–6.

Cohen S, Burns RC. (2002) *Pathways of the pulp*. Mosby: St. Louis.

Croll TP (2003) Commentary on Nightguard Vital bleaching of tetracycline-stained teeth: 90 months post treatment. *J Esthetic Rest Dent* **15**(3):153.

Dodd MA, Dole EJ, Troutman WG, Bennahum DA. (1998) Minocycline-associated tooth staining. *Ann Pharmacother* **32**:887–9.

Gimeno I, Riutord P, Tauler P, Tur JA. (2008) The whitening effect of enzymatic bleaching on tetracycline. *J Dent* **36**(10):795–800.

Good ML, Hussey DL. (2003) Minocycline: stain devil? *Br J Dermatol* **149**:237–9.

Haywood VB, Leonard RH, Dickinson GL. (1997) Efficacy of six months Nightguard Vital Bleaching of tetracycline-stained teeth. *J Esthet Dent* **9**(1):13–9.

Haywood VB, Leonard RH, Nelson CF, Brunson WD. (1994) Effectiveness, side effects and long-term status of Nightguard Vital Bleaching. *J Am Dent Assoc* **125:**1219–26.

Jordan RE, Boksman L. (1984) Conservative vital bleaching treatment of discoloured dentition. *Compend Contin Educ Dent* **V**(10):803–7.

Kinoshita J, Jafarzadeh H, Forghani M. (2009) Vital bleaching of tetracycline-stained teeth by using KTP laser: a case report. *Eur J Dent* **3**(3):229–32.

Kugel G, Aboushala A, Zhou X, Gerlach R. (2002) Daily use of whitening strips on tetracycline stained teeth: comparative results after 2 months. *Compend Contin Educ Den*t 23 (1A):29–34.

Kugel G, Gerlach RW, Aboushala A, Ferreira S. (2011) Long-term use of 6.5% hydrogen peroxide bleaching strips on tetracycline stain: a clinical study. *Compend Contin Educ Dent* **32**(8):50–6.

Leonard RH, Haywood VB, Caplan DJ, Tart ND. (2003) Nightguard Vital Bleaching of tetracycline stained teeth: 90 months post treatment. *J Esthet Restor Dent* **15:** 142–53.

Leonard RH, Haywood VB, Eagle JC, Garland GE. (1999) Nightguard Vital Bleaching of tetracycline-stained teeth: 54 months post treatment. *J Esthet Dent* **11:**265–77.

McKenna BE, Lamely PJ, Kennedy JG, Batten J. (1999) Minocycline-induced staining of the adult permanent dentition: a review of the literature and report of a case. *Dent Update* **24**(4):160–2.Raymond J, Cook D. (2015) Still leaving stains on teeth—the legacy of minocycline? *Australas Med J* **8**(4):139–42.

Sanchez AR, Rogers RS 3rd, Sheridan PJ. (2004) Tetracycline and other tetracycline-derivative staining of the teeth and oral cavity. *Int J Dermatol* **43:**709–15.

Tredwin CJ, Scully C, Bagan-Sebastian JV. (2005) Drug-induced disorders of teeth. *J Dent Res* **84:**596–60.

Walton RE, O'Dell NL, Lake FT, Shimp RG. (1983) Internal bleaching of tetracycline-stained teeth in dogs. *J Endod* **9:** 416–20.

Watts A, Addy M. (2001) Tooth discolouration and staining: a review of the literature. *Br Dent J* **190**(6):309–16.

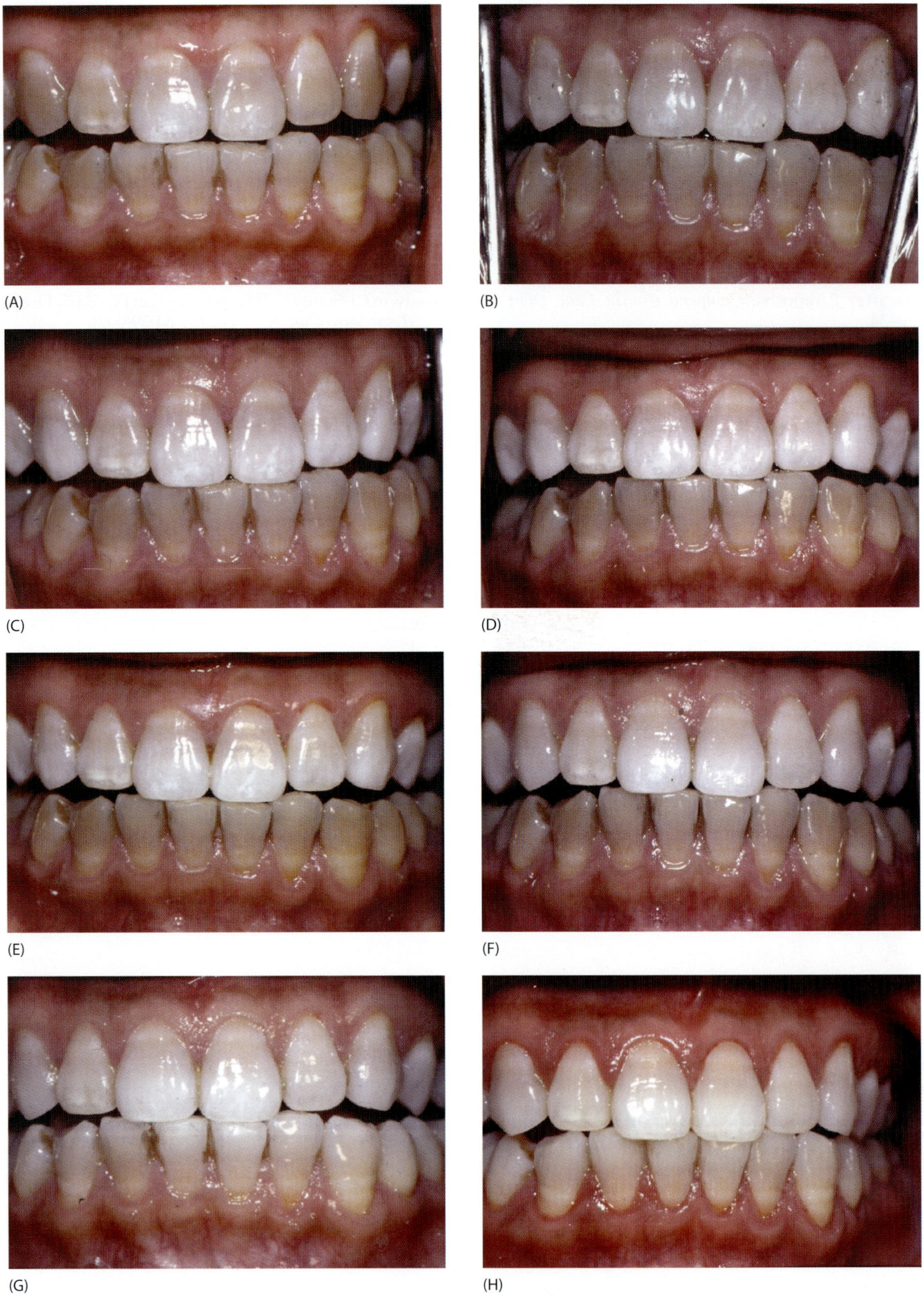

Figure 13.1

A 29-year-old woman who used 10% carbamide peroxide (CP) on the patient's right side and 15% CP on the left side in a custom-made tray with reservoirs, overnight, for 6 months. (A) Baseline; (B) 1 week; (C) 2 weeks; (D) 1 month; (E) 6 months; (F) 3 months postwhitening; (G) 1.5 years postwhitening; (H) 4.5 years postwhitening.

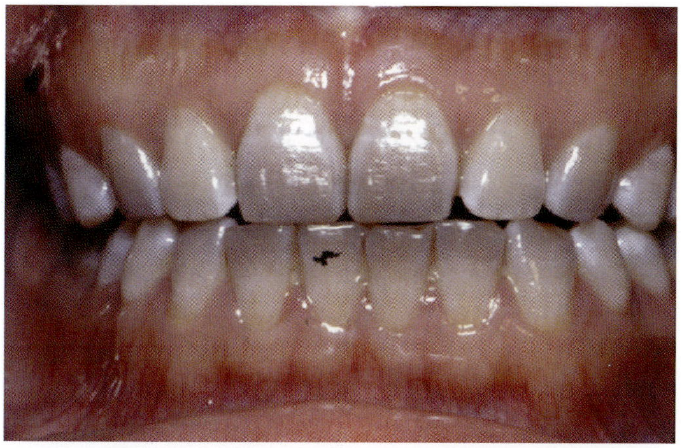
(A)

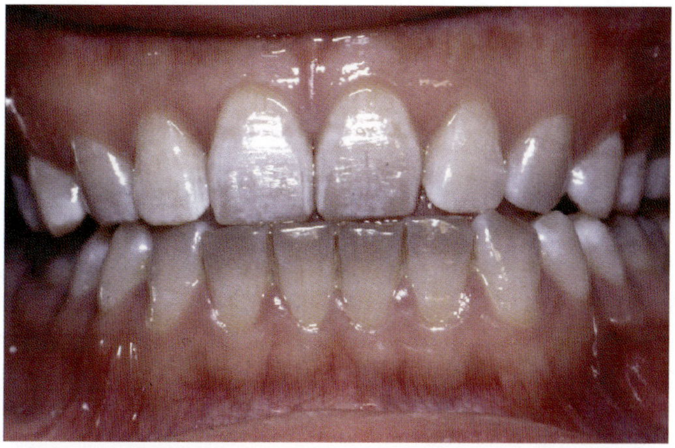
(B)

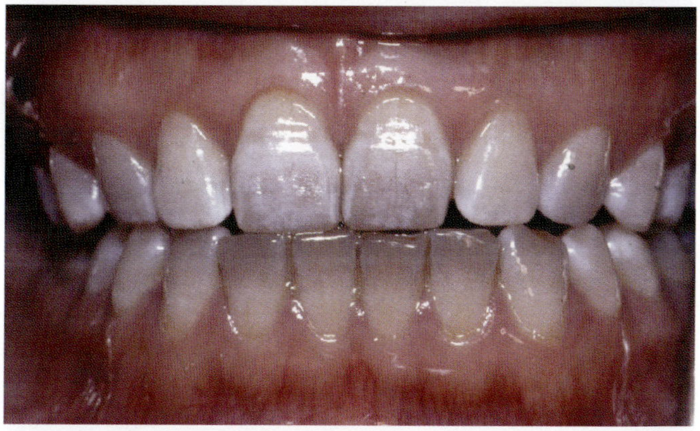
(C)

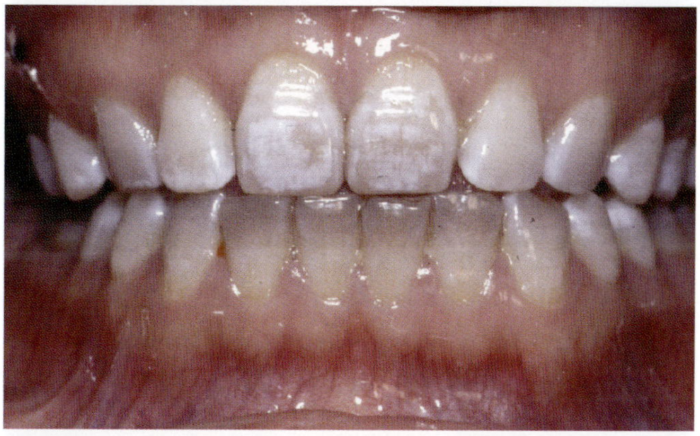
(D)

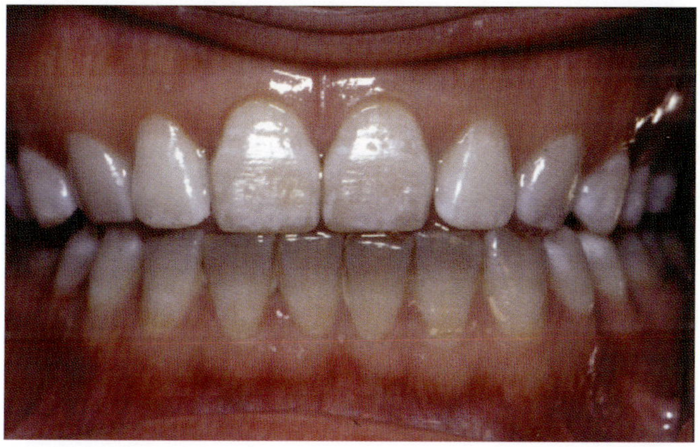
(E)

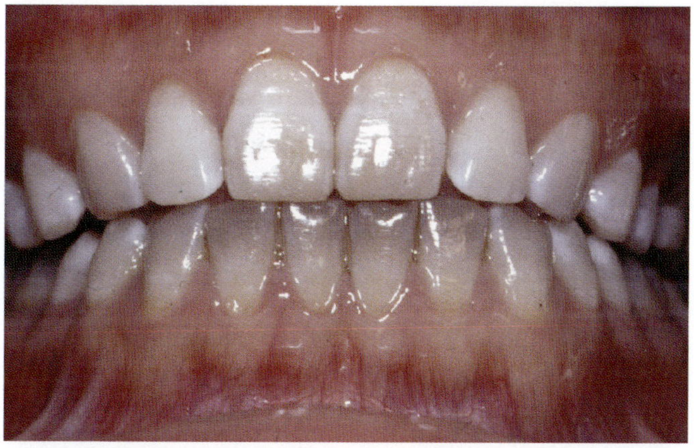
(F)

Figure 13.6

A 21-year-old woman who used 15% carbamide peroxide (CP) on the patient's right side and 10% CP on the left side in a custom-made tray with reservoirs, overnight, for 6 months. (A) Baseline; (B) 1 week; (C) 2 weeks; (D) 1 month; (E) 6 months; (F) 3 months postwhitening.

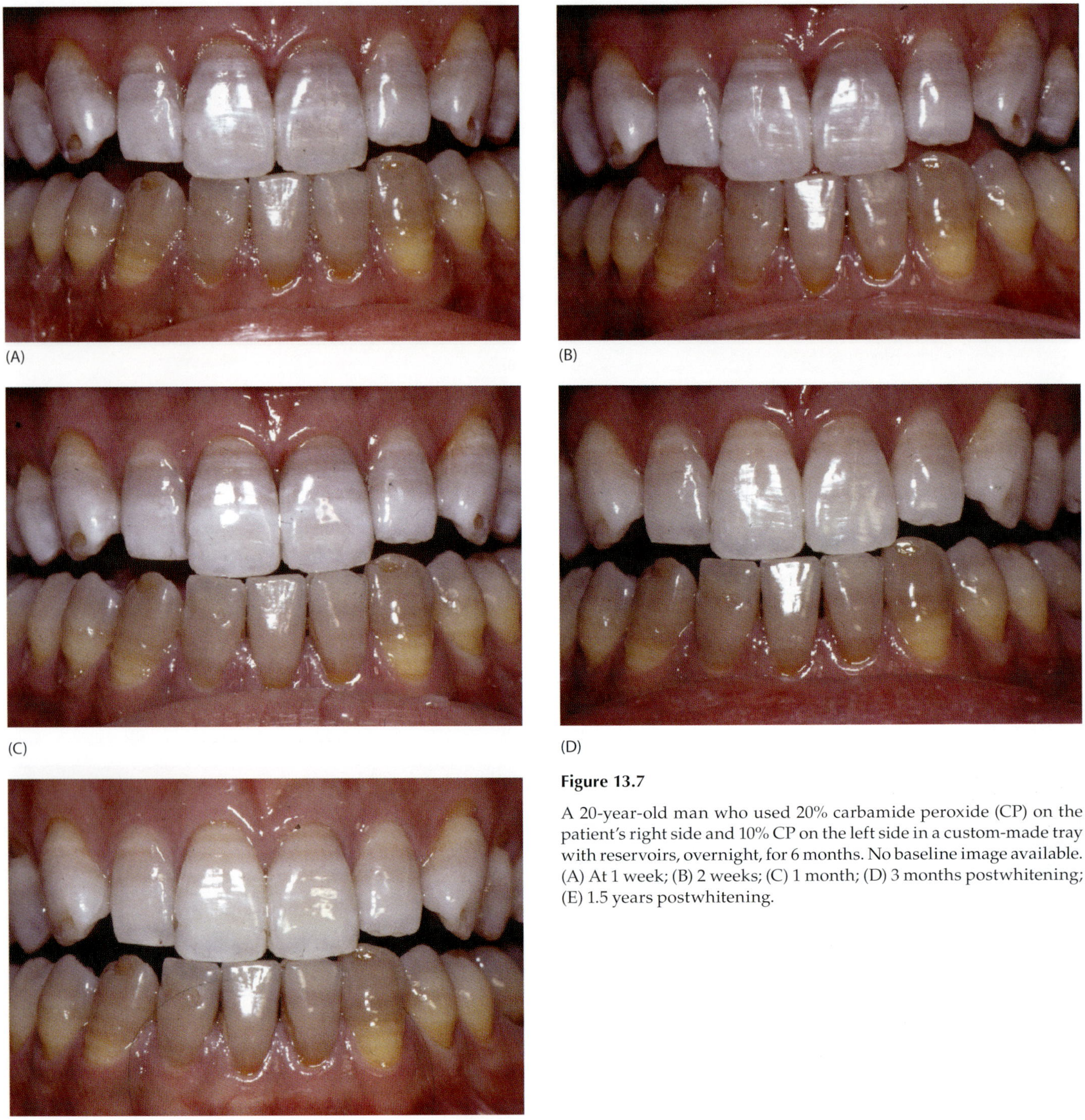

(A) (B) (C) (D) (E)

Figure 13.7

A 20-year-old man who used 20% carbamide peroxide (CP) on the patient's right side and 10% CP on the left side in a custom-made tray with reservoirs, overnight, for 6 months. No baseline image available. (A) At 1 week; (B) 2 weeks; (C) 1 month; (D) 3 months postwhitening; (E) 1.5 years postwhitening.

14 OVER-THE-COUNTER WHITENING STRIPS

Robert W. Gerlach, Britta E. Magnuson, and Gerard Kugel

INTRODUCTION

Whitening strips were introduced to the dental profession in 2000 (Gerlach 2000). The technology behind whitening strips is based on the use of a barrier (in this case, a flexible strip) that holds a peroxide-containing gel (see Figure 14.1). Developed as an easy-to-use option, these strips can be readily self-applied directly to the teeth daily for at-home whitening (see Figure 14.2).

Whitening strips have become a very popular over-the-counter choice for whitening teeth. Patients generally feel comfortable using strips and confident in their success. Since the introduction of these whitening strips, there have been numerous clinical studies on their efficacy and safety demonstrating significant whitening of teeth and minimal side effects (Garcia-Godoy et al. 2004, Swift et al. 2004, Farrell et al. 2008, Gerlach et al. 2009). Studies have generally shown significant whitening even after a few days of use, with the minor occurrence of adverse events mainly consisting of localized irritation or sensitivity (Gerlach et al. 2009).

The literature since the introduction of the strips in 2000 is quite broad. Color change (Swift et al. 2004), side effects and safety (Farrell et al. 2008), color retention (Swift et al. 2009), and special populations, including patients with tetracycline staining (Kugel et al. 2002), pediatric patients (Donly 2005), and patients with xerostomia (Papas et al. 2009), have all been studied. The studies have shown whitening strips to be both safe and effective.

CONSIDERATIONS FOR USE

Indications

Visible tooth discoloration in adults (general discoloration of any origin).

- Intrinsic discoloration caused by aging (Gerlach and Zhou 2001).
- Intrinsic discoloration associated with diet or tobacco use (Gerlach 2004).

Whitening needs in special groups.

- Adolescents (Donly 2005).
- Seniors (Gerlach and Zhou 2001).

Atypical tooth discoloration.

- Mild, fluorosis-related white spots (Donly and Gerlach 2002).
- Postorthodontic discoloration (Donly and Gerlach 2002).
- Staining associated with long-term use of tetracycline (Kugel et al. 2011).

Cases in which other whitening approaches may be contraindicated.

- Recession that could contribute to sensitivity during treatment (Gerlach et al. 2005a).
- Cases in which cost or convenience is a factor (Gerlach 2000).

Contraindications

General areas of caution.

- Existing tooth sensitivity on the anterior facial teeth (compliance).
- Use in young children (primary dentition).

Specific conditions that may affect outcomes.

- Severely misaligned or crowded teeth (strip adaptation).
- Isolated white spot lesions (possible need for microabrasion or restoration).

Preexisting or concurrent dentistry.

- Fixed orthodontic devices on the anterior facial dentition (strip placement).
- Extensive esthetic restorations on the anterior facial surfaces (unless replacement is planned).

Advantages and Disadvantages

There are obvious advantages and disadvantages to the use of whitening strips (Table 14.1). Strips are easy to obtain over the counter or from a dental professional and are easy to use at home (Gerlach 2000, 2007). Cost is likely to be considerably lower than either in-office or tray treatments, and the duration of use is short—anywhere from 5 minutes to 2 hours per day. Another important advantage to whitening strips is that there is less peroxide exposure than with other whitening treatments (Gerlach and Sagel 2004). The newest whitening strips also have the added advantage that patients are able to drink water while wearing the strips.

The primary disadvantage to whitening strips is that they may not be ideal for use in patients with severely misaligned or crowded teeth. Although whitening strips may be adapted to simple misalignment, use in more severe cases may not be optimal. Whitening strips primarily whiten the anterior teeth, which may be problematic for some smile types.

Table 14.1 Summary of advantages and disadvantages of whitening strips versus others

Potential advantages	*Potential disadvantages*
Whitening strips—pretreatment effects	
Convenience and cost	Avoiding routine diagnosis
Easy introduction to esthetic dentistry	Avoiding other dental care
Whitening strips—treatment effects	
Easy in-use experience	Mandibular retention (some strips)
Gentle whitening with few side effects	Strip adaptation with severe malocclusion
Whitening strips—post-treatment effects	
Uniform whitening	Posterior teeth not treated
No persistent, severe problems	Possible mismatch with existing restorations

Finally, use may be initiated and completed without dental supervision—which potentially represents both an advantage and a disadvantage.

Case types and side effects

Clinical research demonstrates that whitening strips may be indicated for the most common case types, including intrinsic discoloration associated with chromogenic foods, smoking, and aging (Swift et al. 2004), and complex case types such as tetracycline staining (Kugel et al. 2002, 2011). Clinical research has also shown safe and effective whitening strip use by adolescents (Donly and Gerlach 2002, Donly 2005, Donly et al. 2006, 2007b) and by individuals with reduced salivary flow (Papas et al. 2009). Unlike trays, which may be contraindicated in patients with bruxism or temporomandibular joint problems (Robinson and Haywood 2000), whitening strips do not typically interfere with occlusion.

For tooth whitening in general, there are relatively few safety concerns with peroxide-containing whitening products (Mahony et al. 2006). The main side effects are transient tooth sensitivity and gingival irritation (Li 1996), which may affect up to two thirds of peroxide tray users (Haywood et al. 1994), and the custom tray alone (without peroxide) may contribute to some discomfort (Leonard et al. 1997). For whitening strips specifically, numerous clinical studies have established in-use safety (Garcia-Godoy et al. 2004, Swift et al. 2004, Farrell et al. 2008, Gerlach et al. 2009). Compared with the literature reports on peroxide-containing custom trays, the side effects with whitening strips are similar in nature but generally fewer in occurrence. For example, in one whitening strip study, side effects were confined to minor local irritation, involving 10% of subjects (Kugel 2004). Side effects (if any) were typically transient in nature, resolved during treatment, and were not different from placebo when evaluated head-to-head over a 12-month continuous-use period (Farrell et al. 2008).

Although many whitening strip applications have been evaluated in clinical trials, other uses are possible.

Table 14.2 Examples of whitening strips used to address specific practice needs

Application	*How whitening strips may be used in the dental practice*
In-office treatment	Instead of a take-home tray after in-office whitening for color stability
Re-treatment	Periodic touch-up to help maintain original whitening
Usage concerns	Option for temporomandibular joint disorder, bruxism, or gagging patients who cannot use trays
Sensitivity	Tooth sensitivity involving the posterior or lingual dentition
Failures	Alternative for patients whose compliance may be limited
Esthetics	Whitening to match existing restorations (that are not being replaced)
Patient relations	Patient recognition for milestones (e.g., graduations, weddings)

Examples include cases of touch-up or follow-up care, or other specialized use situations (Table 14.2). Other applications are possible, but because the evidence may not include controlled clinical testing, the potential risks and benefits should be carefully evaluated.

PRODUCT DESIGN

Whitening strips were originally introduced in the United States by the Procter and Gamble Company (Cincinnati, OH) in 2000 under the brand name Crest Whitestrips. Subsequently, this technology has been modified through research and development and expanded to various geographic locations (sometimes under different brand names tied to Whitestrips) (Gerlach 2007). In total, there are approximately a dozen marketed variations of the Whitestrips technology that were designed to address different aspects of the desired whitening experience.

In general, there are three main variations of Whitestrips that may be encountered in the marketplace and/or the academic literature. All three rely on a common flexible barrier approach to maintain peroxide contact with teeth over a sufficient period for diffusion and intrinsic whitening (Table 14.3). In brief, the three major variations include (1) original strips, (2) very thin gel strips, and (3) high-adhesive strips.

Original whitening strips

The Whitestrips technology was introduced via a supplement to *Compendium of Continuing Education in Dentistry*. This 2000 supplement ambitiously characterized Whitestrips as a paradigm shift in vital whitening (Gerlach 2000). Therein, whitening strips were described as the first major discontinuity and technologic upgrade since the introduction of overnight, tray-based whitening over a decade earlier (Haywood and to the maxillary anterior teeth, ensuring that the strip overlapped the gingival margin, and to limit contact time to 30 minutes daily. Approximately 1 month later, the subject returned for recall having completed treatment at home, and at that time tooth whitening was apparent (see Figure 14.13D). Gingival health in the areas of whitening strip application was exceptional, as evidenced by tissue color and form and the absence of bleeding, especially when compared with the untreated mandibular arch (see Figure 14.13E). Tooth color improvement was evident in the contrasting treated and untreated arches, and, of note, whitening included those teeth with prominent pretreatment cervical defects (see Figure 14.13F). After mandibular whitening, prophylaxis, and hygiene instruction, this patient was ready for definitive esthetic restorative care.

Overall, this is a useful case study with respect to whitening strip implications for dental practice. Whitening was suggested early in treatment. This approach affords the maximum flexibility in scheduling, and early whitening may help build patient confidence in the overall treatment plan. Single arch treatment can play a role in first-person visualization and compliance, and this in turn may promote oral hygiene behavior and gingival health. Use of very thin hydrogen peroxide whitening strips improved tooth color across the visible arch, not just a few teeth, and, importantly, included teeth with severe cervical defects. This in turn allowed initiation of whitening without preceding desensitizing treatment or placement of provisional restorations, thereby reducing the overall treatment plan.

Summarizing the evidence on whitening strips

Overall, the whitening strip clinical research has been diverse in scope, global in scale, and extensive in number of studies (Gerlach 2006, 2007, 2010), with more than a hundred other controlled clinical trials not described here for brevity. Independent reviews similarly identify the whitening strip research as providing a disproportional body of evidence on tooth whitening safety and effectiveness (Hasson et al. 2006). Accordingly, the whitening strip research represents perhaps the most comprehensive oral care product evaluation undertaken in a decade. Although the evidence is comprehensive, it is largely confined to the whitening strip technology developed and marketed under the brand name Whitestrips. Practitioners need to be aware that other easy-to-use products have occasionally been marketed, and factors relating to peroxide concentration, dose, kinetics, stability, and other issues may affect clinical response. There may be little to no clinical trial evidence on the effectiveness and safety of such alternative products. Practitioners may need to consider such evidence (or the lack thereof) when assessing various options for treatment.

SUMMARY

One of the authors (RWG) first introduced whitening strips to the world at the second Loma Linda University School of Dentistry symposium on tooth whitening, held in Orlando, Florida in June 2000. This second edition of *Tooth Whitening Techniques* affords a unique opportunity to (1) look back on the state of tooth whitening before Crest Whitestrips, and (2) look forward to anticipate the numerous changes in whitening and dentistry that are likely directly or indirectly attributable to the Whitestrips introduction.

Looking back is enabled by a supplement to *Compendium of Continuing Education in Dentistry* that was published just before the surprise Crest Whitestrips announcement in Orlando in June 2000. Some of the research remains consistent with the evidence available today. For example, early research on peroxide kinetics during tray-based whitening showed peroxide retention over 2 hours or more, even without use of reservoirs (Matis 2000), whereas other studies showed tray-based whitening to be safe and positively received, even under conditions of extended use (Leonard 2000). Other reports seem archaic. For example, use of tooth whitening products in children was described via an unpublished case report (Haywood 2000), reports of unsafe whitening were confined to two minor case studies without adequate peer review (Li 2000), and some credentialing guidelines advocated use of subjective shade guides plus plaque and gingivitis measurements (Siew 2000). In one of the most telling reports, prognosticators did not anticipate easy-to-use whitening strips, forecasting instead use of surfactants, anticalculus agents, and other ingredients in whitening toothpastes as a future whitening technology to maintain clean teeth between dental prophylaxis visits (Viscio et al. 2000).

Looking forward carries the same risks faced by the authors of the pre-Whitestrips 2000 supplement. Nonetheless, a few observations are merited. Overall, whitening strips continue to be a market leader and demonstrable business success in various geographic areas. Since the introduction of whitening strips, there has been a dramatic increase in the focus on esthetic dentistry, increased awareness, and new options for care that cross social and economic groups (Gerlach 2007). Since the introduction of whitening strips in the United States, there has been an increase in dental school applications, new dental schools have been established, and the profession has generally experienced renewed prominence. The potential impact of marketing in raising awareness of esthetic dentistry was recognized at the time of whitening strip introduction (Gerlach 2000). Whether some of these changes in the profession are directly or indirectly attributable to the marketing campaigns that occasionally accompany a whitening strip launch is a subject of some speculation.

At the time of introduction, whitening strips were immediately recognized as paradigm-shifting, affording the first easy-to-use, broadly available option for treatment (Gerlach 2000). Three major variants of whitening strips have been introduced to date. Each has been supported by an extensive clinical research program that, in total, is virtually unprecedented in esthetic dentistry. As such, whitening strips represent one standard that may be sustained for many years to come.

ACKNOWLEDGMENTS

Dr. Chad J. Anderson, a clinician in the practice-based research network of Tufts University School of Dental Medicine, provided the case study and related clinical photography described in this chapter. All other clinical photography was provided by the Procter and Gamble Company. We recognize these efforts, plus the innumerable staff and study subjects who participated in the extensive research reported herein.

REFERENCES

Bizhang M, Muller M, Phark JH, Barker ML et al. (2007) Clinical trial of long-term color stability of hydrogen peroxide strips and sodium percarbonate film. *Am J Dent* **20**(Spec No A):23A–7A.

Carlsson J. (1987) Salivary peroxidase: an important part of our defense against oxygen toxicity. *J Oral Pathol* **16**:412–6.

Croll TP. (1994) Tooth bleaching for children and teens: a protocol and examples. *Quintessence Int* **25**:811–7.

Donly K, Kennedy P, Anastasia MK, Barker ML. (2007a) Meta-analysis of adolescent tooth whitening clinical trials. *J Dent Res* **86**(Spec Issue A):Abstract No. 2032.

Donly K, Henson, T, Jamison D, Gerlach RW. (2006) Clinical trial evaluating two peroxide whitening strips used by teenagers. *Gen Dent* **54**:110–2.

Donly KJ. (2005) Critical appraisal: tooth whitening in children and adolescents. *J Esthet Restor Dent* **17**:380–3.

Donly KJ, Donly AS, Baharloo, L, Rojas-Candelas E. (2002) Tooth whitening in children. *Compend Contin Educ Dent* **23**:22–8.

Donly KJ, Gerlach RW. (2002) Clinical trials on the use of whitening strips in children and adolescents. *Gen Dent* **50**:242–5.

Donly KJ, Kennedy P, Segura A, Gerlach RW. (2005) Effectiveness and safety of tooth bleaching in teenagers. *Pediatr Dent* **27**:298–302.

Donly KJ, Segura A, Henson T, Barker ML. (2007b) Randomized controlled trial of professional at-home tooth whitening in teenagers. *Gen Dent* **55**:669–74.

Donly KJ, Segura A, Sasa I, Perez E. (2010) A controlled clinical trial to evaluate the safety and whitening efficacy of a 9.5% hydrogen peroxide high-adhesion whitening strip in a teen population. *Am J Dent* **23**:292–6.

Duschner H, Gotz H, White DJ, Kozak KM. (2004) Effects of hydrogen peroxide bleaching strip gels on dental restorative materials in vitro: surface microhardness and surface morphology. *J Clin Dent* **15**:105–11.

Farrell S, Barker, ML, McMillan DA, Gerlach RW. (2008) Placebo-controlled trial evaluating safety with 12-months continuous use of 6% hydrogen peroxide whitening strips. *J Dent* **36**:726–30.

Farrell S, Ovando B, Ralston C, Fiedler SK. (2009) Kinetics of experimental 9.5% hydrogen peroxide whitening strips. *J Dent Res* **88**(Spec Issue A):Abstract 2199.

Ferrari M, Cagidiaco, MC, Monticelli F, Kugel G. (2007) Daytime use of a custom bleaching tray or whitening strips: initial and sustained color improvement. *Am J Dent* **20**(Spec Issue A):19A–22A.

Ferrari M, Kugel G, Cagidiaco MC, Barker ML. (2004) Clinical trial evaluating the peroxide concentration response of whitening strips over 28 days. *Am J Dent* **17**:291–4.

Garcia-Godoy F, Villalta P, Barker ML, Gerlach RW. (2004) Placebo-controlled, 6-week clinical trial on the safety and efficacy of a low-gel, 14% hydrogen-peroxide whitening strip. *Compend Contin Educ Dent* **25**:21–6.

Gerlach RW. (2000) Shifting paradigms in whitening: introduction of a novel system for vital tooth bleaching. *Compend Contin Educ Dent Suppl* **29**:S4–9.

Gerlach RW. (2004) Whitening paradigms revisited: introduction of a thin and concentrated peroxide gel technology for professional tooth whitening. *Compend Contin Educ Dent* **25**:4–8.

Gerlach RW. (2006) Clinical trials and oral care R&D. *J Am Coll Dent* **73**:26–31.

Gerlach RW. (2007) Tooth whitening clinical trials: a global perspective. *Am J Dent* **20**(Spec Issue A):3A–6A.

Gerlach RW. (2010) Clinical trials, case studies, and oral care R&D: inclusivity, consistency, and other atypical evidence. *J Evid Based Dent Pract* **10**:10–2.

Gerlach RW, Barker ML. (2004) Professional vital bleaching using a thin and concentrated peroxide gel on whitening strips: an integrated clinical summary. *J Contemp Dent Pract* **5**:1–17.

Gerlach RW, Zhou X. (2001) Vital bleaching with whitening strips: summary of clinical research on effectiveness and tolerability. *J Contemp Dent Pract* **2**:1–16.

Gerlach RW, Zhou X. (2004a) Meta-analysis of factors contributing to whitening strip effectiveness and safety. *J Dent Res* **83**(Spec Issue A):Abstract No. 0048.

Gerlach RW, Zhou X. (2004b) Clinical trial comparing two daytime hydrogen-peroxide professional vital-bleaching systems. *Compend Contin Educ Dent* **25**:33–40.

Gerlach RW, Barker ML, Anastasia MK, Bsoul S. (2005a) Gingival recession and clinical response with extended whitening strip use. *J Dent Res* **84**(Spec Issue A):Abstract No. 2124.

Gerlach RW, Barker ML, Karpinia, K, Magnusson I. (2009) Single site meta-analysis of 6% hydrogen peroxide whitening strip effectiveness and safety over 2 weeks. *J Dent* **37**:360–365.

Gerlach RW, Barker ML, McMillan DA, Sagel PA. (2004a) In-use comparative kinetics of professional whitening strips: peroxide recovery from strips, teeth, gingiva, and saliva. *Compend Contin Educ Dent* **25**:14–20.

Gerlach RW, Barker ML, Sagel PA. (2002a) Objective and subjective whitening response of two self-directed bleaching systems. *Am J Dent* **15**(Spec Issue):7A–12A.

Gerlach RW, Barker ML, Sagel PA, Ralston CA. (2008) In-use peroxide kinetics of 10% hydrogen peroxide whitening strips. *J Clin Dent* **19**:59–63.

Gerlach RW, Gibb RD, Sagel PA. (2000) A randomized clinical trial comparing a novel 5.3% hydrogen peroxide whitening strip to 10%, 15%, and 20% carbamide peroxide tray-based bleaching systems. *Compend Contin Educ Dent Suppl* **29**:S22–8; quiz S42–3.

Gerlach RW, Sagel PA. (2004) Vital bleaching with a thin peroxide gel: the safety and efficacy of a professional-strength hydrogen peroxide whitening strip. *J Am Dent Assoc* **135**:98–100.

Gerlach RW, Sagel PA, Barker ML, Karpinia K. (2004b) Placebo-controlled clinical trial evaluating a 10% hydrogen peroxide whitening strip. *J Clin Dent* **15**:118–22.

Gerlach RW, Sagel PA, Jeffers ME, Zhou X. (2002b) Effect of peroxide concentration and brushing on whitening clinical response. *Compend Contin Educ Dent* **23**:16–21.

Gerlach RW, Tucker HL, Anastasia MK, Barker ML. (2005b) Clinical trial comparing 2 hydrogen peroxide tooth whitening systems: strips vs pre-rinse. *Compend Contin Educ Dent* **26**:874–8.

Guerrero JC, Jimenez-Farfan MD, Lopez-Salgado A, Barker ML. (2007) Professional whitening strips in a university population. *Am J Dent* **20**(Spec Issue A):15A–8A.

Hasson H, Ismail AI, Neiva G. (2006) Home-based chemically-induced whitening of teeth in adults. *Cochrane Database Syst Rev* **4**:CD006202.

Haywood VB. (2000) Current status of Nightguard Vital Bleaching. *Compend Contin Educ Dent Suppl* **28:**S10–7.

Haywood VB, Heymann HO. (1989) Nightguard Vital Bleaching. *Quintessence Int* **20:**173–6.

Haywood VB, Leonard RH, Nelson CF, Brunson WD. (1994) Effectiveness, side effects and long-term status of Nightguard Vital Bleaching. *J Am Dent Assoc* **125:**1219–26.

Kugel G. (2000) Nontray whitening. *Compend Contin Educ Dent* **21:**524–6, 528.

Kugel G. (2004) *A study of tooth whitening: safety, efficacy and mechanism of action.* PhD Dissertation. University of Siena, Siena, Italy, pp. 25–35.

Kugel G, Aboushala A, Zhou X, Gerlach RW. (2002) Daily use of whitening strips on tetracycline-stained teeth: comparative results after 2 months. *Compend Contin Educ Dent* **23:**29–34.

Kugel G, Ferreira S, Sharma S, Barker ML. (2009) Clinical trial assessing light enhancement of in-office tooth whitening. *J Esthet Restor Dent* **21:**336-47.

Kugel G, Ferreira S, Sharma S, Gerlach RW. (2006) Randomized placebo-controlled clinical trial of 6% hydrogen peroxide whitening strips. *J Dent Res* **85**(Spec Issue A):Abstract No. 1375.

Kugel G, Ferreira S, Towers J, Gerlach RW. (2007) At-home professional bleaching of tetracycline stain: five year recall. *J Dent Res* **86**(Spec Issue A):Abstract No. 123.

Kugel G, Gerlach RW, Aboushala A, Ferreira S. (2011) Long-term use of 6.5% hydrogen peroxide bleaching strips on tetracycline stain: a clinical study. *Compend Contin Educ Dent* **32:**50–56.

Kugel G, Kastali S. (2000) Tooth-whitening efficacy and safety: a randomized and controlled clinical trial. *Compend Contin Educ Dent Suppl* **29:**S16–21.

Leonard RH Jr. (2000) Nightguard Vital Bleaching: dark stains and long-term results. *Compend Contin Educ Dent Suppl* **28:**S18-27.

Leonard RH Jr, Haywood VB, Eagle JC, Garland GE. (1999) Nightguard Vital Bleaching of tetracycline-stained teeth: 54 months post treatment. *J Esthet Dent* **11:**265–77.

Leonard RH Jr, Haywood VB, Phillips C. (1997) Risk factors for developing tooth sensitivity and gingival irritation associated with Nightguard Vital Bleaching. *Quintessence Int* **28:**527–34.

Li Y. (1996) Biological properties of peroxide-containing tooth whiteners. *Food Chem Toxicol* **34:**887–904.

Li Y. (2000) Peroxide-containing tooth whiteners: an update on safety. *Compend Contin Educ Dent Suppl* **28:**S4–9.

Loe H, Silness J. (1963) Periodontal disease in pregnancy. I. Prevalence and severity. *Acta Odontol Scand* **21:**533–51.

Mahony C, Felter SP, McMillan DA. (2006) An exposure-based risk assessment approach to confirm the safety of hydrogen peroxide for use in home tooth bleaching. *Regul Toxicol Pharmacol* **44:**75–82.

Marshall MV, Cancro LP, Fischman SL. (1995) Hydrogen peroxide: a review of its use in dentistry. *J Periodontol* **66:**786–96.

Marshall MV, Gragg PP, Packman EW, Wright PB. (2001) Hydrogen peroxide decomposition in the oral cavity. *Am J Dent* **14:**39–45.

Matis BA. (2000) Degradation of gel in tray whitening. *Compend Contin Educ Dent Suppl* **28:**S31–5.

Odioso LL, Gibb RD, Gerlach RW. (2000) Impact of demographic, behavioral, and dental care utilization parameters on tooth color and personal satisfaction. *Compend Contin Educ Dent Suppl* **29:**S35–41.

Papas AS, Kugel G, Singh M, Barker ML. (2009) Placebo-controlled clinical trial of use of 10% hydrogen peroxide whitening strips for medication-induced xerostomia. *Gerontology* **55:**511–6.

Perry, R, Kugel G, Conde EE, Farrell S. (2013) Comparative performance of two whitening systems in a dental practice. *Compend Contin Educ Dent* **34**(Spec Issue 8):15–8.

Robinson FG, Haywood VB. (2000) Bleaching and temporomandibular disorder using a half tray design: a clinical report. *J Prosthet Dent* **83:**501–3.

Sagel PA, Gerlach RW. (2007) Application of digital imaging in tooth whitening randomized controlled trials. *Am J Dent* **20**(Spec Issue A):7A–14A.

Sagel PA, Landrigan WF. (2004) A new approach to strip-based tooth whitening: 14% hydrogen peroxide delivered via controlled low dose. *Compend Contin Educ Dent* **25:**9–13.

Sagel PA, Odioso LL, McMillan DA, Gerlach RW. (2000) Vital tooth whitening with a novel hydrogen peroxide strip system: design, kinetics, and clinical response. *Compend Contin Educ Dent Suppl* **29:**S10–5.

Shahidi, H, Barker ML, Sagel PA, Gerlach RW. (2005) Randomized controlled trial of 10% hydrogen peroxide whitening strips. *J Clin Dent* **16:**91-5.

Siew C. (2000) ADA guidelines for the acceptance of tooth-whitening products. *Compend Contin Educ Dent Suppl* **28:** S44–7.

Silness, J, Loe H. (1964) Periodontal disease in pregnancy. II. Correlation between oral hygiene and periodontal condition. *Acta Odontol Scand* **22:**121–35.

Simon J, Braxton A, George L, Wilson N. (2012) Comparative whitening efficacy of 2-hour strips and professional laser treatment. *J Dent Res* **91**(Spec Issue A):Abstract No. 1063.

Swift, EJ Jr, Heymann HO, Wilder AD Jr, Barker ML. (2009) Effects of duration of whitening strip treatment on tooth color: a randomized, placebo-controlled clinical trial. *J Dent* **37**(Suppl 1):e51–6.

Swift EJ Jr, Miguez PA, Barker ML, Gerlach RW. (2004) Three-week clinical trial of a 14% hydrogen-peroxide, strip-based bleaching system. *Compend Contin Educ Dent* **25:**27–32.

Viscio D, Gaffar A, Fakhry-Smith S, Xu T. (2000) Present and future technologies of tooth whitening. *Compend Contin Educ Dent Suppl* **28:**S36–43.

White DJ, Kozak KM, Zoladz JR, Duschner H. (2000) Effects of tooth-whitening gels on enamel and dentin ultrastructure—a confocal laser scanning microscopy pilot study. *Compend Contin Educ Dent Suppl* **29:**S29–34.

White DJ, Kozak KM, Zoladz JR, Duschner H. (2002) Peroxide interactions with hard tissues: effects on surface hardness and surface/subsurface ultrastructural properties. *Compend Contin Educ Dent* **23:**42–8.

Xu X, Zhu L, Tang Y, Wang Y. (2007) Randomized clinical trial comparing whitening strips, paint-on gel and negative control. *Am J Dent* **20**(Spec Issue A):28A–31A.

Yudhira R, Peumans M, Barker ML, Gerlach RW. (2007) Clinical trial of tooth whitening with 6% hydrogen peroxide whitening strips and two whitening dentifrices. *Am J Dent* **20**(Spec Issue A):32A–6A.

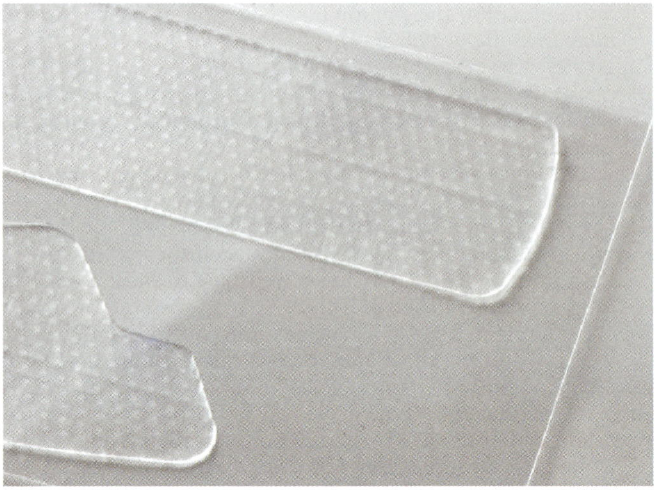

Figure 14.1

Close-up of whitening strips.

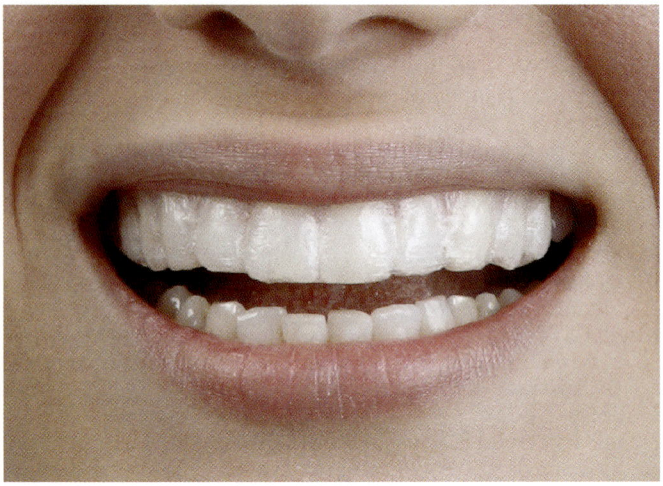

Figure 14.2

Whitening strip worn on the maxillary arch.

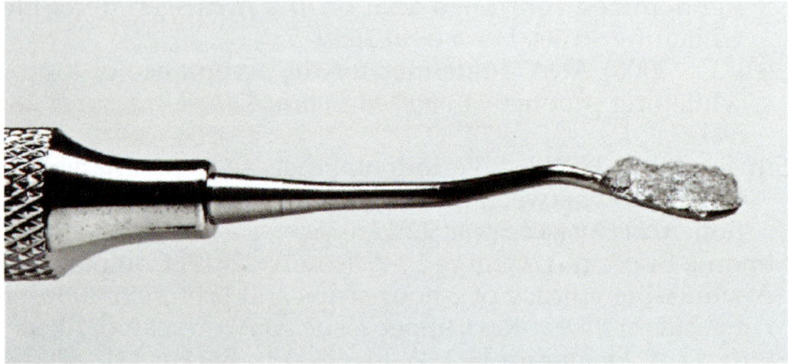

Figure 14.3

Amount of whitening gel on a "very thin" maxillary strip.

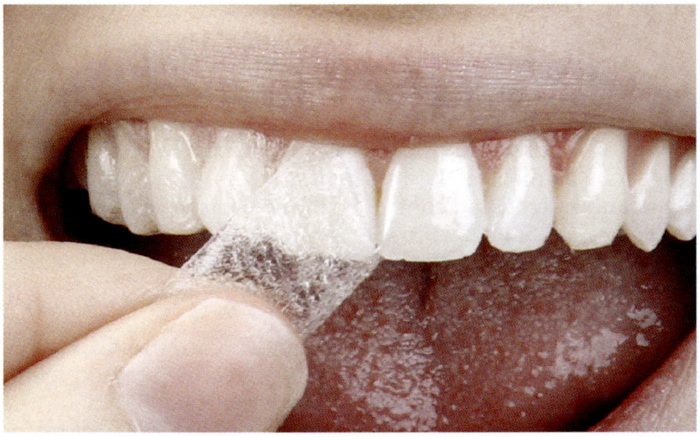

Figure 14.4

Close up of "clean" removal of a high-adhesive maxillary strip.

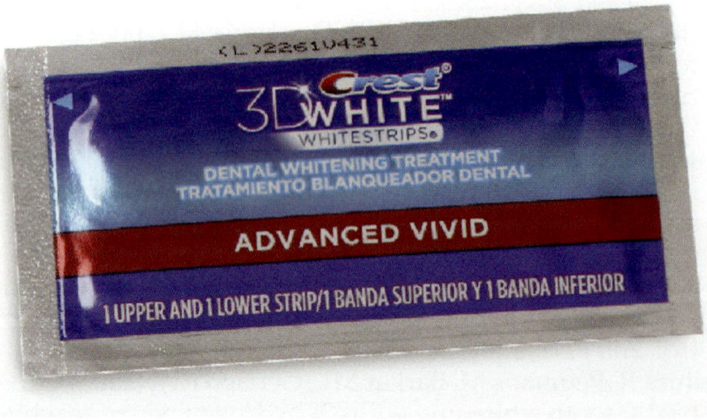

(A)

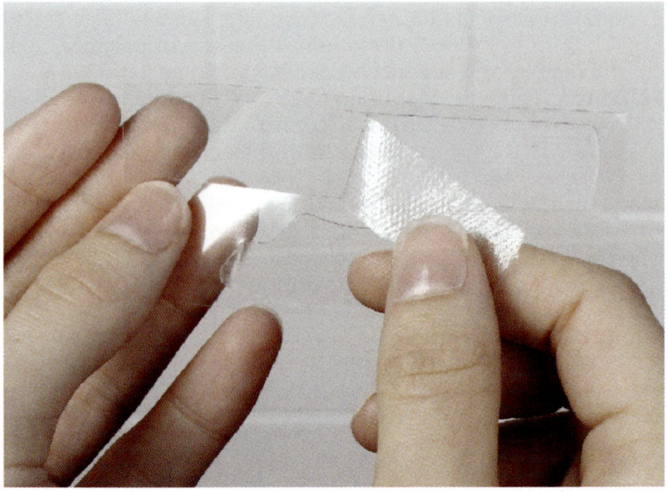

(B)

Figure 14.5

(A) Foil pouch containing whitening strips. (B) Peeling maxillary whitening strip from liner.

continued on the next page

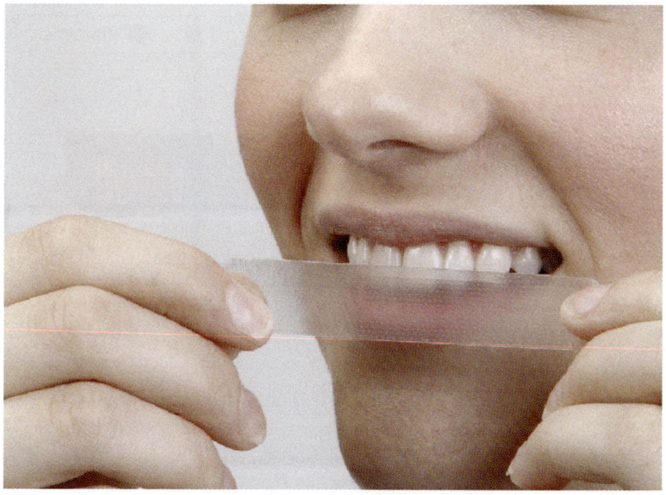

(C)

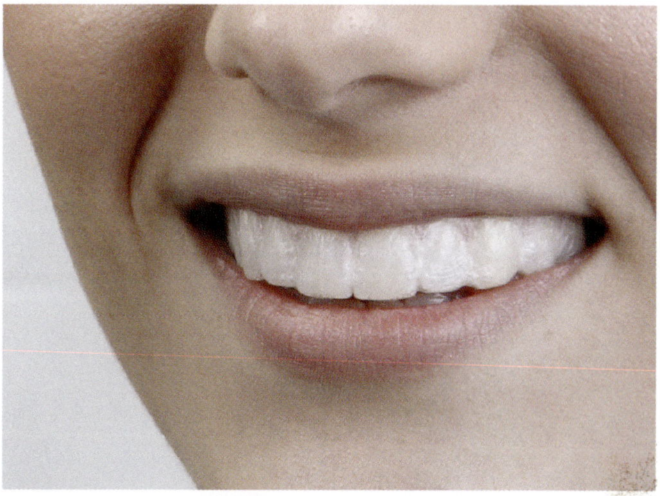

(D)

Figure 14.5 continued

(C) Whitening strip application. (D) Whitening strip in place. (E) Whitening strip removal.

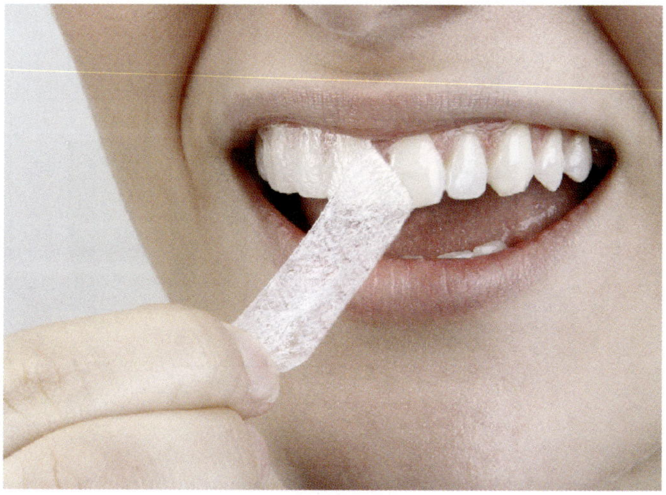

(E)

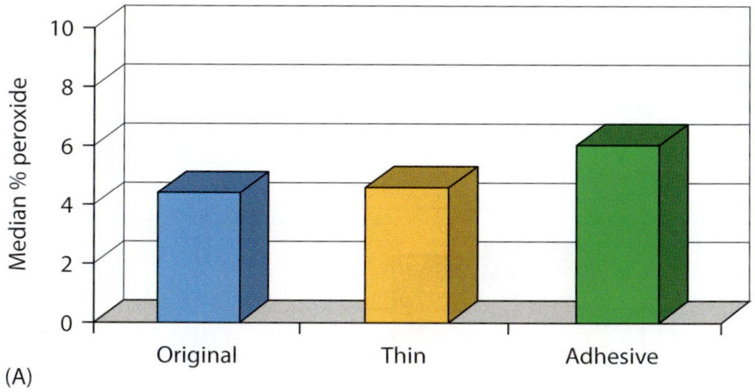

(A)

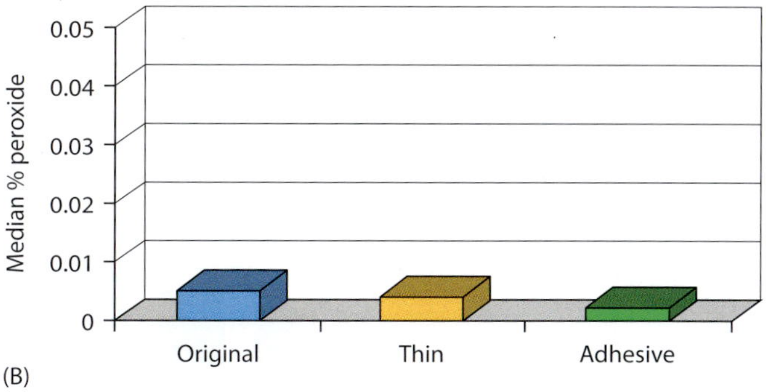

(B)

Figure 14.6

(A) Peroxide concentration on strip (30 minutes after application, three peroxide gels). (B) Peroxide concentration in saliva (30 minutes after application, three peroxide gels).

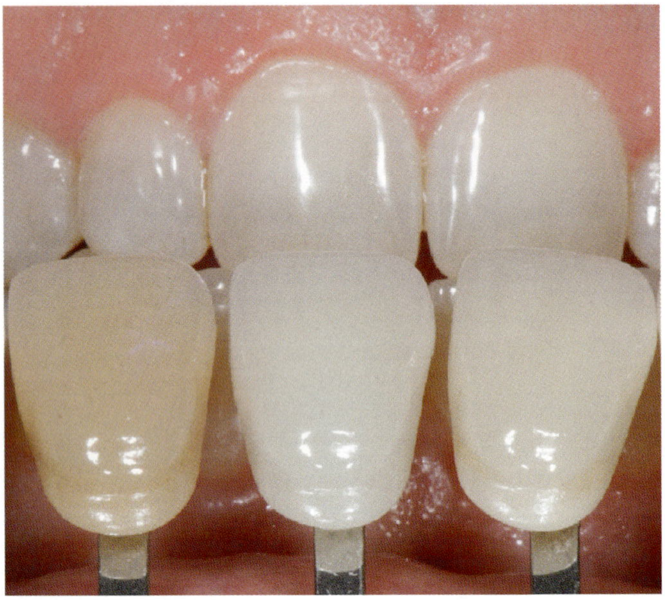

FIGURE 14.7

Whitening strip treatment response with shade tabs.

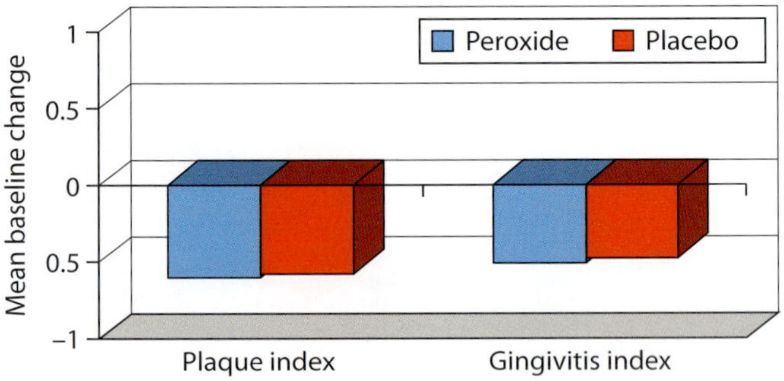

Figure 14.8

Strip effects on plaque and gingivitis (peroxide versus placebo strips).

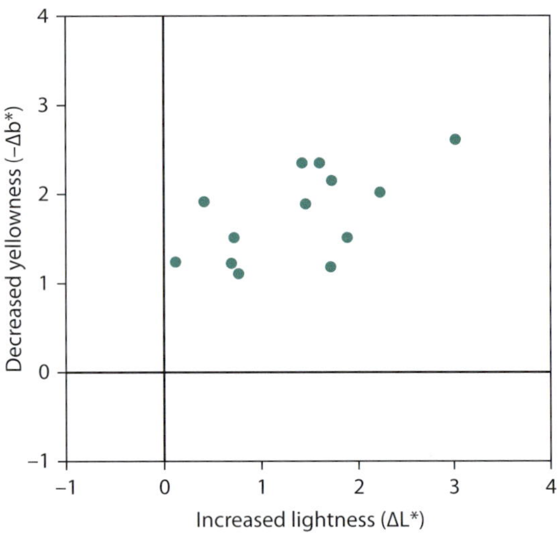

Figure 14.9

Whitening response by subject (peroxide strips).

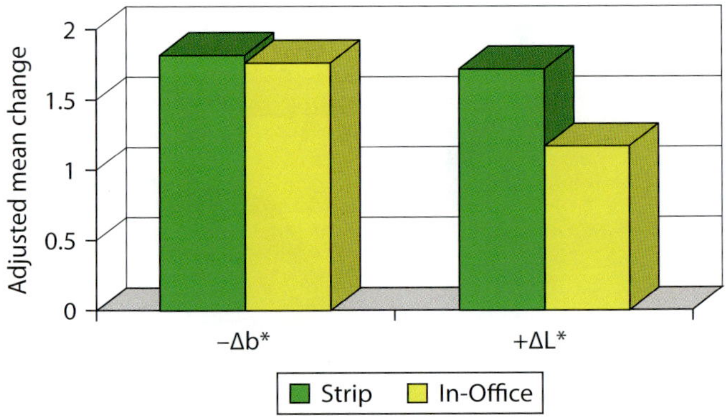

Figure 14.10

Comparative whitening versus a professional control (peroxide strip versus in-office peroxide/light combination).

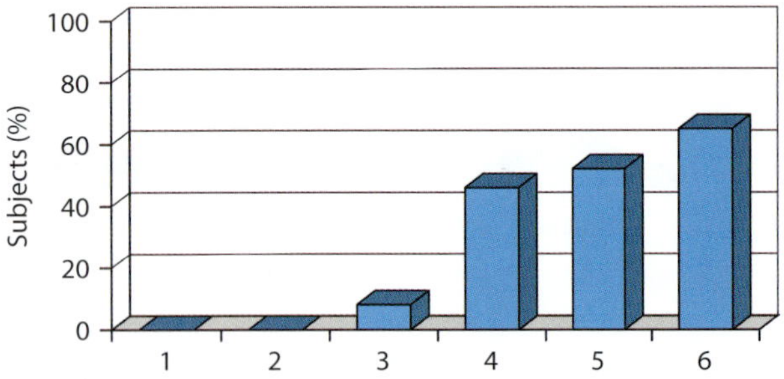

Figure 14.11

Whitening strips and tetracycline stain (percent of subjects improving to shade B1 by month).

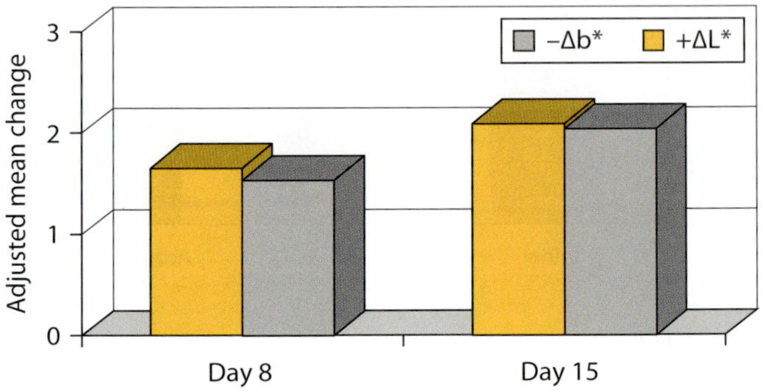

Figure 14.12

Whitening strips and xerostomia (mean tooth color improvement for peroxide strips).

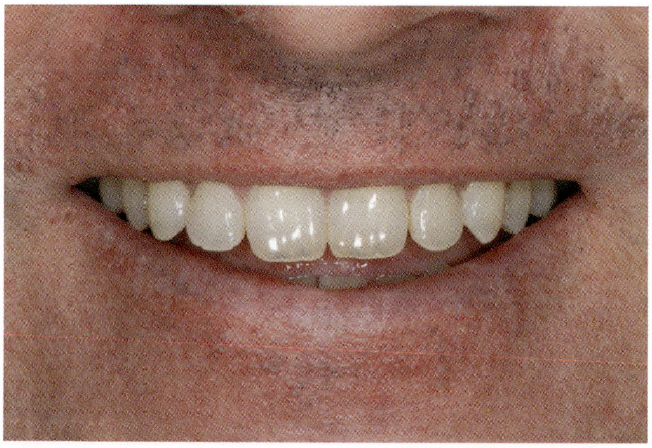

(A)

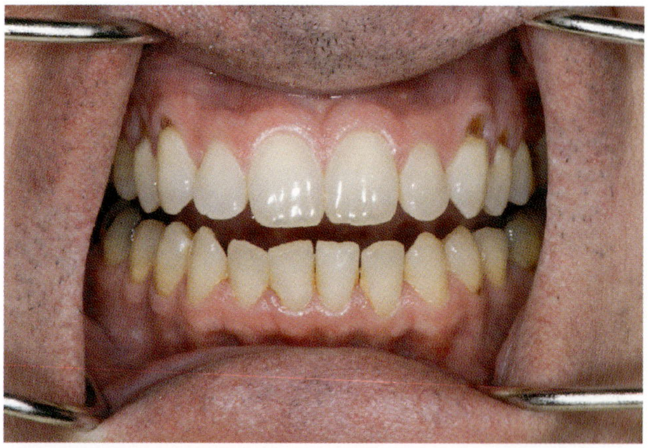

(B)

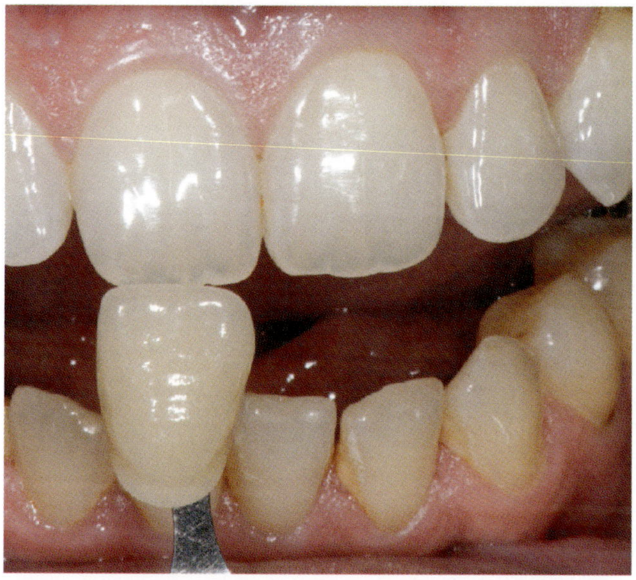

(C)

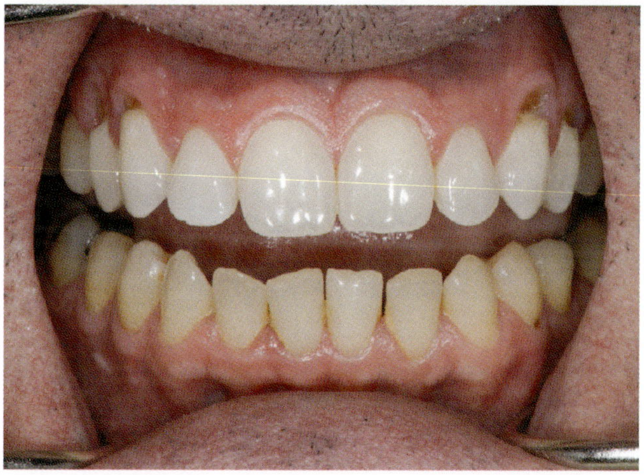

(D)

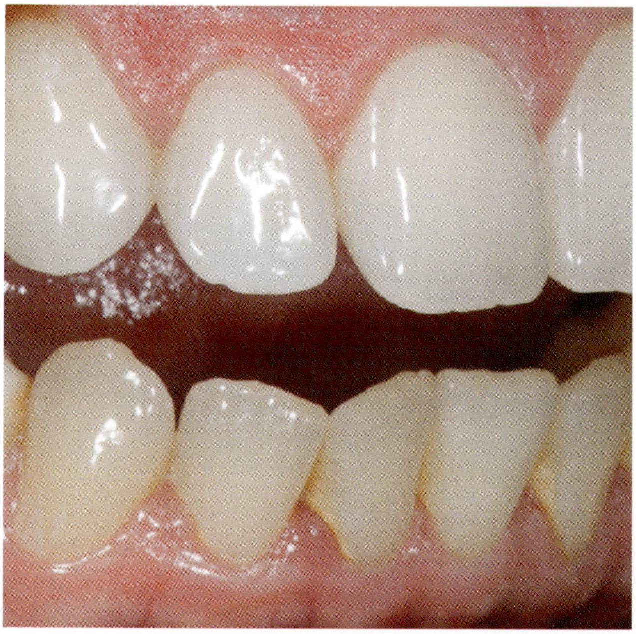

(E)

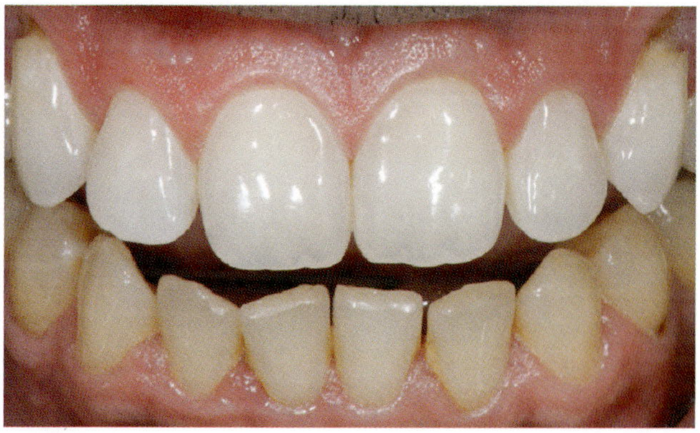

(F)

Figure 14.13

(A) Smile appearance before whitening. (B) Bilateral gingival recession before whitening. (C) Tooth shade collection before whitening. (D) Color contrast after maxillary arch whitening. (E) Gingival response (maxillary arch treated, mandibular arch untreated). (F) Overall color improvement (maxillary arch) before cervical esthetic restorations.

15 COMBINING WHITENING TECHNIQUES AND MINIMALLY INVASIVE TREATMENTS

Linda Greenwall

INTRODUCTION

During the last quarter century, there has been a large increase in the whitening techniques and treatments that are available to patients, which has led to a huge paradigm shift away from the existing philosophy of undertaking mechanical dentistry and towards minimally invasive dentistry. The success of the whitening treatments has shown that enamel treatments and dentin bonding are preferable to cutting healthy tooth structure. There are more opportunities to combine whitening treatments and more techniques for more effective whitening. Combination treatments have been recommended to speed up the whitening process and allow for shorter treatment times. This is also significant when treating single teeth for whitening. Further combinations involve whitening and minimally invasive dentistry (see Tables 15.1 and 15.2).

Types of whitening treatments that can be combined are as follows:

1. Home and power whitening.
2. Internal and external whitening or nonvital and home whitening together.
3. Sectional whitening of specific teeth and full-arch whitening treatment.
4. Chairside whitening treatments using the patient's whitening trays (to speed up the whitening process and make the treatment more effective).
5. Home whitening, microabrasion, and/or resin infiltration.
6. Home whitening and air abrasion, cleaning, and surface preparation.

Although many stains can be treated successfully with a single agent, some may need to be treated using a combination of approaches. Whitening treatments can be combined in various ways depending on the nature of the discoloration. Table 15.3 shows the different options for different levels of discoloration. When one agent fails to remove a stain completely, or when multiple stains of different origins are present in the same tooth, a combination of whitening techniques can be used. Power whitening can be combined with a home whitening program (Garber et al. 1991). Combinations of whitening agents in different concentrations can be used. The microabrasion technique can be combined with home or power whitening. Teeth can even be brightened using pumice and a 10% carbamide peroxide slurry (Baker et al. 1992). In addition, combinations of increasing concentrations of hydrochloric acid and resin infiltration can reduce the effects of white spots.

It is the aim of this chapter to demonstrate how different whitening techniques can be used in combination by showing various case presentations. A modification of the intracoronal technique will be described.

TOOTH SURFACE AND ENAMEL CONDITIONING

Some patients have extensive staining of multiple origins present on the teeth. Some stains are tenacious, such as the stains derived from smoking. It may be useful to use air scaling or enamel conditioning, cleansing, or air abrasion techniques directly on the surface of the teeth before whitening. The surface cleaning approach will eliminate the extrinsic stains so that the intrinsic stains can be examined and plans made to treat the stain or discoloration. The surface treatment involves the following:

1. Cleaning the tooth with pumice and Hibiscrub before whitening.
2. Air scaling to remove some simple stain.
3. Sylc treatment using the Aquacut machine (Velopex International, London). Sylc powder is applied. This is a bioglass similar to Novamin; it contains calcium and phosphate and is used as a cleansing agent and a desensitizer. These materials can clean, seal, and soothe the tooth in preparation for the whitening treatment.
4. The surface cleaning and conditioning may help in treating cariogenic white spots and other superficial stains.

WHY COMBINE WHITENING TREATMENTS?

- To make the whitening program more effective.
- To motivate patients to continue the whitening program at home.
- To treat a specific problem such as a single dark vital tooth or a single nonvital tooth.
- To sequence and stage whitening treatment in a complex treatment plan.

Table 15.1 Treatment options for minimally invasive dentistry

Old		
Mechanical intervention		
Current		
Minimally invasive dentistry	→	Chemical dentistry
	→	Therapeutic dentistry
	→	Resin infiltration
	→	Preservation of the enamel
	→	No cutting or tooth preparation

- To treat difficult stains, such as those caused by tetracycline, which may respond better to a combination approach.
- To treat stains of different origins that exist in the same tooth such as white spots.

Nonvital whitening is a common procedure and has been used as a technique for over 200 years (Abbot and Heah 2009). The most common tooth to be whitened is the upper central incisor (69%; Abbot and Heah 2009), followed by the lateral incisor (20.4%).

Reasons for undertaking nonvital whitening

The reasons for nonvital whitening are as follows, according to Abbot and Heah (2009) and Plotino et al. (2008):

1. Trauma (the most common cause; 58.8%).
2. Previous dental treatment (23.9%).
3. Pulp necrosis (13.7%).
4. Pulp canal calcification (3.6%). Dark-yellow and black teeth require more applications of whitening agent than light-yellow and gray teeth.
5. Intrapulpal hemorrhage, carious tooth.
6. Defects on teeth, calcification.
7. Genetic issues (hyperbilirubinemia, fibrosis of the pancreas, amelogenesis imperfecta, cystic endodontic treatment).
8. Residual pulp tissue after endodontic treatment.
9. Endodontic materials (medications, irrigants, root or canal sealer).
10. Root resorption.

Expected outcome of this technique

The range of expected outcomes for nonvital whitening technique for color modification is as follows:

1. "Good" (87.1%; study by Abbot and Heah 2009)
2. "Acceptable" (12.9%)
3. Unacceptable.
4. No change (rare)

The outside-inside whitening technique: a variation of the nonvital whitening technique

This has also been called *internal/external bleaching* (Settembrini et al. 1997), *patient-administered intracoronal bleaching,* and *modified walking bleach technique* (Liebenberg 1997). The technique combines the intracoronal whitening technique with the home whitening technique. It is used to whiten nonvital teeth in a simple manner and to improve the expected outcomes listed earlier. After barrier placement the access cavity is left open so that the whitening material, which is normally

Table 15.2 Decision making process for combinations of treatments

Home whitening ⟶ Power whitening ⟶ Combination whitening ⟵ Internal whitening ⟶ Outside-inside whitening

Home whitening ↓	Combination whitening ↓	Internal whitening ↓	Internal whitening ↓
Enzymatic whitening 5% Lactoperoxidase	Microabrasion 5% HCL	Sealed in 6% HP = 20% CPS	In addition use of home whitening 10% CPS

Table 15.3 Options for combination treatments including whitening combinations

Surface treatments of enamel	
Direct application	Varnish application
Cleaning	Air polishing, air abrasion, sandblasting, Sylc (Novamin)
Microabrasion	Reduction and elimination of white spots
Slightly deeper treatments	
Therapeutic	Application of amorphous calcium phosphate, fluoride, potassium nitrate into tray
Infiltration	Resin infiltration (Icon)
Deeper treatments	
Penetration from the enamel into the tooth	Whitening
Dentin	Whitening the dentin, air abrasion, Sylc treatment
Pulp	Discoloration from trauma, nonvital whitening, outside-inside whitening

10% or 16% carbamide peroxide or 6% hydrogen peroxide, can be placed into the pulp chamber while the whitening tray is applied to the tooth to retain the material on the tooth. Whitening can thus take place internally and externally at the same time. The higher the concentration of carbamide or hydrogen peroxide, the higher the concentration will be in the pulp chamber, especially if the tooth has been previously restored (Benetti et al. 2004). This technique is a modification of the sealed-in, intracoronal whitening technique (see Chapter 8) and can be used as an alternative technique. Its simplicity and effectiveness warrant description and discussion.

THE PROCEDURE

1. Preparation of the barrier

The nonvital tooth is prepared in the same manner described in Chapter 8 on intracoronal whitening. It is essential to take a pretreatment radiograph to verify the presence of an acceptable root canal treatment and the absence of apical pathology.

Isolation methods

The tooth can be isolated with a rubber dam in preparation for the meticulous removal of the existing extracoronal restoration; however, use of the dental dam is not mandatory because the whitening material is not caustic (Liebenberg 1997).

Gutta-percha removal

As in the intracoronal technique, the gutta-percha is removed to 2–3 mm below the cementoenamel junction (CEJ). The object of the gutta-percha removal is to provide space for the barrier.

Placement of the barrier

A protective barrier is placed over the gutta-percha to prevent the whitening gel from escaping into the root canal system at the CEJ. Conventional glass ionomer or a resin-modified glass ionomer can be used as a barrier (Settembrini et al. 1997).

Protect the gutta-percha

It has been suggested that a calcium hydroxide plug approximately 1 mm in thickness be placed over the exposed gutta-percha. This prophylactic step aims to maintain an alkaline medium because cervical resorption has been associated with a drop in pH at the cervical level (Liebenberg 1997). A periapical radiograph can be taken at this stage to check that the barrier has been well placed, but this is not mandatory.

2. Cleaning of the access cavity

The access cavity is cleaned and any remaining pulp horn constituents are removed. The access cavity can be etched merely to clean the internal surface. It does not enhance the whitening effect. A cotton pellet or pellet of polytetrafluoroethylene (PTFE) tape shaped into a ball is placed into the access cavity to prevent food from packing into it.

3. Shade assessment

The pretreatment shades of both the nonvital tooth and the surrounding teeth are taken and noted in the patient's record or on the whitening record sheet (see Chapter 4).

4. Instructions for home whitening

The whitening tray is checked for fit and comfort (Zimmerli et al. 2010). The patient is instructed not to bite with the anterior tooth for the duration of the treatment (Carillo et al. 1998). The patient is sent home with the whitening instructions and enough whitening materials to lighten the tooth. The cotton pellet in the access cavity is removed with a toothpick before whitening. The whitening syringe can be applied directly into the open chamber before the whitening tray is seated, or the whitening material can be applied into the tray with extra material in the space for the tooth with the open chamber. The patient is instructed to remove the excess with a toothbrush or paper tissue. After the whitening session, the tooth is irrigated with a water syringe and a fresh cotton pellet is inserted back into the tooth. After a meal, the tooth is again irrigated with water to ensure the absence of debris, and a fresh cotton pellet is inserted.

Alternative technique methods

- Alternatively, the access cavity is syringed with whitening gel and the rest is placed into the whitening tray in a thick layer and the rest of the tray is seated in the mouth. The access cavity can be replenished every 2 hours to speed up the whitening process.
- Otherwise the access cavity is filled each evening and the tray is worn overnight
- Another method is to use the sectional whitening tray with windows cut out for the adjacent teeth so that the lighter adjacent teeth do not whiten too quickly before the darker, nonvital tooth has had time to whiten.
- Alternatively, the material can be sealed into the access cavity as described in Chapter 8.

5. Treatment timing

If the patient can change the solution every 2 hours, five to eight applications may be all that it is necessary to achieve the desired lightening. This may take a matter of days (Poyser et al. 2004). The more often the solution is changed, the more quickly the whitening will take place. because the tooth is nonvital, this will not lead to sensitivity.

Nightly application will be slower than twice-daily application.

Daily application: It has been advised that unless the tooth is severely discolored, the whitening agent should be applied during the day so that the lightening can be better controlled.

6. Reassessment of the shade and results

The patient returns in 3–7 days. The shade changes are assessed. If sufficient lightening has occurred, the whitening procedure may be terminated. The longer the tooth has been discolored, the longer it can take for the whitening treatment to remove the discoloration (Carillo et al. 1998). Similarly, the darker the tooth, the longer it will take to lighten. The patient is instructed to return if he or she notices that the shade of the nonvital tooth is fully matching that of the adjacent teeth.

7. Sealing of the access cavity

The access cavity is then sealed with a glass ionomer restoration (Zimmerli et al. 2010). Placement of the final composite restoration may need to be delayed for 2 weeks to allow the oxygen to dissipate from the tooth and to allow the strength of the enamel-composite bond to improve (Carillo et al. 1998). If it is not possible to wait 2 weeks to place the final restoration, catalase or sodium ascorbate (Khoroushi et al. 2010) (hydrogel and vitamin C) can be placed into the access cavity using a sponge pledget for 3 minutes (Liebenberg 1997). The catalase acts to remove any latent hydrogen peroxide by promoting the decomposition of hydrogen peroxide into water and oxygen (Rotstein 1993). The use of sodium ascorbate, which is an antioxidizing agent, has reversed or decreased fracture resistance of the nonvital tooth in in vitro studies (Khoroushi et al. 2010).

Cleaning the access cavity first

The access cavity is first irrigated with sodium hypochlorite to flush out any remaining debris. The access cavity can then be cleaned using catalase. The cavosurface margin, the enamel surrounding the access cavity, and the pulp chamber dentin are etched for 15 seconds with 37% phosphoric acid according to a chosen adhesive protocol. Immediate dentin sealing can be used to seal the dentin surrounding the access cavity (e.g., HurriSeal Bisco). Dentin bonding agents are then applied. Acetone-containing bonding agents are preferred in this situation because they have been shown to reverse the effects of whitening on enamel bond strengths. The access cavity is sealed as follows in the next section.

8. Restoration of the access cavity

- Glass ionomer restoration as a final restoration.
- Composite restorations can be placed 2 weeks after completion of the final whitening treatment. A composite restoration involves use of incremental buildups of composite and a flowable composite at the base, over the glass ionomer.
- Sandwich technique: a condensable glass ionomer restoration can be placed immediately (Settembrini et al. 1997) over the barrier and a cut-back of glass ionomer can be undertaken 2 weeks later. A shallower composite restoration is placed after 2 weeks. The thicker base of glass ionomer can sometimes mask the residual discoloration if the nonvital tooth has not fully whitened to match the adjacent teeth.

9. Review

The tooth should be periodically reviewed and a radiograph taken every 2–3 years to check for any signs of a cervical inflammatory process.

BENEFITS OF THE OUTSIDE-INSIDE WHITENING TECHNIQUE

The benefits of the technique are as follows:

1. More surface area is available both internally and externally for the whitening agent to penetrate.
2. A lower concentration (10% carbamide peroxide with neutral pH) of the whitening agent is used.
3. This technique will, it is hoped, eliminate the incidence of cervical resorption that has been reported with the conventional intracoronal whitening technique, because most of the potential factors for resorption are reduced.
4. The need to change the access cavity dressing is eliminated because the access cavity is left open. (Previously, the oxygen that was released during the whitening process often dislodged the temporary dressing from the tooth. The oxygen can escape normally and there is no buildup of pressure.)
5. Treatment time is reduced to days rather than weeks (Liebenberg 1997) if repeated replenishment is used.
6. The patient can discontinue filling the pulp chamber once the desired color has been achieved.
7. Use of catalase before placement of the restoration can eliminate residual oxygen.
8. No heat is required to activate the whitening material.
9. Treatment is simple and noninvasive, offering an alternative solution for removal of nonvital discoloration.
10. Maintenance treatment is usually undertaken by performing home whitening in trays rather than opening the access cavity and whitening internally. Maintenance is therefore simple.

Risks

The risks of the procedure are as follows:

1. The potential for cervical resorption is reduced but still exists.
2. Noncompliant patients: the technique is patient applied, so it requires the patient to return to have the access cavity filled. Dentists should be careful in their patient selection and education to ensure that the patient returns to have the final restoration placed (Carillo et al. 1998).
3. Although some degree of manual dexterity is required by the patient to place the syringe into the access cavity, the patient's desire to achieve a whiter tooth counteracts this problem.

4. The tooth could be overwhitened through overzealous application of the whitening material by the patient. However, because a matrix is used to apply and retain the whitening material, the color of the other teeth can be lightened evenly to correct the color mismatch. It is thus essential to have regular reviews at frequent intervals to assess the color change taking place.
5. Shade stabilization occurs over a 2-week period (a slight rebound darkening can be expected as with all whitening procedures; 1–2 weeks later the shade can shift by one shade darker).

Indications

The indications for the treatment are as follows:

1. Treatment for adolescents with incomplete gingival maturation.
2. A single dark nonvital tooth where the surrounding teeth are sufficiently light. If this is the case, a window can be cut into the tray over the adjacent teeth to help the patient identify where to place the whitening agent. An oversized provisional crown form (Wahl 1992) can be used where there is difficulty retaining the whitening tray (Carillo et al. 1998).
3. All nonvital indications.

OTHER OPTIONS FOR NONVITAL TEETH

Nonvital teeth can be whitened using the whitening tray at home with 10% carbamide peroxide in a closed-chamber technique (Türkün 2004). This may take longer than with a vital tooth because of the nature of the discoloration and the hemosiderin-stained dentin. The benefits of this technique are that instead of removal of an existing sound restoration, the whitening material is applied to the tooth via the whitening tray (Frazier 1998). This technique may be the treatment of choice when providing a touch-up treatment or a maintenance whitening treatment several years after the initial whitening treatment.

The choice of which whitening agent to use depends on the nature of the discoloration and the severity of the existing discoloration. Previous reports of cervical resorption after internal whitening noted more problems when heat was applied to the tooth and when the tooth had been previously traumatized before revitalization. To avoid cervical resorption, it may be prudent to avoid high concentrations of hydrogen peroxide and heat.

See also Table 15.4.

Table 15.4 Treatment options for whitening nonvital teeth

- Intracoronal whitening: the material is sealed into the access cavity during in-office visits and requires frequent changing of dressings.
- Intracoronal whitening technique (see Chapter 8)
- Sodium perborate and water sealed into the tooth (Rotstein et al. 1991, 1993) (not permitted in Europe).
- Modified intracoronal whitening technique using different products sealed into the tooth such as:
  - Carbamide peroxide 10% and 16%
  - Various increasing hydrogen peroxide concentrations, mainly 3% and 6%
- Intracoronal whitening using the thermocatalytic technique or other forms of heat or heating instruments.
- Open chamber whitening combining intracoronal and extracoronal whitening; the material is applied into the pulp chamber directly and retained with a home whitening matrix.
- Outside-inside technique with whitening tray using:
  - 10% carbamide peroxide in access cavity and whitening tray (Settembrini et al. 1997, Carillo et al. 1998, Caughman et al. 1999)
  - 5%, 16%, 22% concentrations
  - 35% carbamide peroxide–assisted whitening in tray
- Closed chamber whitening—extracoronal. The whitening material is placed on the external surfaces of the tooth.
- Other treatments:
  - Power whitening using hydrogen peroxide
  - Nightguard Vital Whitening using 10%, 15%, or 20% carbamide peroxide applied only to the nonvital tooth in the tray (Frazier 1998)
  - Assisted whitening applied to the external surface on its own or via a whitening tray

Combination of power and home whitening treatments for generalized discoloration

This approach is very commonly used to motivate patients to comply with the home whitening protocol and continue whitening at home. Normally one or two power whitening in-office sessions are undertaken. The patient is then given the home whitening instructions, the tray, and enough material to continue the whitening process at home.

Garber (1997) favors this approach and advises his patients to use the matrix system for only 30–45 minutes at night instead of the longer times proposed for conventional home whitening. He advises using this on alternative days for the first week and thereafter only once per week until the color remains stable.

Benefits of the power and home whitening combination

The benefits of the combined treatments are as follows:

1. It eliminates the tedium of repeated office visits and rubber dam applications; instead, only one rubber dam application is used (Garber 1997).
2. The patient can get the best from the different whitening techniques.
3. The procedure can be adapted to suit the patient's whitening needs, requirements, and lifestyle.
4. It reduces the expense of prolonged office visits.
5. Power whitening provides a "jump-start" and demonstrates some improvement while the tray is being made. This can motivate the patient to continue with the home whitening treatment each night.

Table 15.5 Factors to consider when selecting the sequence of whitening treatment

Treatment choices are based on the following factors:
• Safety
• Effectiveness
• Permanence
• Efficiency
• Time factor—office time or chairtime
• Patient lifestyle
• Patient preference
• Depth, location, and nature of the stain

Which technique should be used first?

It is essential when planning treatment for patients to discuss that a combination of approaches may be necessary, depending on the severity of the staining. There are few reports in the dental literature that offer suggestions about which agent might be the agent of first choice in cases of superficial enamel discoloration (McEvoy 1998). Safety, effectiveness, permanence, and efficiency are all factors to consider when deciding which agent should be used first. Matching agents to stains is only part of the treatment planning; matching the technique to be used with which agent affects the sequence of care and the final result (McEvoy 1998). However, which technique to use first can often depend on the patient's wishes, time demands, and finances. Normally, whitening is carried out first followed by microabrasion. However, for a single isolated lesion, microabrasion can be undertaken first followed by whitening when the child is older. See also Table 15.5.

As the dentist becomes more experienced at using the different techniques, the efficiency and effectiveness of the application can be enhanced. Knowledge of the techniques associated with each agent can help in case selection, treatment planning, and overall success of the whitening treatment. Approaches may need to be different for different cases.

Fluorosis

A combination of whitening techniques may be necessary to remove the discoloration and improve the appearance of the teeth. Normally, home whitening is carried out first so that the results can be assessed; less microabrasion or resin infiltration may be needed. The whitening treatment typically will ensure that brown, orange, yellow, and some white marks are removed first. Microabrasion and whitening may also be used in combination. In some cases of fluorosis, the yellow-brown stains may be removed with the microabrasion technique, but it may fail to remove all the white stains. Power whitening can be undertaken while the rubber dam is still in place. This can be followed by home whitening for 2–5 weeks. An alternative whitening regimen can use home whitening techniques first to see what color change can be achieved. After 2–4 weeks, the patient can be reassessed to see if other whitening techniques are required.

Stains of multiple origins

Stains that have fluorosis, tetracycline, and age-related staining can also have discoloration from a previous endodontic treatment, a traumatic incident, or orthodontic bands. Different teeth in the same mouth can have stains from different causes. Patients who have teeth requiring a combination of different whitening treatments will need to have treatment carefully planned and be charged accordingly for the different techniques used. Success with whitening these stains of multiple origin is not always predictable and the patient should be told before commencing treatment that a combination of different approaches may need to be tried. It is only by undergoing the sequence of whitening treatments that success may be determined toward the end of the process. Alternatives to whitening such as veneers and direct composite bondings should also be discussed with patients before commencing the whitening treatments.

It has also been suggested that for tetracycline-stained teeth, veneers be prepared and then whitened after preparation (Sadan and Lemon 1998). However, the whitening treatment may lighten the shade of the teeth so well that veneers may not be necessary. It is customary to whiten the teeth first, which may eliminate the need for veneers altogether.

Patients have a "threshold of acceptability" wherein although the teeth are severely stained, a moderate improvement may be sufficient to improve the patient's appearance and self-esteem.

CONCLUSION

Dentists should have a thorough knowledge of the chemical agents used for whitening and lightening teeth so that they can determine which agents or techniques used in combination are most likely to achieve the desired result. The combination approach to whitening teeth should incorporate the ability to use agents and techniques in the proper sequence to achieve an excellent esthetic result. It is best to start with the least invasive, most cost-effective option first, unless other circumstances such as time and compliance are factors.

REFERENCES

Abbot P, Heah S. (2009) Internal bleaching of teeth: an analysis of 255 teeth. *Aust Dental J* **54**(4):326–33.

Baker FL, Guillen GE, Frysh H, Rivera Hildago A. (1992) Tooth colour alterations secondary to polishing. *J Dent Res* **71**:540. [Abstract No. 202.]

Benetti AR, Valer MC, Mancini MN, Miranda CB. (2004) In vitro penetration of bleaching agents into the pulp chamber. *Int Endod J* **37**(2):120–4.

Carillo A, Trevino MV, Haywood VB. (1998) Simultaneous bleaching of vital teeth and an open-chamber nonvital tooth with 10% carbamide peroxide. *Quintessence Int* **29**(10):643–8.

Caughman WF, Frazier KB, Haywood VB. (1999) Carbamide peroxide whitening on nonvital single discoloured teeth: case reports. *Quintessence Int* **30**(3):155–61.

Frazier KB. (1998) Nightguard Vital Bleaching to lighten a restored, nonvital discoloured tooth. *Compend Contin Educ Dent* **9**(8):810–13.

Garber DA. (1997) Dentist-monitored bleaching: a discussion of combination and laser bleaching. *J Am Dent Assoc Suppl* **128**(4):26S–30S.

Garber DA, Goldstein R, Goldstein C, Schwartz C. (1991) Dentist monitored bleaching. A combined approach. *Prac Periodont Aesthet Dent* **3**(2):22–6.

Haywood VB. (1992) Bleaching of vital and nonvital teeth. *Curr Opin Dent* **2:**142–9.

Khoroushi M, Feiz A, Khodamoradi R. (2010) Fracture resistance of endodontically-treated teeth: effect of combination bleaching and an antioxidant. *Oper Dent* **35**(5):530–7.

Liebenberg WH. (1997) Intracoronal lightening of discoloured pulpless teeth: a modified walking bleach technique. *Quintessence Int* **28:**771–7.

McEvoy SA. (1998) Combining chemical agents and techniques to remove intrinsic stains from vital teeth. *Gen Dent* **46**(2):168–72.

Miller MB, editor. (2000). *Reality: the information source for esthetic dentistry*. Vol 14. Reality Publishing: Houston, TX.

Plotino G, Buono G, Grande NM, Pameier CH. (2008) Nonvital tooth bleaching: a review of the literature and clinical procedures. *J Endod* **34:**394–407.

Poyser NJ, Kelleher MG, Briggs PF. (2004) Managing discoloured non-vital teeth: the inside/outside bleaching technique. *Dent Update* **31:**204–10, 213–4.

Rotstein I. (1993) Role of catalase in the elimination of residual hydrogen peroxide following tooth bleaching. *J Endod* **19:**567–9.

Rotstein I, Mor C, Friedman S. (1993) Prognosis of intracoronal bleaching with sodium perborate preparations in vitro: 1 year study. *J Endod* **19:**10–4.

Rotstein I, Zalkind M, Mor C, et al. (1991) In-vitro efficacy of sodium perborate preparations used for intracoronal bleaching of discoloured non-vital teeth. *Endod Dent Traumatol* **7**(4):177–80.

Sadan A, Lemon RR. (1998) Combining treatment modalities for tetracycline-discoloured teeth. *Int J Periodont Restor Dent* **18**(6):564–71.

Settembrini L, Gultz J, Kaim J, Scherer W. (1997) A technique for bleaching nonvital teeth: inside/outside bleaching. *J Am Dent Assoc* **128:**1283–4.

Türkün M, LS Türkün. (2004) Effect of nonvital bleaching with 10% carbamide peroxide on sealing ability of resin composite restorations. *Int Endod J* **3**(1):52–60.

Vachon C, Vanek P, Friedman S. (1998) Internal bleaching with 10% carbamide peroxide in vitro. *Pract Periodont Aesthet Dent* **10**(9):1145–54.

Wahl MJ. (1992) At home bleaching of a single tooth. *J Prosthet Dent* **67**(2):281–2.

Zimmerli B, Jeger F, Lussi A. (2010) Bleaching of nonvital teeth. A clinically relevant literature review. *Schweiz Monatsschr Zahnmed* **120**(4):306–20.

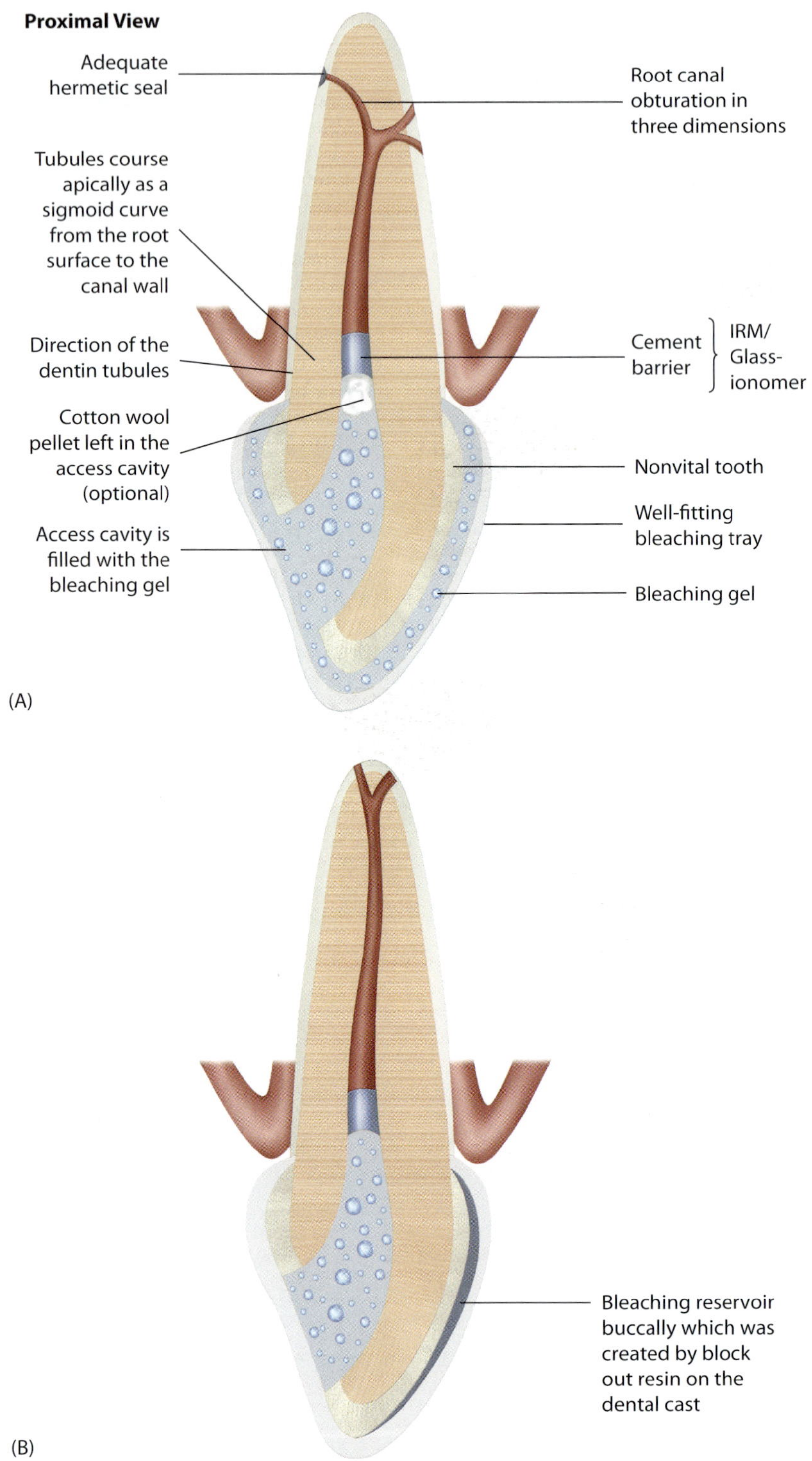

Figure 15.1

The outside-inside technique. (A) Full tooth in cross section. (B) Sectional close-up of anterior tooth with whitening tray seated over an open internal access cavity. The glass ionomer forms a base and barrier and seals the gutta-percha from the oral environment during treatment with the carbamide peroxide whitening material.

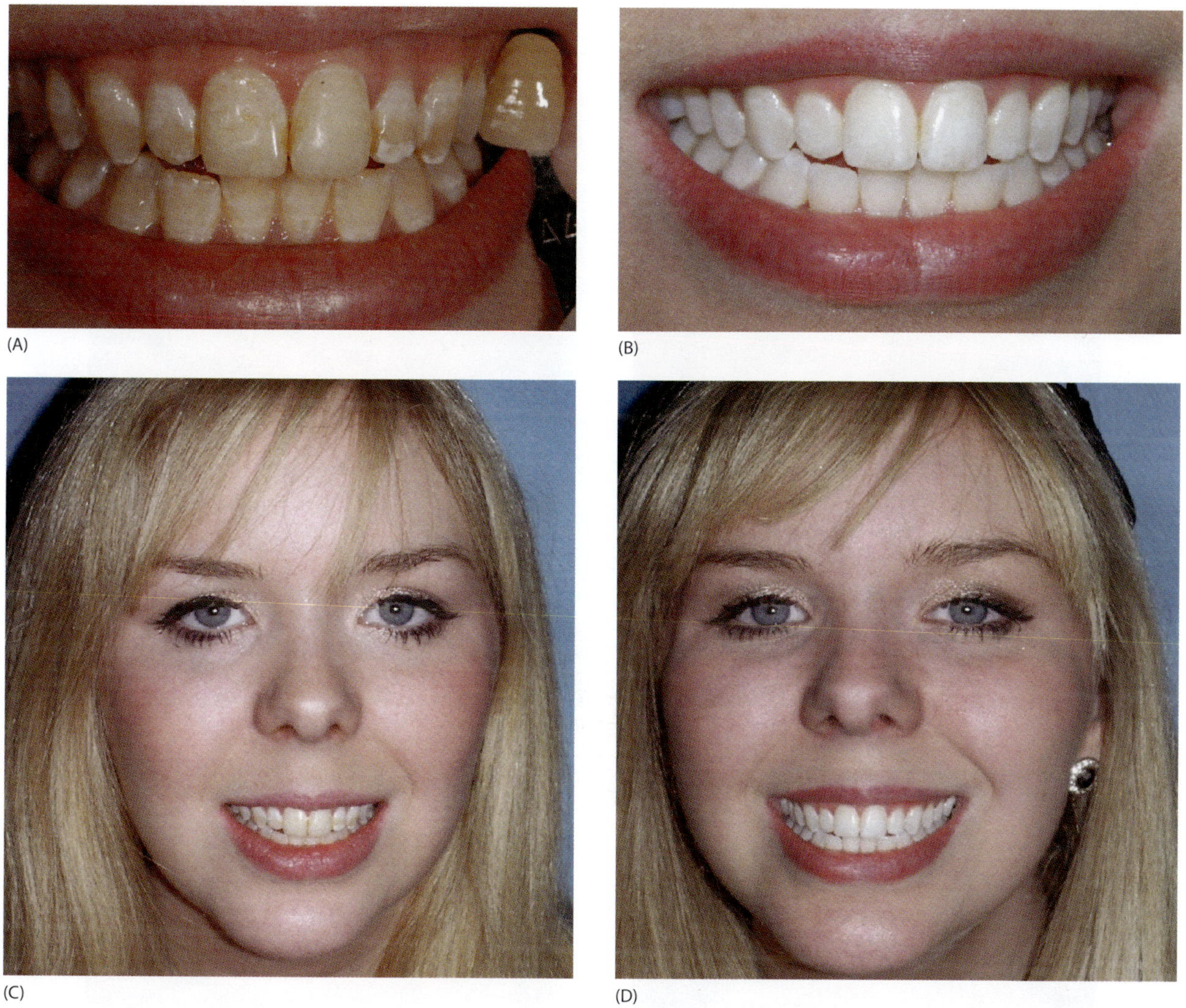

Figure 15.2

(A) Smile view of patient with stains of multiple origin. Patient has fluorosis stain. The two central incisors were covered with direct bonding resin. The resin is discolored as well. There are brown, orange, yellow, and white stains. The direct composite restorations that were placed on the upper central incisors were removed so that the natural enamel was exposed. (B) Final result of whitening the upper and lower teeth in combination with two sessions of microabrasion to remove the white discolorations. (C and D) Portrait views before and after treatment.

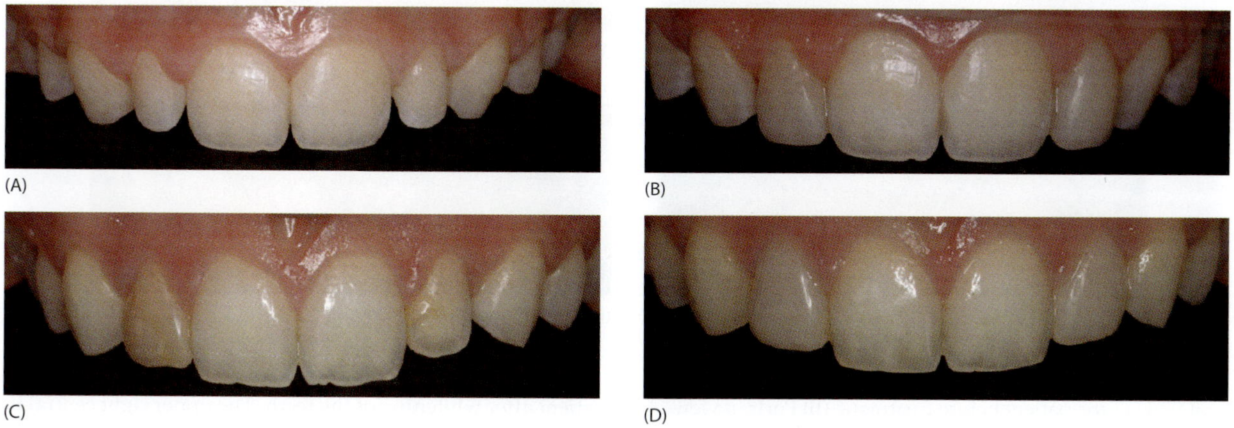

Figure 15.3

(A) Two sisters who both had peg-shaped laterals were both treated with whitening and different restorative treatment. (B) One sister had direct bonding to correct the peg-shaped laterals. (C) The other sister had whitening then some bonding, which was poorly maintained and unsatisfactory. (D) This was followed by direct preformed composite veneers (Edelweiss, Switzerland). The preformed veneers have porcelain on the outside and composite on the internal surface, which is suitable for bonding with a composite cement. The treatment of this patient involved whitening and composite bonding to correct the shapes and contours of the teeth.

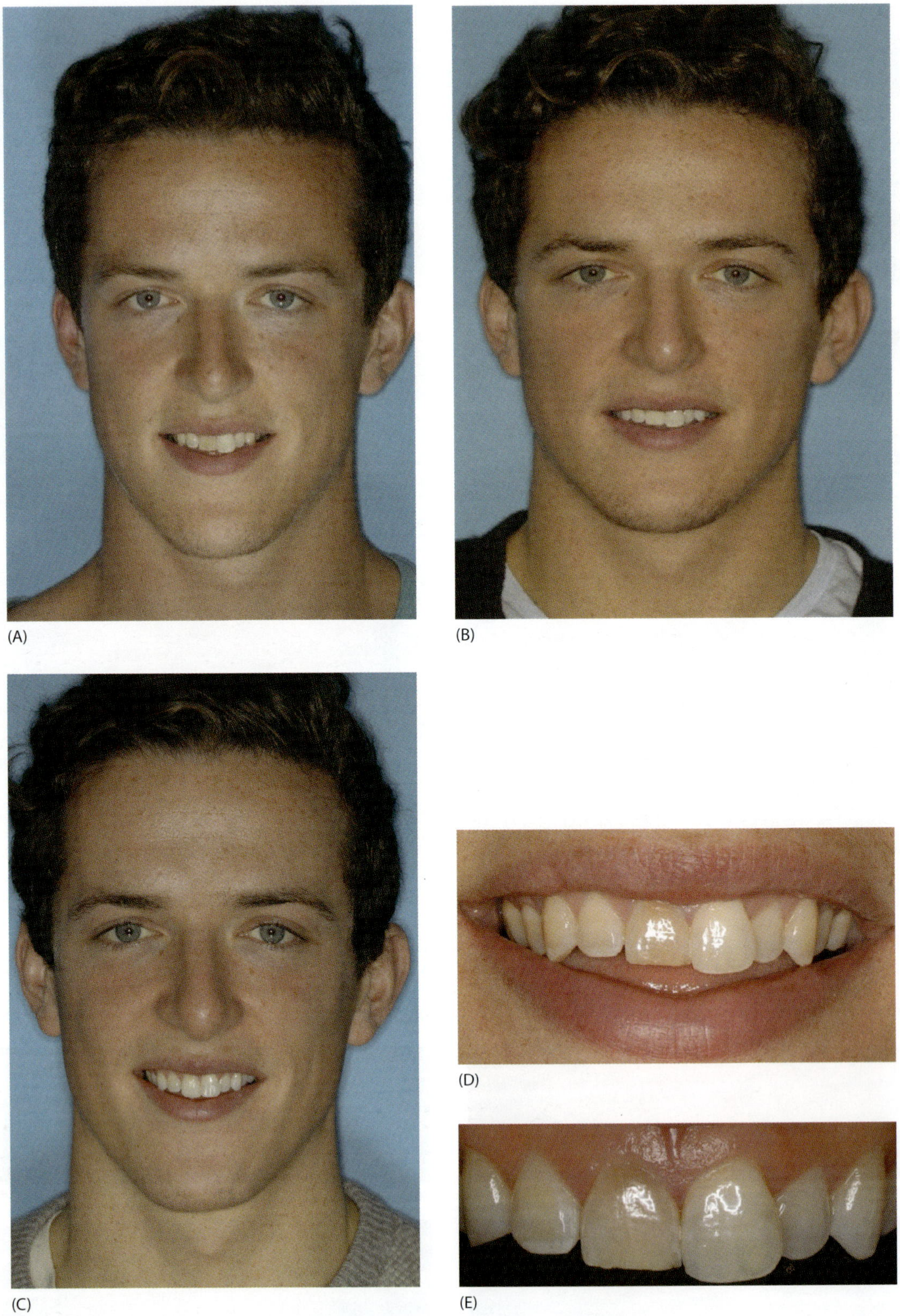

(A) (B) (C) (D) (E)

Figure 15.4

(A) Portrait view of the patient before treatment. (B) Portrait view of the patient after whitening of the teeth. The upper right central incisor is much shorter than the left. This is related to a previous injury sustained by the tooth. (C) Portrait view of the patient after whitening and completion of the composite bonding to restore the shape of the tooth. (D) Smile view of the patient at presentation; the upper right central incisor is brown as a result of previous trauma. The incisal edge (2 mm) was knocked off the tooth. Treatment planning involved options including outside-inside whitening of the upper central incisor. A special whitening tray was made to cut back the tooth on either side. Bonding was planned, and to prevent further loss of the incisal edge as a result of the patient's bruxing habit, a Michigan bite splint was made. Treatment involved combination nonvital whitening using 16% carbamide peroxide sealed into the access cavity and then outside whitening using the specially designed segmental whitening tray. (E) Retracted view of the upper central incisor tooth. *continued on the next page*

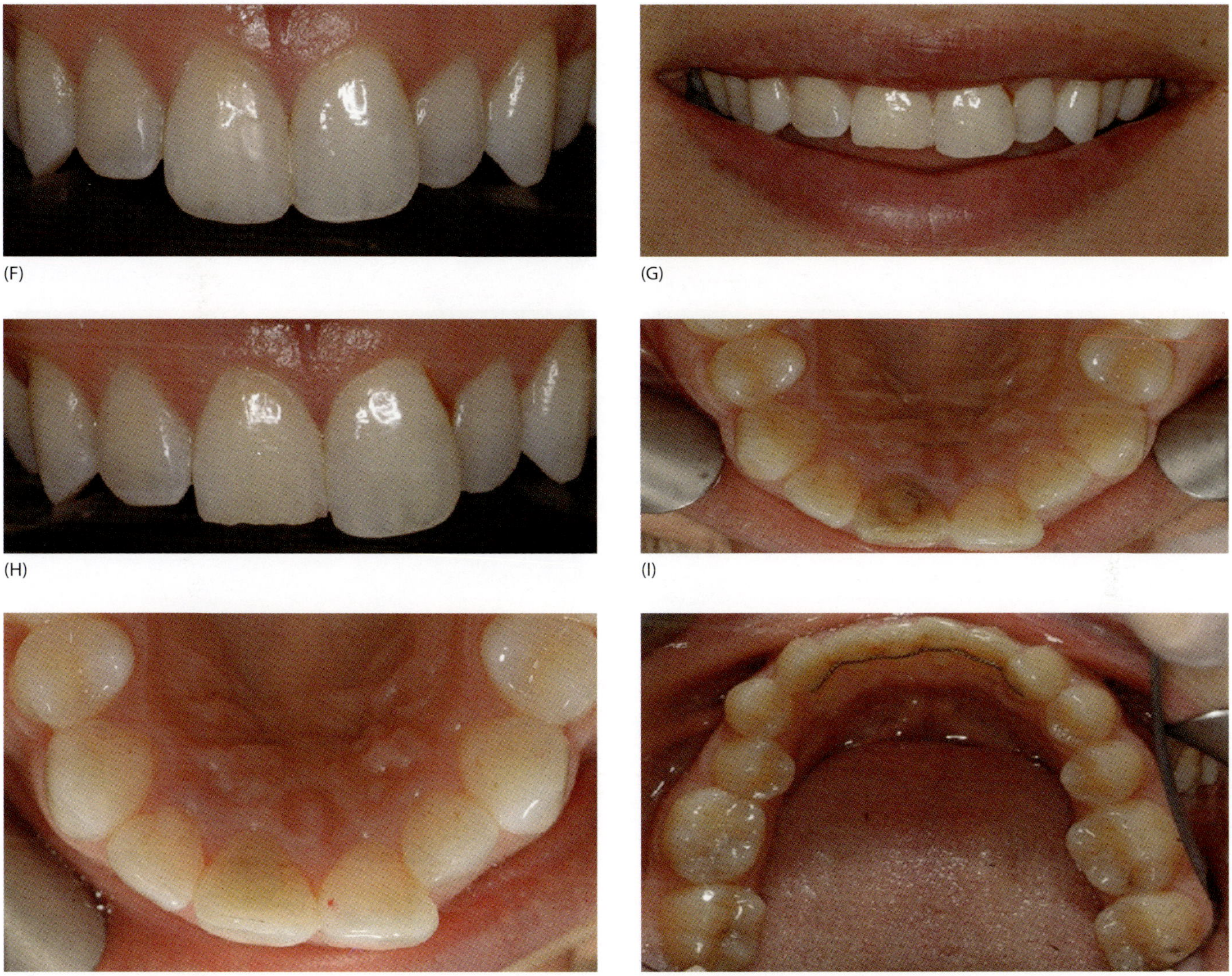

Figure 15.4 continued

(F and G) Smile view and retracted view of the patient after whitening and before bonding. (H) Retracted view of the teeth after final treatment and composite bonding onto the upper right central incisor. (I) Palatal view on presentation. The restoration in the access cavity is poorly contoured and the filling is leaking. This is a very common reason for the shade to regress after whitening if the access cavity is not filled properly. After home whitening and internal whitening, there is residual oxygen inside the tooth. It takes 2 weeks for the bond strength to reach normal levels. It is best after completion of the internal whitening to clean the tooth with catalase or hydrogel or ascorbic acid to restore the bond strength to normal levels. It is not advisable to place a composite restoration directly into the access cavity immediately after completion of internal whitening because it will not be able to bond effectively with the adjacent tooth structure. (J) It is better to place a glass ionomer in the palatal access cavity because there is minimal leakage of the restoration. (K) Lingual view of the lower teeth before whitening treatment. This shows a lingual bonded wire retainer to prevent relapse of the crowding.

continued on the next page

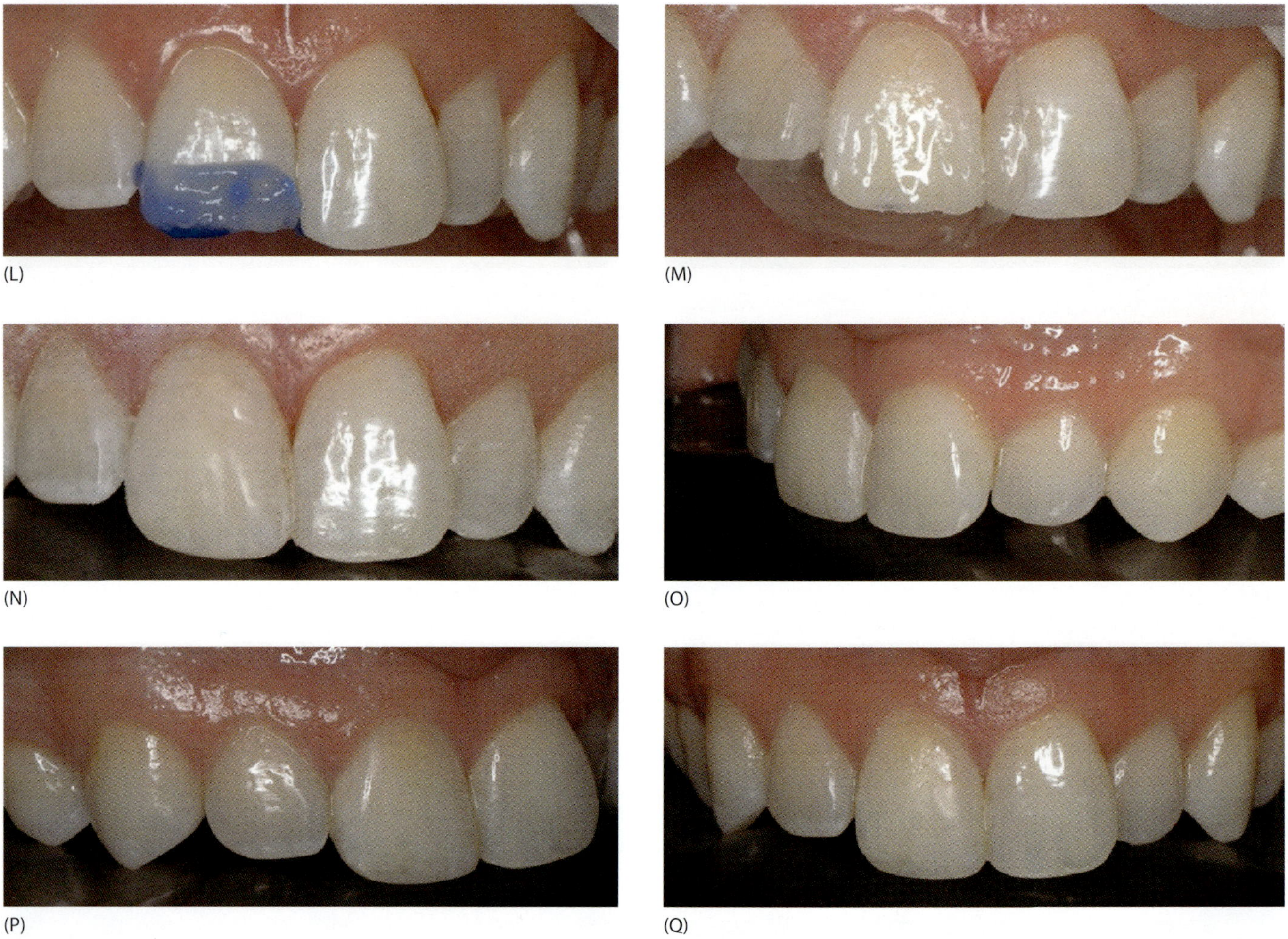

Figure 15.4 continued

(L) Restoration of the tooth commenced 3 weeks after completion of the whitening treatment. Etching of the upper right central incisor. (M) Placement of the curved matrix strip to help with the placement of the palatal composite, which is placed with segmental layering. The enamel layer was placed first to build the natural appearance of the tooth and create translucency from the palatal section forward. (N) Retracted view of the final composite restoration. (O) Left lateral retracted view after treatment was completed. (P) Right lateral view of the completed restoration. (Q) Retracted view of the completed restoration and whitening treatment.

continued on the next page

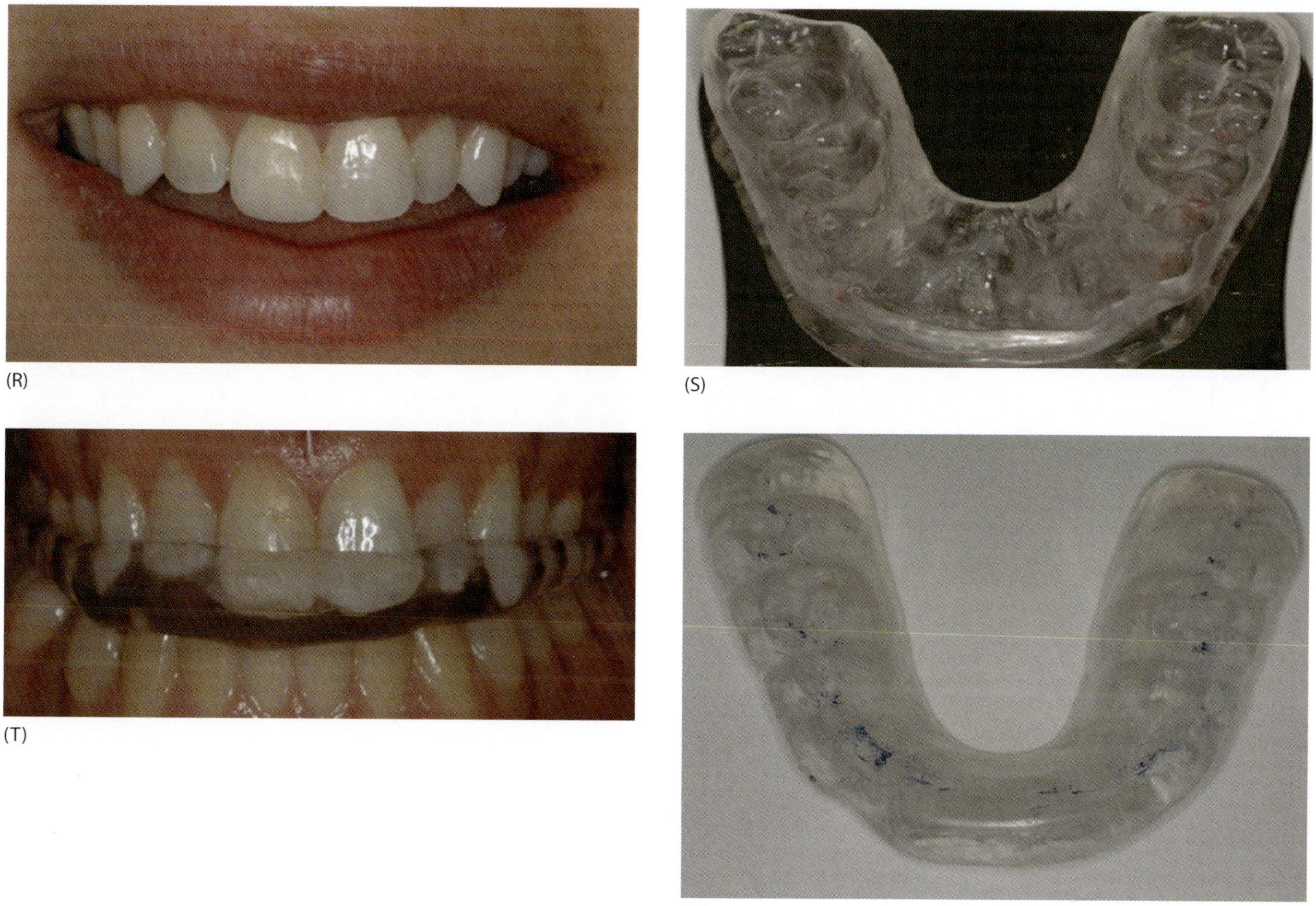

(R) (S) (T) (U)

Figure 15.4 continued

(R) Smile view of the result after whitening and bonding. (S) Acrylic full upper arch bite plate (Michigan splint) made for the patient to reduce the bite force on the upper central incisor and prevent further bruxing of the teeth and also to protect the upper right central incisor from fracturing. This is the view of the internal fitting surface of the bite plate. (T) The retracted view of the Michigan bite splint in position. (U) The external surface of the bite splint showing occlusal markings.

16 THE EFFECT OF WHITENING ON RESTORATIVE MATERIALS

Thomas Attin and Linda Greenwall

INTRODUCTION

The purpose of this chapter is to summarize and discuss the available information concerning the effects of peroxide-releasing whitening agents on composite restorative materials and restorations. All original scientific full papers or reviews listed in PubMed or ISI Web of Science (search terms included *bleaching*, plus *composite* or *resin* or *compomer* or *adhesive*) were screened and included.

The influence of various whitening agents on physical properties, surface morphology, and color of composite restorative materials has been investigated in several in vitro studies simulating the clinical situation as closely as possible. In those studies, home whitening products (10–16% carbamide peroxide) were generally used within a 2- to 4-week whitening simulation with application intervals of 4–8 hours per day. Tooth whiteners designed for in-office application (30–35% hydrogen or carbamide peroxide) were applied in treatment intervals of 15–60 minutes (as recommended by the manufacturers). These different whitening regimens were preferably used in the studies reviewed and are therefore not repeatedly mentioned in describing and discussing the results of the respective studies. Most of the studies did not show differences among these different whitening regimens with regard to their influence on dental restorative materials. However, it should be borne in mind that the total time period of application was much higher for the low-concentration regimens than for the high-concentration ones.

In the literature, the greatest focus has been on the impact of whitening agents on composite restorations and dental adhesives. Therefore this chapter will deal preferentially with these interactions, although it should also be noted that whitening agents may also exert some effects on other restorative materials, such as glass ionomer cements, metal alloys, amalgam, or ceramics (Attin et al. 2004, El-Murr et al. 2011). Because the chemistry of polyacid-modified composite resin materials (i.e., compomers) is very close to that of composites, the influence of whitening regimens on this type of restorative material is also included in this chapter.

INFLUENCE OF WHITENING AGENTS ON PHYSICAL AND OPTICAL PROPERTIES OF COMPOSITE MATERIALS

Surface roughness

Some studies that did not simulate a salivary effect have shown that application of whitening agents might lead to a slight increase in surface roughness and amount of porosities of microfilled and hybrid composite resins (Cehreli et al. 2003, Turker and Biskin T 2003, Basting et al. 2005, Rosentritt et al. 2005, Moraes et al. 2006, Dutra et al. 2009, Gurgan and Yalcin 2007, Hafez et al. 2010, Martin et al. 2010, de Andrade et al. 2011, Wang et al. 2011). This increase in surface roughness corresponds to the fact that surface energy of composites is enhanced after whitening, thus increasing surface wettability (Buzoglu et al. 2009). Other studies have reported only minor or negligible effects of whitening gels in terms of resin composite surface roughness (Kim et al. 2004, Wattanapayungkul et al. 2004, Polydorou et al. 2006, Zavanelli et al. 2011). Interestingly, it should be noted that no effect of whitening on composite surface roughness was observed when hydrogen peroxide gels were applied on composites in a cycling protocol with intermittent storage of the samples in pooled human saliva or in a 14-day in situ study (Schemehorn et al. 2004, de A Silva et al. 2006). It was suggested that contact with saliva might have modified or attenuated the hydrogen peroxide impact by formation of a surface-protective salivary layer on the restorative material.

Surface hardness

Previous studies had yielded controversial results with regard to surface hardness changes of composite resins after application of different home whitening regimens ranging from significant softening, through unchanged hardness, to even increased surface hardness (Garcia-Godoy et al. 2002, Turker and Biskin 2002, Mujdeci and Gökay 2005, Mujdeci and Gökay 2006, Okte et al. 2006, Silva Costa et al. 2009, Polydorou et al. 2007a, Polydorou et al. 2007b, Lima et al. 2008, Yu et al. 2008, Briso et al.

2010b, Kwon et al. 2010, Malkondu et al. 2011). It seems that heated whitening agents lead to more pronounced hardness reduction than unheated agents (Yu et al. 2011). However, in all of these studies, salivary impact was not simulated. In contrast, studies with simulation of salivary exposure between the whitening applications did not reveal surface softening of composite restorative materials using different whitening gels and application forms (Campos et al. 2003, White et al. 2003, Duschner et al. 2004, Duschner et al. 2006).

Color stability

It has been suggested that under clinical conditions in the mouth, ΔE^* color differences, as spectroscopically evaluated with the CIE-L*a*b* method, have been reported to be relevant and perceptible only when higher than 3.3 (Ruyter et al. 1987) or 3.6 (Johnston and Kao 1989). Previous studies had shown that application of 10% hydrogen peroxide or heated and unheated 30% (or 35%) hydrogen peroxide resulted in composite color changes that were presumably clinically detectable, with ΔE^* ranging from 2 to 11 for the different materials and shades tested (Monaghan et al. 1992a, Monaghan et al. 1992b, Canay and Cehreli 2003, Hubbezoglu et al. 2008, Rao et al. 2009, Hafez et al. 2010, de Andrade et al. 2011). Also, gloss of composites seems to be reduced after whitening (Anagnostou et al. 2010, Yalcin and Gurgan 2005b). Application of a film type of whitening regimen demonstrated higher color change of composites than a 10% carbamide peroxide control gel (Anagnostou et al. 2010). Only a slight or even negligible color change of composites was reported for a 10% carbamide peroxide gel (Monaghan et al. 1992b, Canay and Cehreli 2003, Li et al. 2009, Silva Costa et al. 2009, Kwon et al. 2010). It was also proved that color change of composite restorative materials resulting from whitening is significantly lower compared with color change of (bovine) enamel (Rosentritt et al. 2005). Moreover, in this study no close correlation could be observed between hydrogen concentration of whitening agents (based on different compositions) from different manufacturers and the changes in ΔE^*.

It should be noted that whitening might increase the propensity of resin composites to staining induced by contact with discoloring solutions (tea, coffee) (Celik et al. 2009, Yu et al. 2009). On the other hand, whitening is also effective in removal of superficial and also intrinsic staining of composites (Villalta et al. 2006, Türkün and Türkün 2004a, Abd Elhamid and Mosallam 2010, Pruthi et al. 2010).

The alterations in color of the restorative materials have been attributed to oxidation of surface pigment texture and amine compounds, with different color changes occurring in different materials as a result of different amounts of resin and different degrees of conversion of the resin matrix (Monaghan et al. 1992b). These negative influences of the oxidizing agents on the resin matrix are also responsible for water uptake of the restorative materials. This may lead to complete or partial debonding of fillers, causing reduced surface integrity and loss of hardness of the materials (Wattanapayungkul and Yap 2003).

Other physical properties

Some studies have shown that fracture toughness of composites seems to be negatively affected by whitening agents, although this has not been proved in all studies dealing with this topic (Yu et al. 2010, Firoozmand and Pagani 2009, Cho et al. 2009).

In addition, it was recently proved that whitening with hydrogen peroxide has an effect on the three-dimensional polymer network in polymerized composites, leading to an increase in the release of unpolymerized monomers, additives, and unspecific oxidative products (Durner et al. 2011). It might be speculated that this effect is material dependent, because another study revealed less leaching of monomers from whitened composites than from unwhitened ones (Polydorou et al. 2009).

Brushing resistance of composite resins seems not be reduced as a result of whitening, as shown in a whitening/brushing cycle performed over a 21-day period (Faraoni-Romano et al. 2009).

Influence of whitening agents on physical and optical properties of polyacid-modified composite resins

Simulated overuse of highly concentrated whitening regimens for 1–5 days showed detrimental effects on surface texture and mechanical properties of polyacid-modified resin-based composites (compomers) (Jung et al. 2002, Lee et al. 2002, Taher 2005). In this sense, a reduction of surface microhardness was also detected in an in situ experiment using 15% carbamide peroxide over a period of 28 days (Yu et al. 2008). In contrast, a total of three 30-minute whitening sessions with highly concentrated whitening agents conducted at 1-week intervals did not result in detrimental effects of the surface finish of compomers (Wattanapayungkul and Yap 2003). Also, with use of highly concentrated whitening regimens, no surface microhardness changes were observed in polyacid-modified resin-based composites (Yap and Wattanapayungkul 2002). Treatment with 10–16% carbamide peroxide whitening gels resulted in either an increased surface roughness or a decreased surface roughness, suggesting that the effects of the gels seem to be material dependent (Cehreli et al. 2003, Turker and Biskin 2003).

The occurrence of visible color changes in compomers treated with 10–16% carbamide peroxide were, as with the changes in surface texture, dependent on the compomer brand tested, whereas treatment with either film type (6.5% H_2O_2) whitening regimens or 10% and 30% hydrogen peroxide resulted in noticeable color change irrespective of the compomer material evaluated (Canay and Cehreli 2003, Kwon et al. 2003, Rosentritt et al. 2005). It should be noted that color changes resulting from whitening seem to be more pronounced in compomers than in composite materials (Yalcin and Gurgan 2005a, Li et al. 2009, Yu et al. 2009).

Clinical relevance of impact of whitening agents on physical and optical properties of resin-based restoratives

Unfortunately, none of the aforementioned studies investigated how far the induced changes in surface texture and hardness led to recommendable need for repolishing or even replacement of existing restorations after whitening to ensure longevity of the restorations. Only a single study examined subsurface extension of the impact of bleaching agents in composite and polyacid-modified composites (Hannig et al. 2007). This study revealed significant subsurface softening to an extent of up to 0.4 mm depth as a result of contact with whitening agents. Nevertheless, it remains speculative whether the mentioned changes in surface texture and hardness are relevant under clinical conditions or if they are mainly a surface phenomenon that could be removed by simple polishing of restorations.

BOND STRENGTH OF COMPOSITE RESIN TO WHITENED ENAMEL AND DENTIN

There is a long list of in vitro studies showing that bond strength of composite restorative and composite-based materials is significantly reduced when composite application to dentin or enamel surfaces (including acid-etching pretreatment) is performed immediately—that is, within 1 day—after completion of a whitening regimen with both high- and low-concentration agents (Titley et al. 1988, Torneck et al. 1991, Stokes et al. 1992, Titley et al. 1992, Bishara et al. 1993, Dishman et al. 1994, van der Vyver et al. 1997, Demarco et al. 1998, Spyrides et al. 2000, Far and Ruse 2003, Uysal et al. 2003, Miguel et al. 2004, Miyazaki et al. 2004, Shinohara et al. 2004, Teixeira et al. 2004, Cavalli et al. 2005, Shinohara et al. 2005, Cacciafesta et al. 2006, Montalvan et al. 2006, Adanir et al. 2007, Dadoun and Bartlett 2007, Shinkai et al. 2007, Turkkahraman et al. 2007, Barbosa et al. 2008, Mullins et al. 2009, Uysal et al. 2009, Wilson et al. 2009, Barcellos et al. 2010, Briso et al. 2010a, Can-Karabulut et al. 2010, Dietrich et al. 2010, Abe et al. 2011).

In contrast, only a few studies did not reveal an impact on composite bond strength after enamel or dentin whitening (Basting et al. 2004, Loretto et al. 2004, Arcari et al. 2007, Sasaki et al. 2007, Amaral et al. 2008, Mishima et al. 2009, Lima et al. 2011b). Use of a carbamide peroxide–containing dentifrice before an adhesive restoration does not seem to influence enamel and dentin bond strength of resin composite (da Silva et al. 2007). In terms of bond strength to cavities, a single study was able to show that whitening does not affect bond strength to enamel-dentin cavities in bovine teeth restored with silorane- and dimethacrylate-based restoratives (Lima et al. 2011b).

The influence of whitening agents on enamel and dentin bond strength seems to be more pronounced for highly concentrated agents (Patusco et al. 2009). With respect to intracoronal whitening of nonvital teeth, the application of carbamide peroxide gels or mixtures of sodium perborate mixed with water are less negative than applications containing hydrogen peroxide (Teixeira et al. 2004, Timpawat et al. 2005). Controversy still exists regarding whether fluoride-enriched carbamide peroxide gels exert the same reduction in enamel bond strength as nonfluoridated agents (Metz et al. 2007, Chuang et al. 2009). On the other side, for bond strength to whitened enamel it was shown that etch-and-rinse adhesives seem to perform better than nonrinse, self-etching products (Moule et al. 2007, Gurgan et al. 2009). The kind of light-curing device used (light-emitting diode [LED], quartz-tungsten, or plasma arc) does not affect bond strength to whitened enamel and dentin (Bulucu and Ozsezer 2007, Bulucu et al. 2008).

In vitro studies investigating the appropriate time point for bonding of composites after termination of whitening showed that a delay of at least 1–3 weeks is necessary to allow for optimal bonding to both enamel and dentin (Torneck et al. 1991, Adibfar et al. 1992, Titley et al. 1993, van der Vyver et al. 1997, Cavalli et al. 2001, Basting et al. 2004, Cavalli et al. 2004, Türkün and Kaya 2004, Bishara et al. 2005, Bulut et al. 2006, Da Silva Machado et al. 2007, Barbosa et al. 2008, Can-Karabulut and Karabulut 2011, Souza-Gabriel et al. 2011, Oztaş et al. 2012). A single study showed that a time lapse of only 24 hours should be enough to recover enamel bond strength after whitening (Unlu et al. 2008).

Under simulation of intraoral conditions, conflicting results are given for testing bond strength to whitened dental hard tissue. It was shown that no delay is necessary for establishing common bond strength to enamel using 16% carbamide peroxide for whitening; however, for root dentin a delay of 21 days was suggested to achieve proper bond strength under in situ conditions (Miguel et al. 2004, Barbosa et al. 2009). When a 35% hydrogen peroxide agent was used for enamel whitening in situ, a delay of 7 days was recommended (Bittencourt et al. 2010).

Reasons for reduced bond strength to whitened dental hard tissue

Several factors are responsible for the reduction in composite bond strength to whitened enamel and dentin. It was shown that resin tags in whitened enamel subsequently acid etched with 37% phosphoric were less defined, were more fragmented, and penetrated to a lesser depth than in unwhitened enamel controls (Titley et al. 1991, Sundfeld et al. 2005, Nour El-din et al. 2006). Also, tag formation in whitened dentin is compromised (Ferreir et al. 2011). Bond strength to dentin was even reduced when the whitening agent was applied on the surface enamel covering underlying dentin (Lima et al. 2010).

Moreover, whitening with hydrogen peroxide or hydrogen peroxide–releasing agents may result in significant decrease of enamel calcium and phosphate content and in morphologic alterations in the most superficial enamel crystallites (Ruse et al. 1990, Perdigão et al. 1998). Besides this, acid etching of whitened enamel surface produced loss of prismatic form, resulting in an enamel surface that appeared to be overetched (Josey et al. 1996). In addition, it was suggested that the enamel and dentin organic matrix was altered by the oxidizing effect of hydrogen peroxide (Kodaka et al. 1992, Hegedüs et al. 1999). These factors may have led to enamel and dentin surfaces that did not allow for formation of a strong and stable bond and interaction between the composite applied and the superficial etched enamel layer. Furthermore, reduction in bond strength in hydrogen peroxide–treated enamel and dentin could be caused by the presence of residual oxygen in enamel and dentin pores after completion of the whitening treatment. Liberation of the oxygen could either interfere with resin infiltration into enamel and dentin (Torneck et al. 1990, McGuckin et al. 1992) or inhibit polymerization of resins that cure via a free-radical mechanism (Rueggeberg and Margeson 1990). The latter aspect might result in oxygen-inhibited polymerization of the composite components directly in contact with the dental hard tissues, leading to a soft interface not able to withstand debonding forces sufficiently. The recommendations for a 1- to 3-week delay before placement of composite restorations after termination of whitening therapy are made under the assumption that the residual oxygen may have sufficient time to leach from the dental hard tissues.

Methods to counteract reduced bond strength to dental hard tissues

To dissolve remnants of peroxide, cavities can also be cleaned with antioxidants, such as catalase (Rotstein 1993, Kum et al. 2004), α-tocopherol (Sasaki et al. 2009), grapeseed extract (Vidhy et al. 2011), or 10% sodium ascorbate gel or solution (Lai et al. 2001, Lai et al. 2002, Kum et al. 2004, Türkün and Kaya 2004, Türkün and Türkün 2004b, Bulut et al. 2005, Kimyai and Valizadeh 2006, Muraguchi et al. 2007, Gökçe et al. 2008, Kimyai and Valizadeh 2008, Khoroushi et al. 2009, Türkün et al. 2009, Comlekoglu et al. 2010, May et al. 2010, Uysal et al. 2010, Danesh-Sani and Esmaili 2011, Feiz et al. 2011, Kunt et al. 2011, Mazaheri et al. 2011). Pretreatment with ethanol or calcium hydroxide is not effective for recovering bond strength levels to the level of unwhitened enamel (Kum et al. 2004, Türkün and Kaya 2004, Khoroushi et al. 2009). Most of the recent studies dealt with the application of sodium ascorbate as an antioxidant to reduce waiting time before restoration of whitened teeth. Application of sodium ascorbate is also helpful to restore compromised fracture resistance of whitened enamel and does not affect enamel surface hardness (Khoroushi et al. 2010, Oskoee et al. 2010). Pretreatment of whitened enamel with sodium ascorbate before bonding increases tag formation in enamel (Briso et al. 2012). In most of these studies, the application time of sodium ascorbate amounted to 10 minutes, although Lima et al. (2011a) found a 1-minute period to be sufficient. In contrast to this recommendation, Kaya et al. (2008) revealed a 60-minute application of sodium ascorbate gel to be superior to shorter application times. The length of the application time seems to be positively correlated with the antioxidizing effect and the regaining of bond strength. This was shown in a study in which a 120-minute application of 10% sodium ascorbate was more effective than shorter periods. Moreover, addition of a surfactant to a sodium ascorbate gel might increase its effectivity (Moosavi et al. 2010). In contrast, increasing the concentration of sodium ascorbate from 10% to 20% did not improve effectiveness (Dabas et al. 2011). It was also reported that laser treatment (neodymium:yttrium-aluminum-garnet [Nd:YAG] or erbium:yttrium-aluminum-garnet [Er:YAG]) of the whitened enamel and dentin surface can reverse the bond strength reduction (Lago et al. 2011, Leonetti et al. 2011, Rocha Gomes Torres et al. 2012). However, application of the agents or methods mentioned might be time-consuming or expensive, so further investigations are needed to optimize their use under clinical conditions. It is more feasible to follow the aforementioned recommendations to allow for contact time of at least 7 days with water and saliva to avoid the reduction of adhesion of composites to enamel. Optimum bonding to prewhitened dental hard tissue could be achieved after a period of about 3 weeks (Cavalli et al. 2001, Shinohara et al. 2001). In addition, prolonged polymerization times of up to 60 seconds are advised for better conversion rate of applied adhesives (Cadenaro et al. 2006, Bresch et al. 2007, Hussain and Wang 2010).

Impact of whitening on marginal seal of resin-based restorations

Prerestorative nonvital, intracoronal whitening in the manner of "walking bleach" technique, using mixtures of 37% carbamide peroxide or pastes consisting of 30% hydrogen peroxide and sodium perborate, leads to a higher rate of microleakage in composite restorations of both the access cavity and Class V cavities placed immediately after termination of whitening (Demarco et al. 2001, Shinohara et al. 2001, Barkhordar et al. 1997). In Class V restorations, the increase in microleakage after intracoronal application of 37% carbamide peroxide was detected only in dentin margins and not in enamel margins (Shinohara et al. 2001). Short-term use of an intracoronal calcium hydroxide agent for 7 days after completion of walking bleach therapy was able to reverse the negative influences of the hydrogen peroxide application on microleakage of access cavities (Demarco et al. 2001). Similar findings were reported by other authors, who observed significant reduction in sealing quality of access cavities restored with composite resins up to 1 week after application of 10% carbamide peroxide into the pulp chamber (Türkün and Türkün 2004b).

Controversy still exists regarding whether prerestorative external whitening with 10% carbamide peroxide does impair the marginal seal of Class V restorations (Crim 1992b, Yazici et al. 2010). However, postrestorative whitening of existing restorations with 10–15% carbamide peroxide increased microleakage rates of Class V restorations (Crim 1992a, Ulukapi et al. 2003, Moosavi et al. 2009, Mortazavi et al. 2011). However, this effect was not seen in all studies dealing with this topic, even when whitening was performed with highly concentrated hydrogen peroxide formulations under the use of light activation with a plasma arc device (White et al. 2008, Khoroushi and Fardashtaki 2009, Klukowska et al. 2008). This finding might be attributable to the shorter application time of the light-activated system as compared with the carbamide peroxide system.

Penetration of the pulp chamber by whitening agents in composite-restored teeth

It was observed that during external whitening with 30% hydrogen peroxide or 10–35% carbamide peroxide gel, higher levels of hydrogen penetrated into the pulp chamber in teeth with restorations placed in enamel as compared with sound teeth (Gökay et al. 2000a, 2000b, Camargo et al. 2007). This was true for restorations fabricated with composite materials, polyacid-modified composite resins, or resin-modified glass ionomer cements. Furthermore, it was shown that higher-concentration carbamide peroxide gels (35%) led to distinctly higher levels of peroxide in the pulp chamber compared with low-concentration (10%) gels (Benetti et al. 2004).

CLINICAL CONSEQUENCES OF THE IMPACT OF WHITENING AGENTS ON RESTORATIONS

The aforementioned studies underline that pretreatment and post-treatment whitening procedures may negatively affect marginal seal, surface hardness, and color of composite and polyacid-modified composite restorations. Moreover, restorations and margins of restorations could be regarded as a possible pathway facilitating peroxide penetration into the pulp chamber. Peroxide penetration into the pulp chamber causes pulpal reactions, such as increase in tooth hypersensitivity, during external whitening of vital teeth (Robertson and Melfi 1980, Hanks et al. 1993). Dentists should therefore examine restorations meticulously before starting whitening therapy and renew insufficient fillings before whitening in order to achieve an optimal seal of the pulp chamber and thus reduce the risk of adverse effects. Future studies must investigate the extent to which the higher rate of microleakage observed in vitro leads to problems with existing restorations in the clinical situation. Moreover, it has to be considered that existing tooth-colored fillings might show a mismatch in color to the adjacent dental hard tissue after completion of whitening therapy. This sometimes renders the replacement of the complete filling or at least of the labial part of the restoration necessary. In the case of replacement of parts of composite fillings, guidelines have been published that describe how to handle the surface appropriately to get a tight adhesion of the repair filling to the remaining restoration. For composite materials it is recommended to grind the surface of the existing filling and the margins of the dental hard tissue first with a bur, then to condition the composite material by sandblasting with aluminum oxide powder, followed by application of a silane coupling agent and of an adhesive system before final placement of the new composite filling material (Foitzik and Attin 2004).

RECOMMENDATIONS

It is recommended to delay placement of restorations after termination of whitening therapy for at least 1–3 weeks because bonding of adhesively attached restorations to prewhitened dental hard tissue is reduced. Alternatively, a 10% sodium ascorbate gel or solution could be applied for at least 10 minutes to accelerate the deoxidization of the whitened dental hard tissues responsible for reduced bond strength. Moreover, whitening with hydrogen peroxide or hydrogen peroxide–releasing preparations may have a negative effect on restorations and restorative materials. The extent to which these factors may result in significant deterioration of restorations under clinical conditions remains unclear. However, there are no reports in the literature indicating that whitening exerted such a strong negative impact on existing restorations that renewal of the restorations was required. In case of mismatch of color of the restoration with the color of the tooth after whitening, partial or complete renewal of an already existing filling might be advisable.

REFERENCES

Abd Elhamid M, Mosallam R. (2010) Effect of bleaching versus repolishing on colour and surface topography of stained resin composite. *Aust Dent J* **55**:390–8.

Abe R, Endo T, Shimooka S. (2011) Effects of tooth bleaching on shear bond strength of brackets rebonded with a self-etching adhesive system. *Odontology* **99**:83–7.

Adanir N, Turkkahraman H, Gungor AY. (2007) Effects of fluorosis and bleaching on shear bond strengths of orthodontic brackets. *Eur J Dent* **1**:230–5.

Adibfar A, Steele A, Torneck CD, Titley KC. (1992) Leaching of hydrogen peroxide from bleached bovine enamel. *J Endod* **18**:488–91.

Amaral C, Jorge A, Veloso K, Erhardt M. (2008) The effect of in-office in combination with intracoronal bleaching on enamel and dentin bond strength and dentin morphology. *J Contemp Dent Pract* **9**:17–24.

Anagnostou M, Chelioti G, Chioti S, Kakaboura A. (2010) Effect of tooth-bleaching methods on gloss and color of resin composites. *J Dent* **38**(Suppl 2):e129–36.

Arcari GM, Araujo E, Baratieri LN, Lopes GC. (2007) Microtensile bond strength of a nanofilled composite resin to human dentin after nonvital tooth bleaching. *J Adhes Dent* **9**:333–40.

Attin T, Hannig C, Wiegand A, Attin R. (2004) Effect of bleaching on restorative materials and restorations—a systematic review. *Dent Mater* **20**:852–61.

Barbosa CM, Sasaki RT, Florio FM, Basting RT. (2008) Influence of time on bond strength after bleaching with 35% hydrogen peroxide. *J Contemp Dent Pract* **9**:81–8.

Barbosa CM, Sasaki RT, Florio FM, Basting RT. (2009) Influence of in situ post-bleaching times on resin composite shear bond strength to enamel and dentin. *Am J Dent* **22**:387–92.

Barcellos DC, Benetti P, Fernandes VV, Valera MC. (2010) Effect of carbamide peroxide bleaching gel concentration on the bond strength of dental substrates and resin composite. *Oper Dent* **35**:463–9.

Barkhordar RA, Kempler D, Plesh O. (1997) Effect of nonvital tooth bleaching on microleakage of resin composite restorations. *Quintessence Int* **28**:341–4.

Basting RT, Fernandez YF, Ambrosano GM, de Campos IT. (2005) Effects of a 10% carbamide peroxide bleaching agent on roughness and microhardness of packable composite resins. *J Esthet Restor Dent* **17**:256–62; discussion 263.

Basting RT, Freitas PM, Pimenta LA, Serra MC. (2004) Shear bond strength after dentin bleaching with 10% carbamide peroxide agents. *Braz Oral Res* **18**:162–7.

Benetti AR, Valera MC, Mancini MN, Miranda CB. (2004) In vitro penetration of bleaching agents into the pulp chamber. *Int Endod J* **37**:120–4.

Bishara SE, Oonsombat C, Soliman MM, Ajlouni R. (2005) The effect of tooth bleaching on the shear bond strength of orthodontic brackets. *Am J Orthod Dentofacial Orthop* **128**: 755–60.

Bishara SE, Sulieman AH, Olson M. (1993) Effect of enamel bleaching on the bonding strength of orthodontic brackets. *Am J Orthod Dentofacial Orthop* **104**:444–7.

Bittencourt ME, Trentin MS, Linden MS et al. (2010) Influence of in situ postbleaching times on shear bond strength of resin-based composite restorations. *J Am Dent Assoc* **141**: 300–6.

Breschi L, Cadenaro M, Antoniolli F, Visintini E. (2007) Extent of polymerization of dental bonding systems on bleached enamel. *Am J Dent* **20**:275–80.

Briso AL, Toseto RM, de Arruda AM, Tolentino PR. (2010a) Evaluating the bonding of two adhesive systems to enamel submitted to whitening dentifrices. *Acta Odontol Latinoam* **23**:111–6.

Briso AL, Toseto RM, Rahal V, dos Santos PH. (2012) Effect of sodium ascorbate on tag formation in bleached enamel. *J Adhes Dent* **14**(1):19–23.

Briso AL, Tuñas IT, de Almeida LC, Rahal V. (2010b) Effects of five carbamide peroxide bleaching gels on composite resin microhardness. *Acta Odontol Latinoam* **23**:27–31.

Bulucu B, Ozsezer E. (2007) Influence of light-curing units on dentin bond strength after bleaching. *J Adhes Dent* **9**:183–7.

Bulucu B, Ozsezer E, Ertas E, Yuksel G. (2008) The effect of different light sources on microleakage of bleached enamel. *Dent Mater J* **27**:598–604.

Bulut H, Kaya AD, Türkün M. (2005) Tensile bond strength of brackets after antioxidant treatment on bleached teeth. *Eur J Orthod* **27**:466–71.

Bulut H, Türkün M, Kaya AD. (2006) Effect of an antioxidizing agent on the shear bond strength of brackets bonded to bleached human enamel. *Am J Orthod Dentofacial Orthop* **129**:266–72.

Buzoglu HD, Gumusderelioglu M, Rotstein I. (2009) Effect of bleaching agents on surface free energy parameters of resin composite coated with saliva biofilm. *Am J Dent* **22**:223–7.

Cacciafesta V, Sfondrini MF, Stifanelli P, Scribante A. (2006) The effect of bleaching on shear bond strength of brackets bonded with a resin-modified glass ionomer. *Am J Orthod Dentofacial Orthop* **130**:83–7.

Cadenaro M, Breschi L, Antoniolli F, Mazzoni A. (2006) Influence of whitening on the degree of conversion of dental adhesives on dentin. *Eur J Oral Sci* **114**:257–62.

Camargo SE, Valera MC, Camargo CH, Gasparoto Mancini MN. (2007) Penetration of 38% hydrogen peroxide into the pulp chamber in bovine and human teeth submitted to office bleach technique. *J Endod* **33**:1074–7.

Campos I, Briso AL, Pimenta LA, Ambrosano G. (2003) Effects of bleaching with carbamide peroxide gels on microhardness of restoration materials. *J Esthet Restor Dent* **15**:175–82.

Canay S, Cehreli MC. (2003) The effect of current bleaching agents on the color of light-polymerized composites in vitro. *J Prosthet Dent* **89**:474–8.

Can-Karabulut DC, Karabulut B. (2010) Shear bond strength to enamel after power bleaching activated by different sources. *Eur J Esthet Dent* **5**:382–96.

Can-Karabulut DC, Karabulut B. (2011) Influence of activated bleaching on various adhesive restorative systems. *J Esthet Restor Dent* **23**:399–408.

Cavalli V, de Carvalho RM, Giannini M. (2005) Influence of carbamide peroxide-based bleaching agents on the bond strength of resin-enamel/dentin interfaces. *Braz Oral Res* **19**:23–9.

Cavalli V, Giannini M, Carvalho RM. (2004) Effect of carbamide peroxide bleaching agents on tensile strength of human enamel. *Dent Mater* **20**:733–9.

Cavalli V, Reis AF, Giannini M, Ambrosano GM. (2001) The effect of elapsed time following bleaching on enamel bond strength of resin composite. *Oper Dent* **26**:597–602.

Cehreli ZC, Yazici R, Garcia-Godoy F. (2003) Effect of home-use bleaching gels on fluoride releasing restorative materials. *Oper Dent* **28**:605–9.

Celik C, Yuzugullu B, Erkut S, Yazici AR. (2009) Effect of bleaching on staining susceptibility of resin composite restorative materials. *J Esthet Restor Dent* **21**:407–14.

Cho SD, Bulpakdi P, Matis BA, Platt JA. (2009) Effect of bleaching on fracture toughness of resin composites. *Oper Dent* **34**:703–8.

Chuang SF, Chen HP, Chang CH, Liu JK. (2009) Effect of fluoridated carbamide peroxide gels on enamel microtensile bond strength. *Eur J Oral Sci* **117**:435–41.

Comlekoglu ME, Gökçe B, Kaya AD, Türkün M. (2010) Reversal of reduced bond strength after bleaching. *Gen Dent* **58**:258–63; quiz 264–5.

Crim GA. (1992a) Post-operative bleaching: effect on microleakage. *Am J Dent* **5**:109–12.

Crim GA. (1992b) Prerestorative bleaching: effect on microleakage of Class V cavities. *Quintessence Int* **23**:823–5.

Dabas D, Patil AC, Uppin VM. (2011) Evaluation of the effect of concentration and duration of application of sodium ascorbate hydrogel on the bond strength of composite resin to bleached enamel. *J Conserv Dent* **14**:356–60.

Dadoun MP, Bartlett DW. (2007) The microhardness of bleached dentine and its bond strength to a dentine bonding agent. *Eur J Prosthodont Restor Dent* **15**:131–4.

Danesh-Sani SA, Esmaili M. (2011) Effect of 10% sodium ascorbate hydrogel and delayed bonding on shear bond strength of composite resin and resin-modified glass ionomer to bleached enamel. *J Conserv Dent* **14**:241–6.

da Silva BM, Florio FM, Basting RT. (2007) Shear bond strength of resin composite to enamel and dentin submitted to a carbamide peroxide dentifrice. *Am J Dent* **20**:319–23.

Da Silva Machado J, Cândido MS, Sundfeld RH, De Alexandre RS. (2007) The influence of time interval between bleaching and enamel bonding. *J Esthet Restor Dent* **19**:111–8; discussion 119.

de A Silva MF, Davies RM, Stewart B, DeVizio W. (2006) Effect of whitening gels on the surface roughness of restorative materials in situ. *Dent Mater* **22:**919–24.

de Andrade IC, Basting RT, Lima-Arsati YB, do Amaral FL. (2011) Surface roughness evaluation and shade changes of a nanofilled resin composite after bleaching and immersion in staining solutions. *Am J Dent* **24:**245–9.

Demarco FF, Freitas JM, Silva MP, Justino LM. (2001) Microleakage in endodontically treated teeth: influence of calcium hydroxide dressing following bleaching. *Int Endod J* **34:**495–500.

Demarco FF, Turbino ML, Jorge AG, Matson E. (1998) Influence of bleaching on dentin bond strength. *Am J Dent* **11:**78–82.

Dietrich AM, English J, McGrory K, Ontiveros J. (2010) A comparison of shear bond strengths on bleached and unbleached bovine enamel. *Tex Dent J* **127:**285–91.

Dishman MV, Covey DA, Baughan LW. (1994) The effects of peroxide bleaching on composite to enamel bond strength. *Dent Mater* **10:**33–6.

Durner J, Stojanovic M, Urcan E, Spahl W. (2011) Effect of hydrogen peroxide on the three-dimensional polymer network in composites. *Dent Mater* **27:**573–80.

Duschner H, Götz H, White DJ, Kozak KM. (2004) Effects of hydrogen peroxide bleaching strip gels on dental restorative materials in vitro: surface microhardness and surface morphology. *J Clin Dent* **15:**105–11.

Duschner H, Götz H, White DJ, Kozak KM. (2006) Effects of hydrogen peroxide bleaching strips on tooth surface color, surface microhardness, surface and subsurface ultrastructure, and microchemical (Raman spectroscopic) composition. *J Clin Dent* **17:**72–8.

Dutra RA, Branco JR, Alvim HH, Poletto LT. (2009) Effect of hydrogen peroxide topical application on the enamel and composite resin surfaces and interface. *Indian J Dent Res* **20:**65–70.

El-Murr J, Ruel D, St-Georges AJ. (2011) Effects of external bleaching on restorative materials: a review. *J Can Dent Assoc* **77:**b59.

Far C, Ruse D. (2003) Effect of bleaching on fracture toughness of composite-dentin bonds. *J Adhes Dent* **5:**175–82.

Faraoni-Romano JJ, Turssi CP, Serra MC. (2009) Effect of a bleaching agent on abrasion of resin-based restoratives. *Am J Dent* **22:**171–4.

Feiz A, Khoroushi M, Gheisarifar M. (2011) Bond strength of composite resin to bleached dentin: effect of using antioxidant versus buffering agent. *J Dent (Tehran)* **8:**60–6.

Ferreira EA, Souza-Gabriel AE, Silva-Sousa YT, Sousa-Neto MD. (2011) Shear bond strength and ultrastructural interface analysis of different adhesive systems to bleached dentin. *Microsc Res Tech* **74**(3):244–50.

Firoozmand LM, Pagani C. (2009) Influence of bleaching treatment on flexural resistance of hybrid materials. *Acta Odontol Latinoam* **22:**75–80.

Foitzik M, Attin T. (2004) [Filling revision—possibilities and execution]. *Schweiz Monatsschr Zahnmed* **114:**1003–11.

Garcia-Godoy F, Garcia-Godoy A, Garcia-Godoy F. (2002) Effect of bleaching gels on the surface roughness, hardness, and micromorphology of composites. *Gen Dent* **50:**247–50.

Gökay O, Tunçbilek M, Ertan R. (2000a) Penetration of the pulp chamber by carbamide peroxide bleaching agents on teeth restored with a composite resin. *J Oral Rehabil* **27:**428–31.

Gökay O, Yilmaz F, Akin S, Tunçbìlek M. (2000b) Penetration of the pulp chamber by bleaching agents in teeth restored with various restorative materials. *J Endod* **26:**92–4.

Gökçe B, Cömlekoğlu ME, Ozpinar B, Türkün M. (2008) Effect of antioxidant treatment on bond strength of a luting resin to bleached enamel. *J Dent* **36:**780–5.

Gurgan S, Alpaslan T, Kiremitci A, Cakir FY. (2009) Effect of different adhesive systems and laser treatment on the shear bond strength of bleached enamel. *J Dent* **37:**527–34.

Gurgan S, Yalcin F. (2007) The effect of 2 different bleaching regimens on the surface roughness and hardness of tooth-colored restorative materials. *Quintessence Int* **38:**83–7.

Hafez R, Ahmed D, Yousry M, El-Badrawy W. (2010) Effect of in-office bleaching on color and surface roughness of composite restoratives. *Eur J Dent* **4:**118–27.

Hanks CT, Fat JC, Wataha JC, Corcoran JF. (1993) Cytotoxicity and dentin permeability of carbamide peroxide and hydrogen-peroxide vital bleaching materials, in vitro. *J Dent Res* **72:**931–8.

Hannig C, Duong S, Becker K, Brunner E. (2007) Effect of bleaching on subsurface micro-hardness of composite and a polyacid modified composite. *Dent Mater* **23:**198–203.

Hegedüs C, Bistey T, Flóra-Nagy E, Keszthelyi G. (1999) An atomic force microscopy study on the effect of bleaching agents on enamel surface. *J Dent* **27:**509–15.

Hubbezoglu I, Akaoğlu B, Dogan A, Keskin S. (2008) Effect of bleaching on color change and refractive index of dental composite resins. *Dent Mater J* **27:**105–16.

Hussain M, Wang Y. (2010) Influence of prolonged light-curing time on the shear bonding strength of resin to bleached enamel. *Oper Dent* **35:**672–81.

Johnston WM, Kao EC. (1989) Assessment of appearance match by visual observation and clinical colorimetry. *J Dent Res* **68:**819–22.

Josey AL, Meyers IA, Romaniuk K, Symons AL. (1996) The effect of a vital bleaching technique on enamel surface morphology and the bonding of composite resin to enamel. *J Oral Rehabil* **23:**244–50.

Jung CB, Kim HI, Kim KH, Kwon YH. (2002) Influence of 30% hydrogen peroxide bleaching on compomers in their surface modifications and thermal expansion. *Dent Mater J* **21:**396–403.

Kaya AD, Türkün M, Arici M. (2008) Reversal of compromised bonding in bleached enamel using antioxidant gel. *Oper Dent* **33:**441–7.

Khoroushi M, Fardashtaki SR. (2009) Effect of light-activated bleaching on the microleakage of Class V tooth-colored restorations. *Oper Dent* **34:**565–70.

Khoroushi M, Feiz A, Ebadi M. (2009) Influence of intermediary filling material on microleakage of intracoronally bleached and restored teeth. *Dent Res J (Isfahan)* **6:**17–22.

Khoroushi M, Feiz A, Khodamoradi R. (2010) Fracture resistance of endodontically-treated teeth: effect of combination bleaching and an antioxidant. *Oper Dent* **35:**530–37.

Kim JH, Lee YK, Lim BS, Rhee SH. (2004) Effect of tooth-whitening strips and films on changes in color and surface roughness of resin composites. *Clin Oral Investig* **8:**118–22.

Kimyai S, Valizadeh H. (2006) The effect of hydrogel and solution of sodium ascorbate on bond strength in bleached enamel. *Oper Dent* **31:**496–9.

Kimyai S, Valizadeh H. (2008) Comparison of the effect of hydrogel and a solution of sodium ascorbate on dentin-composite bond strength after bleaching. *J Contemp Dent Pract* **9:**105–12.

Klukowska MA, White DJ, Gibb RD, Garcia-Godoy F. (2008) The effects of high concentration tooth whitening bleaches on microleakage of Class V composite restorations. *J Clin Dent* **19:**14–7.

Kodaka T, Toko T, Debari K, Hisamitsu H. (1992) Application of the environmental SEM in human dentin bleached with hydrogen-peroxide in vitro. *J Electron Microsc (Tokyo)* **41**:381–6.

Kum KY, Lim KR, Lee CY, Park KH. (2004) Effects of removing residual peroxide and other oxygen radicals on the shear bond strength and failure modes at resin-tooth interface after tooth bleaching. *Am J Dent* **17**:267–70.

Kunt GE, Yilmaz N, Sen S, Dede DO. (2011) Effect of antioxidant treatment on the shear bond strength of composite resin to bleached enamel. *Acta Odontol Scand* **69**:287–91.

Kwon YH, Kwon TY, Kim HI, Kim KH. (2003) The effect of 30% hydrogen peroxide on the color of compomers. *J Biomed Mater Res* **66B**:306–10.

Kwon YH, Shin DH, Yun DI, Heo YJ. (2010) Effect of hydrogen peroxide on microhardness and color change of resin nanocomposites. *Am J Dent* **23**:19–22.

Lago AD, de Freitas PM, Netto NG. (2011) Evaluation of the bond strength between a composite resin and enamel submitted to bleaching treatment and etched with Er:YAG laser. *Photomed Laser Surg* **29**:91–5.

Lai SC, Mak YF, Cheung GS, Osorio R. (2001) Reversal of compromised bonding to oxidized etched dentin. *J Dent Res* **80**:1919–24.

Lai SC, Tay FR, Cheung GS, Mak YF. (2002) Reversal of compromised bonding in bleached enamel. *J Dent Res* **81**:477–81.

Lee JH, Kim HI, Kim KH, Kwon YH. (2002) Effect of bleaching agents on the fluoride release and microhardness of dental materials. *J Biomed Mater Res* **63**:535–41.

Leonetti Edos S, Rodrigues JA, Reis AF, Navarro RS. (2011) Effects of Er:YAG laser irradiation on the microtensile bond strength to bleached enamel. *Photomed Laser Surg* **29**:551–8.

Li Q, Yu H, Wang Y. (2009) Colour and surface analysis of carbamide peroxide bleaching effects on the dental restorative materials in situ. *J Dent* **37**:348–56.

Lima AF, Fonseca FM, Cavalcanti AN, Aguiar FH. (2010) Effect of the diffusion of bleaching agents through enamel on dentin bonding at different depths. *Am J Dent* **23**:113–5.

Lima AF, Fonseca FM, Freitas MS, Palialol AR. (2011a) Effect of bleaching treatment and reduced application time of an antioxidant on bond strength to bleached enamel and subjacent dentin. *J Adhes Dent* **13**:537–42.

Lima AF, Sasaki RT, Araújo LS, Gaglianone LA. (2011b) Effect of tooth bleaching on bond strength of enamel-dentin cavities restored with silorane- and dimethacrylate-based materials. *Oper Dent* **36**:390–6.

Lima DA, De Alexandre RS, Martins AC, Aguiar FH. (2008) Effect of curing lights and bleaching agents on physical properties of a hybrid composite resin. *J Esthet Restor Dent* **20**:266–73; discussion 274–5.

Loretto SC, Braz R, Lyra AM, Lopes LM. (2004) Influence of photopolymerization light source on enamel shear bond strength after bleaching. *Braz Dent J* **15**:133–7.

Malkondu Ö, Yurdagüven H, Say EC, Kazazoğlu E. (2011) Effect of bleaching on microhardness of esthetic restorative materials. *Oper Dent* **36**:177–86.

Martin JM, de Almeida JB, Rosa EA, Soares P. (2010) Effect of fluoride therapies on the surface roughness of human enamel exposed to bleaching agents. *Quintessence Int* **1**:71–8.

May LG, Salvia AC, Souza RO, Michida SM. (2010) Effect of sodium ascorbate and the time lapse before cementation after internal bleaching on bond strength between dentin and ceramic. *J Prosthodont* **19**:374–80.

Mazaheri H, Khoroushi M, Shafiei E, Ghorbanipour R. (2011) Bond strength of composite-resin and resin-modified glass ionomer to bleached enamel: delay bonding versus an antioxidant agent. *Indian J Dent Res* **22**:432–5.

McGuckin RS, Thurmond BA, Osovitz S. (1992) Enamel shear bond strengths after vital bleaching. *Am J Dent* **5**:216–22.

Metz MJ, Cochran MA, Matis BA, Gonzalez C. (2007) Clinical evaluation of 15% carbamide peroxide on the surface microhardness and shear bond strength of human enamel. *Oper Dent* **32**:427–36.

Miguel LC, Baratieri LN, Monteiro SJ, Ritter AV. (2004) In situ effect of 10% carbamide peroxide on resin-dentin bond strengths: a novel pilot study. *J Esthet Restor Dent* **16**:235–41; discussion 241–2.

Mishima FD, Valentim RG, Araújo MT, Ruellas AC. (2009) The effect of tooth bleaching on the enamel surface and the tensile force to debond orthodontic brackets. *J Orthod* **36**:236–42.

Miyazaki M, Sato H, Sato T, Moore BK. (2004) Effect of a whitening agent application on enamel bond strength of self-etching primer systems. *Am J Dent* **17**:151–5.

Monaghan P, Lim E, Lautenschlager E. (1992a) Effects of home bleaching preparations on composite resin color. *J Prosthet Dent* **68**:575–8.

Monaghan P, Trowbridge T, Lautenschlager E. (1992b) Composite resin color-change after vital tooth bleaching. *J Prosthet Dent* **67**:778–81.

Montalvan E, Vaidyanathan TK, Shey Z, Janal MN. (2006) The shear bond strength of acetone and ethanol-based bonding agents to bleached teeth. *Pediatr Dent* **28**:531–6.

Moosavi H, Ghavamnasiri M, Manari V. (2009) Effect of postoperative bleaching on marginal leakage of resin composite and resin-modified glass ionomer restorations at different delayed periods of exposure to carbamide peroxide. *J Contemp Dent Pract* **10**:E009–16.

Moosavi H, Moghaddas MJ, Ghoddusi J, Rajabi O. (2010) Effects of two antioxidants on the microleakage of resin-based composite restorations after nonvital bleaching. *J Contemp Dent Pract* **11**:E033–40.

Moraes RR, Marimon JL, Schneider LF, Correr Sobrinho L. (2006) Carbamide peroxide bleaching agents: effects on surface roughness of enamel, composite and porcelain. *Clin Oral Investig* **10**:23–8.

Mortazavi V, Fathi M, Soltani F. (2011) Effect of postoperative bleaching on microleakage of etch-and-rinse and self-etch adhesives. *Dent Res J (Isfahan)* **8**:16–21.

Moule CA, Angelis F, Kim GH, Le S. (2007) Resin bonding using an all-etch or self-etch adhesive to enamel after carbamide peroxide and/or CPP-ACP treatment. *Aust Dent J* **52**:133–7.

Mujdeci A, Gökay O. (2005) Dental effects of home bleaching gels and whitening strips on the surface hardness of resin composites. *Am J Dent* **18**:323–6.

Mujdeci A, Gökay O. (2006) Effect of bleaching agents on the microhardness of tooth-colored restorative materials. *J Prosthet Dent* **95**:286–9.

Mullins JM, Kao EC, Martin CA, Gunel E. (2009) Tooth whitening effects on bracket bond strength in vivo. *Angle Orthod* **79**:777–83.

Muraguchi K, Shigenobu S, Suzuki S, Tanaka T. (2007) Improvement of bonding to bleached bovine tooth surfaces by ascorbic acid treatment. *Dent Mater J* **26**:875–81.

Nour El-din AK, Miller BH, Griggs JA, Wakefield C. (2006) Immediate bonding to bleached enamel. *Oper Dent* **31**:106–14.

Okte Z, Villalta P, García-Godoy F, Lu H. (2006) Surface hardness of resin composites after staining and bleaching. *Oper Dent* **31:**623–8.

Oskoee PA, Navimipour EJ, Oskoee SS, Moosavi N. (2010) Effect of 10% sodium ascorbate on bleached bovine enamel surface morphology and microhardness. *Open Dent J* **4:**207–10.

Oztaş E, Bağdelen G, Kiliçoğlu H, Ulukapi H. (2012) The effect of enamel bleaching on the shear bond strengths of metal and ceramic brackets. *Eur J Orthod* **34**(2):232–7.

Patusco VC, Montenegro G, Lenza MA, Alves de Carvalho A. (2009) Bond strength of metallic brackets after dental bleaching. *Angle Orthod* **79:**122–6.

Perdigão J, Francci C, Swift EJ Jr, Ambrose WW. (1998) Ultramorphological study of the interaction of dental adhesives with carbamide peroxide-bleached enamel. *Am J Dent* **11:**291–301.

Polydorou O, Beiter J, König A, Hellwig E. (2009) Effect of bleaching on the elution of monomers from modern dental composite materials. *Dent Mater* **25:**254–60.

Polydorou O, Hellwig E, Auschill TM. (2006) The effect of different bleaching agents on the surface texture of restorative materials. *Oper Dent* **31:**473–80.

Polydorou O, Hellwig E, Auschill TM. (2007a)The effect of at-home bleaching on the microhardness of six esthetic restorative materials. *J Am Dent Assoc* **138:**978–84; quiz 1022.

Polydorou O, Monting JS, Hellwig E, Auschill TM. (2007b) Effect of in-office tooth bleaching on the microhardness of six dental esthetic restorative materials. *Dent Mater* **23:**153–8.

Pruthi G, Jain V, Kandpal HC, Mathur VP. (2010) Effect of bleaching on color change and surface topography of composite restorations. *Int J Dent* **2010:**695748.

Rao YM, Srilakshmi V, Vinayagam KK, Narayanan LL. (2009) An evaluation of the color stability of tooth-colored restorative materials after bleaching using CIELAB color technique. *Indian J Dent Res* **20:**60–4.

Robertson WD, Melfi RC. (1980) Pulpal response to vital bleaching procedures. *J Endod* **6:**645–9.

Rocha Gomes Torres C, Caneppele TM, Del Moral de Lazari R, Ribeiro CF. (2012) Effect of dental surface treatment with Nd:YAG and Er:YAG lasers on bond strength of resin composite to recently bleached enamel. *Lasers Med Sci* **27**(4):755–60.

Rosentritt M, Lang R, Plein T, Behr M. (2005) Discoloration of restorative materials after bleaching application. *Quintessence Int* **36:**33–9.

Rotstein I. (1993) Role of catalase in the elimination of residual hydrogen-peroxide following tooth bleaching. *J Endod* **19:**567–9.

Rueggeberg FA, Margeson DH. (1990) The effect of oxygen inhibition on an unfilled/filled composite system. *J Dent Res* **69:**1652–8.

Ruse ND, Smith DC, Torneck CD, Titley KC. (1990) Preliminary surface analysis of etched, bleached, and normal bovine enamel. *J Dent Res* **69:**1610–3.

Ruyter IE, Nilner K, Moller B. (1987) Color stability of dental composite resin materials for crown and bridge veneers. *Dent Mater* **3:**246–51.

Sasaki RT, Barbosa MC, Florio FM, Basting RT. (2007) Enamel microhardness and shear bond strength after treatment with an 18% carbamide peroxide bleaching varnish. *Am J Dent* **20:**324–8.

Sasaki RT, Florio FM, Basting RT. (2009) Effect of 10% sodium ascorbate and 10% alpha-tocopherol in different formulations on the shear bond strength of enamel and dentin submitted to a home-use bleaching treatment. *Oper Dent* **34:**746–52.

Schemehorn B, Gonzalez-Cabezas C, Joiner A. (2004) A SEM evaluation of a 6% hydrogen peroxide tooth whitening gel on dental materials in vitro. *J Dent* **32**(Suppl 1):35–9.

Shinkai K, Wakaki S, Suzuki S, Katoh Y. (2007) The effect of tooth bleaching on the bond strength of an experimental primer to enamel. *Odontology* **95:**38–43.

Shinohara MS, Peris AR, Pimenta LA, Ambrosano GM. (2005) Shear bond strength evaluation of composite resin on enamel and dentin after nonvital bleaching. *J Esthet Restor Dent* **17:**22–9; discussion 29.

Shinohara MS, Peris AR, Rodrigues JA, Pimenta LA. (2004) The effect of nonvital bleaching on the shear bond strength of composite resin using three adhesive systems. *J Adhes Dent* **6:**205–9.

Shinohara MS, Rodrigues JA, Pimenta LA. (2001) In vitro microleakage of composite restorations after nonvital bleaching. *Quintessence Int* **32:**413–17.

Silva Costa SX, Becker AB, de Souza Rastelli AN, de Castro Monteiro Loffredo L. (2009) Effect of four bleaching regimens on color changes and microhardness of dental nanofilled composite. *Int J Dent* **2009:**313845.

Souza-Gabriel AE, Vitussi LO, Milani C, Alfredo E. (2011) Effect of bleaching protocols with 38% hydrogen peroxide and post-bleaching times on dentin bond strength. *Braz Dent J* **22:**317–21.

Spyrides GM, Perdigão J, Pagani C, Araújo MA. (2000) Effect of whitening agents on dentin bonding. *J Esthet Dent* **12:**264–70.

Stokes AN, Hood JA, Dhariwal D, Patel K. (1992) Effect of peroxide bleaches on resin-enamel bonds. *Quintessence Int* **23:**769–771.

Sundfeld RH, Briso AL, De Sá PM, Sundfeld ML. (2005) Effect of time interval between bleaching and bonding on tag formation. *Bull Tokyo Dent Coll* **46:**1–6.

Taher NM. (2005) The effect of bleaching agents on the surface hardness of tooth colored restorative materials. *J Contemp Dent Pract* **6:**18–26.

Teixeira EC, Turssi CP, Hara AT, Serra MC. (2004) Influence of post-bleaching time intervals on dentin bond strength. *Pesqui Odontol Bras* **18:**75–9.

Timpawat S, Nipattamanon C, Kijsamanmith K, Messer HH. (2005) Effect of bleaching agents on bonding to pulp chamber dentine. *Int Endod J* **38:**211–7.

Titley KC, Torneck CD, Ruse ND, Krmec D. (1993) Adhesion of a resin composite to bleached and unbleached human enamel. *J Endod* **19:**112–5.

Titley KC, Torneck CD, Ruse ND. (1992) The effect of carbamide-peroxide gel on the shear bond strength of a microfil resin to bovine enamel. *J Dent Res* **71:**20–4.

Titley KC, Torneck CD, Smith DC, Chernecky R. (1991) Scanning electron microscopy observations on the penetration and structure of resin tags in bleached and unbleached bovine enamel. *J Endod* **17:**72–5.

Titley KC, Torneck CD, Smith DC, Adibfar A. (1988) Adhesion of composite resin to bleached and unbleached bovine enamel. *J Dent Res* **67:**1523–8.

Torneck CD, Titley KC, Smith DC, Adibfar A. (1990) Adhesion of light-cured composite resin to bleached and unbleached bovine dentin. *Endod Dent Traumatol* **6:**97–103.

Torneck CD, Titley KC, Smith DO, Adibfar A. (1991) Effect of water leaching on the adhesion of composite resin to bleached and unbleached bovine enamel. *J Endod* **17:**156–60.

Turker SB, Biskin T. (2002) The effect of bleaching agents on the microhardness of dental aesthetic restorative materials. *J Oral Rehabil* **29:**657–61.

Turker SB, Biskin T. (2003) Effect of three bleaching agents on the surface properties of three different esthetic restorative materials. *J Prosthet Dent* **89**:466–73.

Turkkahraman H, Adanir N, Gungor AY. (2007) Bleaching and desensitizer application effects on shear bond strengths of orthodontic brackets. *Angle Orthod* **77**:489–93.

Türkün LS, Türkün M. (2004a) Effect of bleaching and repolishing procedures on coffee and tea stain removal from three anterior composite veneering materials. *J Esthet Restor Dent* **16**:290–301.

Türkün M, Celik EU, Kaya AD, Arici M. (2009) Can the hydrogel form of sodium ascorbate be used to reverse compromised bond strength after bleaching? *J Adhes Dent* **11**:35–40.

Türkün M, Kaya AD. (2004) Effect of 10% sodium ascorbate on the shear bond strength of composite resin to bleached bovine enamel. *J Oral Rehabil* **31**:1184–1191.

Türkün M, Türkün LS. (2004b) Effect of nonvital bleaching with 10% carbamide peroxide on sealing ability of resin composite restorations. *Int Endod J* **37**:52–60.

Ulukapi H, Benderli Y, Ulukapi I. (2003) Effect of pre- and postoperative bleaching on marginal effect of leakage of amalgam and composite restorations. *Quintessence Int* **34**:505–8.

Unlu N, Cobankara FK, Ozer F. (2008) Effect of elapsed time following bleaching on the shear bond strength of composite resin to enamel. *J Biomed Mater Res B Appl Biomater* **84**:363–8.

Uysal T, Basciftci FA, Uşümez S, Sari Z. (2003) Can previously bleached teeth be bonded safely? *Am J Orthod Dentofacial Orthop* **123**:628–32.

Uysal T, Er O, Sagsen B, Ustdal A. (2009) Can intracoronally bleached teeth be bonded safely? *Am J Orthod Dentofacial Orthop* **136**:689–94.

Uysal T, Ertas H, Sagsen B, Bulut H (2010). Can intra-coronally bleached teeth be bonded safely after antioxidant treatment? *Dent Mater* J **29**:47–52.

van der Vyver PJ, Lewis SB, Marais JT. (1997) The effect of bleaching agent on composite/enamel bonding. *J Dent Assoc S Afr* **52**:601–3.

Vidhya S, Srinivasulu S, Sujatha M, Mahalaxmi S. (2011) Effect of grape seed extract on the bond strength of bleached enamel. *Oper Dent* **36**:433–8.

Villalta P, Lu H, Okte Z, Garcia-Godoy F. (2006) Effects of staining and bleaching on color change of dental composite resins. *J Prosthet Dent* **95**:137–42.

Wang L, Francisconi LF, Atta MT, Dos Santos JR. (2011) Effect of bleaching gels on surface roughness of nanofilled composite resins. *Eur J Dent* **5**:173–9.

Wattanapayungkul P, Yap AU. (2003) Effects of in-office bleaching products on surface finish of tooth-colored restorations. *Oper Dent* **28**:15–9.

Wattanapayungkul P, Yap AU, Chooi KW, Lee MF. (2004) The effect of home bleaching agents on the surface roughness of tooth-colored restoratives with time. *Oper Dent* **29**:398–403.

White DJ, Duschner H, Pioch T. (2008) Effect of bleaching treatments on microleakage of Class I restorations. *J Clin Dent* **19**:33–36.

White DJ, Kozak KM, Zoladz JR, Duschner HJ. (2003) Effects of Crest Whitestrips bleaching on surface morphology and fracture susceptibility of teeth in vitro. *J Clin Dent* **14**:82–7.

Wilson D, Xu C, Hong L, Wang Y. (2009) Effects of different preparation procedures during tooth whitening on enamel bonding. *J Mater Sci Mater Med* **20**:1001–7.

Yalcin F, Gurgan S. (2005a) Bleaching-induced colour change in plastic filling materials. *J Biomater Appl* **19**:187–95.

Yalcin F, Gurgan S. (2005b) Effect of two different bleaching regimens on the gloss of tooth colored restorative materials. *Dent Mater* **21**:464–8.

Yap AU, Wattanapayungkul P. (2002) Effects of in-office tooth whiteners on hardness of tooth-colored restoratives. *Oper Dent* **27**:137–41.

Yazici AR, Keles A, Tuncer D, Baseren M. (2010) Effect of prerestorative home-bleaching on microleakage of self-etch adhesives. *J Esthet Restor Dent* **22**:186–192.

Yu H, Li Q, Cheng H, Wang Y. (2011) The effects of temperature and bleaching gels on the properties of tooth-colored restorative materials. *J Prosthet Dent* **105**:100–7.

Yu H, Li Q, Hussain M, Wang Y. (2008) Effects of bleaching gels on the surface microhardness of tooth-colored restorative materials in situ. *J Dent* **36**:261–7.

Yu H, Li Q, Lin Y, Buchalla W. (2010) Influence of carbamide peroxide on the flexural strength of tooth-colored restorative materials: an in vitro study at different environmental temperatures. *Oper Dent* **35**:300–7.

Yu H, Pan X, Lin Y, Li Q. (2009) Effects of carbamide peroxide on the staining susceptibility of tooth-colored restorative materials. *Oper Dent* **34**:72–82.

Zavanelli AC, Mazaro VQ, Silva CR, Zavanelli RA. (2011) Surface roughness analysis of four restorative materials exposed to 10% and 15% carbamide peroxide. *Int J Prosthodont* **24**:155–7.

5. Vitamin E (10% α-tocopherol)—VitE (Fleming Pharmacy, Ponta Grossa, PR, Brazil). With a pH of 6.8, this is a lipid-soluble antioxidant that has shown good results in dentin and enamel (Torres et al. 2006). However, it may have been the presence of alcohol that improved the surface properties, resulting in reversal of the bond strength.
6. Ascorbic acid.
7. Butylhydroxyanisole.
8. Catalase alone—catalase at 1.25% (Neutralize, FGM Dental Products, Joinville, SC, Brazil).
9. Five percent potassium nitrate and 2% sodium fluoride (Dessensibilize KF 2%; FGM Dental Products).
10. Ethanol.
11. Acetone.
12. Glutathione peroxidase.
13. Sodium bicarbonate. Sodium bicarbonate is sold along with in-office whitening products for use as a neutralizer when hydrogen peroxide accidentally contacts oral mucosa. The antioxidant activity of sodium bicarbonate was higher than both types of catalase (CAT and NE), and they had similar behavior in reverting bond strength decrease (Garcia et al. 2012).

CLINICAL APPROACH TO ESTHETIC TREATMENT

It is essential to base clinical treatment decisions on the evidence when planning clinical protocols for patients. This can be undertaken very simply by understanding the research and evidence and designing appropriate clinical protocols. In developing appropriate treatment plans, dentists should combine the patient's treatment needs and preferences with the best available scientific evidence, in conjunction with the dentist's clinical expertise (Ismail and Bader 2004).

It is essential that all the correct protocols be followed during the patient's journey from new patient consultation through the treatment planning discussion and explanation of the risks, benefits, advantages, and disadvantages of the procedures.

COMPOSITE BONDING AFTER WHITENING

Despite the reduction in bond strength, composite bonding is the most common procedure undertaken. This procedure can normally be undertaken 2–3 weeks after completion of whitening treatment. After whitening, some of the enamel and dentin may appear more opaque. This is useful when selecting whitening shade composites to undertake segmental layering (Table 17.3). Most manufacturers make whitening shade composites, and this material is often used as the dentin layer, followed by the enamel layer, which is more translucent.

There are various multiple stages in undertaking composite bonding. Selection of the composite shade is essential as the first step in the bonding stage. It is often useful to do a test selection of a few different composite shades first before undertaking the bonding treatment. When undertaking composite bonding after whitening, the use of isolation techniques quickly causes the tooth to dehydrate, so the tooth rapidly becomes lighter.

Dentists differ vastly in their preparation and bonding techniques, but a suggested phased approach is listed here. The stages are as follows:

1. Isolating the tooth (rubber dam: OptraGate, OptraGam Plus [Ivoclar Vivadent).
2. Selecting the shade of composite, using two different color combinations of enamel, dentin, and whitened shades.
3. Cleaning the tooth and preparing the surface. This can involve the following:
   - A combination of pumice and chlorhexidine soap (Hibiscrub, 4% chlorhexidine, Consepsis 2% chlorhexidine antibacterial solution or slurry). This is polished onto the surface of the tooth with a Mini Brush (Ultradent).
   - Air abrasion using powder in different diameter widths, such as aluminum oxide, sodium bicarbonate, or bioglass (Sylc containing calcium and phosphate). This is used in an application machine such as Aquacut (Veloplex International; see Figure 17.3G) or an applicator.
4. Etching the tooth. This can be done in two phases (see Figures 17.3M and 17.3N). The first layer is applied, then rinsed off, and a check is made to see that the tooth is fully etched. This step can be repeated.
5. Intermediate dentin sealing (HurriSeal [Beutlich Pharmaceuticals, Patterson Dental])—an optional step.
6. Bonding.
7. Composite layering. Depending on the shape of the cavity and the tooth surface, the dentin layer is placed first. This is more opaque, and the whitened shade composite may be used. This is then light cured. Checks are made to see if further modification of the color is needed. The layers are placed from darkest to lightest shade to mimic the natural opalescence and translucency of the tooth. The final layer is the enamel layer. If the tooth has a dark cervical root area, this can be opaqued using an opaque white or an opaque pink composite tint before bonding (see Figure 17.8).
8. The composite is then completed by undertaking the final shaping, finishing, and polishing with rubber wheels and polishing paste (SDI [Southern Dental Industries], Bayswater, Melbourne, Australia) and/or with Astropol (Ivoclar Vivadent) (see Figure 14.10).

WHITENING SHADES OF COMPOSITE

The manufacturers of composite materials have responded to requests for providing lighter and whiter shades of composites to match the new shades of whiter teeth. To do so, manufacturers have had to make some changes to the composite formulations. It may be that to achieve bright white or translucent shades of resins, some manufacturers find it necessary to use less camphorquinone or another photoinitiator altogether (Neumann et al. 2005). Photoinitiators such as 1-phenyl-1,2-propanedione (PPD) are photosensitizers of potential value in reducing color problems associated with visible light-cured dental resins. In combination with camphorquinone, they act synergistically to produce a more efficient photoinitiation reaction. Other composite-related factors in the whitener shade composites include shade, translucency, and filler particle size, load, and distribution. Light-related factors include light intensity, spectral distribution, and exposure time. In a study by Gomes et al. (2006), different light-emitting diode (LED) lights were used to polymerize a whitening shade resin composite, and compared with a conventional Optilux 501 light. It was hypothesized that the LED lights would not be able to effectively polymerize this specific resin composite. According to the results, the hardness values of LED 2 were similar to the values observed when the halogen light was used. There appears to be a good correlation between decreasing degree of conversion and decreasing hardness, fracture toughness, and abrasive wear resistance. To compensate for the lower hardness values found, the duration of exposure can be increased, within practical limits determined by the properties of the material and light source, providing enhanced opportunity for creation of free radicals.

In an in vitro study (Farah and Elwi 2014) to assess the effect of the whitening shade composites, whitening shade composite disks were immersed in coffee and tea solutions. Whitening shade composites showed significant discoloration ($\Delta E > 3.3$) after being immersed into coffee and tea solutions. Nanofilled composites discolored more than nanohybrid composites, and carbamide peroxide–based whitening agents were effective in reducing the discoloration to a clinically acceptable value ($\Delta E > 3.3$).

RESURFACING AND REPOLISHING

Although there is little effect on composite restorations during whitening, there is much debate and controversy surrounding the effect on their surface. However, after whitening, as part of the patient request to improve the smile, some restorations can be renewed and refreshed. Some composite restorations can be resurfaced with air abrasion; some may be etched and bonded; further flowable composite may be added; or enamel or dentin whitening shades may be added. Some composites that have marginal defects can be resurfaced after whitening. This is a method of renewing the restoration and maintaining its longevity of the restoration. Repolishing the restoration will remove some of the surface discoloration (Garoushi et al. 2013). This can be done with a rubber wheel and polishing paste.

CONCLUSION

Esthetic treatment after whitening has become routine. The most common procedure is composite bonding treatment. It is essential that the dentist know the side effects of bonding immediately after whitening and have a strategy to deal with the bonding treatments before commencing esthetic treatment after whitening.

REFERENCES

Alqahtani MQ. (2014) Tooth-bleaching procedures and their controversial effects: a literature review. *Saudi Dent J* **26**(2):33–46.

da Costa JB, McPharlin R, Paravina RD, Ferracane JL. (2010) Comparison of at-home and in-office tooth whitening using a novel shade guide. *Oper Dent* **35:**381–8

da Cunha LF, Furuse AY, Mondelli RF, Mondelli J. (2010) Compromised bond strength after root dentin deproteinization reversed with ascorbic acid. *J Endod* **36**(1): 130–4.

Dishman MV, Covey DA, Baughan LW. (1994) The effects of peroxide bleaching on composite to enamel bond strength. *Dent Mater* **10:**33–6.

Farah RI, Elwi H. (2014) Spectrophotometric evaluation of color changes of bleach-shade resin-based composites after staining and bleaching. *J Contemp Dent Pract* **15**(5):587–94.

Garcia EJ, Oldoni TL, Alencar SM, Reis A. (2012) Antioxidant activity by DPPH assay of potential solutions to be applied on bleached teeth. *Braz Dent J* 23(1):22–7.

Garoushi S, Lassila L, Hatem M, Shembesh M. (2013) Influence of staining solutions and whitening procedures on discoloration of hybrid composite resins. *Acta Odontol Scand* **71**(1):144–50.

Gomes GM, Calixto AL, Santos FA, Gomes OM. (2006) Hardness of a bleaching-shade resin composite polymerized with different light-curing sources. *Braz Oral Res* 20(4):337–41.

Han Y, Mo S, Jiang L, Zhu Y. (2014) Effects of antioxidants on the microleakage of composite resin restorations after external tooth bleaching. *Eur J Dent* **8**(2):147–53.

Hansen JR, Frick KJ, Walker MP. (2014) Effect of 35% sodium ascorbate treatment on microtensile bond strength after nonvital bleaching. *J Endod* **40**(10):1668–70.

Ismail AI, Bader JD. (2004) Evidence-based dentistry in clinical practice. *J Am Dent Assoc* **135**(1):78–83.

Kaya AD Türkün M. (2003) Reversal of dentin bonding to bleached teeth. *Oper Dent* **28**(6):825–9.

Kaya AD, Türkün M, Arici M. (2008). Reversal of compromised bonding in bleached enamel using antioxidant gel. *Oper Dent* **33:**441–7.

Khoroushi M, Feiz A, Khodamoradi R. (2010) Fracture resistance of endodontically treated teeth: effect of combination bleaching and an antioxidant. *Oper Dent* **35**(5):530–7.

Kimyai S, Valizadeh H. (2008) Comparison of the effect of hydrogel and a solution of sodium ascorbate on dentin-composite bond strength after bleaching. *J Contemp Dent Pract* **9**(2):105–12.

Neumann MG, Miranda WG Jr, Schmitt CC, Rueggeberg FA. (2005) Molar extinction coefficients and the photon absorption efficiency of dental photoinitiators and light curing units. *J Dent* **33**(6):525–32.

Perdigão J, Francci C, Swift EJ Jr, Ambrose WW. (1998) Ultramorphological study of the interaction of dental adhesives with carbamide peroxide-bleached enamel. *Am J Dent* **11:**291–301.

Rotstein I. (1993) Role of catalase in the elimination of residual hydrogen-peroxide following tooth bleaching. *J Endod* **19:** 567–9.

Soeno K, Taira Y, Jimbo R, Sawase T (2008) Surface treatment with ascorbic acid and ferric chloride improves the micro-tensile bond strength of 4-META/MMA-TBB resin to dentin. *J Dent* **36**(11):940–944.

Stokes AN, Hood JA, Dhariwal D, Patel D. (1992) Effect of peroxide bleaches on resin-enamel bonds. *Quintessence Int* **23**(11):769-71.

Subramonian R, Mathai V, Angelo JB, Ravi J. (2015) Effect of three different antioxidants on the shear bond strength of composite resin to bleached enamel: an in vitro study. *J Conserv Dent* **18**(2):144–8.

Titley KC, Torneck CD, Ruse ND. (1992) The effect of carbamide-peroxide gel on the shear bond strength of a microfil resin to bovine enamel. *J Dent Res* **71**(1):20–4.

Titley KC, Torneck CD, Smith DC, Chernecky R. (1991). Scanning electron microscopy observations on the penetration and structure of resin tags in bleached and unbleached bovine enamel. *J Endod* **17**:72–5.

Torres CR, Koga AF, Borges AB. (2006) The effects of antioxidant agents as neutralizers of bleaching agents on enamel bond strength. *Braz J Oral Sci* **5**:971–6.

Türkün M, Celik EU, Kaya AD, Arici M. (2000). Can the hydrogel form of sodium ascorbate be used to reverse compromised bond strength after bleaching? *J Adhes Dent* **11**(1): 35–40.

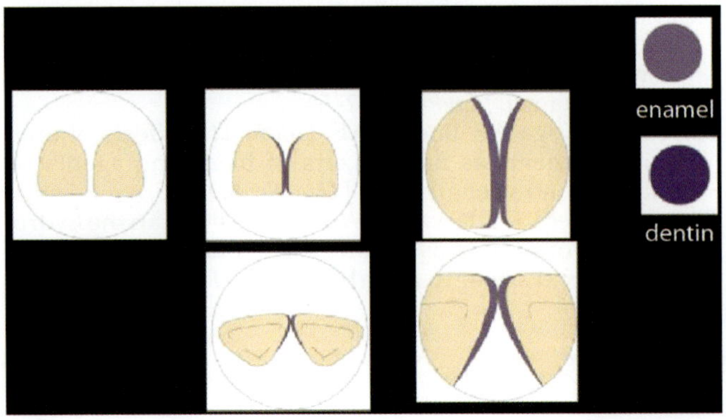

(A)

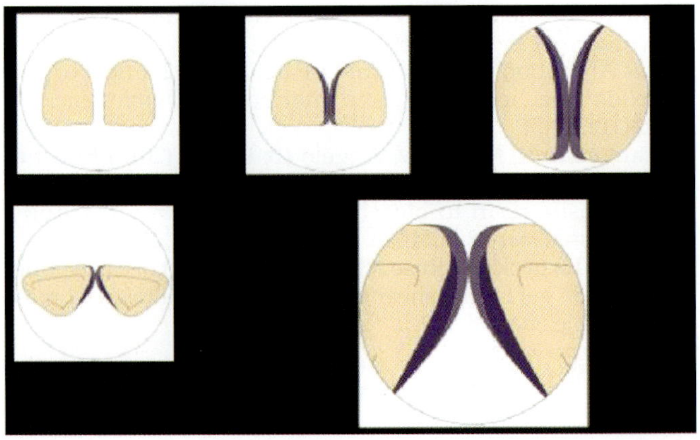

(B)

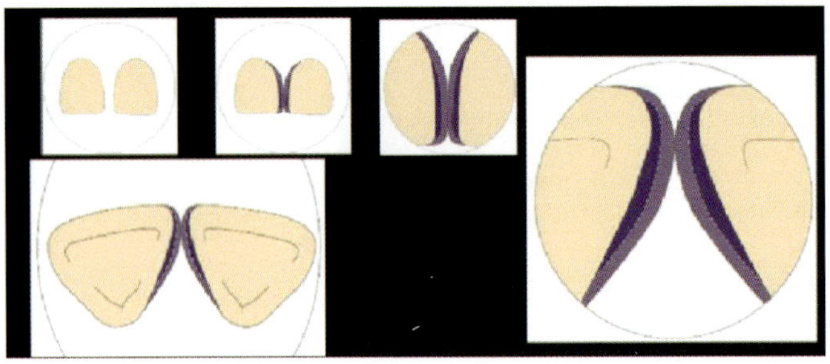

(C)

Figure 17.1

(A) Steps involved in closing a small diastema using enamel composite only. First, classify the size of the diastema. If small, use enamel only depending on the tooth anatomy. (B) Steps involved in diastema closure for a medium-sized diastema (0.5–1 mm). Using dentin and enamel composite in layers, start from the palatal dentin and layer forward with enamel. (C) Steps involved in layering of composite with a large diastema (1–2 mm). Layer with dentin first, then enamel (dentin to wrap over the tooth, blended composite, enamel wrapped over the entire restoration).

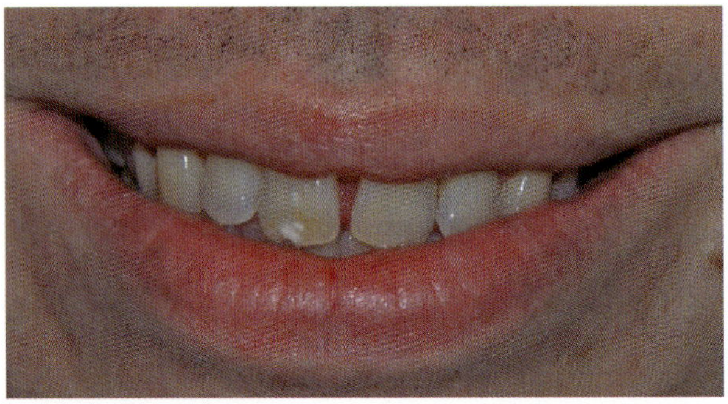

(A)

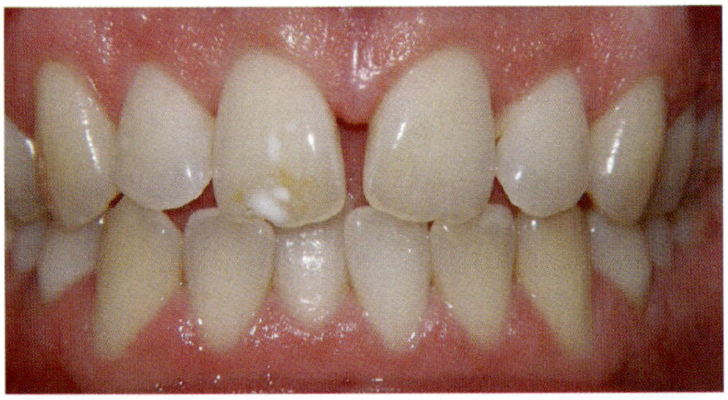

(B)

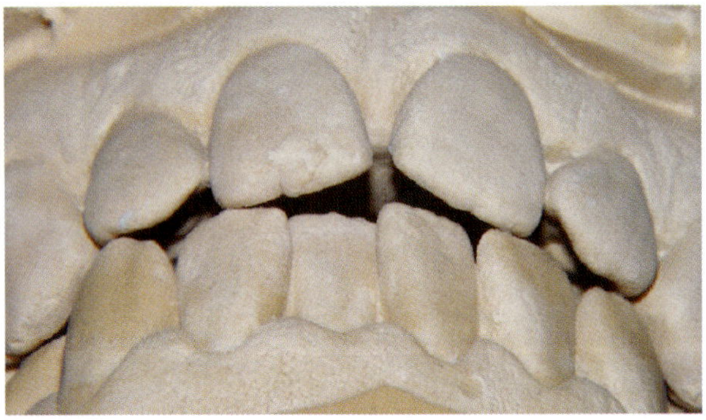

(C)

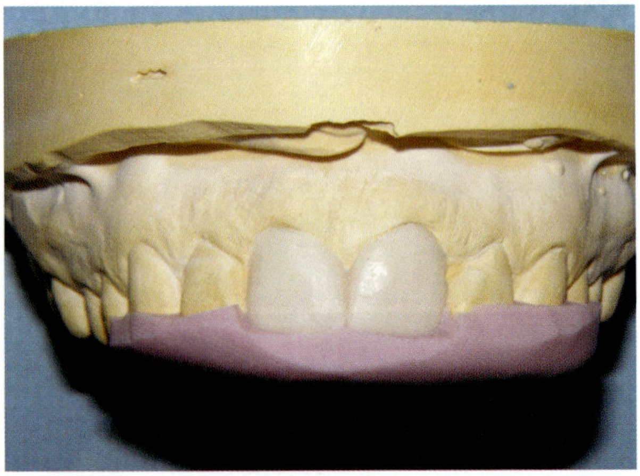

(D)

Figure 17.2

(A) Appearance of the teeth before whitening (smile view). The patient had brown and white marks on his upper right central incisor. (B) Retracted view of the patient before whitening. (C) Study models to analyze occlusion before bonding assessment. (D) Diagnostic tooth-colored wax-up model showing how the teeth would look before any bonding treatment. This allows the patient to visualize the appearance of the teeth with the diastema closed.

continued on the next page

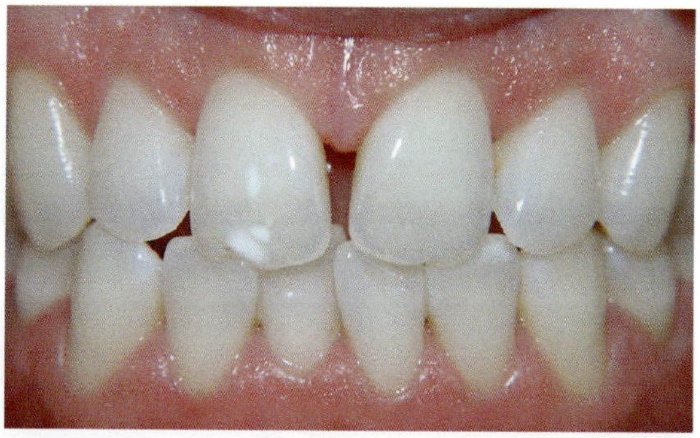

(E)

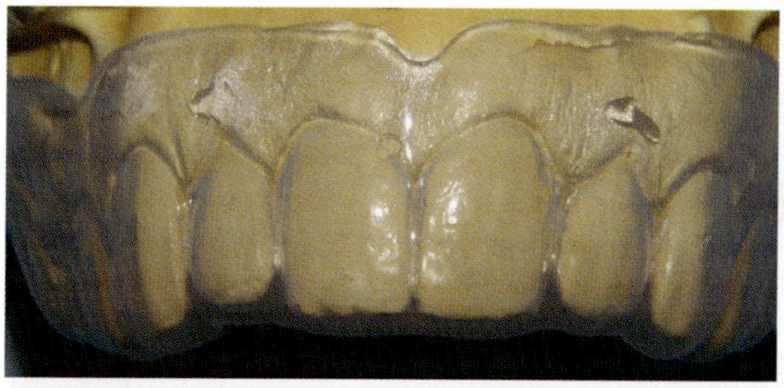

(F)

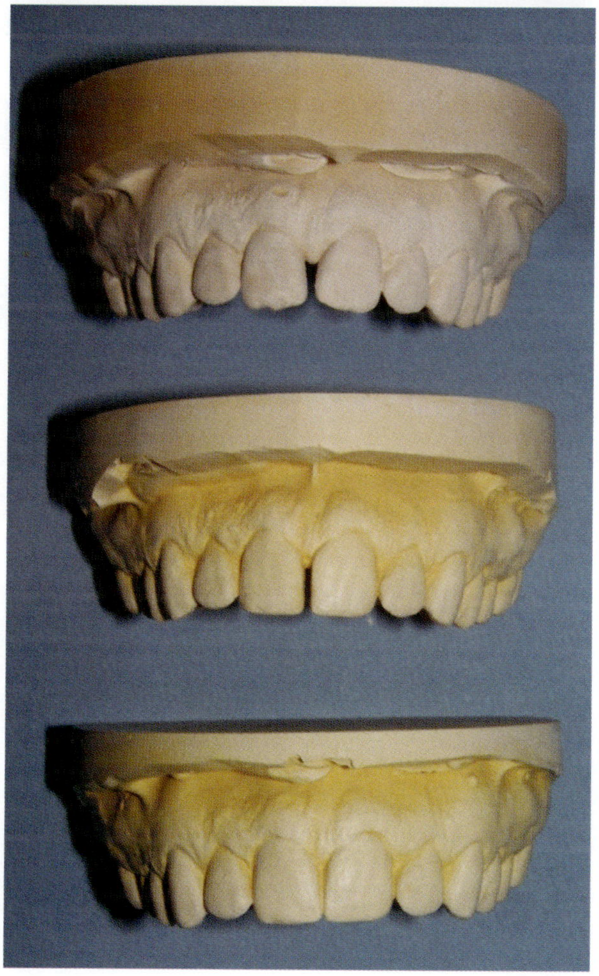

(G)

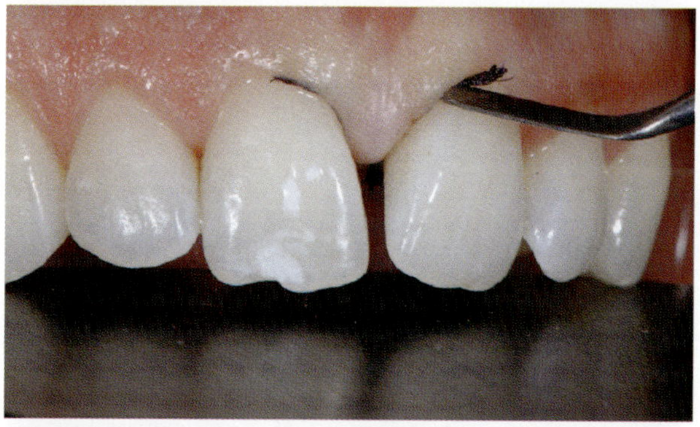

(H)

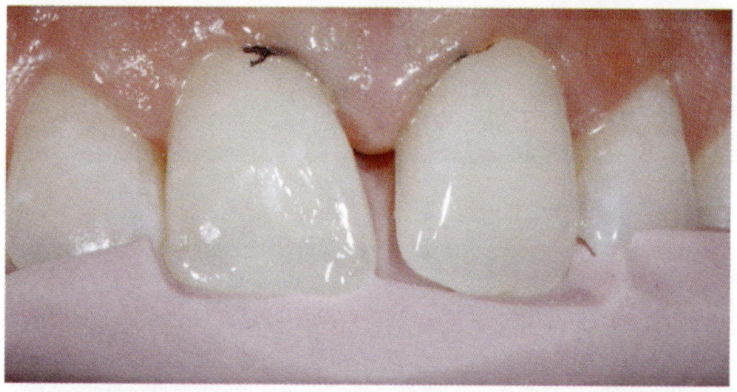

(I)

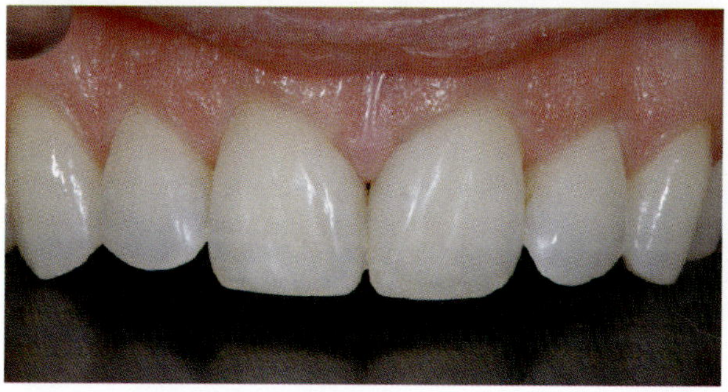

(J)

Figure 17.2 continued

(E) Appearance of the teeth after whitening and microabrasion treatment. (F) Blow-down model to help with composite bonding from the buccal surface, which is made from a duplicate copy of the wax-up. (G) Three sets of study casts showing the preoperative model, the diastema closed halfway, and the diastema fully closed. This helps the patient to visualize the appearance of the teeth after bonding. The patient took these study casts home to show his family to help him decide on the final appearance of the teeth. (H) In preparation for bonding, retraction cords are placed. (I) The first layer of enamel composite is placed from the palatal surface using the silicone matrix. This helps for accurate placement. (J) Final result after bonding.

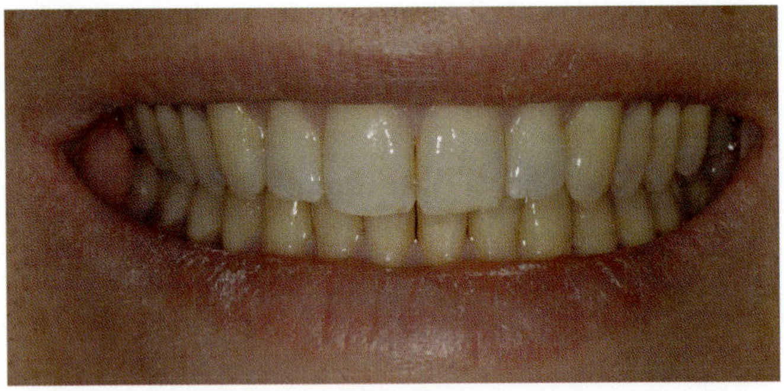

(A)

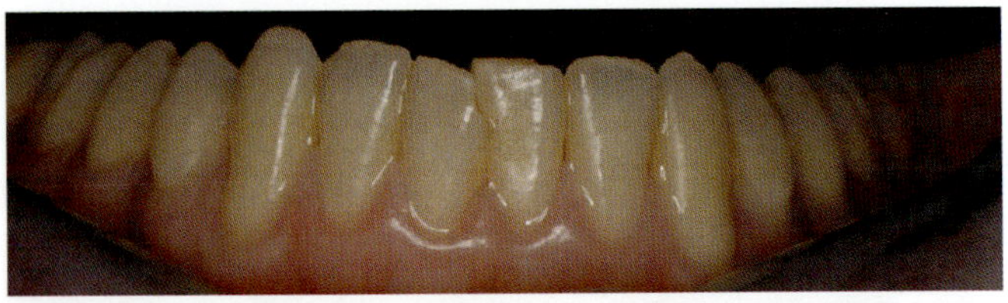

(B)

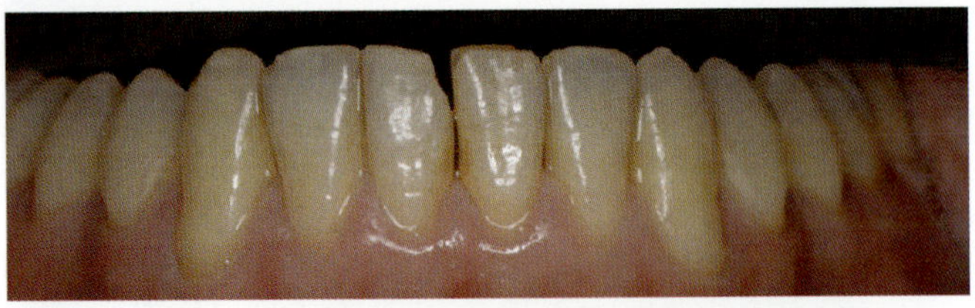

(D)

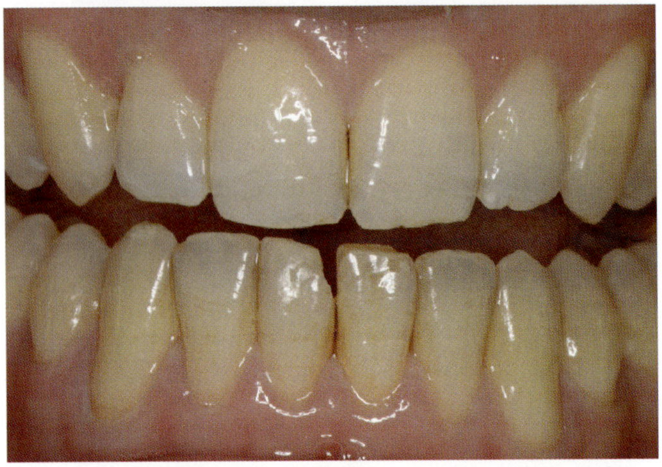

(C)

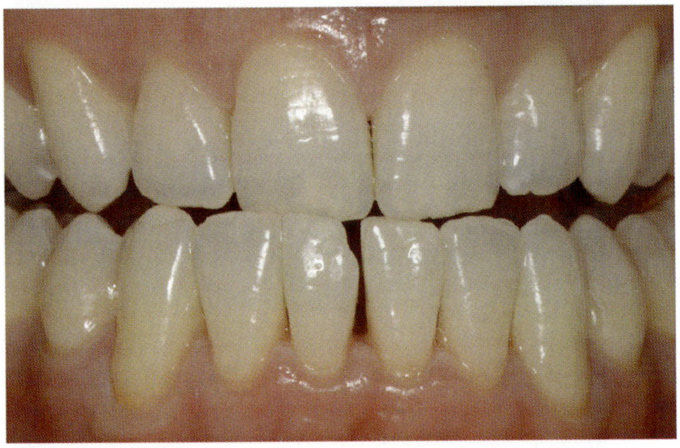

(F)

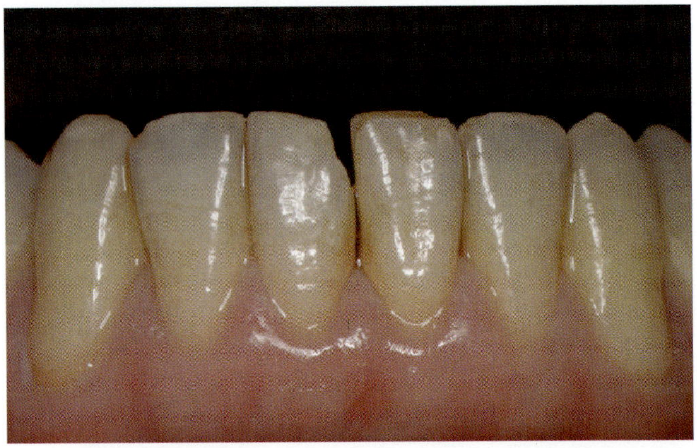

(E)

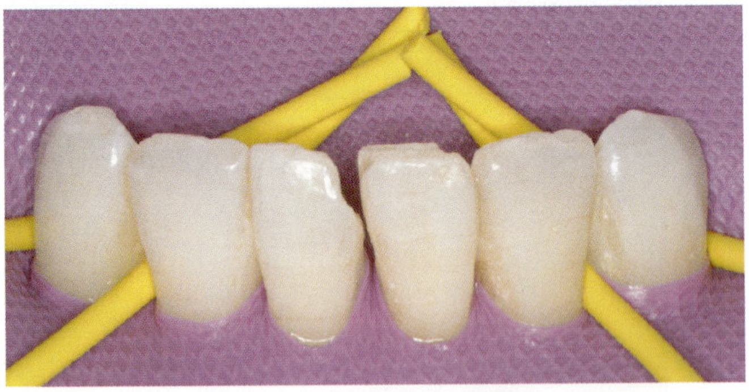

(G)

Figure 17.3

(A) Appearance of the teeth before any whitening treatment. This patient underwent a course of orthodontic treatment first. This was followed by whitening treatment and then composite bonding treatment. (B) Appearance of the lower teeth before orthodontic treatment. The two lower central incisors are crowded because there is insufficient space. (C) Appearance of the teeth after orthodontic treatment. (D) Appearance of the lower teeth after completion of orthodontic treatment. (E) Close-up view of the lower central incisors after orthodontic treatment. (F) Appearance of the teeth after whitening treatment to the upper and lower teeth. (G) In preparation for bonding, the teeth were isolated and cleaned using the Aquacut Sylc setting. This is a bioglass that contains calcium and phosphate. It cleans and conditions the teeth before bonding. The surface stains are removed and the enamel margins of the restoration are cleaned and sandblasted using the Aquacut machine on the abrasion Sylc setting.

continued on the next page

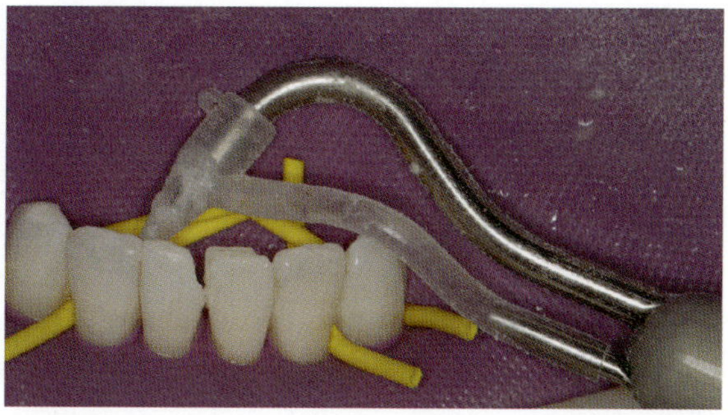

(H)

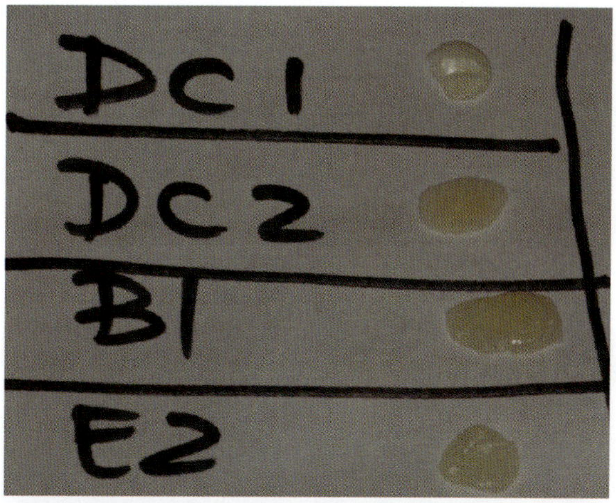

(I)

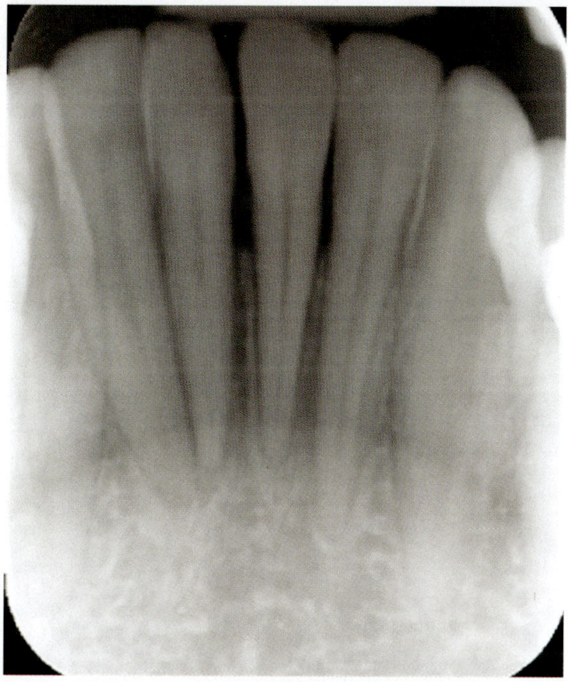

(J)

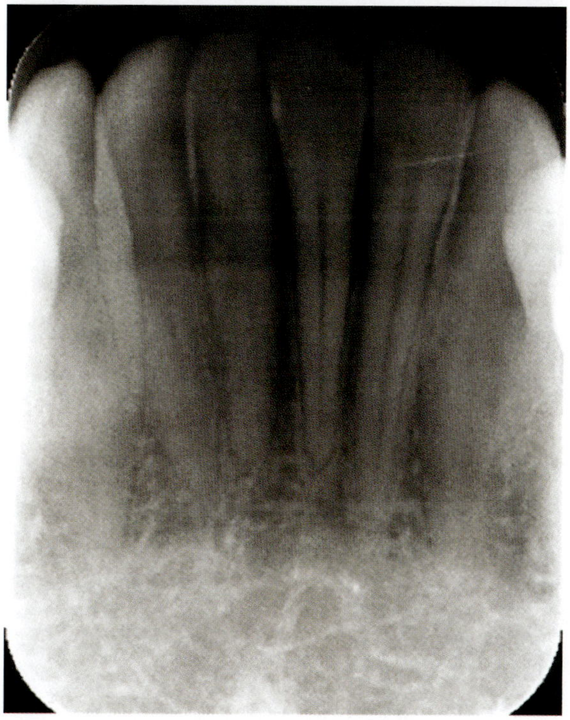

(K)

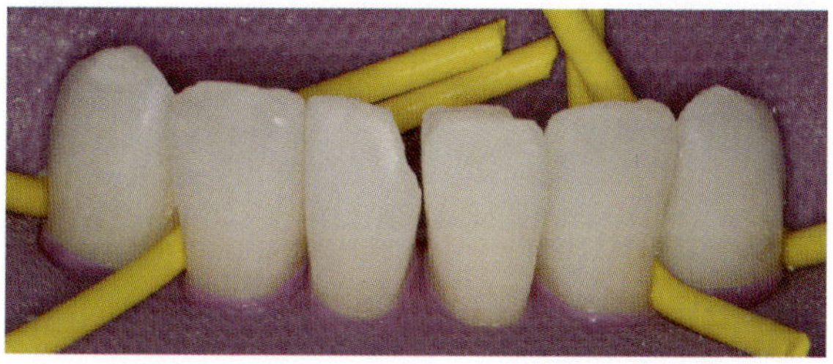

(L)

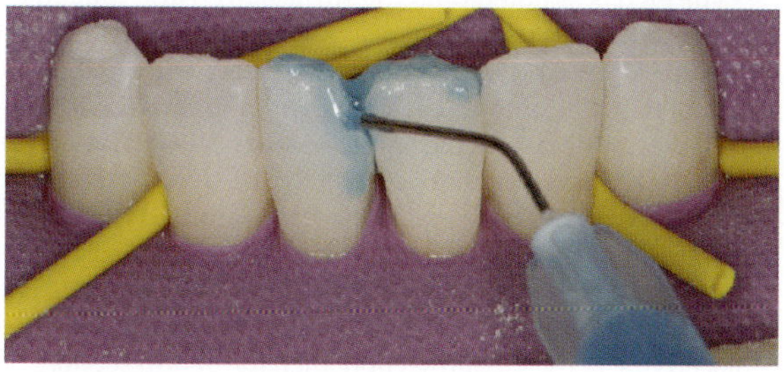

(M)

Figure 17.3 continued

(H) Applicator has a water jet to help clean all the surfaces of the teeth. (I) The shade selection of the teeth is undertaken before isolation to ensure that the teeth are not dehydrated and thus lighter. Composite shade selection is one of the first stages to be undertaken before full bonding. The shades are mapped out on a sheet of nonstick bonding paper. The restoration was undertaken using Aura composite, which is a layering composite from SDI Australia. (J) Anterior periapical radiograph before orthodontic treatment. (K) Anterior periapical radiograph after completion of orthodontic treatment. (L) Appearance of the teeth once they are fully clean and the stain has been removed. (M) Once the teeth are fully clean and air abraded, the 37% phosphoric acid etching gel is placed on the tooth to be bonded.

continued on the next page

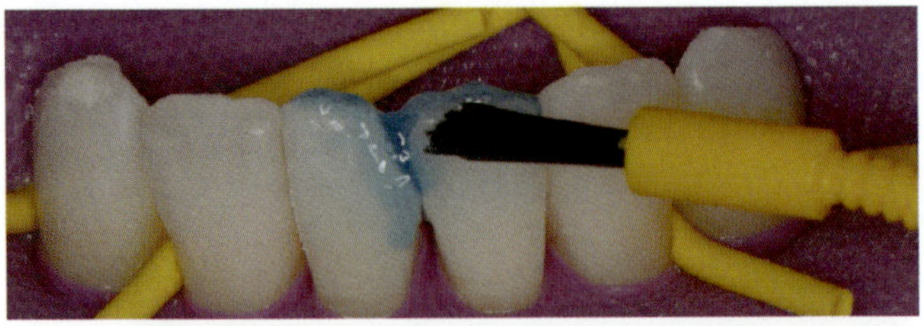
(N)

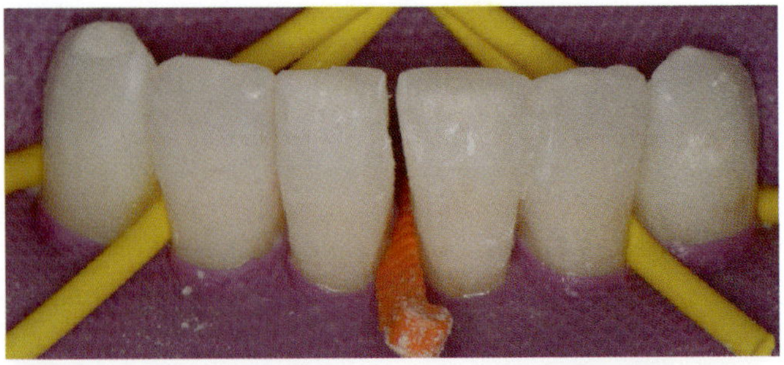
(O)

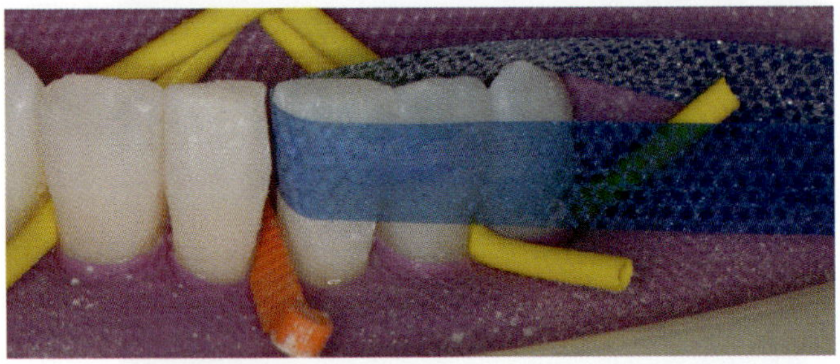
(P)

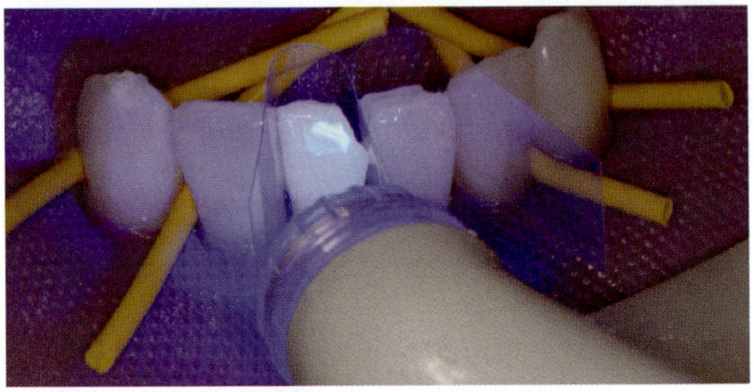
(Q)

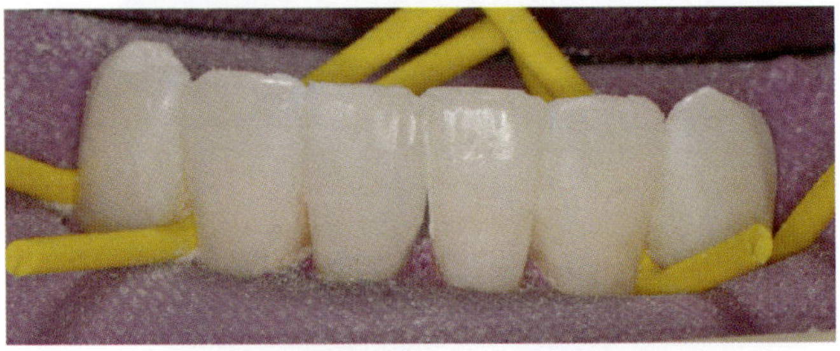
(R)

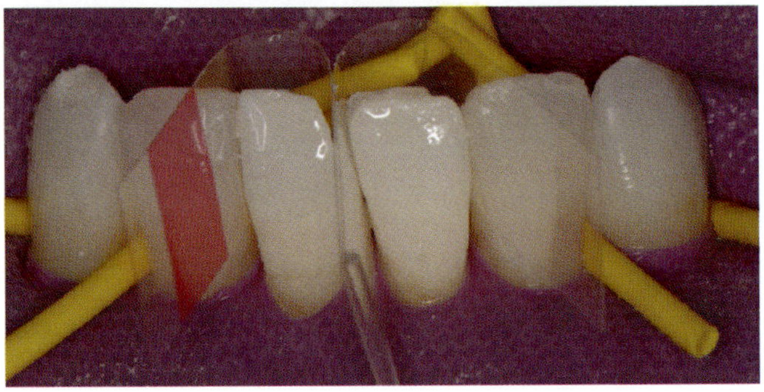
(S)

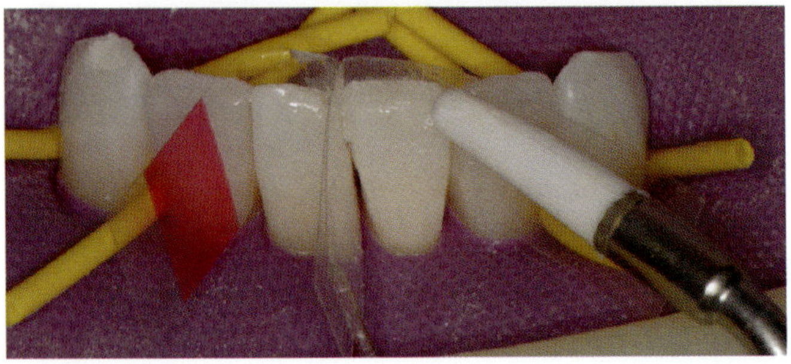
(T)

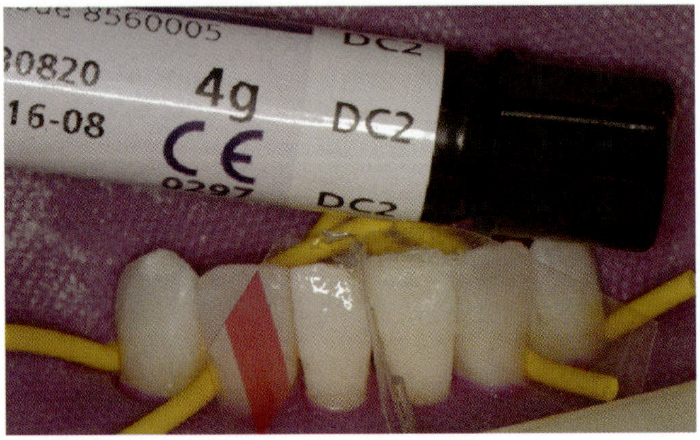

(U)

Figure 17.3 continued

(N) The etch is agitated onto the surface to ensure that all the etching gel penetrates the tooth. (O) A plastic wedge is placed between the teeth to ensure no overhangs of composite occur. (P) When bonding, it is essential that the contours of the teeth are symmetric. Excess composite is removed with an Epitec sandpaper strip. (Q) The dentin layer of composite is placed and light cured. (R) The layering is almost complete at this stage. (S) The matrix strips are contoured for easy composite placement. The matrices are rounded and then bonded gently into place for ease of placement of the composite. (T) The composite is contoured with a rubber sculpting instrument. (U) The dentin is layered. Enamel is placed first at the palatal section, then the dentin section. Shade DC1, Aura nanohybrid composite. *continued on the next page*

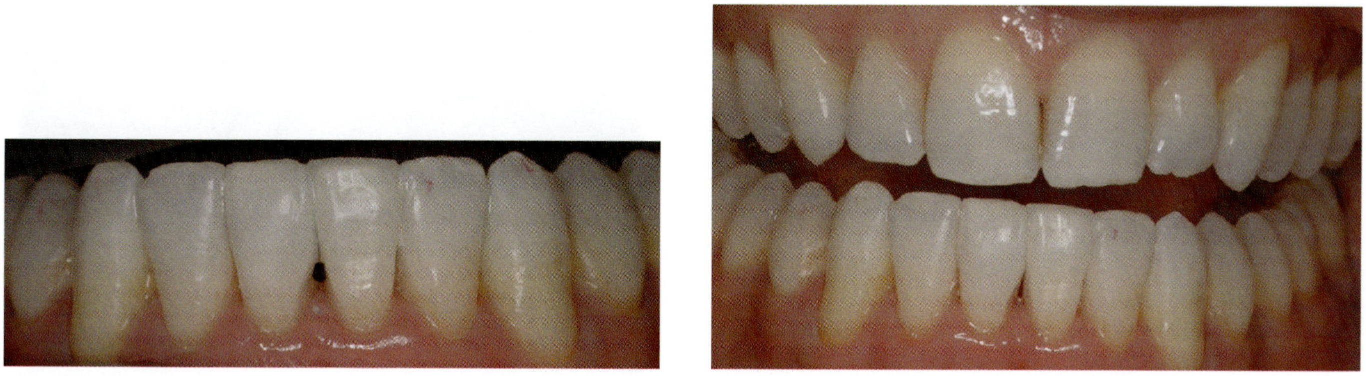

(V) (W)

Figure 17.3 continued

(V) Final shape of the Class IV restoration. (W) Appearance of the teeth after bonding.

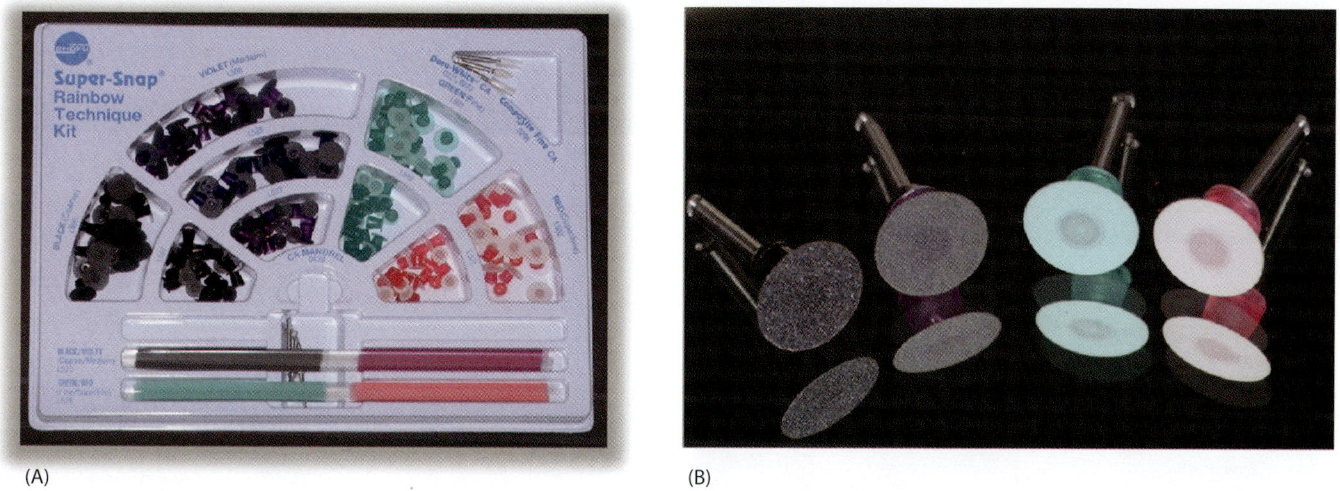

(A) (B)

Figure 17.4

(A) Shofu finishing kit contains sandpaper disks and sandpaper strips for final contouring. (B) Close-up view of the sandpaper disks in increasing coarseness, left to right.

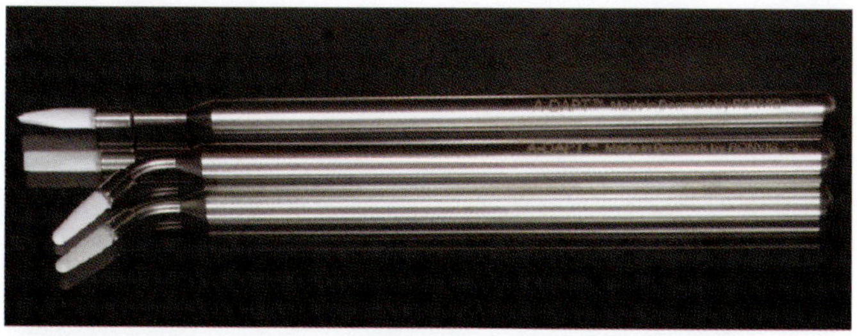

Figure 17.5

Rubber-tipped nonstick sculpting instruments (Optident).

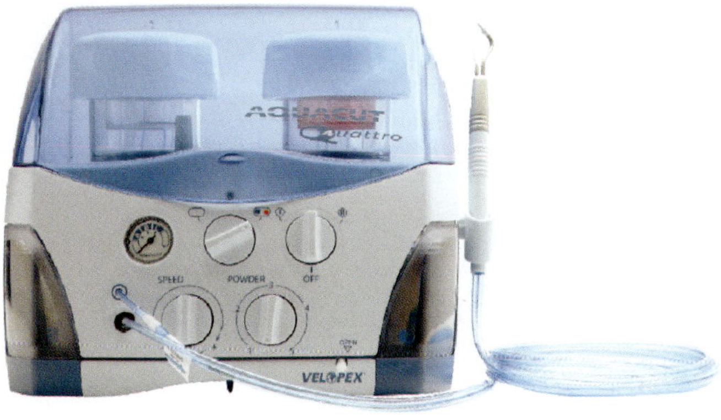

Figure 17.6

Aquacut air abrasion unit (Velopex International).

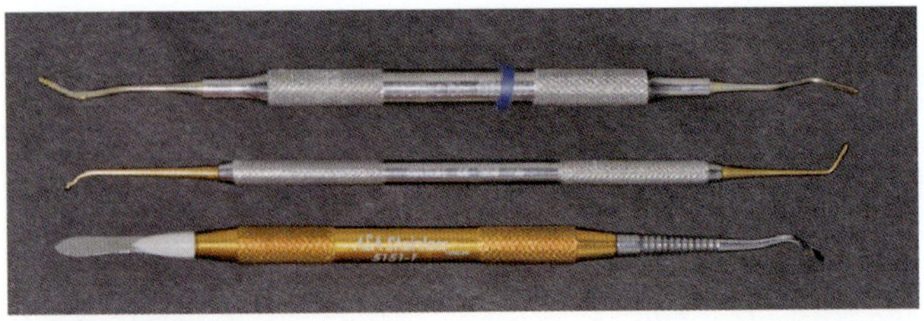

Figure 17.7

Composite placement instruments that are frequently used for composite bonding after whitening (www.enlightensmiles.co.uk, www.cosmedent.com).

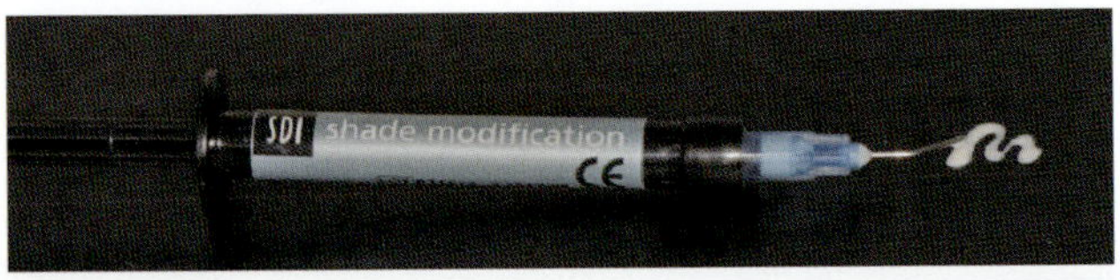

(A)

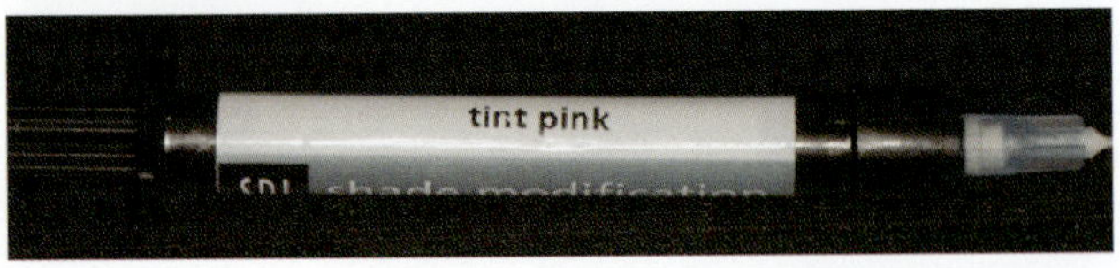

(B)

Figure 17.8

(A) Opaquing material used to block dark cervical areas. (B) Pink opaquer is effective in masking dark root areas.

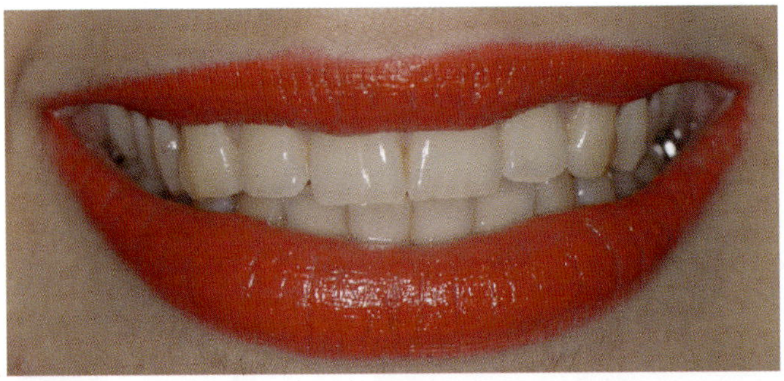

(A)

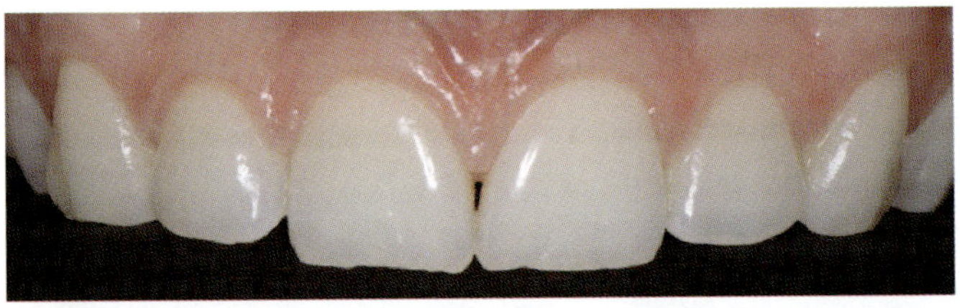

(B)

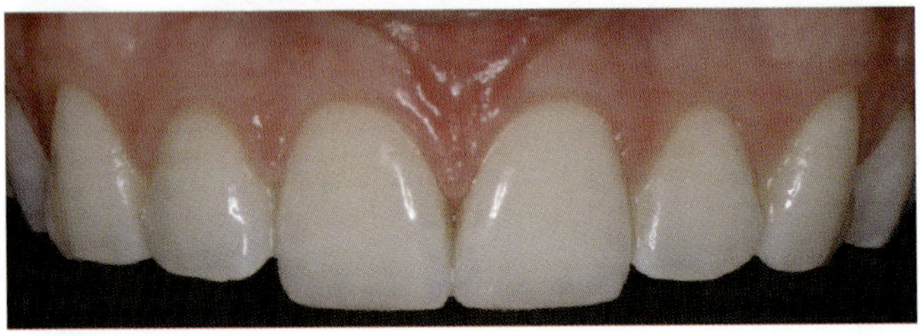

(C)

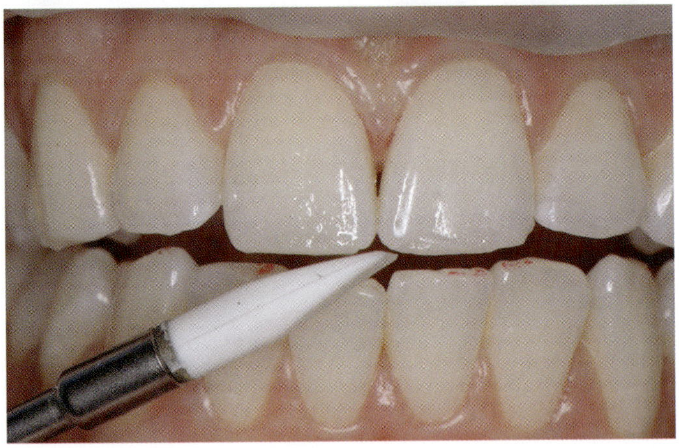

(D)

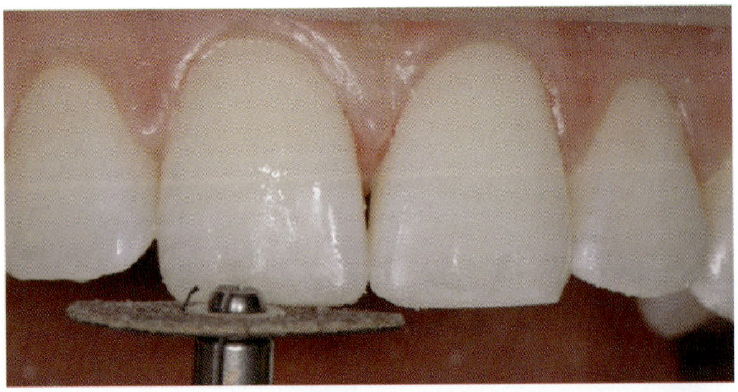

(E)

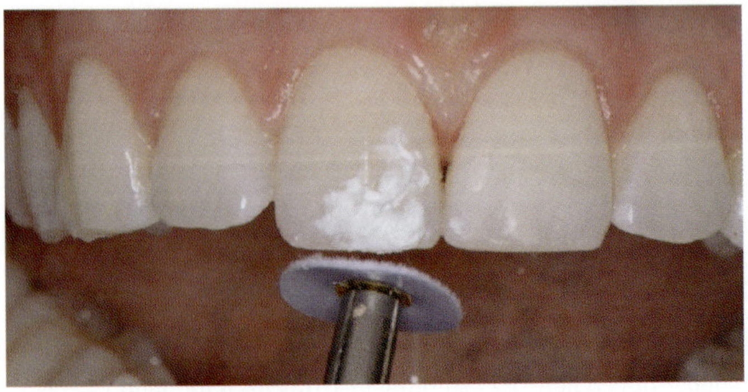

(F)

Figure 17.9

(A) Appearance of the teeth before whitening. (B) Appearance of the teeth after whitening; the incisal edges are worn from grinding. (C) Final appearance of the teeth after incisal edge bonding. (D) Sculpting the incisal edges. (E) Smoothening the incisal edge with a Sof-Lex disk (3M, St. Paul, MN). (F) Final polishing of the incisal edge with a felt disk and polishing paste.

18 COMPARISON OF TOOTH BLEACHING RESULTS

Brian Millar

VITAL TOOTH BLEACHING

Tooth bleaching is considered to be the treatment of choice for discolored teeth, provided the patient has realistic expectations and the teeth are acceptably shaped and intact. Tooth bleaching is noninvasive and less expensive than porcelain or composite veneers. It also has a place as a prerestorative treatment before other noninvasive esthetic procedures such as edge bonding and after tooth realignment. However, it can be unpredictable in outcome, particularly in the longer term as color regression occurs.

Methods

The main bleaching techniques are as follows:

1. Dentist-administered bleaching—in-office bleaching using high-concentration hydrogen peroxide or high-concentration (e.g., 35%) carbamide peroxide.
2. Dentist-provided and patient-applied bleaching—home bleaching or Nightguard Vital Bleaching (NGVB) using lower concentrations, typically 10–22% carbamide peroxide or 1–10% hydrogen peroxide.
3. Over-the-counter (OTC) products—these products typically contain low levels of bleaching agent (e.g., 3–8% hydrogen peroxide) that are self-applied to the teeth via gum shields, strips, paint-on products, or toothpaste.

IN-OFFICE VITAL TOOTH BLEACHING TECHNIQUES

In-office vital bleaching is usually performed using high concentrations (35–37%) of hydrogen peroxide in conjunction with heat and/or light (Haywood 1998), often referred to as "power bleaching." Activation can be by halogen curing lights, light-emitting diodes (LEDs), diode lasers, argon lasers, and plasma arc lamps. The advantage of this method for the patient is questionable, because the more rapid color change observed is largely a result of dehydration, but the disadvantages of in-office bleaching are significant:

1. The caustic nature of the 35–50% hydrogen peroxide, with the potential for soft tissue damage to patient and provider.
2. The discomfort of the rubber dam and drying of the oral cavity during treatment, and higher incidence of pain after treatment.
3. The effect of temperature on the pulp and the resultant post-treatment sensitivity.
4. If etching is performed, polishing is required after each visit, with some enamel loss (Leonard et al. 1998).
5. The treatment time required, which makes this procedure more expensive than home bleaching.
6. The unpredictable nature of the result and greater risk of irreversible damage (see Figure 18.1).
7. The unknown duration of the treatment (Ritter et al. 2002).
8. Significant and rapid relapse and the need to repeat the entire procedure.

TRAY-APPLIED BLEACHING

Originally termed *Nightguard Vital Bleaching* (Haywood and Heymann 1989), this type of bleaching typically involves the application of a 10% carbamide peroxide solution in a custom-fitted nightguard for 6–8 hours at night. Nowadays, shorter bleaching cycles can be used to avoid overnight wear, and hence *home bleaching* is a more accurate term. Results are typically seen in 2–3 weeks, and the final outcome is complete in 5–6 weeks (Haywood 1998). Some patients prefer daytime wearing of the tray, which has the advantage of more frequent replenishment of the bleaching gel for maximum bleaching effect (Dunn 1998).

Advantages of at-home vital tooth bleaching include a lower cost to patient and clinician with minimal in-office chair time, less post-treatment discomfort, a high percentage of successful treatments, and ease of touch-up re-treatments at low cost. However, the disadvantage with home bleaching is poor compliance because the procedure takes weeks to complete.

COMPARISON OF CARBAMIDE PEROXIDE AND HYDROGEN PEROXIDE

Bleaching with carbamide peroxide differs from use of hydrogen peroxide (Haywood 2006a) because hydrogen peroxide breaks down in minutes into a perhydroxyl free radical (HO_2) and then into $H_2O + O_2$ (Zantnera et al. 2007). On the other hand, carbamide peroxide breaks down into urea and hydrogen peroxide, which then follows the same path. A 10% carbamide peroxide solution is equivalent to 3.5% hydrogen peroxide and 6.5% urea. The effect of the urea is partly to increase the pH during treatment and give the bleaching medium a longer period of release of peroxide (Haywood 2006b). The urea also converts to carbon dioxide and ammonia, which further raises the pH to facilitate bleaching, explaining why carbamide peroxide is more effective than hydrogen peroxide (Goldstein and Garber 1995).

COLOR REGRESSION AFTER IN-OFFICE BLEACHING

Several in vitro and in vivo studies have demonstrated the efficacy of in-office bleaching procedures with various concentrations of hydrogen peroxide or carbamide peroxide. However, although immediate effects after bleaching were good, color stability was poor. Rosenstiel et al. (1991) measured color and its stability after a single 30-minute session of in-office bleaching with 35% hydrogen peroxide activated with light. The initial color change decreased considerably shortly after treatment, with more than half the color change reversed 1 week after bleaching. Further relapse reduced the color change to only 28% of the original change by 6 to 9 months. Interestingly, repeated in-office bleaching did not significantly increase the immediate or long-term bleaching result (Rosenstiel et al. 1991b).

Gottardi et al. (2006) showed that the number of in-office treatments using 35% hydrogen peroxide with light may influence patients' satisfaction and color retention. One to four sessions were performed and each session resulted in improvement of 2.1 to 3.7 Vita shade units. A significant color relapse, typically of two units, was observed at the 2-week postbleaching evaluation. Not surprisingly, more relapse was recorded for the patients who had fewer bleaching sessions.

Tooth dehydration associated with in-office treatment could lead to false evaluation of the actual shade change; the new shade regresses quickly as teeth rehydrate (Jones et al. 1999). Kugel et al. (2006) showed greater rebound with a light-activated product than a chemically activated gel despite greater initial color improvement. To allow rehydration of teeth, Al Shethri et al. (2003) postponed color evaluation until 1 week after bleaching. The results showed that relapse began after the bleaching treatments were finished and continued until the fifth week, after which no further significant changes appeared. Other studies have shown similar relapse patterns wherein the color stabilized by 6 weeks at a level still significantly different from the baseline color (Matis et al. 2007).

ACTIVATION METHOD

An evaluation of eight different in-office light-activated products with hydrogen peroxide concentrations of 15–35% found no statistical differences among groups (Matis et al. 2007). As in other reports, there was a significant bleaching immediately after treatment, followed by a sudden drop by week 1 with a mean reversal of 51% of the original gain. This increased to a 65% reversal by 6 weeks after bleaching. Although the sample size was small, the pattern among all the products was similar, with sudden improvement followed by a significant relapse. Fortunately for most products the relapse is to a final color that is lighter than the original.

In a comparison among (1) 25% hydrogen peroxide gel with light enhancement, (2) hydrogen peroxide gel alone, and (3) light alone with no peroxide, improved bleaching was observed when the light was used, but the color rebound was extensive in all groups, with 41–51% of initial gains lost over 30 days (Kugel 2009). This study showed that light activation increased in-office bleaching although the magnitude of the color improvement was relatively small and the improvement was followed by extensive relapse.

Tavares et al. (2003) showed that on average the peroxide-and-light treatment resulted in significantly greater color change (over eight shades) than peroxide alone (under six shades) in shades taken immediately after treatment by one examiner using a shade guide only. However, this is unlikely to be observed after the inevitable rebound has taken place and indicates the importance of measuring shade at least 1 week after bleaching. Also, the accuracy and validity of measuring by a single operator using a shade guide has to be questioned.

Marson et al. (2008) found no statistically significant differences observed with or without the use of a curing light in relation to color change after in-office bleaching treatment. There was a slight color relapse after 6 months, but there were no statistically significant differences between the groups.

Another study reported no statistical difference between results obtained with light irradiation and those obtained without light and proposed that the use of a light source should be considered optional for this technique when using high-concentration hydrogen peroxide (Bernardon et al. 2010). An evaluation of the efficacy of two bleaching agents (35% hydrogen peroxide and 37% carbamide peroxide) with a range of light sources (halogen lamp and plasma arc lamp, LED/diode laser, argon laser) and no light source in a short in vitro study showed that carbamide peroxide significantly differed from hydrogen peroxide and was less effective in color change but provided a more stable outcome (Lima et al. 2009).

COLOR REGRESSION AFTER NIGHTGUARD VITAL BLEACHING

The substantial increase in color value (lightness) and decrease in chroma observed directly after bleaching is often followed by a decrease in bleaching, indicating that the initial bleaching effect is not stable (Wiegand et al. 2008). Initial color relapse can occur because the residual peroxide in the tooth changes its optical qualities (Haywood 2000), then further color regression toward baseline shades can occur (Wiegand et al. 2008). Shade regression is a common problem that can be affected by a number of factors including the bleaching agent, method and duration of treatment, initial color, and cause of discoloration (Burrows 2009).

The process of color reversion toward darker shades is poorly described but is suspected to be the opposite of the bleaching events (Heymann et al. 1998). Some previously oxidized substances may become chemically reduced and so cause the tooth to return to the original discoloration. Also, the enamel may become remineralized with the staining molecule of the original systemic stain (Lyons and Ng 1998). This has been correlated with the presence of the remineralization processes within the tooth tissue (Li et al. 2010). In addition, external chromogens (coffee, wine, nicotine, metallic ions) might contribute to the color regression of bleached teeth. An in vitro study (Berger et al. 2008) suggested that 35% hydrogen peroxide promoted alterations in the enamel surface, which increased wine staining susceptibility up to 1 week after the bleaching when compared with unbleached enamel surfaces. Figure 18.1 illustrates an extreme example of this.

NIGHTGUARD VITAL BLEACHING WITH 10% CARBAMIDE PEROXIDE

This simple technique is popular for bleaching teeth both as a definitive treatment and before reshaping with composite resin (see Figure 18.2). Note that bleaching alone (see Figure 18.2B) does not improve the overall esthetics of the smile because the extreme "white" accentuates the contrasting shape and space defects, the "black" components. Retaining some natural color in the teeth and providing shape correction provides a more natural esthetic appearance (see Figure 18.2C). Even after many years of service, this completely noninvasive therapy looks acceptable (see Figure 18.2D) with no damage to the teeth or surrounding tissues, unlike most esthetic treatments.

Gels vary in efficacy, and one study (Cibirka et al. 1999) that compared two 10% carbamide peroxide gels overnight for 2 weeks found statistically significant lightening for both products (90% and 93% lightening) after 1 week of treatment. A study investigating 3 weeks of overnight bleaching resulted in significant lightening in 96% of the tested group immediately after treatment, and the improvement in lightness was maintained for 6 months in 88% of this group (Dos Santos Medeiros and de Lima 2008). Only 4% of participants had a one-unit reduction on the Vita classical shade guide from day 21 to day 30, and only 12% color reversal was observed at 6 months. It was concluded that NGVB was effective for lightening tooth color both for the period immediately after treatment and for the 6-month follow-up period, with no difference observed in the tooth color immediately after bleaching and after 30 days.

Immediate results are usually impressive, and in some studies all patients had at least a two-shade lightening effect when evaluated immediately after the 2 weeks of bleaching (Swift et al. 1997). However, some loss of the bleaching effect was observed in time, with 97% and 89.6% of patients having teeth lighter than at baseline at the 3-month and 6-month reviews, respectively.

Most studies have reported that color stabilization takes a few weeks, and so studies that record the final shade immediately after the bleaching period will obtain falsely optimistic results. Color relapse begins after bleaching treatment is completed and continues until the sixth week, after which it tends to remain stable for 3 months (Zekonis et al. 2003). Other studies report that color relapse after at-home treatment occurs mainly during the first month after bleaching (Matis et al. 1998). The colors at weeks 6, 12, and 24 were not significantly different from one another, which shows that the main color loss occurred between weeks 2 and 6 of the study.

The type of tooth and the initial tooth color appear to influence the relapse: the yellower the teeth at baseline, the greater the magnitude of the bleaching response (Matis et al. 1998). Canine teeth are usually more chromatic than the adjacent lateral incisors, which can be a concern in some patients in whom the contrast is marked (see Figure 18.3).

Canines show significantly greater color changes immediately after bleaching compared with incisors (Gegauff et al. 1993). However, greater initial bleaching effects often result in greater color relapse. After 5 days of bleaching in a group of 20 young patients, the canines showed the greatest color change (Gegauff et al. 1993). Most of the color relapse occurred by 1 week after treatment, with little difference between 1-month and 3-month measurements, indicating that the color had stabilized. Rosenstiel et al. (1996) conducted a 6-month study in a larger group of older subjects and found that the greatest color change was obtained after 1 week for the canines. The older patients showed less bleaching but also less color reversal. This is in agreement with others, who have reported higher levels of color change for canines than for lateral and central incisors at all points after treatment (Gegauff et al. 1993). Initial color regression occurred sooner for incisors (4 weeks) and took longer for canines (10 weeks), but neither regressed back to baseline for the duration of this 6-month study. Color can therefore be considered to have stabilized by 4 weeks after treatment in incisor teeth and by 10 weeks after treatment in canine teeth.

A particular problem is managing the missing lateral incisor tooth when the canine color is particularly dark (see Figure 18.4). Single-tooth color correction can easily be achieved through the use of a 10% carbamide peroxide gel on a single tooth (Millar 1994).

TOUCH-UPS

Longitudinal studies report satisfactory shade retention once the color stabilizes after the initial relapse. In addition, rebleaching may improve shade stability after active treatment. Among studies, controversy exists over the time period necessary before rebleaching.

Grobler et al. (2010) found that 10% carbamide peroxide used for a period of 14 days provided significant esthetic results for up to 6 months after bleaching. It was suggested that rebleaching after 6 months is not necessary but should be carried out about 14 months after treatment. Better color retention was reported in another small study at 2 years after the initial bleaching treatment (Swift et al. 1999). Although some relapse from the original lightening effect occurred, the median shade measured at 2 years was the same as that measured at 6 months after bleaching. This is in agreement with Small (1994), who indicated that the longevity of the bleaching effect seems to be acceptable and maintained well for 18 months with little or no relapse.

Leonard et al. (2001) reported that 10% carbamide peroxide was effective in lightening teeth in 98% of the patients, with this effect being sustained for 47 months after treatment in 82% of the participants. Leonard et al. reported that 92% of the participants in the active group had at least a two-shade change from baseline after 2 weeks of treatment, whereas at 6 months after treatment 88% still showed at least a two-shade change. At least 82% of the combined group had a two-shade change from baseline 47 months after treatment. Six of the participants had re-treated their teeth at 32 months.

Leonard (2000) stated that 42% of the patients, who had not had additional treatment during the post-treatment period, were satisfied with the shade of their teeth at approximately 7 years after treatment. No patient felt that the teeth had regressed to the original shade. Another study reported shade stability in 43% of the participants at approximately 10 years after treatment (Ritter et al. 2002).

It should be noted that in many studies the data on shade stability were collected from the participants' responses and so accuracy could be questionable. Although many participants indicated no change in color, the actual color might have relapsed after the original treatment.

NIGHTGUARD VITAL BLEACHING WITH DIFFERENT CONCENTRATIONS OF CARBAMIDE PEROXIDE

Several studies compared the efficacy and shade stability after bleaching with different carbamide peroxide concentrations in a tray system, and different findings were reported. Some studies reported faster color changes with higher concentrations of carbamide peroxide (Leonard et al. 1998).

In a comparison of 10% carbamide peroxide and 17% carbamide peroxide, noticeable changes of shade values were observed after 3 days in the 17% group and after 7 days in the 10% group. After 1 week, in both the 17% group and the 10% group, values for lightness and chroma were significantly different from the control with no statistical difference between the test groups. Two weeks after treatment, a rebound of shade values was observed in both test groups, with a statistically significant decrease in the values for lightness and chroma. Because there was a similar decrease in the 17% group and in the 10% group, final values did not differ. Major changes in shade values were found for canines as reported earlier in this chapter. Figure 18.3 shows a typical outcome for canines. Changes in lightness, chroma, and hue in canines were statistically different from those observed for incisors at each assessment after treatment.

A study comparing 10% carbamide peroxide and 15% carbamide peroxide over 4 weeks found that the difference in shade change from baseline between the two groups (10% and 15% carbamide peroxide) after 1 week of treatment was nonsignificant (Kihn et al. 2000). However, continuation of treatment for a week more revealed a significant difference in the two groups at the end of active treatment (2 weeks) and at the 2-week post-treatment evaluation. The 15% product was associated with significantly more color change than the 10% product (mean ± standard deviation [SD], 9.4 ± 2.3 and 7.7 ± 3.0, respectively). There was no color relapse observed at the end of active treatment or at the 2-week post-treatment evaluation in both groups.

However, the decision to perform the final color evaluation immediately after treatment or to wait 2 weeks is debatable. In studies that included postbleaching color evaluations after the teeth had an adequate time for color rebound, there were no significant differences in efficacy between lower and higher concentration products at the final evaluation, but different rates of color relapse can be observed (Browning and Swift 2007). Matis et al. (2000) reported color relapse for both 10% and 15% concentrations of carbamide peroxide as soon as subjects discontinued use of the bleaching material, with 15% showing greater relapse at 2 and 6 weeks; by the end of the study they reached almost identical values as in the 10% group. Although the post-treatment evaluation period in both studies was short, longer clinical trials of both concentrations seem to be in agreement with these findings.

Meireles (2008) conducted a clinical trial to evaluate two custom tray bleaching systems (10% and 16% carbamide peroxide) at 1 week after 3 weeks of active bleaching (Meireles 2008), at 6-month follow-up (Meireles et al. 2008), and at 1-year follow-up (Meireles et al. 2009). The studies also investigated aspects related to participants' diet and oral hygiene behaviors to evaluate their influence on the longevity of the bleaching effect of the bleaching treatment. The results of the study 1 year after bleaching showed that the teeth in both treatment groups remained at least 5.7 Vita classical shade guide units lighter than at baseline. Although the participants treated with 16% carbamide peroxide had median tooth shade values lower than those in the 10% carbamide peroxide group at the 1-week and 6-month evaluations, this difference was not present 1 year later. The bleaching effect obtained 1 week after bleaching was maintained in the 10% carbamide peroxide group but was decreased in the 16% carbamide peroxide group.

DIFFERENT CONCENTRATIONS OF CARBAMIDE PEROXIDE AND HYDROGEN PEROXIDE DURING DAYTIME USE

Most studies have agreed that the faster the rate of bleaching, the greater the relapse and the longer the time for the color to become stable. One study found that 20% carbamide peroxide demonstrated faster and greater color change compared with 7.5% hydrogen peroxide during a 2-week bleaching period (Mokhlis et al. 2000). Results obtained using a colorimeter also indicated that for both products, lightness increased rapidly during the first week and continued to increase at a slower rate through the second week. Both products exhibited relatively fast color relapse during the third week of the study. Color relapse continued at a slower rate until 6 weeks (4 weeks after bleaching), after which there was no significant change for either product. The teeth in the 20% carbamide peroxide group reflected color relapses at a higher rate than that for teeth in the 7.5% hydrogen peroxide group during the first 4 weeks after bleaching was discontinued. Use of the 20% carbamide peroxide resulted in significantly more lightness than the 7.5% hydrogen peroxide during the first 14 days of the study, but at the end of the study there was no significant difference between the two products.

EFFECT OF TRAY DESIGN

An evaluation of the effect of tray design on degree of color change using 15% carbamide peroxide suggested that trays with reservoirs had significantly higher amounts of color change initially than trays without reservoirs; however, the reservoir group then showed relapses at a higher rate when compared with the non-reservoir group, with no significant clinical difference (Matis et al. 2002a), in agreement with the findings of others (Javaheri and Janis 2000).

HIGH-CONCENTRATION CARBAMIDE PEROXIDE

Türkün et al. (2010) compared daytime at-home bleaching (28% carbamide peroxide) with the overnight application of 10% carbamide peroxide. The overnight application of 10% carbamide peroxide revealed a greater bleaching response immediately after treatment, and this difference remained significant at 1 year after treatment. Surprisingly, no significant difference was detected between post-treatment and 1-year follow-up. The bleaching effect remained similar 1 year after the bleaching treatment for both at-home bleaching systems, with little relapse occurring during this time, which suggests that touching up was being carried out.

The use of 35% carbamide peroxide in a close-fitting tray fitted by the clinician gives a useful low-cost option to boosting an NGVB regimen during treatment. An in vitro study (Patel et al. 2008) showed this material to be highly effective, and this can be used for single or multiple teeth.

NIGHTGUARD VITAL BLEACHING FOR SPECIFIC COLOR PROBLEMS

Bleaching works particularly well for teeth with a yellow hue (Ishikawa-Nagai et al. 2004). Treatment is less successful in teeth with a yellow-gray tone, and even less with a gray color. Particularly difficult are teeth with a brown-yellow color (Seale and Thrash 1985). For blue-gray stains the prognosis is probably the worst owing to poor bleaching and more frequent and faster relapse (Christensen 1998). Reports of color improvement in teeth having deep dentinal discoloration, such as tetracycline staining or brown staining from dentinogenesis imperfecta, reveal that some degree of color correction is possible and that persistence is the key to success (Haywood 1997). Studies report that longer active treatment is usually followed by a longer color relapse. Figure 18.5 illustrates the outcome of a 10-week regimen for a tetracycline case.

Haywood showed that bleaching with 10% carbamide peroxide in a custom-fitted tray for an extended period of 6 months produces variable amounts of lightening on tetracycline-stained teeth (Haywood et al. 1997). Stable color has been seen in 84% of the teeth treated at the 1-year recall without touch-ups. Most color relapse occurred in the first 6 months after treatment.

Leonard et al. (1999) conducted a longitudinal study to determine the color stability and patient satisfaction after 6 months of active treatment of tetracycline-stained teeth with 10% carbamide peroxide. Eighty-five percent of patients reported no obvious change at 6 and 12 months after treatment. At 54 months after treatment, at least 83% of the participants perceived no obvious change in tooth color or only a slight darkening from immediately after treatment. This had dropped to 60% at the 90-month post-treatment appointment. In this study, no one thought that the shade of his or her teeth was back to the original shade at any time point.

Matis et al. (2002b) compared the effectiveness of 6 months of overnight bleaching with different concentrations (10%, 15%, and 20% carbamide peroxide) in treating tetracycline discoloration. Tooth color changed rapidly in the first month and at 3 and 9 months. Although color lightening continued through 24 weeks for all three products, the teeth bleached with 10%, 15%, and 20% concentrations attained 54%, 60%, and 62% of the maximum lightness, respectively, after 1 month of bleaching.

The color change stabilized 2 months after bleaching for teeth treated with the 10% carbamide peroxide and 1 month after bleaching for teeth bleached with 15% carbamide peroxide. The color change had not stabilized by 3 months after bleaching for teeth treated with 20% carbamide peroxide. At 4.5 years after bleaching (Matis 2006), teeth treated with all three concentrations of bleaching agents had retained more than 65% of their original color change (the 10%, 15%, and 20% concentrations had retained 68%, 67%, and 66% of the total color change, respectively). In summary, it seems that those who bleach to remove stain caused by tetracycline might need to rebleach within 5 years.

White spots can also be managed through the use of tooth bleaching to reduce the color contrast (see Figure 18.6).

COMPARISON OF IN-OFFICE BLEACHING VERSUS NIGHTGUARD VITAL BLEACHING

Matis et al. (2007) reported that some in-office products lightened teeth immediately to the same degree after bleaching as occurs with at-home tray-based bleaching agents, but the color reversal in most of the products occurred more rapidly than was found in at-home tray-based bleaching products. Many opinion leaders agree that the efficacy of in-office bleaching is not as favorable as at-home bleaching treatment.

In a study by Zekonis et al. (2003), at 2 weeks the average ΔE (a measure of color change) reached 12.32 for at-home treatment and 5.32 for in-office treatment. For both groups the color relapse began after bleaching treatments were finished and continued until the sixth week. By 6 weeks, ΔE had decreased to 6.64 for at-home treatment and as low as just 3.63 for in-office treatment. In-office treatment color change and color relapse occurred at a lower rate compared with the at-home treatment. Color stabilized by 6 weeks for both at-home and in-office treatments at a level significantly different from baseline and between the treatments. In addition, 84% of the subjects reported the at-home treatment to be more efficient. None of the subjects reported the in-office bleaching treatment to be superior to the at-home bleaching treatment.

Similar observations were reported by Gottardi et al. (2006). Among patients who had two or three in-office appointments and were recorded as satisfied, 24 asked for at-home bleaching treatment. This indicated that even though results could be seen in one appointment for patients who had lighter teeth, more appointments were necessary to improve shade stability. These results agree with the findings of some researchers who have stated that teeth need more bleaching to achieve stabilization of shade (Goldstein and Garber 1995, Al Shethri et al. 2003).

An in vitro study comparing the different treatments showed that 10% carbamide peroxide was significantly more effective than all other treatments except 35% hydrogen peroxide with halogen activation (Patel et al. 2008). The effect of each treatment regimen over time showed that 10% carbamide peroxide gave a significant gain immediately and 1 week later; however, all the bleaching effects were lost over time after these single treatments.

In-office Bleaching Followed by Nightguard Vital Bleaching

To promote better color stability, the use of both in-office and at-home treatments has been recommended (Matis et al. 2009b). This is based on the understanding that in-office bleaching lightens teeth rapidly but is followed by a considerable relapse within 2 weeks of bleaching. In contrast, at-home bleaching usually requires several weeks of treatment but is followed by less reversal.

Bernardon et al. (2010) found that the technique associating one session of in-office bleaching with the home bleaching technique obtained higher ΔE values at the 1-week period only. After the second week, ΔE obtained for the hemi-arches bleached with this combination were not statistically different from ΔE obtained for teeth bleached using custom trays with 10% carbamide peroxide. Both techniques in this group presented color stability for up to 16 weeks. It has been shown that one session of in-office bleaching associated with home bleaching does not influence the maintenance of color with time.

The combination of in-office and at-home bleaching treatments has been reported as responsible for dramatic changes in tooth shade (Matis et al. 2009a), although there are no long-term studies of its efficacy. Figure 18.2 shows an example of this. The combination of 10% carbamide peroxide at home for 3 days after in-office 35% hydrogen peroxide gel resulted in 8.5 shade changes, and use of in-office 38% hydrogen peroxide gel resulted in nine shade changes. Both treatments resulted in an average shade rebound of two shades at 7 days after bleaching cessation.

In-office tooth bleaching followed by at-home bleaching with trays has been shown to be significantly more effective than in-office bleaching without at-home bleaching (Matis et al. 2009b). A review of nine published studies comparing the effectiveness of overnight, daytime, in-office, and OTC bleaching methods using meta-analysis showed that ΔE* values were 9.7 and 6.6 for overnight and daytime bleaching groups immediately after treatment (Matis et al. 2009a). Ten weeks after treatment the ΔE* value was 4.7 for the overnight bleaching group and 3.4 for the daytime bleaching group. For in-office bleaching the ΔE* value was 5.4 immediately after treatment and 2.1 10 weeks after bleaching. This favors the use of at-home bleaching over in-office bleaching, particularly when trays can be worn overnight.

CONCLUSION

The popularity of tooth bleaching has resulted in a dramatic rise in the number of bleaching products and procedures. Despite claims made in advertising, the scientific literature supports the use of at-home techniques (Table 18.1). Most studies have indicated that color improvement should be determined at least 2 weeks after the termination of active treatment and possibly as long as 6 weeks with higher concentrations of materials. This delay allows the oxygen generated from bleaching to dissipate from the tooth and avoids the misinterpretation of the effect of dehydration as true bleaching. Many commercials measure color too early and quote erroneous data.

Bleaching with carbamide peroxide is followed by a color relapse in 4 to 6 weeks, and this time differs for different concentrations. Higher concentrations have demonstrated faster and greater color change initially but also longer and greater color rebound. The color usually stabilizes by 6 weeks at a level still significantly different from baseline, but the reversal can reach 65% 6 weeks after bleaching.

Light use during in-office procedures does not seem to improve the longevity of bleaching. It was observed that the immediate change in the light-activated material seemed to be related to the dehydration effect of the isolation and heat of the light rather than any improvement in bleaching efficacy. There is a noticeable lack of studies

Table 18.1 Comparison of different bleaching techniques

	Technique	*Advantages*	*Disadvantages*
Home bleaching (Nightguard Vital Bleaching [NGVB])	Trays made and worn with the bleaching material inside for more than 2 hours (mainly worn overnight)	Minimal chair time; low cost for touch-up treatments	Poor compliance can mean the treatment takes weeks to complete.
In-office bleaching (power bleaching)	In-office bleaching with light or gel applied into trays and worn in office	More rapid color change; good for quick touch-up treatments	Color stability can be poor. Post-treatment sensitivity from temperature of light. Potential soft tissue damage. Long in-office treatment time.
Combined bleaching (NGVB and power bleaching)	In-office bleaching combined with NGVB (bleaching trays at home)	Better color stability; more effective results than in-office treatment alone	More in-office time. Not as cost-effective for patients.

showing benefit of the in-office techniques over at-home methods.

The yellower the teeth at baseline, the greater the magnitude of the bleaching response. This means a significant relationship between the patient's age and the magnitude of bleaching response. Younger subjects experience greater tooth bleaching but more relapse. Nevertheless, most of the initial shade improvement remains at 6 months after treatment.

Darker teeth such as canines have greater potential color change, which is followed by a longer time of color relapse. The relapse occurs at the same rate as for lighter incisors but it takes longer for the color to stabilize. This may explain the discrepancy in color relapse between studies.

The type of the initial discoloration significantly affects bleaching effectiveness and shade retention. Discoloration caused by aging or fluorosis changes shade more quickly than discoloration from trauma or tetracycline. Studies have concluded that teeth in the yellow range are easier to lighten than those stained gray. Teeth stained by tetracycline do not lighten as much as teeth stained by other means, requiring long and persistent treatment; this is followed by a color relapse for up to 6 months, after which the results may last 5 years.

The method of measuring color changes after bleaching may affect the results. Less relapse is usually reported when only shade guides and/or the patient's perception are used to evaluate the color retention.

However, despite shade relapse, numerous studies report good longevity of tooth bleaching with satisfactory retention of the shade change without re-treatment. Unfortunately, there are no similar reports in the literature about long-term results for in-office bleaching.

In summary:

- In-office bleaching results in greater relapse.
- Faster bleaching gives more relapse.
- Yellow teeth bleach more than gray teeth.
- Carbamide peroxide is the more effective product.
- Relapse slows by 6 weeks.

ACKNOWLEDGMENTS

I thank Dr. Magdalena Owen, BDS, MClinDent for assisting with the literature review.

REFERENCES

Al Shethri S, Matis BA, Cochran MA, Zekonis R. (2003) A clinical evaluation of two in-office bleaching products. *Oper Dent* **28:**488–95.

Berger SB, Coelho AS, Oliveira VA, Cavalli V. (2008) Enamel susceptibility to red wine staining after 35% hydrogen peroxide bleaching. *J Appl Oral Sci* **16:**201–4.

Bernardon JK, Sartori N, Ballarin A, Perdigão J. (2010) Clinical performance of vital bleaching techniques. *Oper Dent* **35:**3–10.

Browning WD, Swift EJ. (2007) Critical appraisal: comparison of the effectiveness and safety of carbamide peroxide whitening agents at different concentrations. *J Esthet Restor Dent* **19:**289–96.

Burrows S. (2009) A review of the efficacy of tooth bleaching. *Dent Update* **36:**537–51.

Christensen GJ. (1998) Bleaching teeth: report of a survey, 1997. *J Esthet Restor Dent* **10:**16–20.

Cibirka RM, Myers M, Downey MC, Nelson SK. (1999) Clinical study of tooth shade lightening from dentist-supervised, patient-applied treatment with two 10% carbamide peroxide gels. *J Esthet Restor Dent* **11:**325–31.

Dos Santos Medeiros MC, De Lima KC. (2008) Effectiveness of Nightguard Vital Bleaching with 10% carbamide peroxide—a clinical study. *J Can Dent Assoc* **74:**163–f.

Dunn J. (1998) Dentist-prescribed home bleaching: current status. *Compend Contin Educ Dent* **19:**760–4.

Gegauff AG, Rosenstiel SF, Langhout KJ. (1993) Evaluating tooth color change from carbamide peroxide gel. *J Am Dent Assoc* **124:**65–72.

Goldstein RE, Garber DA. (1995) *Complete dental bleaching.* Quintessence Publishing: Chicago, 6–28.

Gottardi MS, Brackett MG, Haywood VB. (2006) Number of in-office light-activated bleaching treatments needed to achieve patient satisfaction. *Quintessence Int* **7:**115–20.

Grobler SR, Hayward R, Wiese S, Moola MH. (2010) Spectrophotometric assessment of the effectiveness of Opalescence PF 10%: a 14-month clinical study. *J Dent* **38:**113–7.

Haywood VB. (1997) Extended bleaching of tetracycline-stained teeth: a case report. *Contemp Esthet Restor Pract* **1:**14–21.

Haywood VB. (1998) Nightguard Vital Bleaching and in-office bleaching. *Contemp Esthet Restor Pract* **2:**78–81.

Haywood VB. (2000) Current status of Nightguard Vital Bleaching. *Compend Contin Educ Dent* **21**(Suppl 28):S10–7.

Haywood VB. (2006a) Considerations for vital nightguard tooth bleaching with 10% carbamide peroxide after nearly 20 years of proven use. *Inside Dent* **9:**2–5.

Haywood VB. (2006b) Nightguard Vital Bleaching: indications and limitations. *US Dent* **18:**2–8.

Haywood VB, Heymann HO. (1989) Nightguard Vital Bleaching. *Quintessence Int* **20:**173–6.

Haywood VB, Leonard RH, Dickinson GL. (1997) Efficacy of six-months Nightguard Vital Bleaching of tetracycline-stained teeth. *J Esthet Restor Dent* **9:**13–9.

Heymann HO, Swift EJ Jr, Bayne SC, May KN Jr. (1998) Clinical evaluation of two carbamide peroxide tooth-whitening agents. *Compend Contin Educ Dent* **19:**359–76.

Ishikawa-Nagai S, Terui T, Ishibashi K, Weber HP. (2004) Prediction of optical efficacy of vital tooth bleaching using regression analysis. *Color Res Appl* **29:**390–4.

Javaheri DS, Janis JN. (2000) The efficacy of reservoirs in bleaching trays. *Oper Dent* **25:**149–51.

Jones AH, Diaz-Arnold AM, Vargas MA, Cobb DS. (1999) Colorimetric assessment of laser and home bleaching techniques. *J Esthet Restor Dent* **11:**81–4.

Kihn P, Barnes DM, Romberg E, Peterson K. (2000) A clinical evaluation of 10 percent vs 15 percent carbamide peroxide tooth whitening agent. *J Am Dent Assoc* **131:**1478–84.

Kugel G. (2009) Clinical trial assessing light enhancement of in-office tooth whitening. *J Esthet Restor Dent* **21:**336–47.

Kugel G, Papathanasiou A, Williams AJ 3rd, Anderson C. (2006) Clinical evaluation of chemical and light-activated tooth whitening systems. *Compend Contin Educ Dent* **27:**54–62.

Leonard RH Jr. (2000) Nightguard Vital Bleaching: dark stains and long-term results. *Compend Contin Educ Dent* **21**(Suppl 28):S18–27.

Leonard RH, Sharma A, Haywood VB. (1998) Use of different concentrations of carbamide peroxide for bleaching teeth: an in-vitro study. *Quintessence Int* **29:**503–7.

Leonard RH Jr, Bentley C, Eagle JC, Garland GE. (2001) Nightguard Vital Bleaching: a long-term study of efficacy, shade retention, side effects, and patients' perceptions. *J Esthet Restor Dent* **13:**357–69.

Leonard RH Jr, Haywood VB, Eagle JC, Garland GE. (1999) Nightguard Vital Bleaching of tetracycline-stained teeth: 54 months post treatment. *J Esthet Restor Dent* **11:**265–77.

Li Q, Xu BT, Li R, Yu H. (2010) Quantitative evaluation of colour regression and mineral content change of bleached teeth. *J Dent* **38:**253–60.

Lima DA, Aguiar FH, Liporoni PC, Munin E. (2009) In vitro evaluation of the effectiveness of bleaching agents activated by different light sources. *J Prosthodont* **18:**249–54.

Lyons K, Ng B. (1998) Nightguard Vital Bleaching: a review and clinical study. *N Z Dent J* **94:**100–3.

Marson FC, Sensi LG, Vieira LC, Araújo E. (2008) Clinical evaluation of in-office dental bleaching treatments with and without the use of light-activation sources. *Oper Dent* **33:**15–22.

Matis BA. (2006) Extended bleaching of tetracycline-stained teeth: a 5-year study. *Oper Dent* **31:**643–51.

Matis BA, Cochran MA, Eckert G. (2009a) Review of the effectiveness of various tooth whitening systems. *Oper Dent* **34:**230–35.

Matis BA, Cochran MA, Eckert G, Carlson TJ. (1998) The efficacy and safety of a 10% carbamide peroxide bleaching gel. *Quintessence Int* **29:**555–63.

Matis BA, Cochran MA, Franco M, Al-Ammar W. (2007) Eight in-office tooth whitening systems evaluated in vivo: a pilot study. *Oper Dent* **32:**322–7.

Matis BA, Cochran MA, Wang G, Eckert GJ. (2009b) A clinical evaluation of two in-office bleaching regimens with and without tray bleaching. *Oper Dent* **34:**142–9.

Matis BA, Hamdan YS, Cochran MA, Eckert GJ. (2002a) A clinical evaluation of a bleaching agent used with and without reservoirs. *Oper Dent* **27:**5–11.

Matis BA, Mousa HN, Cochran MA, Eckert GJ. (2000) Clinical evaluation of bleaching agents of different concentrations. *Quintessence Int* **31:**303–10.

Matis BA, Wang Y, Jiang T, Eckert GJ. (2002b) Extended at-home bleaching of tetracycline-stained teeth with different concentrations of carbamide peroxide. *Quintessence Int* **33:**645–55.

Meireles SS. (2008) Efficacy and safety of 10% and 16% carbamide peroxide tooth-whitening gels: a randomized clinical trial. *Oper Dent* **33:**606–12.

Meireles SS, Heckmann SS, Santos IS, Della Bona A. (2008) A double blind randomized clinical trial of at-home tooth bleaching using two carbamide peroxide concentrations: 6-month follow-up. *J Dent* **36:**878–84.

Meireles SS, Santos IS, Della Bona A, Demarco FF. (2009) A double-blind randomized controlled clinical trial of 10 percent versus 16 percent carbamide peroxide tooth-bleaching agents: one-year follow-up. *J Am Dent Assoc* **140:**1109–17.

Millar BJ. (1994) Home-bleaching for single tooth color correction. *J Esthet Dent* **6:**1–4.

Mokhlis GR, Matis BA, Cochran MA, Eckert GJ. (2000) A clinical evaluation of carbamide peroxide and hydrogen peroxide whitening agents during daytime use. *J Am Dent Assoc* **131:**1269–77.

Patel A, Louca C, Millar BJ. (2008) An in vitro comparison of tooth whitening techniques on natural tooth colour. *Br Dent J* **204:**1–4.

Ritter AV, Leonard RH Jr, St Georges AJ, Caplan DJ. (2002) Safety and stability of Nightguard Vital Bleaching: 9 to 12 years post-treatment. *J Esthet Restor Dent* **14:**275–85.

Rosenstiel SF, Gegauff AG, Johnston WM. (1991a) Duration of tooth color change after bleaching. *J Am Dent Assoc* **122:** 54–9.

Rosenstiel SF, Gegauff AG, Johnston WM. (1996) Randomized clinical trial of the efficacy of a home bleaching procedure. *Quintessence Int* **27:**413–24.

Rosenstiel SF, Gegauff AG, McCafferty RJ, Johnston WM. (1991b) In vitro tooth color change with repeated bleaching. *Quintessence Int* **22:**7–12.

Seale NS, Thrash WJ. (1985) Systematic assessment of color removal following vital bleaching of intrinsically stained teeth. *J Dent Res* **64:**457–61.

Small BW. (1994) Bleaching with 10% carbamide peroxide: an 18-month study. *Gen Den* **42:**142–6.

Swift EJ, May KN, Wilder AD, Heymann HO. (1997) Six-month clinical evaluation of a tooth whitening system using an innovative design. *J Esthet Restor Dent* **9:**265–74.

Swift EJ, May KN, Wilder AD, Heymann HO. (1999) Two-year clinical evaluation of tooth whitening using an at home bleaching system. *J Esthet Restor Dent* **11:**36–42.

Tavares M, Stultz J, Newman M, Smith V. (2003) Light augments tooth whitening with peroxide. *J Am Dent Assoc* **134:**167–75.

Türkün M, Celik EU, Aladağ A, Gökay N. (2010) One-year clinical evaluation of the efficacy of a new daytime at-home bleaching technique. *J Esthet Restor Dent* **22:**139–46.

Wiegand A, Drebenstedt S, Roos M, Magalhães AC. (2008) 12-Month color stability of enamel, dentine, and enamel–dentine samples after bleaching. *Clin Oral Invest* **12:**303–10.

Zantnera C, Beheim-Schwarzbacha N, Neumannb K, Kielbassaa AM. (2007) Surface microhardness of enamel after different home bleaching procedures. *Dent Mater* **23:**243–50.

Zekonis R, Matis BA, Cochran MA, Al Shetri SE. (2003) Clinical evaluation of in-office and at home bleaching treatments. *Oper Dent* **28:**114–21.

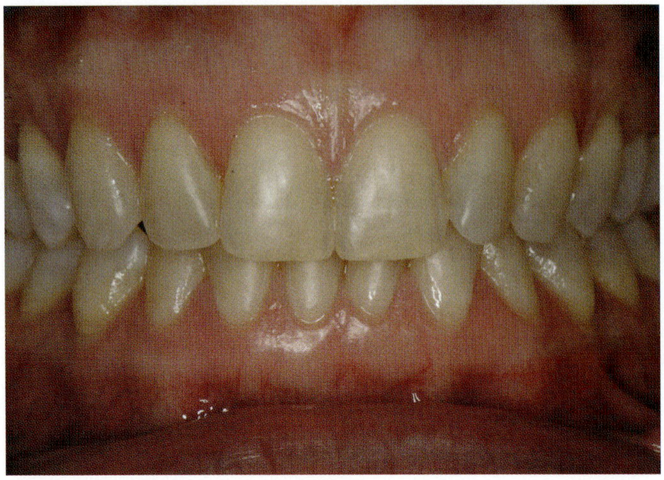

Figure 18.1

Permanent enamel loss on the anterior teeth after aggressive in-office bleaching. Compare the color of the anterior teeth now with the untreated premolar teeth. The anterior teeth have lost the surface luster and now attract stains, making the esthetics even less favorable.

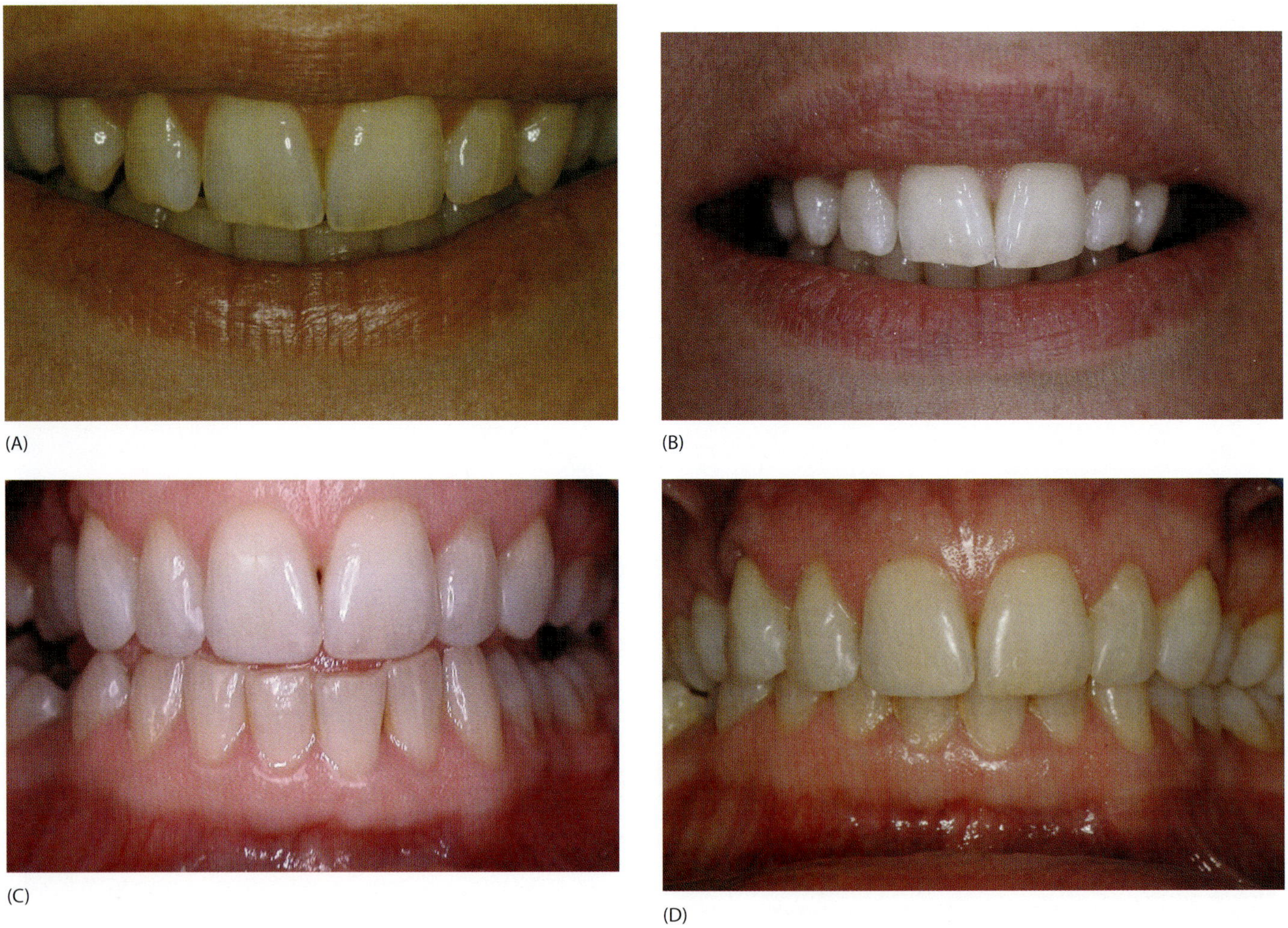

Figure 18.2

Tooth bleaching before edge bonding to provide a 100% noninvasive smile design. (A) Before treatment. (B) Immediately after treatment. (C) Six weeks after treatment, after composite bonding with Miris (Coltene). (D) Twelve years after treatment.

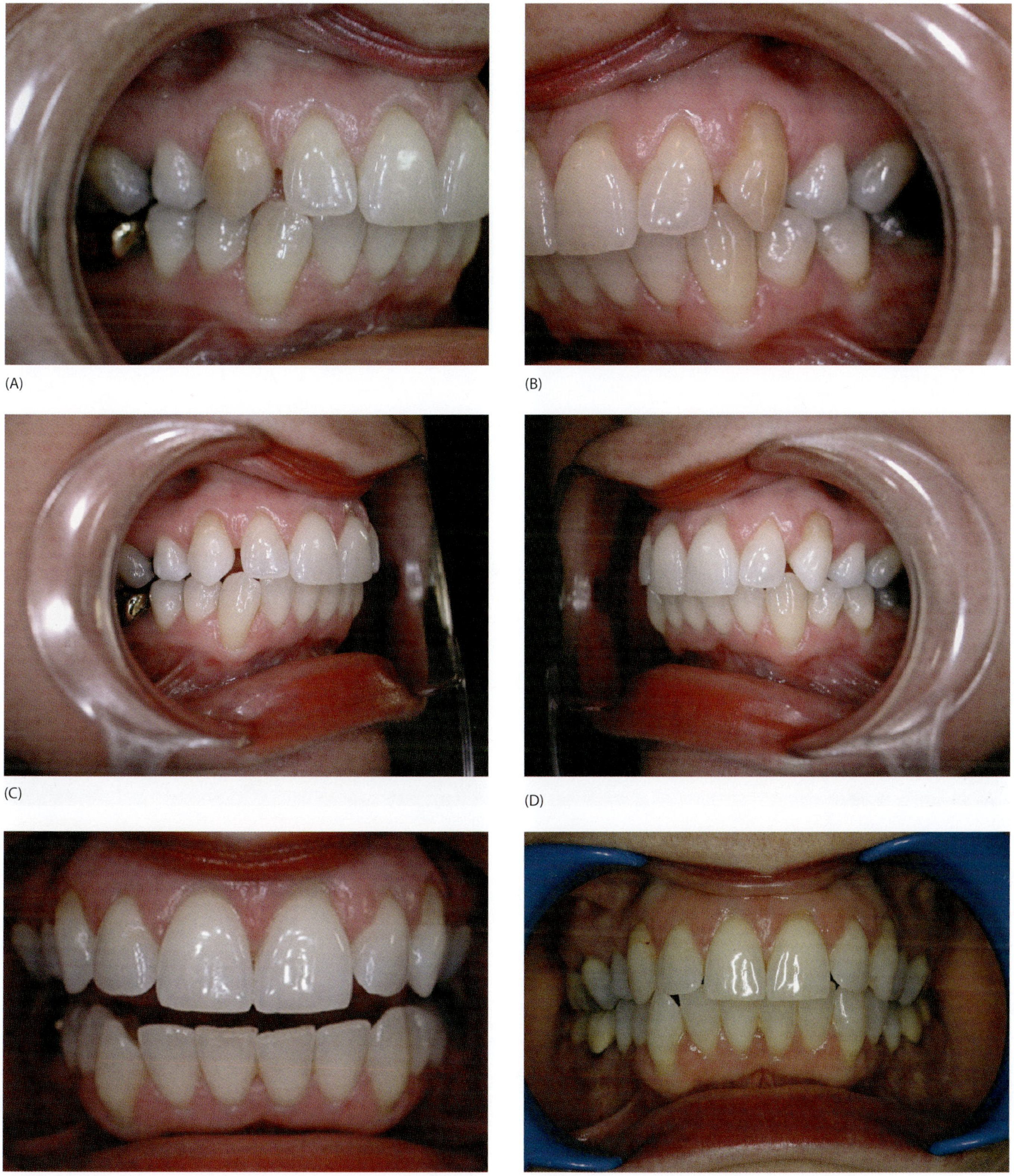

(A) (B) (C) (D) (E) (F)

Figure 18.3

Dark canines (A and B) treated with in-office 35% hydrogen peroxide and halogen light followed by trays and 10% carbamide peroxide (C and D), which provided an excellent result at 6 weeks (E) and 10 years (F).

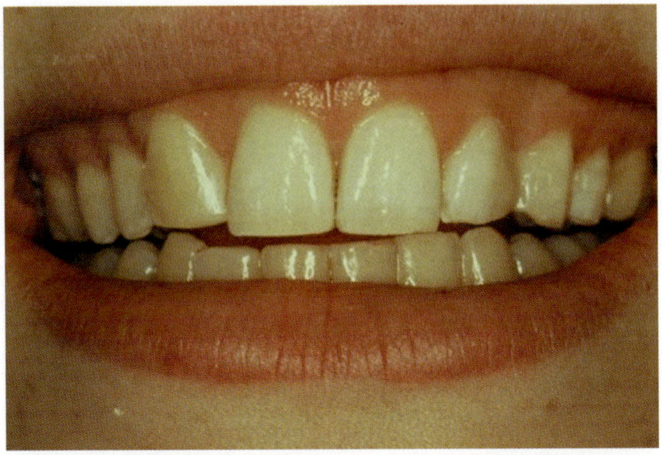

(A)

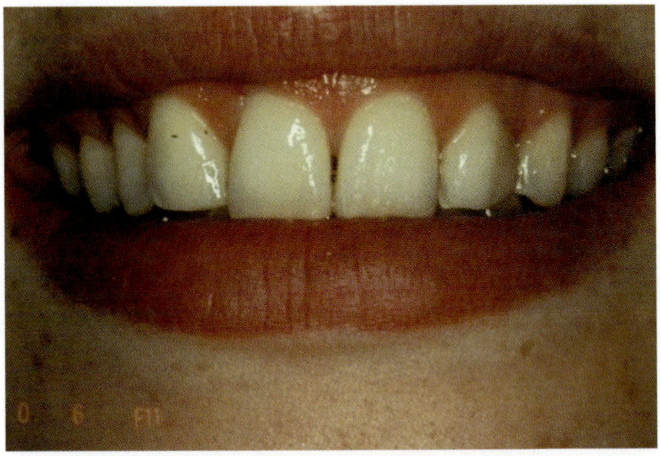

(B)

Figure 18.4

(A) Single-tooth bleaching to modify UR3 to mimic a UR2, (B) after recontouring with composite.

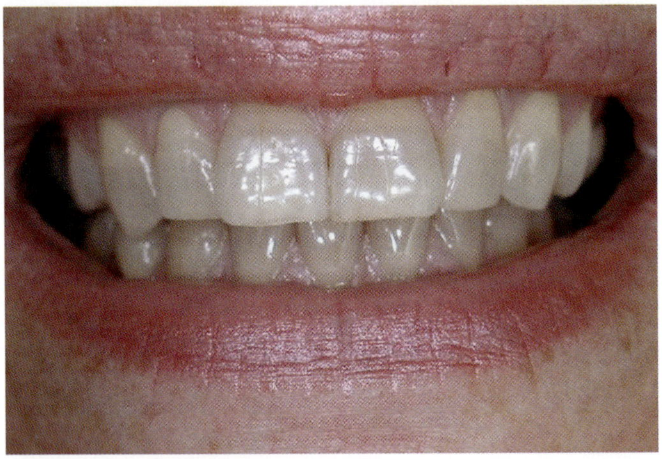

(A)

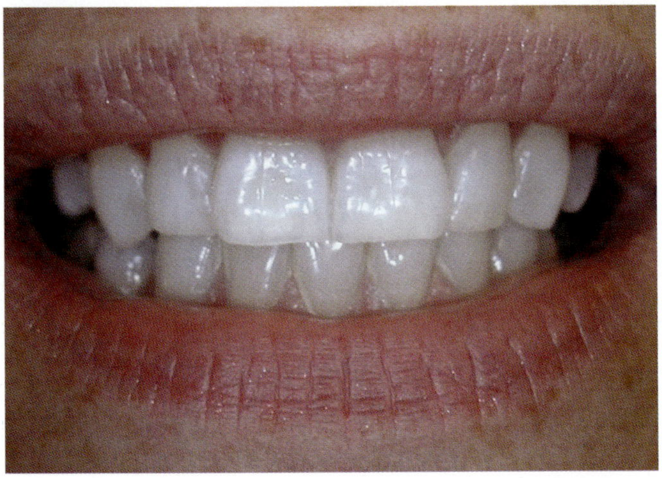

(B)

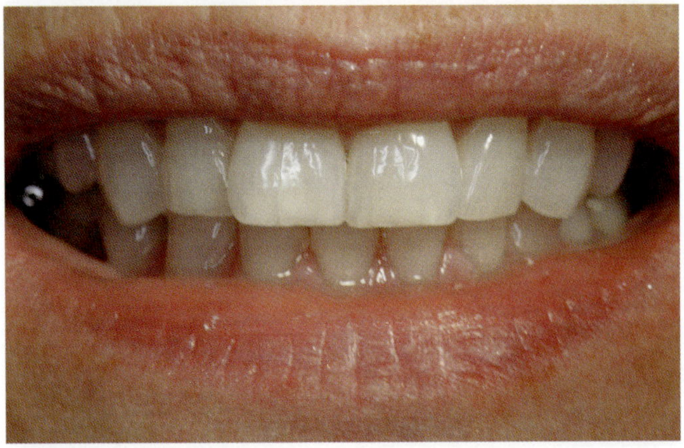

(C)

Figure 18.5

Tetracycline stain treated with 30 minutes of power bleaching (35% hydrogen peroxide plus halogen light) then 10 weeks of Nightguard Vital Bleaching with 10% carbamide peroxide. (A) Pretreatment; (B) 6 weeks after treatment; (C and D) 8 years after treatment.

continued on the next page

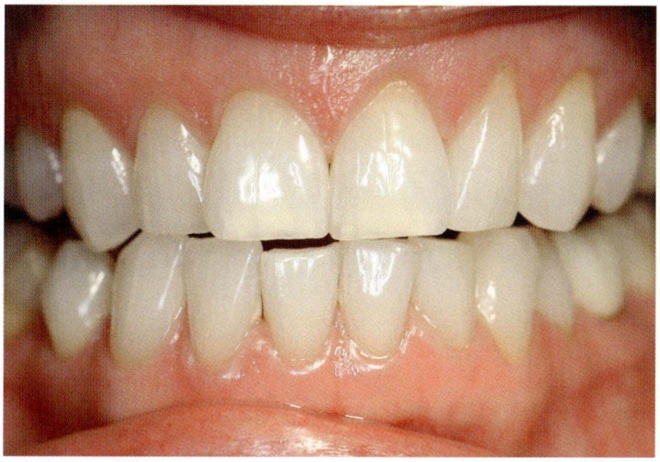

(D)

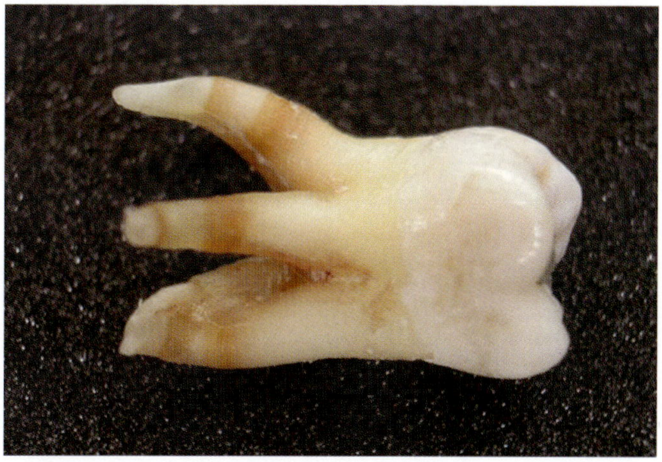

(E)

Figure 18.5 continued

Tetracycline stain treated with 30 minutes of power bleaching (35% hydrogen peroxide plus halogen light) then 10 weeks of Nightguard Vital Bleaching with 10% carbamide peroxide. (C and D) 8 years after treatment. (E) Banding in an extracted third molar from same patient showing the initial dentin discoloration.

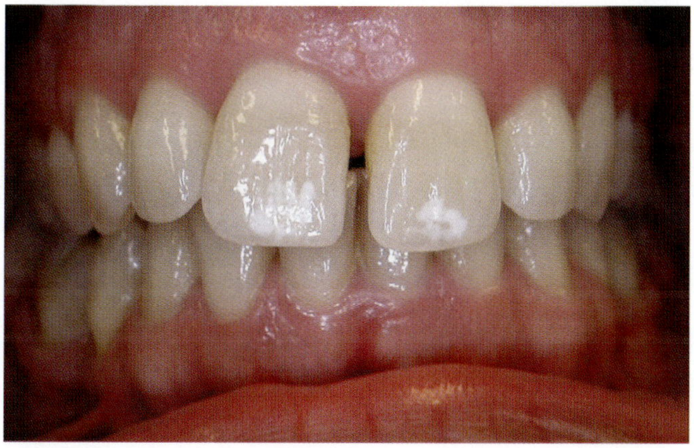

(A)

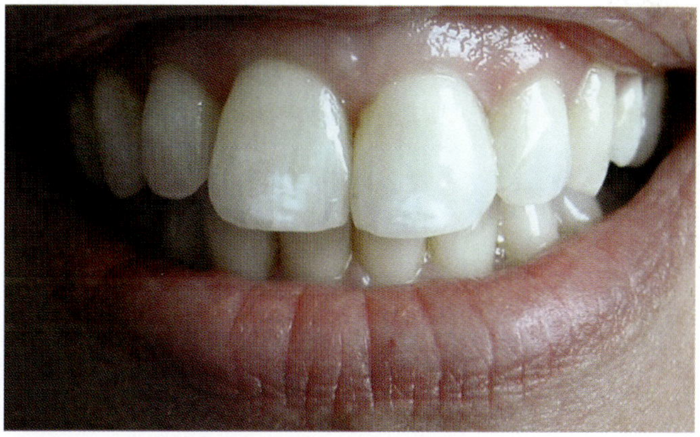

(B)

Figure 18.6

Disguising white spots noninvasively in an adult with white opacities before space closure with composite and nonsurgical papillary growth to eliminate the black triangle.

19

NIGHTGUARD VITAL BLEACHING
Post-Treatment Effects, Longevity, and Long-Term Results

Ralph H. Leonard, Jr.

INTRODUCTION

In 1989, Haywood and Heymann published their landmark article describing a new and revolutionary technique for lightening extrinsically stained or discolored teeth. Originally termed *Nightguard Vital Bleaching* (NGVB), the treatment has also been referred to as *tooth whitening, tooth bleaching,* and *dentist-prescribed, home-applied* (DPHA) *bleaching.* As described in the Haywood and Heymann article, this innovative technique was performed under the supervision of a dentist with respect to tray fabrication, diagnosis of tooth discoloration, and so on, but was implemented by the patient, who applied the treatment solution at home. As word spread about the new technique, acceptance of this simple and effective process to lighten teeth was rapid among dental practitioners as well as patients seeking a simple and effective way to lighten discolored teeth (Christensen 1989, Albers 1991, Haywood 1992) (Figures 19.1–19.3) Thus, manufacturers of dental products saw the interest in and demand for tooth bleaching and soon developed products ranging from simple bleaching solutions to comprehensive bleaching systems. Along with these product lines came the investment of millions of dollars in advertising to enlighten the public about this technique. It was no surprise that NGVB became one of the most sought-after cosmetic dental procedures requested by the public.

As described by Haywood and Heymann, the original technique involved wearing a rigid, nonscalloped treatment tray without reservoirs for 6 weeks and using a medium-viscosity 10% carbamide peroxide treatment solution. The technique has undergone many modifications including changes in tray material and design, different active ingredient concentrations, addition of thickening agents for sustained release of the active ingredient, use of reservoirs, and adjustments in treatment times (Christensen 1989, Darnell and Moore 1990, Freedman 1990, Haywood 1990, Albers 1991, Christensen 1991, Garber et al. 1991, Haywood 1991a, Haywood 1991b, Haywood 1991c, Haywood 1992a, Haywood 1992b, Haywood et al. 1994, Haywood et al. 1997). In addition, a trayless system using strips as the treatment solution delivery mechanism was developed (Sagel et al. 2000).

The use of NGVB generally preceded what the literature was reporting, and patients were asking questions concerning efficacy, longevity, and safety. Early on, the literature did report NGVB as being effective in lightening extrinsically stained or discolored teeth, in many cases up to 98% lighter (Haywood and Heymann 1989, Darnell and Moore 1990, Albers 1991, Christensen 1991, Garber et al. 1991, Haywood 1991c, Haywood 1992a, Ouellet et al. 1992, Williams et al. 1992, Gegauff et al. 1993, Reinhardt et al. 1993, Haywood et al. 1994, Matis et al. 2002). It was also well documented that up to 67% of patients using this procedure were reporting side effects, primarily tooth sensitivity (TS) and/or gingival irritation (Freedman 1990, Haywood 1990, Haywood 1991c, Powell and Bates 1991, Cooper et al. 1992, Howard 1992, Ouellet et al. 1992, Scherer et al. 1992a, Scherer et al. 1992b, Williams et al. 1992, Reinhardt et al. 1993, Schulte et al. 1993, Haywood et al. 1994, Schulte et al. 1994, Matis et al. 2002). These side effects were thought to be minor and transient, disappearing soon after completion of the treatment. At that point, speculation could only be made as to the longevity of NGVB and the long-term sequelae of the side effects associated with this tooth lightening technique.

The purpose of this chapter is to summarize the literature on the long-term effects of NGVB. Efficacy of NGVB using trays and strips and treatment solutions of various concentrations has been discussed elsewhere. Although several clinical studies will be cited, the emphases of this chapter will come from long-term NGVB studies in which I have been involved (Haywood et al. 1994, Leonard et al. 1997a, Leonard et al. 2001, Ritter et al. 2002, Boushell et al. 2012). In all the studies cited, unless otherwise noted, participants used a 10% carbamide peroxide bleaching solution at night for up to 8 hours. Specifically, the purpose of this chapter is to discuss the longevity, post-treatment effects, and long-term results of NGVB using a 10% carbamide peroxide bleaching solution.

LONGEVITY

"How long does bleaching last?" was a question posed by both patients and dental clinicians in the early 1990s. The literature did report the efficacy of NGVB (up to 98%), with a certain percentage of patients reporting side effects (up to two thirds); however, nothing existed in the literature related to longevity (Darnell et al. 1990, Haywood 1991c, Haywood 1992b, Ouellet et al. 1992, Gegauff et al. 1993, Reinhardt et al. 1993, Haywood et al. 1997, Sagel et al. 2000). In 1990 Dr. Van Haywood began an NGVB clinical study to evaluate efficacy, longevity, and occurrence of side effects. This patient cohort was followed for 12 years. As stated by Haywood et al. in their original article, 74% of the patients who initially responded to NGVB treatment and had not re-treated were satisfied with the shade of their teeth at 1.5 years after treatment (Haywood et al. 1994). Satisfaction decreased to 62% at 3 years after treatment. Ritter et al. reported on the same cohort of participants 9–12 years after treatment (mean 10 years). Shade retention and satisfaction at 10 years after treatment was 43% (Ritter et al. 2002). Only one participant at the 10-year recall appointment felt that the teeth had regressed back to the baseline shade.

Two other long-term studies worth consideration have followed patients for 47 months (Leonard et al. 2001) and 90 months (Leonard et al. 1997a). As reported in the 47-month longitudinal study by Leonard et al. (2001), the efficacy rate for the treatment solution used was 98%. The treatment time was 2 weeks using a viscous 10% carbamide peroxide solution. The bleaching effect was observed at 47 months (range 36–55 months) after treatment in 89% of the participants. Eighty-two percent still had at least a two-shade change from baseline, and on average the participants had a mean shade value of five Vita shade units lighter than baseline at 47 months after treatment.

With respect to the 90-month (range 84–100) study using a 6-month extended treatment time for patients with tetracycline-stained teeth, 60% were still satisfied with the shade of their teeth, with no one reporting tooth darkening back to the original shade (Leonard et al. 1997a). Thirty-six percent (four) of the participants had re-treated their teeth between the 54- and 90-month recall appointments. Eighty-eight percent of the participants had at least a two-shade Vita shade tab change from baseline at 90 months after treatment. Overall, the participants had a mean shade value of 10 Vita shade units lighter than baseline. Patients were given a satisfaction survey to complete before their clinical examination. According to the survey, patients were satisfied with the efficacy of the procedure and shade retention after treatment. It was noted in the study that shade regression occurred within the first 6 months after the completion of treatment and that the shade remained stable thereafter and would be consistent if the patient was not exposed to any more tetracycline products.

Boushell et al. (2012) reported on a cohort of patients who had successfully bleached their teeth and were at least 10 years post-treatment and as long as 17 years post-treatment (mean 12.3 years). Thirty-one of approximately 150 participants in various NGVB studies were evaluated clinically and asked to complete a questionnaire regarding their perceptions of the bleaching procedure. In this study it was reported that 35% of the patients who underwent NGVB with no additional retreatment were satisfied with results for up to 17 years post-treatment (Figures 19.1–19.3, Table 19.1).

In summary, longitudinal studies have documented that NGVB can be an effective method to lighten stained or discolored teeth. The longevity and stability as determined by both clinician examination and patient perception have also been documented. The results of these studies are consistent with overall long-term trends in levels of patient satisfaction, indicating that approximately one third of the patients who use NGVB will likely experience long-term satisfactory results.

Another question that patients ask is, "Will I need to re-treat, and if so, how often?" Based on the information that now exists in the literature, patients should be informed that in some cases a touch-up or re-treatment procedure may be needed after treatment (Haywood et al. 1994, Leonard et al. 1997a, Leonard et al. 2001, Burrows 2009). From the data gathered from the aforementioned studies, the re-treatment may take only 1 or 2 days to complete. It is important to point out to patients that, just as with the original treatment, the touch-up bleaching procedures should be done under the direct supervision of a dentist. As reported in the original study by Haywood et al., patients re-treated only after a mean of 25 months post-treatment (Haywood et al. 1994). In Leonard's 47-month study, re-treatment occurred at 32 months (range 24–42), and in the extended treatment time for tetracycline-stained teeth, participants re-treated at least 54 months post-treatment (Leonard et al. 2001). Therefore the shade retention of NGVB can be noted in approximately one third of patients up to 17 years post-treatment without any touch-up treatment during that time. The results of these studies should help strengthen the fact that touch-up bleaching is not routinely needed.

POST-TREATMENT EFFECTS

Side effects

As previously stated, two thirds of patients undergoing NGVB may experience side effects, primarily tooth sensitivity and gingival irritation. Why some patients develop side effects and others do not is not fully understood, especially because all patients are exposed to the same chemical byproducts of carbamide peroxide degradation. Leonard et al. conducted an NGVB clinical study in which 20% of the participants reported sensitivity to wearing the treatment guard without any treatment solution and 36% reported sensitivity to a placebo (Leonard et al. 2002). In a second study by Leonard et al., 7.5% of the participants reported sensitivity to wearing the guard alone (Leonard et al. 2004). It was concluded that factors other than the treatment solution play a major role in the occurrence of side effects as reported by patients. There is no doubt that the cause of tooth

Table 19.1 Questionnaire summary of patients' perception of shade satisfaction and side effects after Nightguard Vital Bleaching, average of 12.3 years post-treatment (range 10–17 years)

Question				*Responses n (%)*	*Participants Responding n (%)*
1. Since completion of bleaching, have you had your teeth re-treated?					
			NO	19 (61)	31 (100)
			YES	12 (39)	
If YES, for what reason? To improve esthetics					
2. Check the item that best describes your satisfaction with the original treatment*:					
Immediately after treatment	**No re-treatment (19)**	**Yes re-treatment (12)**			
Very Satisfied	12/18	5/12		17 (57)	
Partially Satisfied	6/18	7/12		13 (43)	30 (97)
Not Satisfied	0/18	0/12		0 (0)	
Currently					
Very Satisfied	4/13	4/11		8 (33.3)	
Partially Satisfied	7/13	7/11		14 (58.3)	24 (77)
Not Satisfied	2/13	0/11		2 (8.3)	
3. Did you experience any kind of problems during treatment?					
			NO	16 (52)	31 (100)
			YES	15 (48)	
Tooth sensitivity—10 (32)	Gingival sensitivity—5 (16)	Both—2 (6)			
4. Did you experience any kind of problems immediately after treatment that you felt was treatment related?			NO	30 (97)	31 (100)
Tooth Sensitivity—1 (3)			YES	1 (3)	
5. Compared with the un-treated teeth, have you experienced any of the following problems on your treated teeth that you think might be related to the treatment?			Staining	1 (3)	
			Decay	0 (0)	
			Gum (periodontal) problems	0 (0)	31 (100)
			Other problems or concerns	0 (0)	
6. Have you had any of the treated teeth veneered or crowned?					
			NO	25 (81)	31 (100)
			YES	6 (19)	
	Reason: broken tooth†—4 (13), esthetic concerns—2 (6)				
7. Have you had to have a root canal on any of the treated teeth?					
			NO	29 (94)	31 (100)
			YES	2 (6)	
8. Have you had any gum surgery (biopsy) done after ending the bleaching treatment that may be treatment related?			NO	31 (100)	31 (100)
			YES	0 (0)	
9. Would you have your teeth treated (bleached) again?					
			YES	27 (87)	31 (100)
			NO	4 (13)	

* Not all participants responded to various aspects of this question.
† The broken teeth reported were posterior teeth.

sensitivity and/or gingival irritation is multifactorial (Leonard et al. 1997b).

The most likely cause for gingival irritation is the border of the tray extending onto the gingiva and trapping the bleaching solution against the gingival tissue. This can be corrected or avoided by trimming the treatment tray just short of the tissue. Haywood showed that even if the tray did not completely cover the entire tooth, the tooth would still lighten because of the angulation of the enamel rods.

Tooth sensitivity can come from many sources, but orthodontic movement of the teeth caused by the tray as

TABLE 19.2 Questionnaire summary response of patients having undergone a Nightguard Vital Bleaching procedure at least 8 years previously (three studies combined; N = 76)

Since the treatment of your teeth:	*YES*	*NO*
1. Have you had to have any crowns (caps) on any of the teeth you treated?	5%	95%
2. Have you had to have any root canals, or any treatment to the nerve, on any of the teeth you treated?	4%	96%
3. Have you had any sensitivity with any of the teeth you treated since ending the treatment process that may be treatment related?	5%	95%
4. Have you had any gingiva (gum) sensitivity since ending the treatment process that may be treatment related?	3%	97%
5. Are you glad you went through this treatment process?	96%	4%
6. Would you go through this treatment process again?	87%	13%
7. Would you recommend this treatment procedure to a friend?	94%	6%
8. Do you feel that your teeth are lighter now than when you began the Nightguard Vital Bleaching procedure?	84%	16%

well as penetration of the carbamide peroxide through the tooth structure and into the pulp is one likely cause. Increased carbamide peroxide exposure time and carbamide peroxide concentration will also increase the risk of developing tooth sensitivity. On the market today are various bleaching formulations using additives such as amorphous calcium phosphate, fluoride, and/or potassium nitrate that may decrease the risk of tooth sensitivity. Haywood et al. (2005) demonstrated that the use of a potassium nitrate plus fluoride dentifrice for 2 weeks before bleaching as well as throughout the treatment procedure was useful in the management of bleaching-induced tooth sensitivity. Leonard et al. (2004) reported that a 30-minute application of a 3% potassium nitrate and 0.11% fluoride desensitizing agent before bleaching was useful in decreasing tooth sensitivity, especially in a population at risk for developing tooth sensitivity during bleaching.

It should not be construed that the occurrence of tooth sensitivity is an indication of pulpal pathology. Fugaro et al. (2004) evaluated the histologic changes in the dental pulp after NGVB. The study demonstrated that any minor histologic changes, sometimes noted during bleaching, resolved within 2 weeks after treatment. Their conclusion was that a 2-week NGVB procedure using 10% carbamide peroxide was safe for the dental pulp, which can be verified in the digital images in Figures 19.1–19.3. Note the absence of any pulpal pathology or external or internal resorption 12–16 years after treatment.

Occurrence of side effects can be evaluated from two viewpoints: dentist-evaluated clinical parameters and the perception of the patient. The patient's perception can be evaluated by the use of a log form and/or questionnaire completed by the patient during and after treatment. Clinical parameters evaluated by the dentist often include tooth sensitivity to an air blast directed toward the cementoenamel junction (CEJ), sensitivity of the tooth to Endo Ice (Coltène/Whaledent Inc., Cuyahoga Falls, OH) (or other similar products), percussion sensitivity, increased incidence of caries and/or tooth fracture, failure of existing restorations, changes in the gingival and plaque indices, and radiographic changes. When clinical parameters alone are evaluated, the occurrence of side effects may be minimal (Tables 19.1 and 19.2). Interestingly, in some cases the gingival condition and plaque index of patients may improve (Scherer et al. 1992a, Schulte et al. 1993, Curtis et al. 1995, Sterrett et al. 1995, Curtis et al. 1996, Lazarchik et al. 2010).

When patients are asked to give their perspectives concerning side effects, they are likely to report just the opposite of the dentist-evaluated clinical parameters. In several of the previously mentioned longitudinal studies, side effects were reported by as many as two thirds of the patients. Thermal tooth sensitivity and gingival irritation were the most common side effects, although sore throat, tooth pain, tingling of the tissues, and headaches also were reported. Although not statistically significant, it has been clinically observed that patients aged 18–40 tend to have more side effects than patients older than 40 (Leonard et al. 1997b). This certainly seems reasonable because the pulp decreases in size with aging, and thus one would expect less tooth sensitivity. Patients reporting preexisting teeth sensitivity to hot and cold, use of fluoride to relieve tooth sensitivity, restorative treatment for tooth sensitivity, daily use of citrus fruits and juices as well as colas, and increased sensitivity after a prophylaxis are also prone to more side effects (Leonard et al. 2004). All patients should be advised to wait at least 2 weeks after prophylaxis to begin their bleaching procedure.

In the clinical studies cited here, side effects were experienced during active treatment and subsided quickly when treatment ended. In many cases, they disappeared completely within 24 hours. No one in the Haywood et al. longitudinal study reported side effects at 1.5 or 3 years after treatment (Haywood et al. 1997). At the 10-year post-treatment appointment, four patients reported tooth sensitivity and/or gingival irritation (Ritter et al. 2002). Three had had these conditions before treatment, and none of the four reported the symptoms at their 1.5- or 3-year post-treatment appointments.

In the 47-month longitudinal study, no one reported side effects that they felt were treatment related (Leonard et al. 2001). No correlation could be made between the bleaching procedure and tooth sensitivity or gingival irritation because no data existed regarding preexisting tooth sensitivity to hot and cold or after dental prophylaxis.

A similar circumstance occurred in the tetracycline study (Leonard et al. 1997a). One participant reported side effects at 90 months after treatment that the patient felt were treatment related. However, this participant had not reported any side effects after completion of treatment or at 12 months after treatment.

As reported in the 17-year study by Boushell et al., only one of the 31 participants reported any type of post-treatment complication, which in this case was tooth sensitivity (Boushell et al. 2012). Originally, half the study population had reported some type of side effect while undergoing the active treatment (Table 19.1).

Safety issues

Thirty of 38 participants in the 10-year study, 31 of 48 participants in the 47-month study, and 15 of 21 participants in the 90-month tetracycline study, for a total of 76 participants of a possible 107, returned for their post-treatment evaluation. Of these, 5% reported having had a crown placed on a treated tooth and 3% reported having undergone a root canal procedure (Table 19.2). These percentages are within the norm that can be expected. Radiographic evaluation of the participants in all three studies did not reveal evidence of external root resorption or any other endodontic pathology. There was no evidence of caries, bone loss, or any type of pulpal pathology. In addition, the gingival index and percent of treated teeth responding to Endo Ice were within normal limits for what is expected in a population. No soft tissue pathology was noted.

Enamel surface changes were evaluated in all three studies. Post-treatment impressions were taken of the facial surfaces of the anterior teeth and evaluated under a scanning electron microscope (SEM) at 200× and 2000× (Figure 19.4). When compared with untreated mandibular teeth or an untreated extracted tooth, only minimal changes to the enamel surface could be detected in the treated maxillary teeth. Therefore, it can be concluded that a 2-week regimen of NGVB using a 10% carbamide peroxide solution has minimal effect on enamel surface morphology and does not worsen over time.

In Boushell and colleagues' 17-year study, it was reported that side effects and safety issues were minimal for up to 17 years after treatment (mean of 12.3; Table 19.1; Boushell et al. 2012). No one reported dental caries (decay), fractured teeth, or replacement of a restoration for the teeth that were treated. One participant reported staining that the patient felt was treatment related. When Loe's Gingival Index (Loe and Silness 1963) was used to evaluate gingival inflammation, 91% percent of the examined teeth had normal gingivae with no inflammation. Seven percent had mild inflammation, and 2% had moderate inflammation. No one reported needing a gingival biopsy after treatment for any oral pathology abnormality that may have been treatment related. Sixty-nine percent of the treated teeth tested responded positively to Endo Ice. Independent evaluation of the periapical digital images taken of the treatment teeth showed no evidence of external root resorption, and no apical lesions were observed in the teeth examined (Figures 19.1 and 19.2).

In summary, data from long-term studies revealed no evidence of detrimental sequelae or adverse effects to the gingivae or dentition.

PATIENT PERCEPTIONS OF NIGHTGUARD VITAL BLEACHING

In evaluating the patients' perceptions of the NGVB procedure as reflected in their questionnaire responses, one can conclude that patient satisfaction correlates highly with how well the procedure worked. It is paramount that the dentist know what the patient's expectation for success is before initiating NGVB treatment. Often it is the patient's expectations that determine the perception of the success of the treatment. Combining the patient questionnaire responses for the participants in the three longitudinal studies (10 year, 47 months, and 90 months; Table 19.2), 84% felt that their teeth were currently lighter than at baseline. Ninety-six percent said they were glad they had undertaken the bleaching procedure, 87% said they would undertake the bleaching process again, and 94% said they would recommend NGVB to a friend. The patients were glad they had undergone tooth bleaching and were very positive about the bleaching technique. Boushell et al. reported that 87% of the participants were positive about the bleaching procedure at an average of 12.3 years after treatment (range 10–17 years) and would bleach again (Table 19.1; Boushell et al. 2012).

CONCLUSION

Clinical trials overwhelmingly support the efficacy and safety of NGVB with use of a 10% treatment solution. From the earliest reported studies using a medium-viscosity 10% carbamide peroxide solution in a hard tray for 6 weeks to the latest reported data on sustained-release, highly viscous or paste carbamide peroxide agents using a soft tray for 7 to 14 days, the success rate of treating non–tetracycline-stained teeth may be as high as 98% (Haywood et al. 1994, Leonard et al. 2001). By altering the treatment time and/or concentration of the bleaching agent, dentists may reach a success rate for tetracycline-stained teeth of 86% or higher. Satisfactory retention of the shade change can be expected in 74% of patients 1.5 years after treatment, 62% at 3 years, and 43% at 10 years (Ritter et al. 2002). As reported in the 17-year study, 35% of the participants were satisfied with the shade of their teeth (Boushell et al. 2012).

Approximately 66% of patients experience side effects; however, most are minor and transient, disappearing within days after completion of treatment. The most common side effects are tooth sensitivity and gingival irritation. Nonetheless, side effects are easily managed by decreasing wear time, reducing the amount of treatment solution in the tray, and trimming the guard so that it will not infringe on soft tissue. In addition, patients may pretreat with a desensitizing agent before beginning the bleaching treatment or incorporate one if sensitivity occurs during treatment. In the longitudinal post-treatment studies discussed in this chapter, side effects were not noted by patients as a regular occurrence after treatment, nor was an increased incidence of decay, tooth fracture, oral pathology, or endodontic pathology noted on the long-term post-treatment radiographs. As a rule, the only long-term change after tooth bleaching from baseline was the lighter tooth shade noted by both patients and dental examiners, which may last up to 17 years (mean 12.3) after treatment. Patients' perceptions of the bleaching process are positive and they are genuinely glad they underwent the procedure. As stated by Boushell et al., "Assessment of the long-term effects of NGVB on maxillary anterior teeth revealed low risk of the development of gingival inflammation, pulpal inflammation and external cervical root resorption. Additionally, no evidence of malignancy or any other soft tissue pathology was found. NGVB with 10% [carbamide peroxide] was found to be effective with minimal side effects up to 17 years post-treatment" (Boushell et al. 2012). From all the evidence, NGVB appears to be as safe and effective as any procedure that we do in dentistry.

REFERENCES

Albers HF. (1991) Home bleaching. *Adept Rep* **2**(1):9–17.

Boushell LW, Ritter AV, Garland GE, Tiwana KK. (2012) Nightguard Vital Bleaching: side effects and patient satisfaction 10-17 years post-treatment. *J Esthet Restor Dent* **24**(3):211–9.

Burrows S. (2009) A review of the efficacy of tooth bleaching. *Dent Update* **36**(9):541–4.

Christensen GJ. (1989) Tooth bleaching, home-use products. *Clin Res Assoc Newsl* **13**(7):1.

Christensen GJ. (1991) Home-use bleaching survey—1991. *Clin Res Assoc Newsl* **15**(10):2–3.

Cooper JS, Bokmeyer TJ, Bowles WH. (1992) Penetration of the pulp chamber by carbamide peroxide bleaching agents. *J Endod* **18**(7):315–7.

Curtis JW, Dickinson GL, Downey MC, Russell CM. (1996) Assessing the effects of 10 percent carbamide peroxide on oral soft tissue. *J Am Dent Assoc* **127:**1218–23.

Curtis JW Jr, Dickinson GL, Myers ML, Russell CM. (1995) Evaluating the effects of a dentist-supervised, patient-applied carbamide peroxide bleaching agent on oral soft tissues. *J Esthet Dent* **7:**18–25.

Darnell DH, Moore WC. (1990) Vital tooth bleaching: the White and Brite technique. *Compend Contin Educ Dent* **11:**86–94.

Freedman GA. (1990) The safety of tooth whitening. *Dent Today* **April:**32–33.

Fugaro JO, Nordahl I, Fugaro OJ, Matis BA. (2004) Pulp reaction to vital bleaching. *Oper Dent* **29**(4):363–8.

Garber DA, Goldstein RE, Goldstein GE, Schwartz CG. (1991) Dentist monitored bleaching: a combined approach. *Pract Periodontics Aesthet Dent* **3**(2):22–6.

Gegauff AG, Rosenstiel SF, Langhout KJ, Johnston WM. (1993) Evaluating tooth color change from carbamide peroxide gel. *J Am Dent Assoc* **124:**65–72.

Haywood VB. (1990) Nightguard Vital Bleaching: current information and research. *Esthet Dent Update* **1**(2):7–12.

Haywood VB. (1991a) Nightguard Vital Bleaching: a history and products update. Part 1 *Esthet Dent Update* **2**(4):63–6.

Haywood VB. (1991b) Nightguard Vital Bleaching: a history and products update. Part 2. *Esthet Dent Update* **2**(5):82–5.

Haywood VB. (1991c) Overview and status of mouthguard bleaching. *J Esthet Dent* **3:**157–61.

Haywood VB. (1992a) Bleaching of vital and nonvital teeth. *Curr Opin Dent* **2:**142–9.

Haywood VB. (1992b) History, safety, and effectiveness of current techniques and applications of the Nightguard Vital Bleaching technique. *Quintessence Int* **23:**471–88.

Haywood VB, Cordero R, Wright K, Gendreau L. (2005) Brushing with a potassium nitrate dentifrice to reduce bleaching sensitivity. *J Clin Dent* **16**(1):17–22.

Haywood VB, Heymann HO. (1989) Nightguard Vital Bleaching. *Quintessence Int* **20:**173–6.

Haywood VB, Leonard RH, Dickinson GL. (1997) Efficacy of six months of Nightguard Vital Bleaching of tetracycline-stained teeth. *J Esthet Dent* **9**(1):13–9.

Haywood VB, Leonard RH, Nelson CF, Brunson WD. (1994) Effectiveness, side effects, and long-term status of Nightguard Vital Bleaching. *J Am Dent Assoc* **125:**1219–26.

Howard WR. (1992) Patient-applied tooth whiteners: are they safe, effective with supervision? *J Am Dent Assoc* **123**(2):57–60.

Lazarchik DA, Haywood VB. (2010) Use of tray-applied 10 percent carbamide peroxide gels for improving oral health in patients with special-care needs. *J Am Dent Assoc* **141**(6):639–46.

Leonard RH, Haywood VB, Caplan D, Tart ND. (1997a) Nightguard Vital Bleaching of tetracycline stained teeth 7.5 years post-treatment. *J Esthet Restor Dent* **12:**142–153.

Leonard RH, Haywood VB, Phillips C. (1997b) Risk factors for developing tooth sensitivity and gingival irritation associated with Nightguard Vital Bleaching. *Quintessence Int* **28**(8):527–34, 1997.

Leonard RH, Smith LR, Garland GE, Caplan DJ. (2004) Desensitizing agent efficacy during whitening in an at-risk population. *J Esthet Rest Dent* **16**(1):49–56.

Leonard, RH, Garland GE, Eagle JC, Caplan AJ. (2002) Safety issues when using a 16% carbamide peroxide whitening solution. *J Esthet Restor Dent* **14**(6):358–67, 2002.

Leonard RH Jr, Bentley C, Eagle JC, Garland GE. (2001) Nightguard Vital Bleaching: a long-term study on efficacy, shade retention, side effects and patients' perceptions. *J Esthet Rest Dent* **13**(6):357–69.

Loe H, Silness J. (1963) Periodontal disease in pregnancy. I. prevalence and severity. *Acta Odontol Scand* **21:**533–51.

Matis BA, Wang Y, Jiang T, Eckert GJ. (2002) Extended at-home bleaching of tetracycline-stained teeth with different concentrations of carbamide peroxide. *Quintessence Int* **33**(9): 645–55.

Ouellet D, Los S, Case H, Healy R. (1992) Double blind whitening nightguard study using 10 percent carbamide peroxide. *J Esthet Dent* **4:**79–83, 1992.

Powell LV, Bates DJ. (1991) Tooth bleaching: its effect on oral tissues. *J Am Dent Assoc* **122:**50–4.

Reinhardt JW, Eivins SE, Swift EJ Jr, Denehy GE. (1993) A clinical study of Nightguard Vital Bleaching. *Quintessence Int* **24**(6):379–85.

Ritter AV, Leonard RH, St-Georges AJ, Caplan DJ, Haywood VB. (2002) Safety and stability of Nightguard Vital

Bleaching 9 to 12 years post-treatment. *J Esthet Rest Dent* **14**(5):275–85.
Sagel PA, Odioso LL, McMillian DA, Gerlach RW. (2000) Vital tooth whitening with a novel hydrogen peroxide strip system: design, kinetics and clinical response. *Compend Contin Educ Dent* **21**(Suppl 29):S10–5.
Scherer W, Palat M, Hittelman E, Putter H. (1992a) At-home bleaching system: effect on gingival tissue. *J Esthet Dent* **4**(3):86–89.
Scherer W, Penugonda B, Styner D. (1992b) At-home vital bleaching: effects on stained enamel and dentin. *Pract Periodontics Aesthet Dent* **4**(2):11–5.
Schulte JR, Morrissette DB, Gasior EJ, Czajewski MV. (1993) Clinical changes in the gingiva as a result of at-home bleaching. *Compend Contin Educ Dent* **14**(11):1362–72.
Schulte JR, Morrissette DB, Gasior EJ, Czajewski MV. (1994) The effects of bleaching application time on the dental pulp. *J Am Dent Assoc* **125:**1330–5.
Sterrett J, Price RB, Bankey T. (1995) Effects of home bleaching on the tissues of the oral cavity. *J Can Dent Assoc* **61**(5): 412–20.
Williams HA, Rueggeberg FA, Meister LW. (1992) Bleaching the natural dentition to match the color existing restorations: case reports. *Quintessence Int* **23:**673–7.

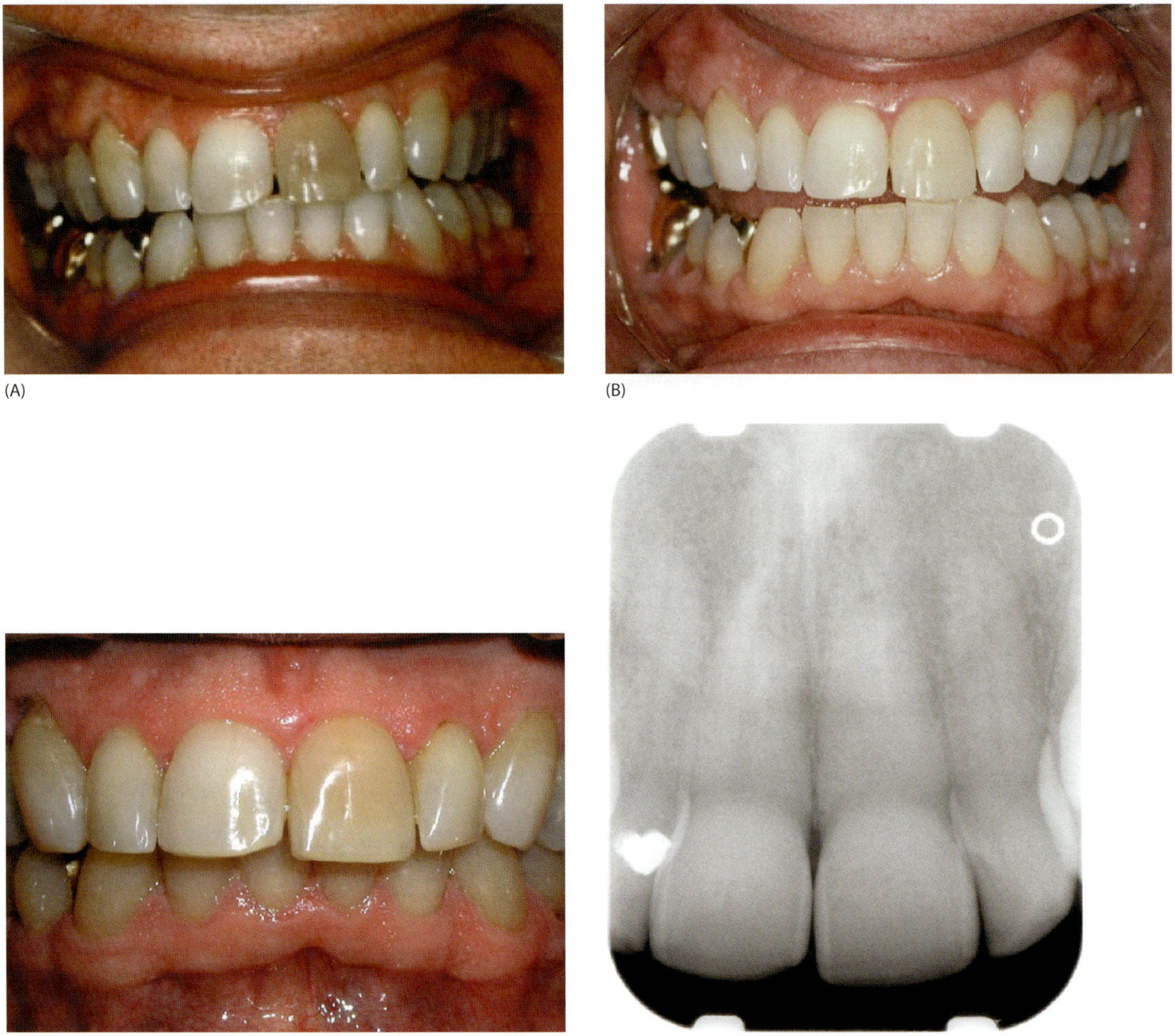

(A) (B) (C) (D)

Figure 19.1

(A) Pretreatment, (B) 3 years post-treatment, and (C) 15 years, 11 months post-treatment. (D) Radiographic images of the teeth examined (6–11) at 15 years, 11 months post-treatment. Note that there is no soft tissue or pulpal pathology (internal or external resorption) at any timeframe. (From Boushell LW, Ritter AV, Garland GE, Tiwana KK. (2012) Nightguard Vital Bleaching: side effects and patient satisfaction 10 to 17 years post-treatment. *J Esthet Restor Dent* **24**[3]:211–9, with permission.)

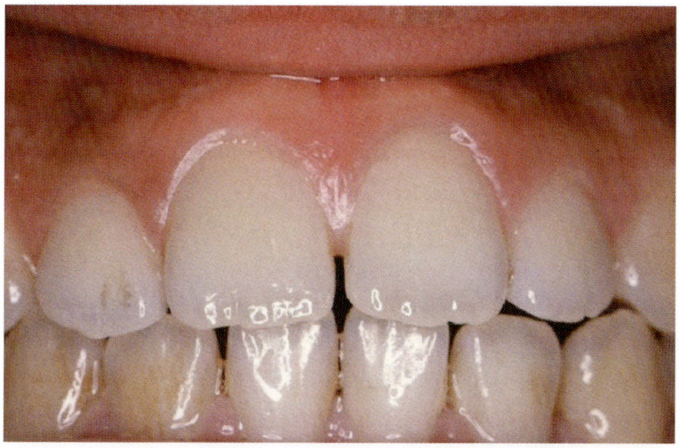
(A)

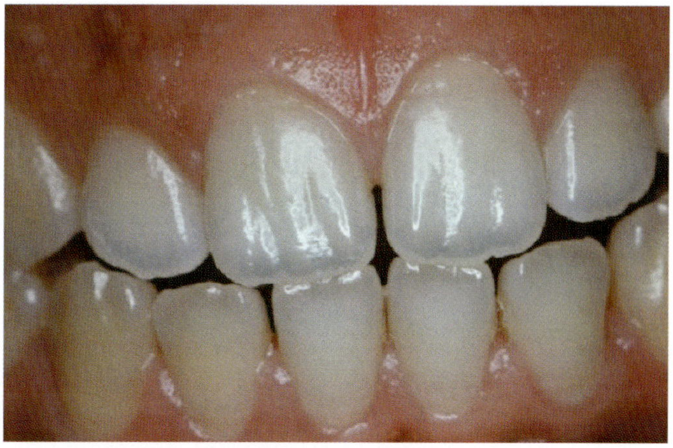
(B)

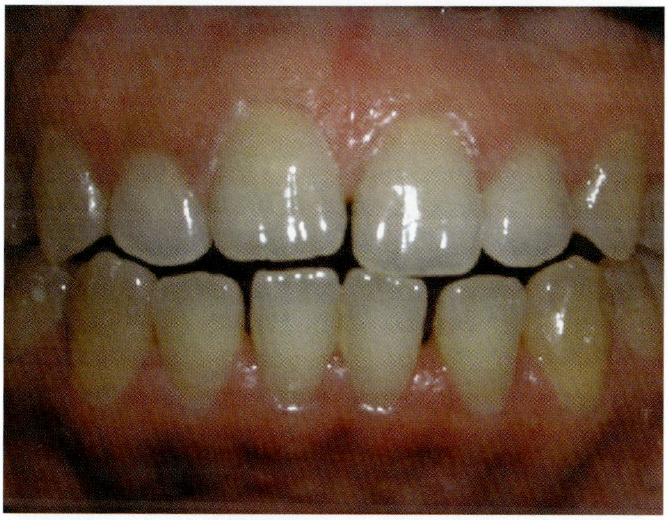
(C)

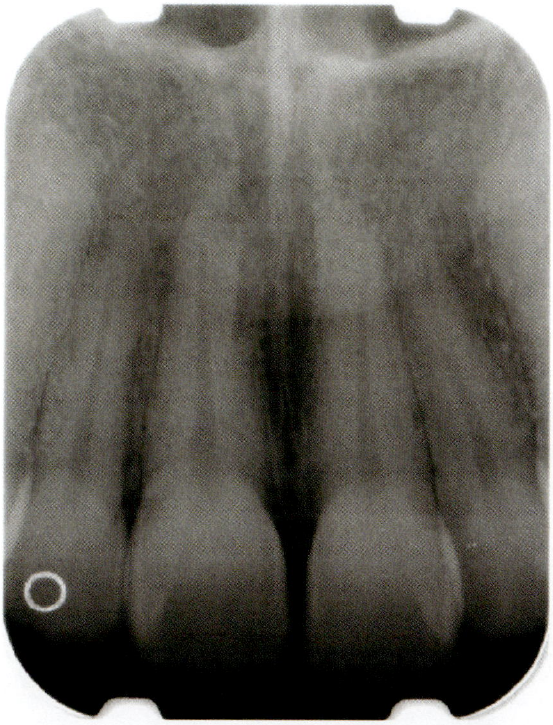
(D)

Figure 19.2

(A) Pretreatment. (B) 0 months post-treatment, and (C) 16 years, 4 months post-treatment. (D) Radiographic images of the teeth examined (6–11) at 16 years, 4 months post-treatment. Note that there is no soft tissue or pulpal pathology (internal or external resorption) at any timeframe. (From Boushell LW, Ritter AV, Garland GE, Tiwana KK. (2012) Nightguard Vital Bleaching: side effects and patient satisfaction 10 to 17 years post-treatment. *J Esthet Restor Dent* **24**[3]: 211–9, with permission.)

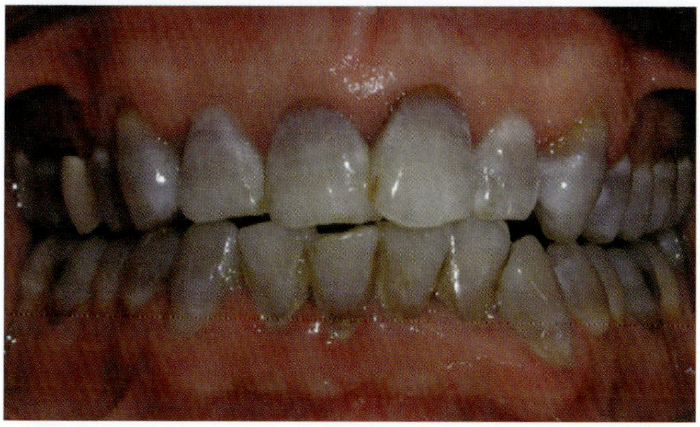
(A)

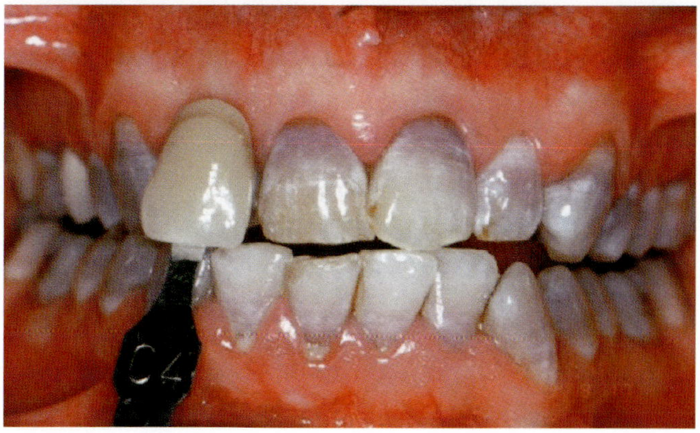
(B)

Figure 19.3

(A) Pretreatment, (B) 0 months post-treatment.

continued on the next page

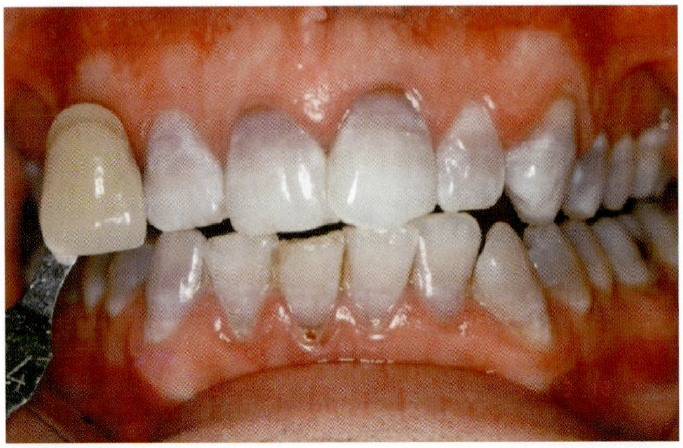

(C)

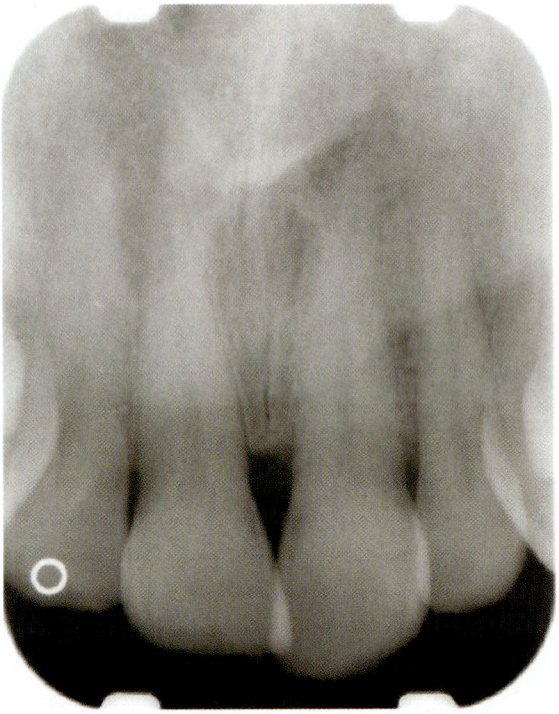

(D)

Figure 19.3 continued

(C) 12 years, 7 months post-treatment, (D) Radiographic images of the teeth examined (6–11) at 12 years, 7 months post-treatment. Note that there is no soft tissue or pulpal pathology (internal or external resorption) at any timeframe. (From Boushell LW, Ritter AV, Garland GE, Tiwana KK. (2012) Nightguard Vital Bleaching: side effects and patient satisfaction 10 to 17 years post-treatment. *J Esthet Restor Dent* **24**[3]:211–9, with permission.)

(A)

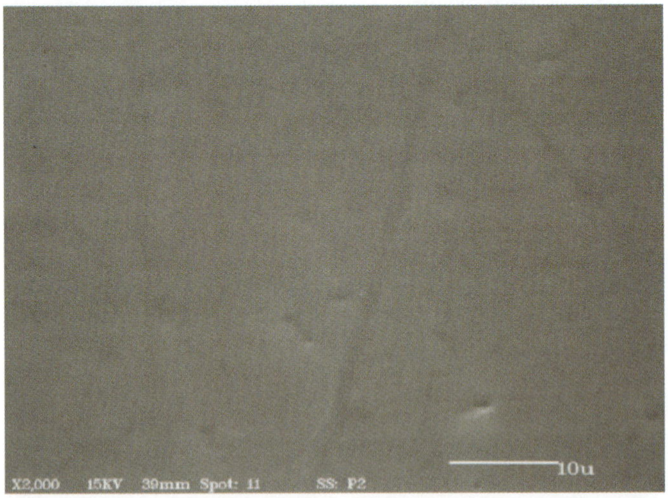

(B)

Figure 19.4

(A) Pretreatment and (B) post-treatment scanning electron microscope (SEM) images showing enamel surface morphology. The active treatment period was 2 weeks. Enamel surface morphology appears similar in both images. (From Boushell LW, Ritter AV, Garland GE, Tiwana KK. (2012) Nightguard Vital Bleaching: side effects and patient satisfaction 10 to 17 years post-treatment. *J Esthet Restor Dent* **24**[3]:211–9, with permission.)

20 TOOTH SENSITIVITY ASSOCIATED WITH TOOTH WHITENING

Linda Greenwall

INTRODUCTION

Tooth sensitivity is common during whitening treatment. Almost all sensitivity experienced during whitening is transient and fades after the whitening treatment is discontinued (Li and Greenwall 2013). Because sensitivity is the most common side effect experienced during whitening, this chapter will look at the etiology of sensitivity, which patients are at risk for experiencing sensitivity, and prevention and reduction strategies.

There is a difference between the severity of the sensitivity experienced during home whitening and that experienced during power whitening. The intensity of the sensitivity experienced during power whitening can be more severe.

HISTORY OF PREEXISTING SENSITIVITY

If a patient has preexisting sensitivity, will he or she be more likely to experience sensitivity during whitening? It is thought that this may be the case and that it is essential to question the patient to obtain an accurate dental history. The patient should be asked about his or her experience with sensitivity to heat, cold, and sweet things; pain on biting; and pain with cold sensations (see Tables 20.1 and 20.2 for the tooth sensitivity algorithm). Each sensitive stimulus will determine whether the pain is from gingival recession or a more severe cause such as acute pulpitis. Sensitivity to cold and pain on biting together can mean the presence of a crack in the tooth, and this should be attended to before any further whitening treatment is undertaken. This is because whitening gels go straight into a crack in a tooth (Kwon et al. 2012) and could make the tooth more sensitive. Use of a desensitizing toothpaste for 2 weeks before the whitening treatment has been shown to be effective in reducing the incidence and severity of pain during whitening.

Another treatment possibility is using a desensitizing toothpaste or a proprietary desensitizing material as a treatment for 1 hour in the tray each evening or placing the desensitizing gel in the tray overnight. This will make the teeth less sensitive, and the patient can then proceed with the normal whitening treatment (see Figure 20.4).

SENSITIVITY ELIMINATION OR REDUCTION

Sensitivity is a common side effect when whitening teeth (Haywood 1999). About 67% of patients may experience some type of sensitivity at some stage during whitening (Haywood et al. 1994, Nathanson 1997). Different levels of sensitivity may be experienced (Thitinanthapan et al. 1999, Albers 2000). Normally patients do not experience any sensitivity for the first three or four nights. It is not known what determines whether or not a patient will experience sensitivity. In a study conducted at the University of North Carolina School of Dentistry, Leonard and coworkers (1997) found that of those patients who changed the solution more than once per night, 55% had sensitivity. This factor was found to be significant ($P < .02$). Two thirds of the patients who demonstrated tooth characteristics such as gingival recession, defective restorations, and enamel-cementum abrasion reported sensitivity, but when these characteristics were statistically evaluated, they were not found to be statistically significant risk factors. No statistical relationship existed between age, sex, allergy, whitening solution used, tooth characteristics, or dental arch lightened and the development of side effects. (For relevant factors see Table 20.2.)

ORIGIN OF SENSITIVITY

The yellow color of dentin contributes to the overall color of the tooth. Dentin consists of millions of round tubules (see Figure 20.1). Movement of fluid in the dentinal tubules is detected by the pain fibers. The movement is triggered by temperature changes, differences in osmotic pressure among different oral solutions, and tactile pressure acting on the exposed dentin surface (Bartlett and Ide 1999). The sensitivity of dentin occurs when the dentinal tubules are open and exposed to the oral cavity. The presence of open tubules has been related to increased activation of the pain fibers within the pulp by cold stimuli when applied to tooth surfaces (Bartlett and Ide 1999). These factors may suggest why patients experience sensitivity during tooth whitening treatment. Treatment is aimed at blocking the tubules (see Figure 20.1).

Table 20.1 Treatment sequence for managing whitening sensitivity

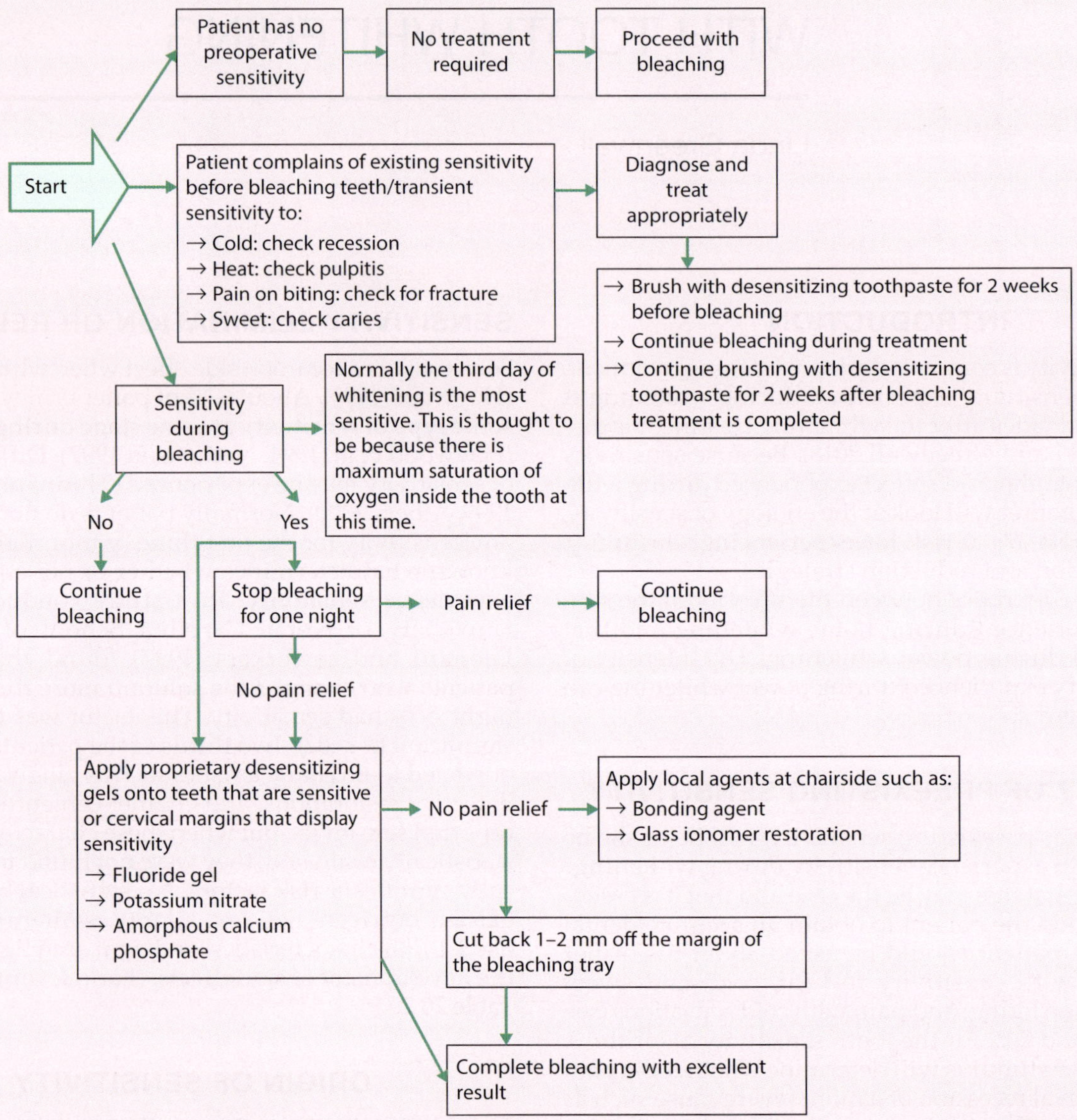

From Greenwall L, Jameson C. Success strategies for the aesthetic dental practice, *Quintessence*: London, 2012, with permission.

Table 20.2 Factors affecting sensitivity

- Inherent patient sensitivity
- Frequency of application (e.g., application twice a day can cause teeth to become sensitive)
- Concentration of the material
- History of sensitivity (assess at consultation)
  - Hot or cold sensitivity?
  - Pain on biting?
  - Pain with sweet items?

TOOTH SENSITIVITY DURING WHITENING

It is common for patients to experience sensitivity during both home and power whitening. There are multiple simple and complex causes of tooth sensitivity experienced during whitening (see Table 20.3). For home whitening treatments, it is extremely important to establish a management strategy that includes a self-management home desensitizing regimen so that the patient can continue the whitening treatment (see Table 20.4). There are multiple treatment options, which are listed in Table 20.5. It is advisable to give the patient an alternative when administering home desensitizing treatments. The patient should brush with a desensitizing toothpaste during the time of whitening. It has also been shown that brushing with a desensitizing toothpaste for 2 weeks before whitening can help eliminate or reduce the sensitivity experienced during whitening. Then the patient is given instructions on how to use the proprietary soothing gels. Figure 20.10 shows a tray that has been set up for explaining the methods of

Table 20.3 Possible causes of tooth sensitivity and gingival irritation

- Addition of Carbopol and other thickening agents.
- Age of the patient (patients younger than age 40 experience more side effects)
- Anhydrous-based whitening products
- Chemical byproducts of carbamide peroxide
- Chemical interaction of the tray
- Concentration of whitening solution
- Dissolving media
- Exposure time
- Flavors added to the whitening solution
- Frequency of application
- Inherent patient sensitivity
- Medical status of the patient
- pH of the whitening solution
- Sex of the patient (women appear to experience more side effects than men)
- Tray material used
- Tray rigidity

Data from Leonard (1998) and Knight et al. (1997).

Table 20.4 Management plan for dealing with sensitivity during whitening

Stage 1	Prevention
Stage 2	Treatment
Stage 3	Avoidance: helping patients self-manage

Table 20.5 Options for sensitivity reduction or elimination

Active treatment

- Cover deep cervical lesions with glass ionomer pretreatment (Class V restorations)
- Apply material into the tray
  - Neutral sodium fluoride gel
  - 5% potassium nitrate
  - Amorphous calcium phosphate (ACP), MI Paste, MI Paste Plus
  - Proprietary desensitizing materials and soothers
- Use new materials that incorporate soothers
- Brush with desensitizing toothpaste or ACP
- Apply soothers directly onto the teeth
  - ACP varnish
  - Immediate dentin sealing agent (e.g., HurriSeal)
  - Dentin bonding agent

Passive treatment

- Modify whitening technique
- Ensure all excess is removed
- Use lower concentration
- Reduce treatment times
- Apply every second or third night
- Trim back tray
- Interrupt treatment
- Stop treatment

soothing during whitening and the vast array of products available for this purpose.

Methods for treating sensitivity (see Table 20.5)

There are two methods to consider for the treatment of sensitivity during whitening treatment: the passive method and the active method.

Passive method

- Altering the whitening time.
- Changing the frequency.
- Reducing concentration to find a comfortable solution for the patient.
- Allowing the patient to skip a night of whitening.
- Using less whitening gel in the tray.
- Trimming back the whitening tray so that it does not impinge on the gingival margins.

Active method

- In the active method, desensitizing materials are applied either directly onto the teeth or inside the whitening tray.
- Products used are fluoride or potassium nitrate applied in the tray as a pretreatment, at the onset of symptoms, or after a course of treatment.
- The use of fluoride and potassium nitrate to treat whitening sensitivity has been clinically researched and seems to work well (Haywood 1999).

Fluoride as a desensitizing material

Fluoride reduces sensitivity by blocking the tubules. This restricts the ingress of fluids according to the hydrodynamic theory of pain (Bartlett and Ide 1999). A neutral fluoride has been recommended for treatment use, such as PreviDent 5000 Plus (Colgate Oral Pharmaceuticals).

Potassium nitrate

Potassium nitrate reduces sensitivity via chemical interference that prevents the pulpal sensory nerve from repolarizing after initial depolarization (Leonard 1998), or it aids the release of nitric oxide (Haywood 1999). Either way, the effect is directly on the nerve, resulting in a calming effect on the tooth. Many desensitizing toothpastes contain potassium nitrate. Brushing with the desensitizing toothpaste will reduce sensitivity after 2 weeks. The U.S. Food and Drug Administration (FDA) allows 5% potassium nitrate as the maximum concentration.

Other materials

Some patients may experience a tissue burn as a side effect of placing the desensitizing toothpaste in the tray.

Options for treatment of sensitivity during whitening

Active treatment

For patients with normally sensitive teeth:

- Fluoride toothpaste can be placed in the trays and worn on alternate nights. (Some whitening agents contain fluoride within the whitening material to reduce the likelihood of sensitivity—e.g., Opalescence F [Ultradent].)

- A desensitizing toothpaste can be brushed on the teeth or massaged into the cervical margins. Or a specific sensitivity-reduction material (e.g., products by Ultradent and Denmat) that contains potassium nitrate is placed in the whitening tray and is worn for 1–2 hours, depending on the amount of sensitivity, or applied in the tray for 10–30 minutes before or after whitening.
- The patient can use a neutral sodium fluoride gel in the trays overnight.
- A specifically manufactured potassium nitrate–fluoride gel for use in the tray can be applied when needed or alternated with the whitening treatment (see Figure 20.7).

For patients with a history of sensitive teeth:

- Two weeks before commencing whitening, the patient can brush regularly with desensitizing toothpaste (e.g., Sensodyne Gentle Whitening, which in the United Kingdom contains potassium chloride instead of potassium nitrate).
- Amorphous calcium phosphate paste can be prescribed for the patient. The patient can use this in three ways: brush with it; apply it to a finger and massage onto the teeth; or place it into the whitening tray (see Figure 20.9) and apply this to the teeth for either 1 hour or an overnight use. This treatment can be used before whitening and after whitening procedures. There are numerous brands of amorphous calcium phosphate (ACP) paste (see Figures 20.7 and 20.8), which can also be applied directly to the teeth or as a varnish to act as a protective coat for the teeth (see Figure 20.14).
- Neutral fluoride in the whitening trays can be applied to the teeth 3 weeks before commencing whitening treatment, to reduce sensitivity.
- A patient can begin to wear the empty tray at night for a few nights, then slowly increase the wear time from 1 hour a day for the first week to overnight on the second week or later (Haywood 1999).
- An immediate dentin sealer can be placed in multiple coats and air dried (see Figure 20.11).
- A dentin bonding agent can be used in the cervical areas (see Figure 20.14).
- A glass ionomer restoration can be placed to cover the deep cervical lesions. This helps with better tray fit and reduces the likelihood of experiencing sensitivity (see Figure 20.5).

Passive treatment

The whitening technique can be modified as follows:

- Ensure that all excess material is removed.
- Patient can use a whitening gel with a lower concentration. If using a 20% carbamide peroxide gel, the patient can change to a 15%, 10%, or 5% gel.
- Patient can reduce daily treatment time (Leonard 1998) or whiten every second or third night.
- Patient should not replenish the whitening solution more than once.
- Patient can use less whitening material in the tray and not overfill it, to avoid extrusion of excess gel.
- Dentist can ensure that the tray is trimmed back further so that it does not impinge on the gingiva (see Figure 20.15).

Single-tooth sensitivity

The type of sensitivity associated with whitening treatment is different from single-tooth sensitivity. If a patient has sensitivity in a single tooth, agents can simply be applied directly to the tooth (e.g., a bonding agent [Bartlett and Ide 1999], fluoride varnish, hydroxyethyl methacrylate [HEMA] or oxylate preparations) or, if necessary, the restoration can be replaced. These approaches will help only if sensitivity can be isolated to one accessible area. It is thus best for the dentist to supervise whitening and to determine the best approach to deal with sensitivity should it arise.

Prevalence of sensitivity during whitening

The prevalence of sensitivity during whitening can be high. Thirty-five percent to 50% of patients experience pain or sensitivity during home whitening. Despite the high incidence of transient sensitivity, the exact mechanism is not clearly understood (Swift 2006).

Treatment strategies

Managing whitening sensitivity

There are many management strategies for reducing the incidence of sensitivity during whitening. It is essential to give the patient choices for managing his or her sensitivity (see Table 20.4). This helps the patient reduce the anxiety related to the possibility that sensitivity will occur during the whitening treatment.

Reasons for the tooth sensitivity

When the whitening gel is applied to the tooth, the gel travels through the enamel, into the dentin, and into the pulp within 5–15 minutes of gel application. This can account for the occurrence of the sensitivity.

In addition, when the gel travels into the tooth it enters into the weakest part of the tooth first. Therefore if there is a crack in the tooth, the whitening gel will travel into the crack first. That is why teeth with cracks may experience more sensitivity. If there is an area of hypocalcification, the whitening gel will travel into this section first, causing the defect area to appear whiter in the beginning. White spots may thus appear whiter at the beginning stage of whitening.

The higher the concentration, the greater the sensitivity.

Treatment strategies for desensitizing during whitening are as follows:

Active method

- Materials used for sensitizing teeth during whitening:
  - Proprietary materials used for desensitizing teeth during whitening.

- Potassium nitrate.
- Fluoride.
- More recently, ACP has been added to some of the tooth whitening products to reduce sensitivity, reduce the demineralization of enamel through a remineralization process after whitening treatments, and add a lustrous shine to teeth (Alqahtani 2014).
- Dentin bonding agents.
- Other options:
  - Cut back the tray.
- Change the treatment sequence.

Passive method

- Reduce concentration of gel.
- Change the whitening regimen.
- Skip a night.

TOOTH SENSITIVITY DURING POWER WHITENING

Tooth sensitivity associated with power whitening is normally reversible and is commonly experienced. The sensitivity experienced can range from mild to considerable or in some cases severe.

Incidence of sensitivity experienced during power whitening

What contributes to sensitivity during power whitening?

- The higher the concentration of the whitening gel, the greater the incidence of sensitivity during whitening, the faster the action of the whitening gel, and the faster the incidence of the sensitivity. Benetti et al. (2004) found that the higher the concentration of the whitening gel, the greater the amount preserved in the pulp.
- The use of heat can contribute to the sensitivity.
- The light can emit heat and contribute to further sensitivity.
- The isolation process and the resulting dehydration effect of the gel on the teeth may also lead to further sensitivity.

Methods of reducing sensitivity during power whitening

The incidence and severity of tooth sensitivity can be reduced by pretreatment with a desensitizer such as potassium nitrate, fluoride, or ACP. Early studies on dogs showed that a transient mild pulpitis may be experienced. However, later histologic studies and clinical studies on long-term pulpal effects are lacking to definitively support the safety of in-office tooth whitening. Future studies on the etiology of tooth sensitivity related to whitening might greatly improve the means of preventing and managing this side effect (Kwon and Swift 2014).

Does a combination of home and power whitening contribute to the increase in sensitivity?

In a randomized clinical study, Dawson et al. (2011) assessed efficacy in terms of color change and production of sensitivity after home whitening alone and home whitening supplemented with in-office whitening. Thirty-six patients (aged 19–58 years) were randomly assigned to one of three different treatment groups: (A) home whitening for 2 weeks with 16% carbamide peroxide in custom-made trays; (B) home whitening for 2 weeks, with 16% carbamide peroxide in custom-made trays supplemented with in-office whitening with 9% hydrogen peroxide (in the same trays); or (C) home whitening for 2 weeks with 16% carbamide peroxide in custom-made trays supplemented with in-office whitening with 27% hydrogen peroxide (in the same trays). The efficacy of tooth whitening was assessed by determining the color change associated with the six upper anterior teeth using a value-ordered shade guide.

Sensitivity was self-assessed with the use of a visual analog scale (VAS). Tooth shade and sensitivity were assessed at the following points: pretreatment; immediately after the home whitening phase; immediately after the in-office phase (groups B and C); and 1 week after active treatment. At the 1-week follow-up visit, subjects in group A had a mean (standard deviation [SD]) color change of 5.9 (1.83) (teeth were lighter) immediately after cessation of treatment ($P < .01$). Subjects in groups B and C experienced a greater change in mean (SD) shade immediately after their respective in-office treatments of 5.1 (1.53) and 5.4 (1.55). However, within 1 week, the shade of these teeth had regressed to a similar degree to that achieved by subjects treated in group A. Overall there was no significant difference in shade change or sensitivity that was produced among the three groups. These investigators concluded that the in-office element of combined whitening produced no significant difference in tooth color or sensitivity when compared with home whitening alone.

TOOTH SENSITIVITY AFTER TREATMENT

Post-treatment sensitivity is usually related to small microscopic enamel defects and subsurface pores, which allow the whitening agent to penetrate into the dental tubules and ultimately the pulp, causing reversible pulpitis and consequent thermal sensitivity in the teeth, but not causing permanent damage to the pulp (Haywood 1999, Berga-Caballero et al. 2006). These responses correlate with the peroxide concentration, time, frequency of gel application, and pulp temperature rise after light activation.

CONCLUSION

Although sensitivity can be experienced before, during, and after whitening, the effects are transient and always disappear a few days after whitening is completed. There are many treatment and management strategies to deal with the sensitivity that patients experience, so this should not deter patients from completing whitening treatment effectively. Most of the current whitening materials contain built-in desensitizers to reduce the likelihood of sensitivity. Patients should be given instruction on how to self-manage their sensitivity during treatment so that they can cope with the transient sensitivity that may be experienced.

REFERENCES

Albers HF. (2000) Dentine and sensitivity. *Adept Rep* **6**:4,10–1.

Alqahtani MQ. (2014) Tooth-bleaching procedures and their controversial effects: a literature review. *Saudi Dent J* **26**(2):33–46.

Auschill TM, Hellwig E, Schmidale S, Sculean A. (2005) Efficacy, side-effects and patients' acceptance of different bleaching techniques (OTC, in-office, at-home). *Oper Dent* **30**(2):156–63.

Bartlett DW, Ide M. (1999) Dealing with sensitive teeth. *Prim Dent Care* **6**(1):25–7.

Benetti AR, Valera MC, Mancini MN, Miranda CB. (2004) In vitro penetration of bleaching agents into the pulp chamber. *Int Endod J* **37**(2) 120–4.

Berga-Caballero A, Forner-Navarro L, Amengual-Lorenzo J. (2006) At-home vital bleaching: a comparison of hydrogen peroxide and carbamide peroxide treatments. *Med Oral Patol Oral Cir Bucal* **11**:E94–9.

Cooper JS, Bokmeyer TJ, Bowles WH. (1992) Penetration of the pulp chamber by carbamide peroxide bleaching agents. *J Endod* **18**:315–7.

Costa CA, Riehl H, Kina JF. (2010) Human pulp responses to in-office tooth bleaching. *Oral Surg Oral Med Oral Pathol Oral Radiol Endod* **109**(4):e59–64.

Dawson PF, Sharif MO, Smith AB. (2011) A clinical study comparing the efficacy and sensitivity of home vs combined whitening. *Oper Dent* **36**(5):460–6.

Haywood VB. (1999) Current status and recommendations for dentist-prescribed, at-home tooth whitening. *Contemp Esthet Restor Pract* **3**(Suppl 1):2–9.

Haywood VB, Caughman WF, Frazier KB, Myers ML. (2001) Tray delivery of potassium nitrate. *Quintessence Int* **32**:105–9.

Haywood VB, Cordero R, Wright K, Gendreau L. (2005) Brushing with potassium nitrate dentifrice to reduce bleaching sensitivity. *J Clin Dent* **16**(1):17–22.

Haywood VB, Leonard RH, Nelson CF. (1994) Effectiveness, side effects and long term status of Nightguard Vital Bleaching. *J Am Dent Assoc* **125**:1219–26.

Hewlett ER. (2007) Etiology and management of whitening-induced tooth hypersensitivity. *J Calif Dent Assoc* **35**(7):499–506.

Knight MC, Leonard RH, Bentley C, et al. (1997) Safety issues of 10% carbamide peroxide in clinical usage. *J Dent Res* 76 [IADR Abstracts No. 2366].

Kwon SR, Swift EJ Jr. (2014) Critical appraisal. In-office tooth whitening: pulpal effects and tooth sensitivity issues. *Esthet Restor Dent* **26**(5):353–8.

Kwon SR, Wertz PW, Li Y, Chan DC. (2012) Penetration pattern of rhodamine dyes into enamel and dentin: confocal laser microscopy observation. *Int J Cosmet Sci* **34**(1):97–101.

Leonard RH. (1998) Efficacy, longevity, side effects and patient perceptions of Nightguard Vital Bleaching. *Compend Contin Educ Dent* **19**(8):776–81.

Leonard RH, Haywood VB, Phillips C. (1997) Risk factors for developing tooth sensitivity and gingival irritation associated with Nightguard Vital Bleaching. *Quintessence Int* **28**(8):527–34.

Leonard RH Jr, Bentley C, Eagle JC, Garland GE. (2001) Nightguard Vital Bleaching: a long-term study on efficacy, shade retention, side effects, and patients' perceptions. *J Esthet Restor Dent* **13**(6):357–69.

Li Y, Greenwall L. (2013) Safety issues of tooth whitening using peroxide-based materials. *Br Dent J* **215**(1):29–34.

Moghadam FV, Majidinia S, Chasteen J, Ghavamnasiri M. (2013) The degree of color change, rebound effect and sensitivity of bleached teeth associated with at-home and power bleaching techniques: a randomized clinical trial. *Eur J Dent* **7**(4):405–11.

Nathanson D. (1997) Vital tooth bleaching: sensitivity and pulpal considerations. *J Am Dent Assoc* **128**:41S–4S.

Ray DS. (2014) Using light to enhance in-office vital bleaching may increase both efficacy and tooth sensitivity. *J Am Dent Assoc* **145**(11):1159–60.

Swift EJ Jr. (2006) At-home bleaching: pulpal effects and tooth sensitivity issues, part II. *Esthet Restor Dent* **18**(5):301–5.

Tay LY, Kose C, Loguercio AD, Reis A. (2009) Assessing the effect of a desensitizing agent used before in-office tooth bleaching. *J Am Dent Assoc* **40**(10):1245–51.

Thiesen CH, Rodrigues Filho R, Prates LH, Sartori N. (2013) The influence of desensitizing dentifrices on pain induced by in-office bleaching. *Braz Oral Res* **27**(6):517–23.

Thitinanthapan W, Satamanont P, Vongsavan N. (1999) In-vitro penetration of the pulp chamber by three brands of carbamide peroxide. *J Esthet Dent* **11**(5):259–63.

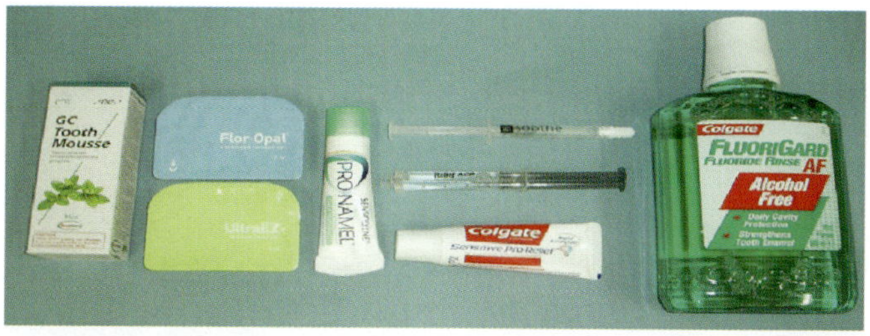

Figure 20.10

A tray set up to undertake desensitizing for a patient and delivery of the home care instructions that are needed for the patient to manage sensitivity. Normally a sample of a tube of desensitizing toothpaste is given to the patient to use during whitening. This will reduce the amount of sensitivity experienced.

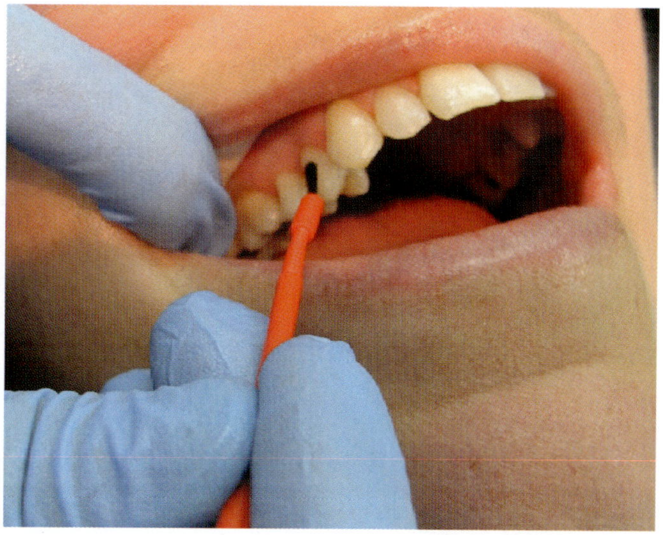

Figure 20.12

Applying dentin bonding agent directly to the cervical areas of the upper teeth.

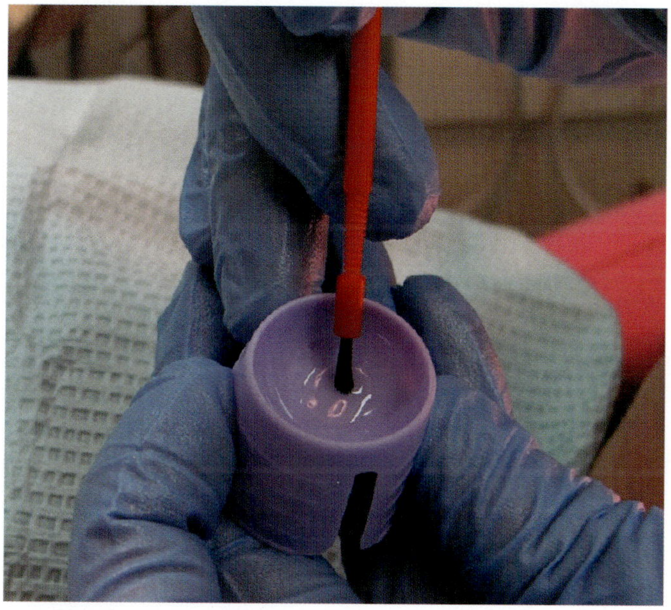

Figure 20.11

The HurriSeal is placed into a dappen dish and then applied in multiple coats directly onto the sensitive area, which is often a cervical erosion area.

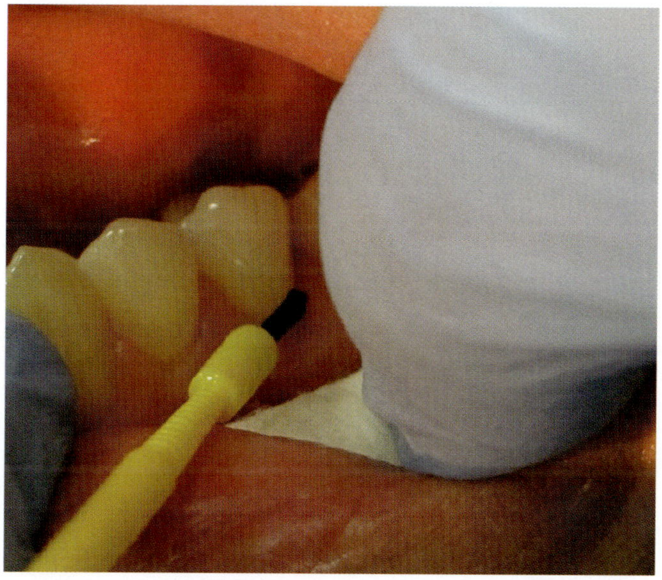

Figure 20.13

Applying HurriSeal to the lower cervical area during whitening treatment.

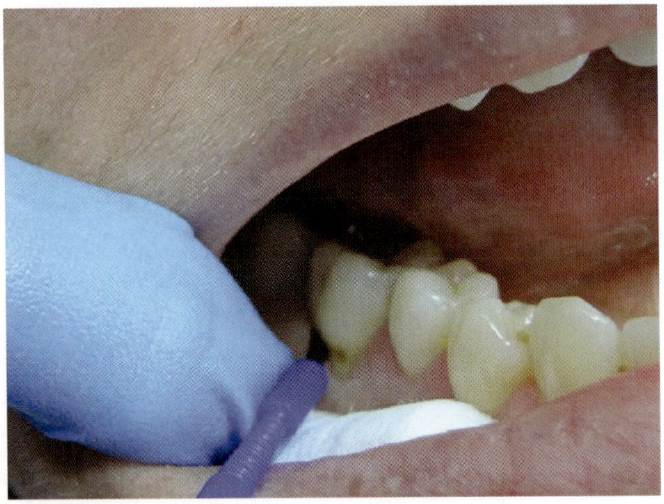

Figure 20.14

Applying fluoride varnish directly onto the cervical area to reduce sensitivity.

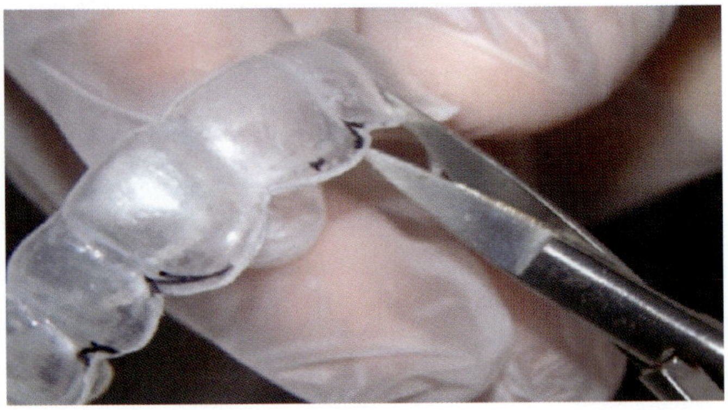

Figure 20.15

Trimming the whitening tray back where it is overextended. The over-extended areas are marked with a marking pen and the excess trimmed with special fine-point scissors (Ultra-Trim [Ultradent Products, South Jordan, UT]).

21 SAFETY AND TOXICOLOGIC CONSIDERATIONS FOR TOOTH BLEACHING

Yiming Li

INTRODUCTION

Tooth bleaching using peroxide compounds has been practiced in dentistry for more than a century. The procedure, which typically involves the use of high concentrations of hydrogen peroxide (H_2O_2, usually 30–35%), was exclusively performed by dentists in their offices (Li 1996). Home bleaching, however, was not available until 1989, when the at-home bleaching procedure was introduced by Haywood and Heymann (Haywood and Heymann 1989). The initial home-use tooth bleaching gel contained 10% carbamide peroxide, which is equivalent to approximately 3.5% H_2O_2, as the active ingredient, and it was available only from dentists. With its demonstrated efficacy, its low cost compared with in-office bleaching, and the convenience of self-application by the user, at-home bleaching quickly gained popularity and has now become an integrated procedure in esthetic dentistry (Kihn 2007). In addition, over-the-counter (OTC) and infomercial home-use bleaching products have now become available directly to consumers without involving dental professionals. In recent years, tooth bleaching using materials and procedures similar to those used for in-office bleaching but performed in nondental settings, such as mall kiosks, spas, and cruise ships, has become available (American Dental Association [ADA] 2009a).

Although attempts have been made to introduce at-home tooth whiteners that claimed to contain no peroxide, such products did not gain acceptance because of the lack of evidence regarding their efficacy and controversy over their nonperoxide claim (Li 2003). Current tooth bleaching materials, regardless of their use for in-office or at-home bleaching, are typically made in the form of a gel and contain a peroxide compound as the active ingredient, with carbamide peroxide and H_2O_2 being the most common (Li 1996, 2003). In general, H_2O_2 in concentrations ranging from 25–40% is the choice for in-office bleaching gels, and at-home bleaching formulations use carbamide peroxide and/or H_2O_2 in concentrations of 10–22% carbamide peroxide or 3–7.5% H_2O_2. In recent years, there has been a trend toward elevating the H_2O_2 concentration in home-use bleaching gels, and products of up to 15% H_2O_2 have now become available directly to consumers.

Throughout the history of tooth bleaching using peroxide-based gels, there has been little dispute regarding the efficacy. However, safety concerns associated with potential toxicologic effects of peroxides used in bleaching gels have been raised. With the accumulation of scientific data over the last two decades, most of the toxicologic concerns with bleaching using peroxide-based gels have diminished. Nevertheless, controversy concerning their safety has continued, and there have been reports of adverse effects of bleaching on oral tissues (see Figures 21.1C and 21.5) and restorative materials (Cubbon and Ore 1991, Hammel 1998, Dahl and Pallesen 2003, Attin et al. 2004, Goldberg et al. 2010).

This chapter provides an overview on safety issues in tooth bleaching in relation to biologic properties of H_2O_2 and discusses proper use of bleaching to maximize the benefits while minimizing the potential risks.

SAFETY CONCERNS WITH TOOTH BLEACHING RELEVANT TO BIOLOGIC PROPERTIES OF H_2O_2

Peroxide compounds typically form H_2O_2 in aqueous solutions. Chemically, carbamide peroxide is composed of approximately 3.5 parts of H_2O_2 and 6.5 parts of urea, so a bleaching gel of 10% carbamide peroxide contains approximately 3.5% H_2O_2. Consequently, H_2O_2 is the active ingredient regardless of whether a bleaching gel contains carbamide peroxide or H_2O_2.

The chemistry of H_2O_2 is well understood. As a chemical, H_2O_2 was first identified in 1818; it was detected in human respiration in 1880. The well-known Fenton reaction was proposed in 1894. Two important enzymes for H_2O_2 metabolism in humans, peroxidase and catalase, were found in 1898 and 1901, respectively. Since 1969 when H_2O_2 was recognized as an important byproduct in oxygen metabolism after the discovery of another important enzyme, superoxide dismutase (SOD), in human physiology and biochemistry, the research efforts on the biologic properties of H_2O_2 have significantly increased (Li 1996). H_2O_2 is now known as a normal intermediate metabolite in the human liver, with a daily production of approximately 6.48 g.

A key characteristic of H_2O_2 is its capability of producing free radicals, which are known to be capable of inducing various toxicities, including hydroxyl radicals that have been implicated in various stages of carcinogenesis. More relevant to safety is that oxidative reactions of free radicals with proteins, lipids, and nucleic acids are believed to be involved in a number of potential pathologic consequences; the damage from oxidative free radicals may be associated with aging, stroke, and other degenerative diseases (Harman 1981, Lutz 1990). H_2O_2 is highly cytotoxic to cultured mammalian cells at concentrations ranging from 1.7–19.7 µg/mL (0.05–0.58 mmol/L) (Li 2003). The oxidative reactions and subsequent damage in cells by free radicals are believed to be the major mechanisms responsible for the observed toxicity of H_2O_2.

On the other hand, there are various defensive mechanisms available at cellular and tissue levels to prevent potential damage to cells during oxidative reactions and to repair any damage sustained. Enzymes such as catalase, SOD, peroxidase, and selenium-dependent glutathione peroxidase, which exist widely in body fluids, tissues, and organs, effectively metabolize H_2O_2 (Floyd 1990). Studies have shown that the cytotoxicity of H_2O_2 can be effectively reduced or eliminated by simply increasing serum concentration in the culture media (Sacks et al. 1978, Rubin and Farber 1984). In a cell culture study, 20 mM H_2O_2 was undetectable after 30 minutes in the culture media alone and after 15 minutes in the media with bone tissues, indicating decomposition and inactivation of H_2O_2 in cell culture systems (Ramp 1987). Human saliva has also been found to contain these enzymes; in fact, salivary peroxidase has been suggested to be the body's most important and effective defense against the potential adverse effects of H_2O_2 (Carlsson 1987).

Because of the known toxicology of H_2O_2, especially the effects of free radicals, there have been concerns regarding potential systemic adverse effects if the bleaching gel is ingested as well as local adverse effects on enamel, pulp, and gingiva when the gel directly contacts the tissues (see Figures 21.1 and 21.6) (Li 1996, 2001, ADA 2009). The safety controversies surrounding peroxide-based tooth bleaching have prompted not only scientific deliberations but also legal challenges to the use of these products in dentistry (Weiner et al. 2000, Scientific Committee on Consumer Products 2005).

POTENTIAL EXPOSURE TO BLEACHING GEL

Exposure is one of the important factors that determine toxicologic consequences of an agent. For in-office bleaching, the exposure to bleaching gel during the treatment appears to be minimal (see Figures 21.1, 21.3, and 21.6) because the soft tissues are adequately protected with use of barrier materials (see Figure 21.5B). In addition, at the end of treatment the gel is first removed with a high-volume evacuator, and the teeth are rinsed thoroughly with water. Little, if any, gel is left behind for possible ingestion. Furthermore, because of its high concentration of H_2O_2, any gel contact with oral soft tissues would immediately cause irritation and signal its presence to the patient and dentist. Accordingly, the actual exposure dose of H_2O_2 during in-office tooth bleaching is minute if the product is used properly.

For at-home bleaching, the initial study estimated that the approximate dose of carbamide peroxide for each at-home application was 90 mg (Haywood and Heymann 1989). This was confirmed in a later report in which the average amount of bleaching gel used clinically for 10 maxillary teeth (full arch) was 502 mg per application (Li 1996). When both arches are being bleached, the average amount of bleach is approximately 1.0 g. For a bleaching gel containing 10% carbamide peroxide, the exposure dose would be 100 mg per application. Dahl and Becher (1995) estimated that approximately 10% of the applied bleaching gel may be consumed during the application. Therefore, for an individual of 60-kg body weight who performs at-home bleaching for both arches once daily, the exposure to the bleaching gel can be calculated at 1.67 mg/kg/day, and the exposure to carbamide peroxide through a gel containing 10% carbamide peroxide will be 0.167 mg/kg/day. Carbamide peroxide contains approximately 3.5% H_2O_2; consequently, the estimated H_2O_2 exposure is 0.058 mg/kg/day, or 3.48 mg H_2O_2 per day for an adult of 60-kg body weight.

This estimation appears conservative, because it assumes a constant concentration of 10% carbamide peroxide in the gel during the whole bleaching period, which usually lasts an hour to overnight. Studies have shown that the H_2O_2 content decreases with the time—particularly significant during the earlier part of the application (Matis 2000, Sagel et al. 2001, Al-Qunaian et al. 2003). The rate of peroxide decomposition appears to be associated with the viscosity of the material. A clinical study found that the human oral cavity, including that of adults, juveniles, infants, and adults with impaired salivary flow, was capable of eliminating 30 mg H_2O_2 in less than 1.5 minutes (Marshall et al.). Consequently, the estimated exposure dose of 3.48 mg H_2O_2 during at-home bleaching does not appear to constitute a significant risk.

SAFETY CONCERNS WITH POTENTIAL SYSTEMIC ADVERSE EFFECTS OF PEROXIDE-BASED TOOTH BLEACHING

Potential systemic toxicity of H_2O_2 and peroxide-based tooth bleaching gels has been the subject of a comprehensive body of literature, which includes topics of acute and subacute systemic toxicity, sensitization or allergic reaction, reproductive toxicity and teratology, genotoxicity, and carcinogenicity (Li 1996). Accidental ingestion of large amounts of concentrated H_2O_2 solution can cause acute toxic consequences including death (Humberston et al. 1990, Rackoff and Merton 1990, Christensen et al. 1992, Cina et al. 1994, Dickson and Caravati 1994). Such incidences appear to be more common in the pediatric population (71% for patients younger than 18 years of age) than adults (Dickson and Caravati 1994). One major factor associated with the toxicity of H_2O_2 is its concentration. Ingestion of H_2O_2 solutions of less than 10% usually produces no significant adverse effects, although it may cause mild irritation to mucous membranes that results in spontaneous emesis or mild abdominal bloating (Humberston et al. 1990, Rackoff and Merton 1990). Exposure to higher concentrations of H_2O_2 (>10%), however, can result in severe tissue burns (see Figure 21.6) and significant systemic toxicity. In addition to the oxidative tissue damage, gas embolism is responsible for various pathologic consequences of H_2O_2 ingestion (Humberston et al. 1990, Rackoff and Merton 1990, Dickson and Caravati 1994).

Subacute systemic toxicities of H_2O_2 and peroxide-based tooth bleaching gels have been investigated in animals only. The no-observed-effect level (NOEL) of H_2O_2 in rats was 30 and 56.2 mg/kg/day for 100 and 90 days, respectively (Kawasaki et al. 1969, Ito et al. 1976). Mice receiving a higher H_2O_2 dose at 150 mg/kg/day for 35 weeks grew normally and showed no visible abnormalities; necropsy results, however, showed changes in the liver, kidney, stomach, and small intestine (U.S. Food and Drug Administration [FDA] 1983). In rats, the dose of H_2O_2 at 506 mg/kg for 90 days caused suppressed body weight gain, decreased food consumption, and changes in hematology, blood chemistry, and organ weights (Ito et al. 1976).

Published research on sensitization potential, reproductive toxicity, and teratology of H_2O_2 and peroxide-based tooth bleaching gels remains sparse. Available data appear to indicate a low risk of sensitization potential because peroxide compounds exist ubiquitously in our environment and diet, and H_2O_2 is a normal intermediate metabolite of humans (Li 1996). A plausible explanation for the negative productive toxicity or teratologic effects of H_2O_2 is that the ingested H_2O_2 is quickly and effectively metabolized before it reaches the target organs (Hankan 1958, Burnett et al. 1976, Korhonen et al. 1984, de Lamirande and Gagnon 1994).

The results of studies on the genotoxicity of H_2O_2 and peroxide-based tooth bleaching gels have been somewhat controversial. The overall data available so far show that H_2O_2 and peroxide-based tooth bleaching gels are genotoxic only in in vitro systems without enzymatic activation; when enzymatic activation is incorporated in in vitro assays or when tested in animals, H_2O_2 and peroxide-based tooth bleaching gels are nongenotoxic (Li 1997, 2000, 2011b). Again, such observations are most likely related to the effective metabolic process of peroxide by microsomes or in vivo defensive systems.

Consequently, with the available toxicologic data on H_2O_2 as well as the research on bleaching gels and their exposure assessment, safety concerns regarding most potential systemic toxicities associated with the use of gels containing 10% carbamide peroxide have largely diminished. When these products are used appropriately, the H_2O_2 exposure from bleaching is essentially limited to the oral cavity, and it is incapable of reaching a systemic level to be toxic because of the effective metabolic defensive mechanisms.

However, the issue of carcinogenicity of H_2O_2 has remained controversial in the literature, and results of some studies are contradictory (Li 2000, 2011b). Most found no evidence of carcinogenicity of H_2O_2; a few showed that H_2O_2 was anticarcinogenic, whereas several investigators reported carcinogenicity or cocarcinogenicity of H_2O_2. The studies that have been cited most frequently as evidence of carcinogenicity and cocarcinogenicity of H_2O_2 were reported by Ito et al. (1981, 1982, 1984) and Weitzman et al. (1986). However, evaluation of these studies found significant deficiencies in design and conduct of the experiments as well as in the assessment of the results; consequently, the findings of these four studies were determined to be inadequate to substantiate their conclusions (Li 1996, 2011b).

It is obvious that any carcinogenicity or cocarcinogenicity of tooth bleaching constitutes a significant health risk. Because of the potential significance of the Weitzman study, which used local application of H_2O_2 on oral mucosa of Syrian golden hamsters, the same study was repeated using proper design and methods; the results found no evidence of carcinogenicity or cocarcinogenicity of 3% H_2O_2 (Marshall et al. 1996). Consequently, bleaching using 10% carbamide peroxide, which is equivalent to 3.5% H_2O_2, is regarded as having no significant carcinogenic or cocarcinogenic risks. The overall data on bleaching obtained from more than 20 years also appear to support this conclusion. However, because of the significance of the carcinogenicity and relatively limited data available on the topic for bleaching, especially for products with more than 10% carbamide peroxide, questions and debates over the carcinogenic risks of bleaching arise periodically. Future research is encouraged to help clarify the controversy and concerns with the topic.

POTENTIAL LOCAL ADVERSE EFFECTS ASSOCIATED WITH PEROXIDE-BASED TOOTH BLEACHING

Tooth bleaching requires continuous direct contact of the gel to enamel surface for half an hour to up to 7 or 8 hours (overnight). The enamel-gel contact may also be repeated within the same day or daily for an extended period. Unlike in-office bleaching, during which oral tissues are protected and procedures are performed by dental professionals, at-home bleaching often involves unintended direct contact of the bleaching gel to gingiva when applied by consumers. For some at-home systems, such as strips, the gingival contact is inevitable. In addition, users of home bleaching systems tend to overuse the product, which may aggravate the tissue contact with the gel (see Figures 21.2 and 21.5). Consequently, possible adverse effects of bleaching on the enamel, gingiva, pulp, and restorations have been raised and investigated.

Potential adverse effects on enamel

The effects of bleaching on enamel were primarily examined in vitro using extracted human or bovine teeth. Bleaching appears to have minimal or no effects on enamel microhardness and mineral content; however, the results on enamel surface change are inconsistent (Potocni et al. 2000, White et al. 2002, Rotstein and Li 2008, Ren et al. 2009). Although several investigators reported significant alteration of enamel surfaces, including depression, porosity, and erosion, after bleaching, a majority of scanning electron microscopy studies showed little or no morphologic change in enamel surfaces associated with bleaching. In most cases, however, the observed enamel surface alterations varied among bleaching products and appeared to be related to those using acidic prerinses or gels of low pH. Questions have also been raised regarding the clinical relevancy of the observed changes in the enamel surface morphology. Studies have shown that some soft drinks and fruit juices are capable of causing comparable or greater demineralization and surface alteration of enamel compared with those reported for bleaching agents (Ren et al. 2009). To date, no clinical evidence of adverse effects of professional at-home bleaching systems on enamel has been reported; however, there have been two clinical cases of significant enamel damage associated with the use of OTC bleaching products (Cubbon and Ore 1991, Hammel 1998).

Potential adverse effects on gingiva

H_2O_2 is highly cytotoxic to cultured mammalian cells, and studies have also reported that peroxide-based bleaching gels induced cytotoxicity, which appears to be dose related according to H_2O_2 content in the gel ((Kawasaki et al. 1969, Ito et al. 1976, U.S. Food and Drug Administration 1983, Dickson and Caravati 1994). At concentrations of 10% or higher, H_2O_2 is potentially corrosive to mucous membranes or skin, causing a burning sensation and tissue damage (see Figures 21.2 and 21.5) (Li 1996, Scientific Committee on Consumer Products 2005).

During the in-office bleaching procedure, which routinely involves the use of a gel with 25% H_2O_2 or greater, adequate barriers are necessary to protect gingiva from mucosal damage. If leakage occurs, serious tissue burn can result. Because of this potential risk, local anesthesia should not be used for in-office bleaching, so that the patient can alert the dentist if the gel seeps through the barriers to cause a burning sensation or pain. However, simply relying on the patient's response is inadequate; clear instructions to the patient to report any discomfort, careful examination of the seal of the barrier after the gel application, and frequent monitoring of the seal throughout the bleaching treatment are all necessary to minimize the risk of gingival damage and irritation.

Gingival irritation is a common side effect of at-home bleaching. A study (Kugel et al. 2002) found a higher (33.3%) prevalence of gingival irritation in patients using strips of 6.5% H_2O_2 compared with those using at-home tray bleaching with 10% carbamide peroxide (10%); the latter is equivalent to 3.5% H_2O_2. A separate study (Gerlach and Zhou 2002) showed that 50% of patients using a 6.5% H_2O_2 strip reported gingival irritation, which was about three times the rate of those using a 5.3% strip (16.7%). These data indicate that the risk of gingival irritation with at-home bleaching is associated with the H_2O_2 concentration in the bleaching gel—that is, a higher prevalence of gingival irritation is associated with bleaching gels of higher peroxide concentrations.

In most cases, the gingival irritation is mild to moderate, tends to be transient, and will dissipate when the application discontinues. So far, studies on professional at-home bleaching have reported no significant or permanent gingival damage.

Potential adverse effects on pulp and the risk of tooth sensitivity

Tooth sensitivity to temperature changes is probably the most commonly observed clinical side effect of bleaching; it has been suggested to be an indication of possible pulp response to H_2O_2 that penetrates through tooth hard tissue and reaches the pulp, although initially its mechanisms were not fully understood. Recent research, most of which used in vitro models, has shown that H_2O_2 in bleaching gel applied on the enamel surface is capable of penetrating through the enamel and dentin to reach the pulp chamber (Thitinanthapan et al. 1999, Slezak et al. 2002, Benetti et al. 2004, Pugh et al. 2005, Camargo et al. 2009). An amount of less than 30 µg of H_2O_2 may reach pulp after the application of gels containing up to 12% H_2O_2 on enamel surface for up to 7 hours. Although the amount of H_2O_2 detected in the pulp chamber tends to increase with the time and H_2O_2 concentration in the gel, such a relationship is not proportional. It has been suggested that an amount of 50,000 µg H_2O_2 would be needed to inhibit pulpal enzymes (Bowles and Ugwuneri 1987), so the detected amount of H_2O_2 penetrating into the pulp chamber appears unlikely to cause significant damage to pulp tissues. This assumption appears to be consistent with the clinical findings; so far there have been no confirmed cases of irreversible pulp damage as a result of tooth bleaching. However, there is a lack of in vivo studies on this topic, and long-term effects of such H_2O_2 exposure on pulp, including subclinical pathologic consequences, have yet to be determined.

Tooth sensitivity may or may not occur with the gingival irritation (Leonard 1998). In some cases, the patient may mistake gingival irritation for tooth sensitivity (see Figure 21.5), or vice versa; therefore, careful examination and differential diagnosis are necessary for appropriate treatment regimens. In general, up to two thirds of people may experience temporary tooth sensitivity as a result of tooth bleaching (Leonard 1998, Jorgensen and Carroll 2002, Hasson et al. 2006, Burrows 2009). The development of tooth sensitivity does not appear to be related to the patient's age or sex, defective restorations, enamel-cementum abrasion, or the dental arch treated; however, the risk increases in patients with the frequency of the daily application. The incidence and severity of the sensitivity may also depend on the quality of the bleaching gel, the techniques used, and an individual's response to the bleaching (American Dental Association 2009a). The sensitivity, usually mild and transient, often occurs during the early stages of tooth bleaching, and for most patients it is tolerable to complete the treatment. Teeth with caries, with exposed dentin, in close proximity to pulp horns, or with suspected cracks are potentially at risk for developing severe sensitivity, and these teeth need to be carefully observed during bleaching. In addition, defective restorations should be replaced before bleaching. It was thought that extra caution should be applied to children and adolescents (Lee et al. 2005) because of their relatively larger pulp chamber; however, this has not been shown to be the case.

Potential adverse effects on restorative materials

A relevant safety concern is the mercury release from amalgam restorations during and after the bleaching (Rotstein et al. 2000, Rotstein et al. 2004, Al-Salehi 2009). Although not much debate exists regarding whether bleaching causes mercury release, the reported amount of mercury release associated with bleaching varies greatly. The issue of potential health implications of the mercury released remains controversial, and these implications have yet to be determined. Because of the known toxicity of mercury, as a general rule it is not advisable to perform bleaching for patients whose teeth have been restored extensively with amalgam (see Figure 21.7).

Although adverse effects of tooth bleaching on resin-based materials are not considered direct health risks, the consequences can be significant to the quality and longevity of such restorations. Numerous studies have reported that tooth bleaching may adversely affect physical and/or chemical properties of restorative materials; such effects include increased surface roughness, crack development, marginal breakdown, release of metallic ions, and decreases in tooth-to-restoration bond strength. Potential adverse effects of bleaching on bonding strength have been well recognized (Attin et al. 2004, Breschi et al. 2007, Lima et al. 2010). A plausible mechanism is the inhibition of adequate polymerization of bonding agent by residual oxygen formed during the bleaching. Similar effects are also applicable to other resin-based restorative materials that require in situ polymerization. The post-bleaching inhibitory effects on the polymerization dissipate with time, and an interval of 2 weeks has been found to be adequate to avoid such adverse effects.

SAFETY CONCERNS WITH BLEACHING NOT INVOLVING DENTAL PROFESSIONALS

Shortly after the introduction of nightguard tray bleaching, which was originally administered by dental professionals, OTC products became available directly to consumers for their use at home. There are a variety of forms of these OTC bleaching products, including gels applied using a tray or paint-on brush, mouthrinses, chewing gums, toothpastes, and strips. Similar products are also available through infomercials and the Internet. More recently, tooth bleaching has become available in mall kiosks, salons, and spas and even on cruise ships, which usually simulates the in-office bleaching settings, often involving the use of a light but being performed by individuals with no formal dental training and not licensed to practice dentistry; such practices have come under scrutiny in several states and jurisdictions, resulting in actions to reserve the delivery of this service to dentists or appropriately supervised allied dental personnel (American Dental Association 2009a). Also of concern is the use of products with chlorine dioxide for tooth bleaching, which has been reported to have significant adverse effects on enamel (see Figure 21.4) (Li and Greenwall 2013).

Basically no scientific research has been conducted on tooth bleaching performed in the settings of mall kiosks, salons, spas, and cruise ships; in contrast, a significant amount of clinical data on the OTC bleaching products are available in the literature (Gerlach and Zhou 2002, Kugel et al. 2002, Li 2003, Hasson et al. 2006). Overall data indicate that adverse effects associated with the use of the OTC bleaching products appear to be rare. However, there is a major issue with the results and conclusions of these OTC bleaching studies—that is, the data were collected in settings typical for clinical trials, including specific inclusion and exclusion criteria, by dental professionals, which are not intended by these OTC products. Consequently, it is unclear whether the low incidence of adverse effects associated with the use of the OTC bleaching is the result of its low risk or the lack of means to detect and report the adverse effects. The only two publications on irreversible enamel damage caused by OTC bleaching were case reports, not clinical studies (Cubbon and Ore 1991, Hammel 1998). In addition, consumers are not generally aware of how to report adverse events through the FDA's MedWatch system (American Dental Association 2009a). It is a reasonable assumption that when an individual purchases and uses an OTC bleaching product, some adverse effects, such as enamel surface changes, may go unnoticed; even those felt or detected by the user most likely remain unreported. More of a concern is the tendency of overusing or abusing an OTC product. Research efforts are needed to define the risks of OTC home bleaching, if any, under relevant scenarios intended for these products.

ROLES OF DENTAL PROFESSIONALS IN TOOTH BLEACHING

The direct major outcome of tooth bleaching is the lightening of tooth shade or color, and it may thus be perceived as a simple cosmetic or esthetic procedure. However, this can be a misconception because a tooth of darker color or discoloration, particularly with intrinsic stains, may not simply be an esthetic problem, and bleaching may not be the appropriate or the best choice for treatment (Shafer et al. 1983, Li 2003, 2011b). Initial evaluation and examination of tooth discoloration are necessary for proper diagnosis and treatment. Bleaching can affect restorative materials and may also result in color mismatch of teeth with existing restorations or crowns. These are just examples of the necessary process of tooth bleaching that cannot be performed or determined by consumers themselves or individuals without dental training. For at-home bleaching using trays, professionally fabricated, custom-fit trays help reduce the amount of gel needed for maximal efficacy and minimize the gel contact with gingiva. In addition, periodic evaluation of bleaching progress by dentists allows early detection of any possible side effects and reduces the risk of use of inferior bleaching materials and inappropriate application procedures as well as any temptation to overuse or abuse the product. A case report illustrates the importance of the role of dental professionals in tooth bleaching treatment (Li 2011a). The authors performed comprehensive clinical examinations of the dentition and gingiva, custom designed at-home bleaching regimen, provided detailed instructions, and conducted monitoring of the bleaching progress with adjustments made accordingly; such careful planning and conduct of the bleaching helped maximize the efficacy while minimizing potential risks, which was obviously the key to ensuring the success of this difficult case. Therefore, it is highly recommended that tooth bleaching involve dental professionals. The ADA encourages all patients interested in tooth bleaching to seek advice from a dental professional (American Dental Association 2009a, 2009b).

SUMMARY AND CONCLUSIONS

In addition to the long history of in-office tooth bleaching, at-home bleaching has become an accepted and integrated procedure in dentistry. Data accumulated over the last 20 years also indicate no significant, long-term oral or systemic health risks associated with professional at-home tooth bleaching using gels of 10% carbamide peroxide, which is equivalent to 3.5% H_2O_2. Therefore, when used appropriately, tooth bleaching is safe and effective.

However, as any dental procedure, bleaching involves risks. Tooth sensitivity and gingival irritation occur in a significant portion of the patients, although in most cases they are mild to moderate and transient. When gels of high H_2O_2 concentrations, such as those for in-office bleaching, are used without adequate gingival protection, severe mucosal damage can occur. Although rare, potential adverse effects are possible with inappropriate application, abuse, or the use of inappropriate at-home bleaching products. H_2O_2 is capable of producing various toxicologic effects, so potential risks exist and need to be recognized. So far, little data are available on the safety of OTC at-home bleaching that simulate the intended application mode of these products, and the safety of bleaching performed at mall kiosks, salons, or spas and on cruise ships is of particular concern because the procedures are similar to in-office bleaching but are performed by individuals without dental training.

Effective and safe tooth bleaching requires correct diagnosis of the problems associated with tooth discoloration or stains. Furthermore, side effects such as tooth sensitivity and gingival irritation may occur during the course of bleaching treatment. To minimize risks and maximize benefits, the involvement of dental professionals in bleaching treatment is necessary.

REFERENCES

Al-Qunaian TA, Matis BA, Cochran MA. (2003) In vivo kinetics of bleaching gel with three-percent hydrogen peroxide within the first hour. *Oper Dent* **28:**236–41.

Al-Salehi SK. (2009) Effects of bleaching on mercury ion release from dental amalgam. *J Dent Res* **88:**239–43.

American Dental Association (ADA). (2009a) *Tooth whitening/bleaching: treatment considerations for dentists and their patients.* ADA Council on Scientific Affairs: Chicago, IL.

American Dental Association (ADA), Journal of the American Dental Association, ADA Division of Science. (2009b) For the dental patient: tooth whitening—what you should know. *J Am Dent Assoc* **40:**384.

Attin T, Hannig C, Wiegand A, Attin R. (2004) Effect of bleaching on restorative materials and restorations—a systematic review. *Dent Mater* **20:**852–61.

Benetti AR, Valera MC, Mancini MN, Miranda CB. (2004) In vitro penetration of bleaching agents into the pulp chamber. *Int Endod J* **37:**120–4.

Bowles WH, Ugwuneri Z. (1987) Pulp chamber penetration of hydrogen peroxide following vital bleaching procedures. *J Endod* **8:**875–7.

Breschi L, Cadenaro M, Antoniolli F, Visintini E. (2007) Extent of polymerization of dental bonding systems on bleached enamel. *Am J Dent* **20:**275–80.

Burnett C, Goldenthal EI, Harris SB, Wazeter FX. (1976) Teratology and percutaneous toxicity studies on hair dyes. *J Toxicol Environ Health* **1:**1027–40.

Burrows S. (2009) A review of the safety of tooth bleaching. *Dent Update* **36:**604–6, 608–10, 612–4.

Camargo SE, Cardoso PE, Valera MC, de Araújo MA. (2009) Penetration of 35% hydrogen peroxide into the pulp chamber in bovine teeth after LED or Nd:YAG laser activation. *Eur J Esthet Dent* **4:**82–8.

Carlsson J. (1987) Salivary peroxidase: an important part of our defense against oxygen toxicity. *J Oral Pathol* **16:**412–6.

Christensen DW, Faught WE, Black RE, Woodward GA. (1992) Fatal oxygen embolization after hydrogen peroxide ingestion. *Crit Care Med* **20:**543–4.

Cina SJ, Downs JC, Conradi SE. (1994) Hydrogen peroxide: a source of lethal oxygen embolism. Case report and review of the literature. *Am J Forensic Med Pathol* **15:**44–50.

Cubbon T, Ore D. (1991) Hard tissue and home tooth whiteners. *CDS Rev* **84:**32–5.

Dahl JE, Becher R. (1995) Acute toxicity of carbamide peroxide and a commercially available tooth-bleaching agent in rat. *J Dent Res* **74:**710–4.

Dahl JE, Pallesen U. (2003) Tooth bleaching—a critical review of the biological aspects. *Crit Rev Oral Biol Med* **14:**292–304.

de Lamirande E, Gagnon C. (1994) Reactive oxygen species (ROS) and reproduction. In Armstrong D, editor. *Free radicals in diagnostic medicine.* Plenum: New York, 185–97.

Dickson KF, Caravati EM. (1994) Hydrogen peroxide—325 exposures reported to a regional poison control center. *J Toxicol Clin Toxicol* **32:**705–14.

Floyd RA. (1990) Role of oxygen free radicals in carcinogenesis and brain ischemia. *FASEB J* **4:**2587–97.

Gerlach RW, Zhou X. (2002) Comparative clinical efficacy of two professional bleaching systems. *Compend Contin Educ Dent* **23:**35–41.

Goldberg M, Grootveld M, Lynch E. (2010) Undesirable and adverse effects of tooth-whitening products: a review. *Clin Oral Invest* **14:**1–10.

Hammel S. (1998) Do-it-yourself tooth whitening is risky. *U.S. News and World Report* 2 April 1998, p. 66.

Hankan L. (1958) Hydrogen peroxide ingestion and the growth of rats. *Nature* **182:**1453.

Harman D. (1981) The aging process. *Proc Natl Acad Sci U S A* **78:**7124–32.

Hasson H, Ismail AI, Neiva G. (2006) Home-based chemically-induced whitening of teeth in adults. *Cochrane Database Syst Rev* **4:**CD006202.

Haywood VB, Heymann HO. (1989) Nightguard vital bleaching. *Quintessence Int* **20:**173–6.

Humberston CL, Dean BS, Krenzelok EP. (1990) Ingestion of 35% hydrogen peroxide. *J Toxicol Clin Toxicol* **28:**95–100.

Ito A, Naito M, Naito Y, Watanabe H. (1982) Induction and characterization of gastro-duodenal lesions in mice given continuous oral administration of hydrogen peroxide. *Gan* **73:**315–22.

Ito A, Watanabe H, Naito M, Naito Y. (1981) Induction of duodenal tumors in mice by oral administration of hydrogen peroxide. *Gan* **72:**174–5.

Ito A, Watanabe H, Naito M, Naito Y. (1984) Correlation between induction of duodenal tumor by hydrogen peroxide and catalase activity in mice. *Gan* **75:**17–21.

Ito R, Kawamura H, Chang HS. (1976) Safety study on hydrogen peroxide: acute and subacute toxicity. *J Med Soc Toho Japan* **23:**531–7.

Jorgensen MG, Carroll WB. (2002) Incidence of tooth sensitivity after home whitening treatment. *J Am Dent Assoc* **133:**1076–82.

Kihn PW. (2007) Vital tooth whitening. *Dent Clin North Am* **51:**319–31.

Korhonen A, Hemminki K, Vainio H. (1984) Embryotoxic effects of eight organic peroxides and hydrogen peroxide on three-day chicken embryos. *Environ Res* **33:**54–61.

Kugel G, Aboushala A, Zhou X, Gerlach RW. (2002) Daily use of whitening strips on tetracycline-stained teeth: comparative results after 2 months. *Compend Contin Educ Dent* **23:**29–34.

Lee SS, Zhang W, Lee DH, Li Y. (2005) Tooth whitening in children and adolescents: a literature review. *Pediatr Dent* **27:**362–8.

Leonard RH. (1998) Efficacy, longevity, side effects, and patient perceptions of Nightguard Vital Bleaching. *Compend Contin Educ Dent* **19:**766–81.

Li Y. (1996) Biological properties of peroxide-containing tooth whiteners. *Food Chem Toxicol* **34:**887–904.

Li Y. (1997) Toxicological considerations of tooth bleaching using peroxide-containing agents. *J Am Dent Assoc* **128:**31S–6S.

Li Y. (2000) Peroxide-containing tooth whiteners: an update on safety. *Compend Contin Educ Dent* **21**(Suppl 28):S4–9.

Li Y. (2003) The safety of peroxide-containing at-home tooth whiteners. *Compend Contin Educ Dent* **24:**384–9.

Li Y. (2011a) Commentary. Successful bleaching of teeth with dentinogenesis imperfecta discoloration: a case report. *J Esthet Restor Dent* **23:**11.

Li Y. (2011b) Safety controversies in tooth bleaching. *Dent Clin North Am* **55:**255–63.

Li Y, Greenwall L. (2013) Safety issues of tooth whitening using peroxide-based materials. *Br Dent J* **215:**29–34.

Lima AF, Fonseca FM, Cavalcanti AN, Aguiar FH. (2010) Effect of the diffusion of bleaching agents through enamel on dentin bonding at different depths. *Am J Dent* **23:**113–5.

Liu XL, Sato S, Dai W, Yamanaka N. (1969) Effect of hydrogen peroxide on the growth of rats. *J Food Hygienic Soc Japan* **10:**68–72.

Lutz WK. (1990) Endogenous genotoxic agents and processes as a basis of spontaneous carcinogenesis. *Mutat Res* **238:**287–95.

Marshall MV, Gragg PP, Packman EW, Wright PB. (2001) Hydrogen peroxide decomposition in the oral cavity. *Am J Dent* **14:**39–45.

Marshall MV, Kuhn JO, Torrey CF. (1996) Hamster cheek pouch bioassay of dentifrices containing hydrogen peroxide and baking soda. *J Am Coll Toxicol* **15:**45–61.

Matis BA. (2000) Degradation of gel in tray whitening. *Compend Contin Educ Dent* **21**(Suppl 28):S28–35.

Potocnik I, Kosec L, Gaspersic D. (2000) Effect of 10% carbamide peroxide bleaching gel on enamel microhardness, microstructure, and mineral content. *J Endod* **26:**203–6.

Pugh G Jr, Zaidel L, Lin N, Stranick M. (2005) High levels of hydrogen peroxide in overnight tooth-whitening formulas: effects on enamel and pulp. *J Esthet Restor Dent* **17:**40–5.

Rackoff WR, Merton DF. (1990) Gas embolism after ingestion of hydrogen peroxide. *Pediatrics* **85:**593–4.

Ramp WK, Arnold RR, Russell JE, Yancey JM. (1987) Hydrogen peroxide inhibits glucose metabolism and collagen synthesis in bone. *J Periodont* **58:**340–4.

Ren YF, Amin A, Malmstrom H. (2009) Effects of tooth whitening and orange juice on surface properties of dental enamel. *J Dent* **37:**424–31.

Rotstein I, Avron Y, Shemesh H, Dogan H. (2004) Factors affecting mercury release from dental amalgam exposed to carbamide peroxide bleaching agent. *Am J Dent* **17:**347–50.

Rotstein I, Dogan H, Avron Y, Shemesh H. (2000) Mercury release from dental amalgam after treatment with 10% carbamide peroxide in vitro. *Oral Surg Oral Med Oral Pathol Oral Radiol* Endod **89:**216–9.

Rotstein I, Li Y. (2008) Tooth discoloration and bleaching. In Ingle JI, Bakland LK, Baumgartner JC, editors. *Ingle's endodontics,* 6th edn. BC Decker: Hamilton, 1383–99.

Rubin R, Farber JL. (1984) Mechanisms of the killing of cultured hepatocytes by hydrogen peroxide. *Arc Biochem Biophys* **228:**450–9.

Sacks T, Moldow CF, Craddock PR, Bowers TK. (1978) Oxygen radicals mediate endothelial cell damage by complement-stimulated granulocytes, an in vitro model of immune vascular damage. *J Clin Invest* **61:**1161–7.

Sagel PA, Odioso LL, McMillan DA, Gerlach RW. (2000) Vital tooth whitening with a novel hydrogen peroxide strip system: design, kinetics, and clinical response. *Compend Contin Educ Dent* **21**(Suppl 29):S10–5.

Scientific Committee on Consumer Products (European Commission). (2005) *Opinion on hydrogen peroxide in tooth whitening products.* Health + Consumer Protection Directorate C–Public Health and Risk Assessment: Brussels. SCCP/0844/04, March 15, 2005.

Shafer WG, Hine MG, Levy BM. (1983) *Textbook of oral pathology,* 4th edn. WB Saunders: Philadelphia, 766–8.

Slezak B, Santarpia P, Xu T, Monsul-Barnes V. (2002) Safety profile of a new liquid whitening gel. *Compend Contin Educ Dent* **23**(Suppl 1): 4–11.

Thitinanthapan W, Satamanont P, Vongsavan N. (1999) In vitro penetration of the pulp chamber by three brands of carbamide peroxide. *Esthet Dent* **11:**259–64.

U.S. Food and Drug Administration (FDA). (1983) Hydrogen peroxide: proposed affirmation of GRAS status as a direct human food ingredient with specific limitations. *Fed Regist* **48:**52323–3333.

Weiner ML, Freeman C, Trochimowicz H, de Gerlache J. (2000) 13-week drinking water toxicity study of hydrogen peroxide with 6-week recovery period in catalase-deficient mice. *Food Chem Toxicol* **38:**607–15.

Weitzman SA, Weitberg AB, Stossel TP, Schwartz J. (1986) Effects of hydrogen peroxide on oral carcinogenesis in hamsters. *J Periodontol* **57:**685–8.

White DJ, Kozak KM, Zoladz JR, Duschner H. (2002) Peroxide interactions with hard tissues: effects on surface hardness and surface/subsurface ultrastructural properties. *Compend Contin Educ Dent* **23:**42–8.

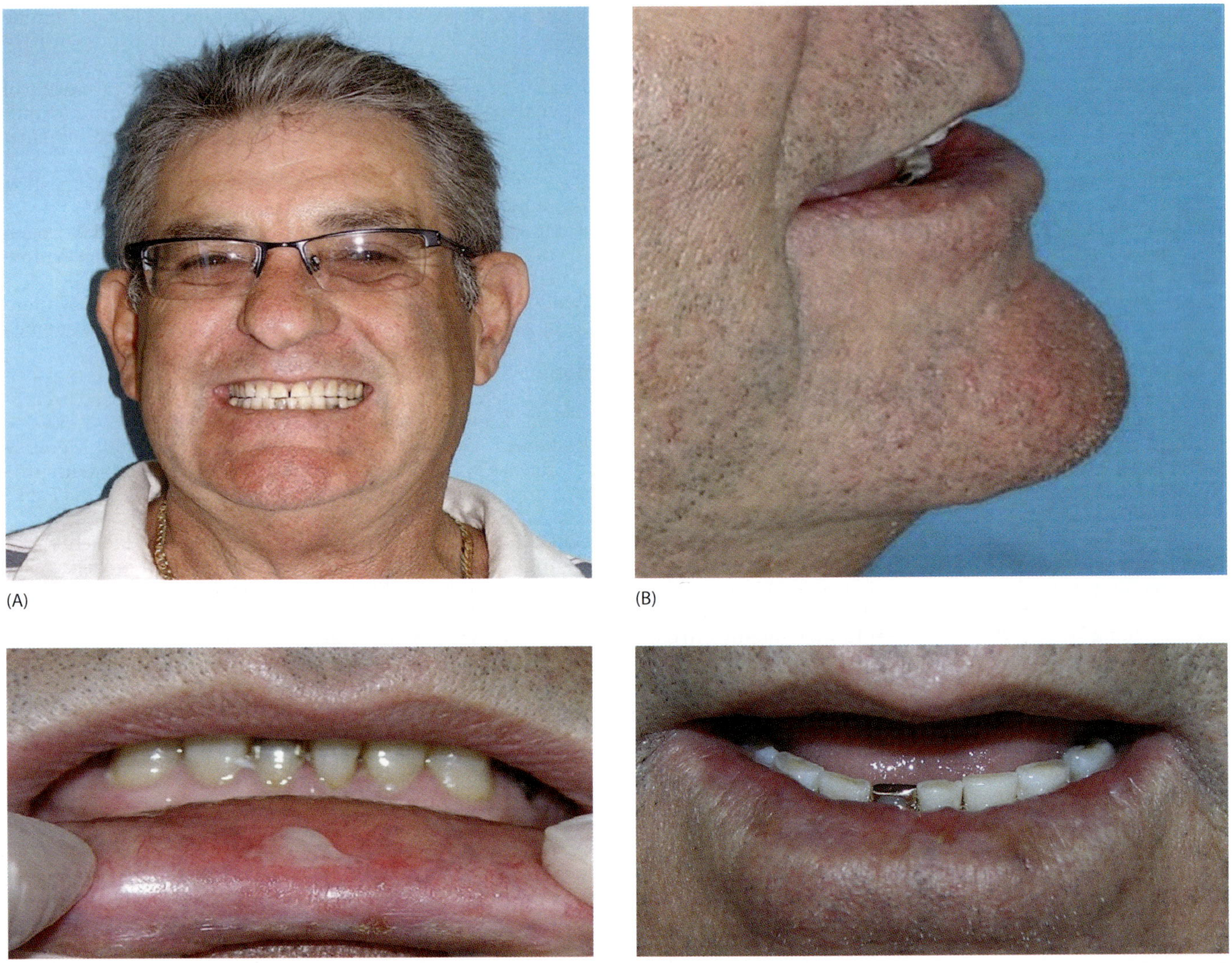

(A) (B) (C) (D)

Figure 21.1

(A) Portrait view of patient 1 day after bleaching procedure. The teeth appear white, but the heat and proximity of the lamp have resulted in a burn on the lower lip. (B) Lip burn. A close-up profile view of the patient, who had an extended swollen lower lip where the bleaching lamp had rested. The ulceration was located on the inside of the vermilion border of the lip. (C) Close-up of the lower lip 1 day after the ulceration had occurred on the lower lip. There is a characteristic white triangular area. It is possible that the chemicals used for bleaching have exacerbated the ulceration. (D) The lower lip showing the swelling.

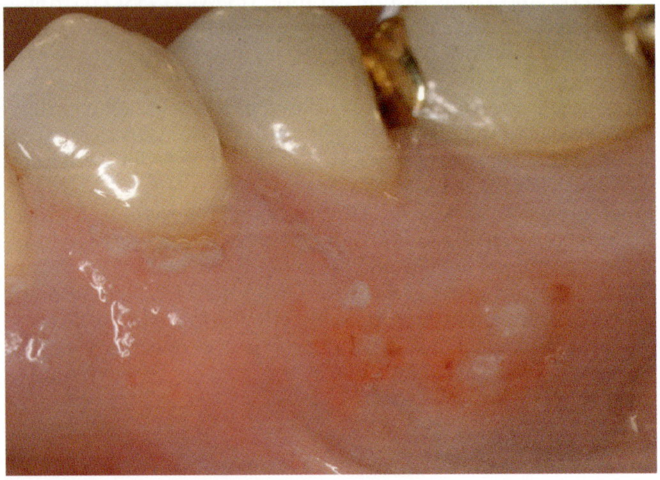

Figure 21.2

Ulceration of the lower gingivae after home bleaching with 10 percent carbamide peroxide in the bleaching tray. The gingival irritation is located on the gingival margin and on the attached and movable mucosa.

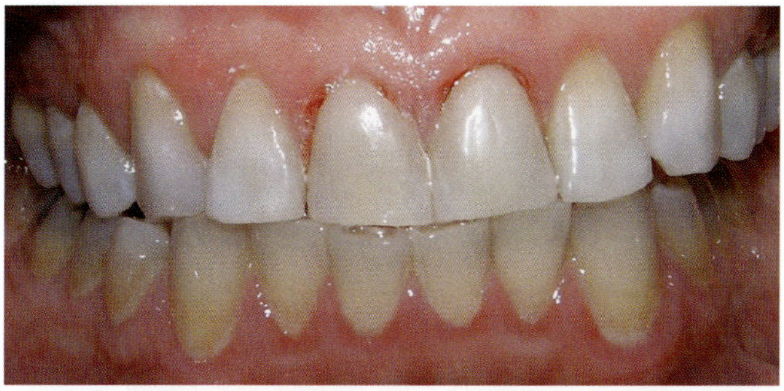

Figure 21.3

Gingival irritation after power bleaching. This figure shows the immediate effect of the bleaching gel when the light-cure dam was removed from the teeth. It was noted that there was an area of gingival irritation on the central incisors.

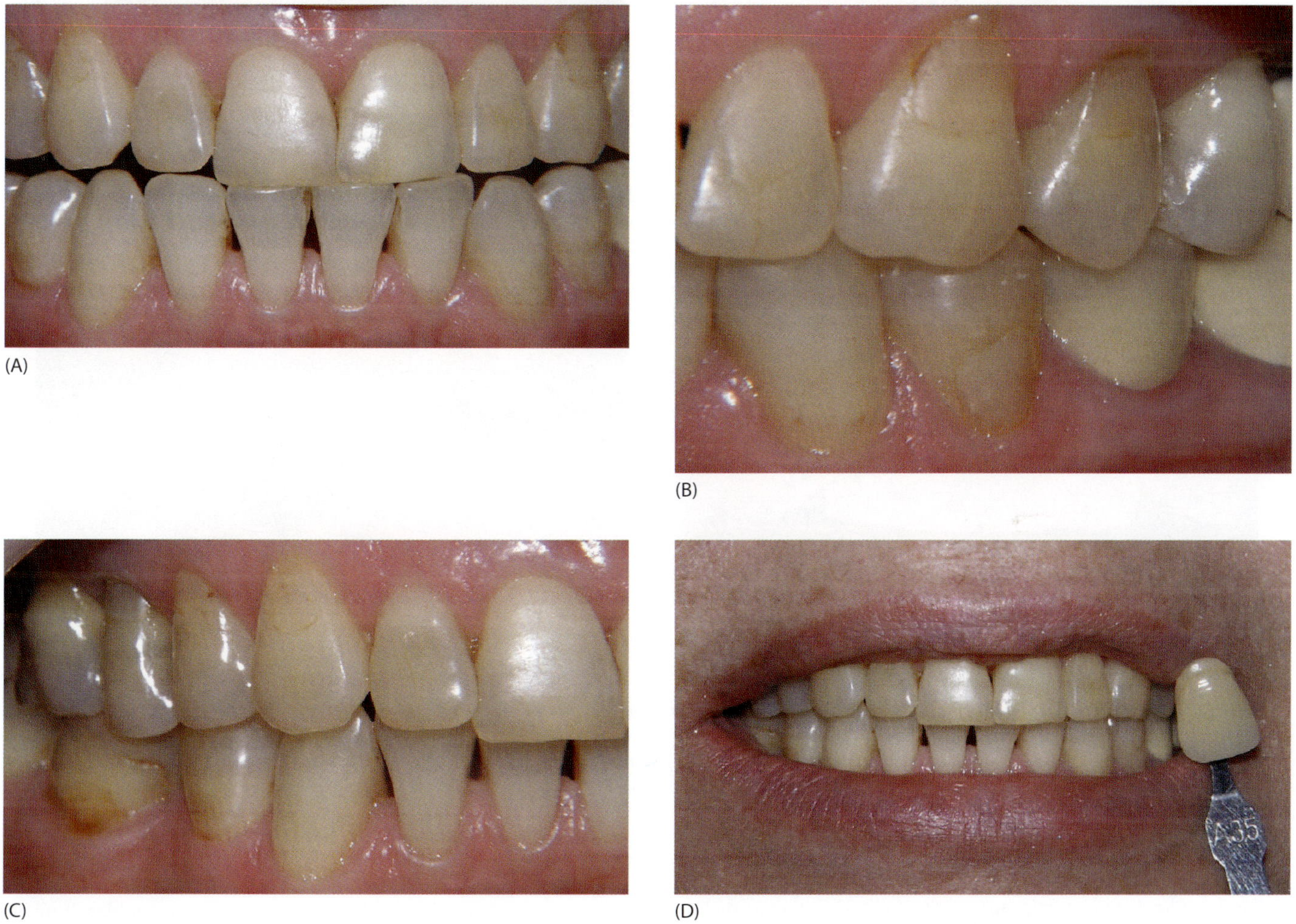

Figure 21.4

(A) Chlorine dioxide bleaching at the beauty therapist. This figure shows the result of use of 0.5% chlorine dioxide gel after application of the gel by a beauty therapist directly onto the surfaces of the teeth. This resulted in the enamel luster being removed from the teeth. The teeth feel rough and are sensitive and tend to pick up more stain because of the etched effect; the teeth appear more gray after the bleaching procedure. (B) The lateral view shows the location where the bleaching gel was placed. The upper left second premolar did not have bleaching gel placed onto the tooth. This area still maintains its enamel luster and is shiny. The etched area is on the first premolar forward. (C) Right lateral view of the patient. It is clear where the chlorine dioxide gel was placed; this area appears dull. The upper right first and second premolar and first molar did not have the gel applied and retain their shiny lustrous sheen. (D) The smile view of the patient showing the shade after bleaching, which matched shade tab A3.5. This is not a light shade and reflects the fact that the etched surface of the chlorine dioxide allows the tooth to pick up further food stains, and the teeth become more yellow.

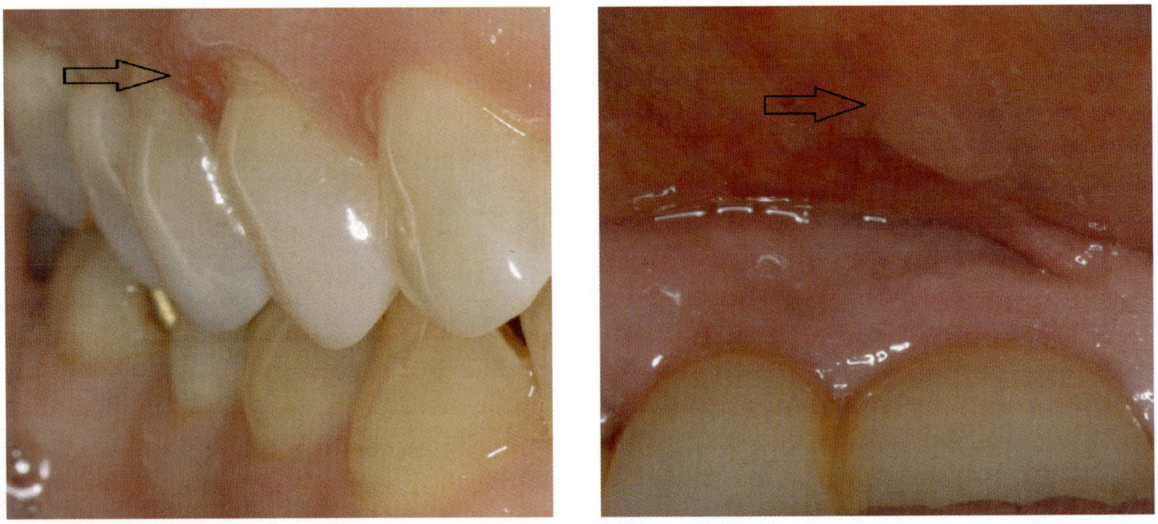

(A) (B)

Figure 21.5

(A) Gingival margin irritation on the upper right first premolar indicated with an arrow. This patient had used too much bleaching gel in the tray. The bleaching tray was cut back by 0.5 mm. The patient had been bleaching her teeth using 10% carbamide peroxide. (B) Blistering on the upper inner lip after power bleaching. See arrow.

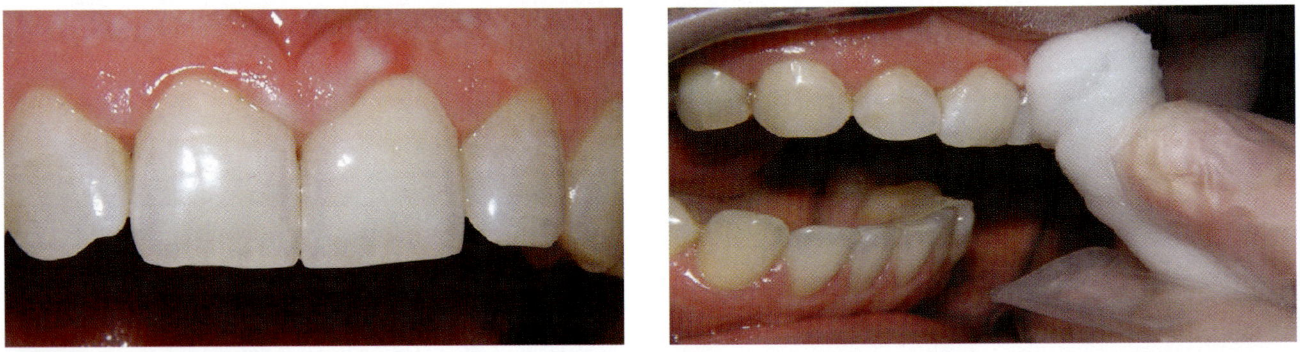

(A) (B)

Figure 21.6

(A) Chemical burn on the central incisor papillae. This shows the result of a chemical burn that occurred when the mouth retractor moved and the power gel leaked underneath the light-cure dam. In this situation close monitoring of the patient and observation are necessary. It is important to act swiftly. The patient is instructed to inform the dental practitioner or assistant if the patient feels any tingling or burning during the power bleaching procedure. If this is the case, then the bleaching procedure is terminated, the power gel is removed from the tooth by wiping it away, and the teeth are rehydrated with water. The light-cure dam is removed to check for any areas of chemical burning. Once these tasks have been attended to, the light-cure dam can be reapplied. It is my opinion that the patient should not have a local anesthetic to undertake power bleaching. That way, if extreme sensitivity is experienced, the dentist can apply materials to sooth the tooth effectively and efficiently. (B) Treatment for a chemical burn occurring on the papillae of the upper central incisors. A wet cotton roll soaked in water is placed over the site of the chemical burn. The chemical burn occurred when the mouth retractor moved and the 25% hydrogen peroxide power bleaching gel leaked under the light-cure dam. When this happens, it is essential to act early and speedily. The first line of defense is water to rehydrate the chemical burn. The wet cotton roll is placed onto the area until the white burn changes to a red area, and then it returns to normal within a few minutes. If the power gel remains for longer, the area will develop into a blister, which can take longer to heal.

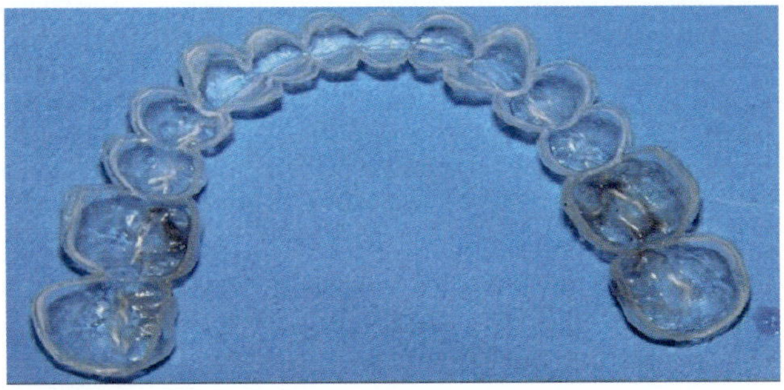

Figure 21.7

A bleaching tray removed from the mouth of a patient with two occlusal amalgam restorations. In the area of the first molars can be seen a black star corresponding to the appearance of the amalgam restoration. This passivation dark oxide layer can be removed from the occlusal amalgam during bleaching.

22 WHITENING FOR PATIENTS YOUNGER THAN 18 *Index of Treatment Need*

Linda Greenwall

INTRODUCTION

There has been controversy related to tooth whitening for patients younger than 18 years since the banning of treatment after a directive issued by the Tooth Whitening Working Group for Europe and the Scientific Committee for Europe in 2012 (European Commission Directive on Cosmetics Products 2012), which said that no whitening can be undertaken for patients younger than 18.

Previously, legislation in the United Kingdom had stated that tooth whitening products were classified as cosmetic products. As a result of the directive, no product that contained more than 0.1% hydrogen peroxide was permitted to be used for tooth whitening. That effectively meant that all dentists in the United Kingdom were practicing dentistry illegally if they were supplying their patients with tooth whitening gel that contained more than 0.1% hydrogen peroxide—and there was no effective product that contained the legal limit of 0.1% hydrogen peroxide. However, before the change in the law, there had been no exclusion of an age group.

There have been further clarifications of the legislation after guidelines were issued by the General Dental Council (GDC) and other professional groups such as the British Society of Paediatric Dentistry (British Dental Bleaching Society (BDBS) 2012, Faculty of Dental Surgery 2014, General Dental Council 2014, General Dental Council 2015).

The European Tooth Whitening Group and the Council of European Dentists Working Group on Tooth Whitening are now considering the research on whitening in patients younger than 18, which has shown that it is safe for patients younger than 18 to whiten their teeth, although it may be some years before the Group reports its findings.

For some children who have tooth discoloration or dyschromia, it is of great concern. Some children have inherently yellow teeth when the secondary teeth erupt as "butter teeth" (Haywood 2006). This deep yellow color affects the child's self-esteem; he or she may be teased or bullied at school and called derogatory names, which can cause psychological harm. Treatment may be sought to whiten the teeth and remove the distressing discoloration. For these and other children, whitening is an essential treatment option. The purpose of this chapter is to examine the need for treatment of patients younger than 18 and to assess who should be exempt from this legislation. An index of whitening need will be introduced to help clarify which children should undergo whitening based on treatment need.

AN INDEX FOR TREATMENT NEED

Over the last few decades, various indices have been devised for treatment need, such as the Index of Orthodontic Treatment Need [IOTN] in orthodontics (Brook and Shaw 1989), Falcon's restorative dentistry index (Falcon et al. 2001), the Dental Aesthetic Index (DAI) (Cons et al. 1986), and the Index of Complexity, Outcome and Need (ICON) (Daniel and Richmond, 2000), which is highly weighted towards esthetics; hence, it is more subjective than objective. The IOTN lists grades in increasing severity, and these are used as guidelines to determine when orthodontic treatment is necessary (Puri et al. 2015). It has been shown to be a valid reproducible index (Siddiqui et al. 2014). The index consists of two components, the Aesthetic Component and the Dental Health Component. The IOTN-AC is the subjective component of the index and consists of a set of 10 intraoral frontal photographs to be rated from 1 to 10, with 1 being the most attractive and 10 being the least attractive. The IOTN-AC provides a measurable, visual assessment regarding the patient's perception of his or her presenting malocclusion and treatment needs (Siddiqui et al. 2014).

It is essential during the assessment to try to give dentists guidelines for when to proceed with treatment based on the severity of the need for treatment. A guideline for restorative dentistry (Falcon et al. 2001) identified that the most important priority for treatment (assessed by clinicians) had three levels; the highest priority was assigned to patients with inherited or developmental defects that justify complex care (e.g., clefts of the lip and palate). Since its initial development, this index has demonstrated some success in a difficult area.

When developing an index for treatment need for whitening, it is important to consider treatment need based on a wide variety of situations including congenital problems such as genetic defects of the teeth or congenital defects such as white or brown markings.

WHEN IS WHITENING NEEDED?

It is essential to clarify whether whitening treatment is needed for patients younger than 18. It would be helpful if an index of treatment need could be established to give further guidance as to who should be able to undergo tooth whitening without contravening the legislation.

According to the Whitening Group, the limit established by the current regulations makes it difficult to easily and cost-effectively treat patients; however, those with the following indications should be given priority:

1. Severe and moderate discoloration
2. Enamel conditions
3. White spots and small white marks
4. Brown, orange and yellow staining
5. Esthetic defects
6. Incisor discrepancies
7. Molar incisor hypoplasia
8. Trauma
9. Hereditary factors e.g., amelogenesis imperfecta
10. Presence of a non-vital discolored anterior tooth

It is essential that treatment options be discussed with patients and their parents and that, where necessary, early intervention—whitening treatment to improve the color of the tooth—be undertaken after explaining all treatment options and the risks and benefits of treating patients younger than 18. All combinations of treatment need to be discussed, such as no treatment, combinations of whitening treatment, and whitening and esthetic or restorative treatment.

Various considerations come into play when evaluating the indications for treatment need:

- The shade of the discoloration (e.g., very dark shades—A4, C4, B4): such discoloration (indication 1) is subdivided into severe, moderate, and mild. Whitening treatment should be undertaken if the type of discoloration can be classified into the severe or moderate category, the child is aware of the discoloration, and the discoloration has an impact on the child's life.
- The nature and extent of the discoloration.
- Whether the discoloration is spread uniformly on the tooth or whether there is mottling on the tooth.
- Whether the tooth is of normal color but with white marks, mottling, or flecks of white.
- The presence of brown discolorations on the labial surface of the tooth, which can be caused by trauma (previous bleeding into the tooth) or fluorosis markings. Occasionally the cause is unknown. Often it is the brown discoloration that is removed first when the whitening treatment commences and is the quickest to lighten. Sometimes it may take longer for the whitening treatment to remove the brown spot entirely. It may just fade to a pale-yellow mark. As the background color is lightened, the mark becomes less noticeable. Brown discolorations can be removed approximately 80% of the time (Haywood 2006). Only a few brown areas have required re-treatment in 1–3 years (Haywood 2006).
- The presence of white markings on the incisors and molar teeth. There is an increasing incidence of white spots on teeth (see Chapter 11). The white spots and markings can be extensive on the anterior teeth as well as the first molars. If this condition is present, early restorative intervention on the molar teeth is indicated as well as whitening treatment to reduce the effect of the white marks on the labial surface of the teeth.
- The impact of the discoloration on the child.
- Whether the discoloration is easily amenable to whitening or may require multiple treatment options such as whitening, enamel surface treatment such as Sylc treatment, sandblasting, microabrasion (12–26 microns of enamel are removed per 5-second application; Haywood 2006), or resin infiltration.
- Whether there is a single tooth discoloration such as a nonvital tooth as a result of trauma.
- Whether multiple discolorations are present throughout the whole dentition.

Patients with the conditions mentioned by the Working Group should have treatment with appropriate treatment planning according to the diagnosis.

Severe discoloration

- Fluorosis.
- Discoloration caused by antibiotics.
- Intrinsic discoloration resulting from a child's complex medical history; deposition of biliverdin or hemosiderin into the tooth.

Moderate discoloration

- The administration of antibiotics at any age can have an impact on the developing dentition; when the teeth erupt they may have moderate discoloration. This may appear as banding, flecks, or patches. This can also manifest as localized or chronic hypoplasia (Wray and Welbury 2001 UK National Guidelines).

Enamel conditions

- Amelogenesis and dentinogenesis imperfecta (DGI).
- Childhood fevers and early antibiotic administration.
- Post-traumatic opacities in the permanent dentition.
- Idiopathic opacity.
- Chronologic hypomineralization or hypoplasia or any other opacity affecting the quality of life of the patient. This can occur because local or systemic factors that interfere with normal matrix formation cause enamel surface defects and irregularities called enamel hypoplasia. The changes can be mild or more extended, such as pitting on the surface. In primary teeth it is unusual to have hypoplasia visible, and this is more evident when the permanent dentition erupts (Dean et al. 2011).
- Hyperplasia of the primary dentition can appear as a halo or ring around the primary tooth.

White spots and small white marks

- Some markings can appear as white lines that develop after the chronologic deposition of enamel—for example, amoxicillin defects. Sometimes the original white spots get more noticeable during the first few days of whitening (called the "splotchy stage") (Haywood 2006). This is because during the whitening process the whitening gel penetrates the weakest part of the tooth first which is the white spot, as it represents a defect. This temporary lightening of white spot is due to the differently formed portions of enamel which are responding to the carbamide peroxide faster. Often this brief whitening can fade the spot entirely and no further adjunctive treatment may be necessary.

Brown and yellow staining

- Normally occurs from fluorosis on the teeth, enamel defects wherein the tooth has erupted with defective areas, or trauma in the primary dentition.

Esthetic defects

- Hypodontia, missing teeth, or teeth that are malformed on eruption—for example, saucer-shaped defects, ridges, and pitted and mottled teeth.
- Incisor discrepancies—a difference in the diameter of the central and lateral incisor teeth. The lateral incisors can often be peg shaped, so the esthetics become more of an issue.

Molar incisor hypoplasia

- The impact on children is significant (see Chapter 11).

Trauma

- Trauma followed by hemorrhage into the tooth during regenerative endodontic procedures.
- Trauma in the primary and secondary teeth.
- Discoloration resulting from endodontic therapy.

Hereditary factors

- See section on primary teeth, ages 2–5, later in the chapter.

Table 22.1 lists the five categories of whitening treatment need.

Table 22.1 Index of whitening treatment need for patients under age 18

Category 1—High
1. Discoloration: severe
2. Location of stain: uniform multiple dark distribution
3. Impact on child: severe
4. Whitening need: high
Category 2—Moderate
1. Discoloration: moderate
2. Location: even distribution
3. Impact on child: has an effect on the child
4. Whitening need: moderate
Category 3—Desirable
1. Discoloration: mild
2. Location: few anterior teeth
3. Impact on child: some impact
4. Whitening need: desirable; this will easily alleviate discoloration issues
Category 4—Advisable
1. Discoloration: isolated areas of discoloration
2. Location: random distribution across the tooth
3. Impact on child: moderate
4. Whitening need: advisable
Category 5—Possible
1. Discoloration: mild discoloration or white spots
2. Location: few teeth or single tooth
3. Impact on child: no effect on the child
4. Whitening need: can be undertaken; may be desirable, but can wait until child is older than 18

WHAT IS THE BEST AGE AT WHICH TO WHITEN TEETH FOR PATIENTS YOUNGER THAN 18?

It is important to assess the amount of discoloration and the cause before planning whitening treatment for a child younger than 18. It seems that the large pulps and the canals promote a good blood supply, which permits effective whitening for patients younger than 18 (Haywood 2006).

Primary teeth, ages 2–5

Causes of discoloration in primary teeth are as follows:

- Genetic conditions:
  - Cystic fibrosis (CF) is an inherited chronic disorder. It is autosomal recessive (Dean et al. 2011). The discoloration is a result of the disease alone or the multiple antibiotics such as tetracycline that are administered. Primosch (1980) studied 86 children with CF and noted that they had high prevalence for tooth discoloration and hypoplasia on their teeth but had fewer caries.
  - Amelogenesis imperfecta.
  - Dentinogenesis imperfecta (DGI) interferes with normal tooth development. It affects approximately one in 6000–8000 people, and dentin dysplasia occurs in 1 in 100,000. It consists of a group of autosomal dominant genetic conditions characterized by abnormal dentin structure affecting either the primary or both the primary and secondary dentitions. Clinically, the teeth are discolored and show structural defects such as bulbous crowns and small pulp chambers radiographically. The underlying defect of mineralization often results in shearing of the overlying enamel, leaving exposed

weakened dentin that is prone to wear, according to the National Institute of Health. There are three types of DGI:

- Type I (DGI-I): This type occurs in individuals who have another inherited disorder called osteogenesis imperfecta (causes brittle bones).
- Type II (DGI-II): The dental features of DGI-II are similar to those of DGI-I but penetrance is virtually complete and osteogenesis imperfecta is not a feature. Bulbous crowns are a typical feature with marked cervical constriction. Normal teeth are never found in DGI-II (Barron et al. 2008).
- Type III (DGI-III): This type occurs in those without other genetic disorders. Some researchers believe types II and III are part of a single disorder along with another condition called dentin dysplasia.
- Dentin dysplasia types I and II: This disorder primarily affects baby teeth more than adult teeth. General symptoms of DGI include tooth discoloration (blue-gray or yellowish-brown), tooth translucency, and teeth that are weaker than normal, which makes them prone to erosion, breakage, and loss.

- Premature birth and low birthweight: the white spots occur because there is insufficient mineralization of the enamel matrix as a result of a mineral deficiency.
- Diseases of the blood:
  - Porphyria: congenital erythropoietic porphyria, Gunther disease. The primary teeth are a purple-brown color. This is a result of the deposition of porphyrin in the developing structures. The permanent dentition may also have staining.
  - Rh incompatibility.
  - Internal hemorrhaging.
  - ABO blood type incompatibility.
- Neonatal jaundice: the teeth erupt with a blue-green discoloration or a brown discoloration. The color can gradually fade, particularly around the anterior teeth, as the child gets older. The blood reorganizes within the tooth structure (Dean et al. 2011).
- Neonatal kidney and liver disease.
- Antibiotics.
  - Tetracyclines administered to children. The tetracycline chelates with the calcium salts. The location of the discoloration corresponds to the chronologic development of the tooth according to when the tetracycline was administered (Haywood 2012). The tetracycline is deposited into the dentin structure of the tooth. When the tetracycline staining darkens from brown to yellow, the fluorescence decreases. The exposure of the teeth to light results in the slow oxidation with a change of the pigment from yellow to brown. The larger the dose, the deeper the pigmentation. The duration of exposure of the drug may be less important than the total dose relative to the body weight. The sensitive period for tetracycline exposure is 3–5 months after birth or up to 7 years of age. Tetracycline can transfer through the placenta, which can affect the primary dentition.
  - Amoxicillin (Amoxil)
  - Ciprofloxacin (Ciproxin)
- Trauma to the primary dentition: discoloration of primary teeth can be caused by trauma and sometimes subsequent devitalization of the tooth, or by mild trauma after which the primary tooth remains vital. Primary teeth can erupt with discoloration.

Whitening of primary teeth at age 2–5 in cases of trauma can be undertaken when there is a specific need (e.g., if the central incisors are darkened by trauma), when the child is aware of the discoloration, and when this has an impact on the child (Haywood 2000). The whitening treatment can be undertaken in a tray. Whitening should be done only if all other reasons for discoloration have been eliminated (e.g., abscessed teeth, caries, resorption) (Haywood 2006). Whitening is an easier, a more esthetic, and a more cost-effective treatment than bonding or placing composite or stainless steel crowns with esthetic facings, given the short life of the primary tooth.

It is best that the parents supervise the treatment application and treatment time and the wear schedule for the child. If the child's chronic medical condition is unstable, then whitening treatment should be delayed until the child is stable and in better health.

Mixed dentition, ages 6–10

During the mixed dentition stage, whitening can be undertaken and may require a specific tray design: the tray is scalloped to include primary and secondary teeth but it should not impinge on the gingivae in any way that interferes with the eruption of the teeth. Orthodontists have indicated that the whitening tray will not impede the eruption of the permanent teeth (Haywood 2006).

At age 6–10, specific markings on teeth may be treated with whitening, microabrasion, or resin infiltration. If the tooth erupts with a specific discolored area or a white mark or fleck that concerns the child, then limited treatment can be undertaken on the isolated lesion. It is best to wait for eruption of all the permanent teeth.

Lower limit: 10–14 years

Normally, 10–14 years of age is the lower limit because of the mixed dentition phase, but whitening can be undertaken in patients of this age group. In the mixed dentition stage, several whitening trays may need to be made because of different eruptions of permanent teeth.

Age 15

Age 15 is a cornerstone in the child's development. Children undergo a change in their appearance and develop a sense of self, body awareness, and self-perception including other issues concerning their social development. Body dysmorphic issues, anorexia, acid diets, poor diets, and fad dieting can develop at this age. If the appearance of the teeth concerns the child and the discoloration is severe or moderate, it is advisable to undertake whitening of the teeth. Whitening at this age may be straightforward and simple and may have a massive impact on the child's self-confidence, which is an important attribute at this age.

Quite apart from issues of awareness of body image, these teenagers become acutely aware of any defects or discoloration on their teeth.

After orthodontic treatment

At age 15 many children complete their orthodontic treatment and become aware that their teeth have discolored significantly. In addition, the gingivae initially after removal of the braces are hypoplastic; once the gingivae have returned to good health, more of the labial surface of the enamel is visible and the discoloration may become more evident. The carbamide peroxide can be used for improving the gingival health as well as whitening the teeth using the patient's existing orthodontic retainer.

When the braces are removed, many children notice that their teeth have severely discolored during the 18 months to 2 years that the braces have been on their teeth. This may occur because the fixed braces cause plaque to accumulate and the plaque retention, together with poor oral hygiene, causes discoloration. If this is the case and the teeth appear an orange shade after the removal of the braces, then it is appropriate to whiten the child's teeth. In addition, when the braces are removed white spot lesions may be detectable. There is a specific protocol to follow for the white spot lesions, but if the child's oral hygiene is well controlled then whitening may be an ideal treatment to reduce the effect of the white spots. This may be followed by whitening in the orthodontic retainer and microabrasion or resin infiltration. Whitening may be undertaken in the clear retainers or stabilizing aligners that are fitted during or after orthodontic treatment. These rigid trays allow for the whitening material to be retained well within the tray, and whitening is quick and effective.

Impact of medication

Some children with complex medical histories such as chronic gastric problems may take multiple courses of antibiotics, which may cause severe tooth discoloration such as orange markings.

Ages 16–18

If specifically indicated as detailed earlier, this is a good age at which to undertake whitening treatment. The dentition is more stable, the gingivae are maturing, and the outcomes can be predictable.

OTHER FACTORS TO CONSIDER WHEN UNDERTAKING WHITENING FOR PATIENTS YOUNGER THAN 18

The severity of discoloration. The darker the teeth, the longer they will take to whiten.

Patient's medical history. This will play a significant part in the discoloration and subsequent whitening treatment.

Antibiotic intake. See earlier.

Amount of restorative treatment. This depends on the decay risk of the child. If the decay is severe, restorative treatment should be undertaken first before any whitening treatment. If the decay risk is low, whitening treatment can be undertaken first, followed by preventive measures such as varnish and tooth mousse. A new whitening varnish has been introduced that uses the same adhesive technology as the varnish treatment (Philips Oral Care).

Decay risk—whether the child is at high risk for tooth decay. If the discoloration is more of an issue for the child and there is early evidence of demineralization caused by decay, it is best to whiten first because the whitening gel reduces the effect of the tooth and root decay.

Presence of sensitivity. This may be related to molar incisor hypoplasia, in which the teeth are hypersensitive.

Compliance. Taste can be a factor in the child's compliance with the whitening treatment. There are normally several flavors to select from, and this should not be a major factor in restricting whitening treatment.

Supervision. Parental supervision is necessary during the whitening treatment for patients younger than 18. Parents should be actively involved in the decision making and compliance with the whitening protocol.

CONCLUSION

Tooth whitening treatment can be undertaken for patients younger than 18 years. Tooth whitening treatments are safe and predictable for this age group. In some cases after orthodontic treatment, when the gingivae are swollen, the whitening treatment may be desirable to help heal the mouth.

REFERENCES

American Academy on Pediatric Dentistry Council on Clinical Affairs. (2009) Policy on dental bleaching for child and adolescent patients. *Pediatr Dent* **30**(7 Suppl):61–3.

Attal JP, Atlan A, Denis M, Vennat E. (2014) White spots on enamel: treatment protocol by superficial or deep infiltration (part 2). *Int Orthod* **12**(1):1–31.

Barron MJ, McDonnell ST, MacKie I, Dixon MJ. (2008) Hereditary dentine disorders: dentinogenesis imperfecta and dentine dysplasia. *Orphanet J Rare Dis* **3**:31.

British Dental Bleaching Society (BDBS). (2012) *BDBS advice sheet on the changes in the cosmetic products regulations which take effect on 31st October 2012.* Available at: www.bdbs.co.uk/news_26_451581864.pdf. [Accessed 3 June 2016].

Brook PH, Shaw WC. (1989) The development of an index of orthodontic treatment priority. *Eur J Orthodontics* **11:** 309–20.

Castro KS, de Araújo Ferreira AC, Duarte RM, Sampaio FC. (2014) Acceptability, efficacy and safety of two treatment protocols for dental fluorosis: a randomized clinical trial. *J Dent* **42**(8):938–44.

Cons NC, Jenny J, Kohout FJ. (1986) *DAI: the Dental Aesthetic Index.* College of Dentistry, University of Iowa: Iowa City, Iowa.

Croll TP, Sasa IS. (1995) Carbamide peroxide bleaching of teeth with dentinogenesis imperfecta discoloration: report of a case. *Quintessence Int* **26**(10):683–6.

Daniel C, Richmond S. (2000) The development of Index Complexity, Outcome and Need (ICON). *J Orthod* **27**:149–62.

Dean JA, Avery DR, McDonald RE. (2011) Acquired and developmental disturbances of the teeth and associated oral structures. In *McDonald and Avery's dentistry for the child and adolescent*, 9th edn. Elsevier: Maryland Heights, Missouri.

Donly KJ. (1995) The adolescent patient: special whitening challenges. *Compend Contin Educ Dent* **24**(4A):390–6.

European Commission Directive on Cosmetics Products. (2012) 76/768/EEC. Available at: ec.europe.eu/health/scientific_committees/consumer_safety/docs/sccs_s_006.pdf (3 June 2016).

Faculty of Dental Surgery. (2014) We did it! GDC changes position on tooth bleaching in under 18s. *Fac Dent J* 5(3):102–3. Available at http://publishing.rcseng.ac.uk/doi/pdf/10.1308/204268514X14017784505691.

Falcon HC, Richardson P, Shaw MJ, Bulman JS. (2001) Restorative dentistry: developing an index of restorative dental treatment need. *Br Dent J* **190**:479–86.

General Dental Council (GDC). (2014) GDC letter, 29 May 2014. Available at www.gdc-uk.org/Membersofpublic/Illegal practice/Documents/Position%20Statement%20on%20Tooth%20Whitening%20UD%2029.05.pdf.

General Dental Council (GDC). (2015) *Tooth whitening Q & As*. Available at www.gdc-uk.org/dentalprofessionals/standards/pages/tooth-whitening.aspx.

Haywood VB. (1992) History, safety, and effectiveness of current bleaching techniques and applications of the Nightguard Vital Bleaching technique. *Quintessence Int* **23**(3):471–88.

Haywood VB. (2000) The current status of Nightguard Vital Bleaching. *Compend Contin Educ Dent* **21**:S18–S27.

Haywood VB. (2006) Bleaching children's teeth: questions and answers. *GAGD Explorer*, 4-7. Available at http://vanhaywood.com/uploads/articlespage/GAGDSummer06.pdf.

Haywood VB. (2012) Pre-bleaching exam vital for optimum whitening. *Compend Contin Educ Dent* **33**:76–7.

Kelleher M. (2010) The 'daughter test' in aesthetic or cosmetic dentistry. *Dent Update* **37**:5–11.

Kelleher M. (2014) The law is an ass: legal and ethical issues surrounding the bleaching of younger patients discoloured teeth. *Fac Dent J* **5**(2):56–67.

Kugel G, Gerlach RW, Aboushala A, Ferreira S. (2011) Long-term use of 6.5% hydrogen peroxide bleaching strips on tetracycline stain: a clinical study. *Compend Contin Educ Dent* **32**(8):506–7.

Lee SS, Zhang W, Lee DH, Li Y. (2005) Tooth whitening in children and adolescents: a literature review. *Pediatr Dent* **27**(5):362–8.

Mangan T. (2011) Genetic diseases of the teeth. Available at www.livestrong.com/article/79449-genetic-diseases-teeth.

Primosch RE. (1980) Tetracycline discolouration, enamel defects and dental caries in patients with cystic fibrosis. *Oral Surg Oral Med Oral Pathol* **50**(4):301–8, 1980.

Puri A, Ho-A-Yun J, McGuinness NJ. (2015) Use and knowledge of IOTN among GDPs in Scotland. *Br Dent J* **218**(7): 399–404.

Siddiqui TA, Shaikh A, Fida M. (2014) Agreement between orthodontist and patient perception using Index of Orthodontic Treatment Need. *Saudi Dent J* **26**:156–65.

Sujak SL, Abdul Kadir R, Dom TN. (2004) Esthetic perception and psychosocial impact of developmental enamel defects among Malaysian adolescents. *J Oral Sci* **46**(4):221–6.

Sundfeld RH, Rahal V, Croll TP, De Aalexandre RS. (2007) Enamel microabrasion followed by dental bleaching for patients after orthodontic treatment—case reports. *J Esthet Restor Dent* **19**(2):71–7; discussion 78.

Wong MC, Glenny AM, Tsang BW, Lo EC. (2010) Topical fluoride as a cause of dental fluorosis in children. *Cochrane Database Syst Rev* **1**:CD007693.

Wray A, Welbury R. (2001) *Treatment of intrinsic discoloration in permanent anterior teeth in children and adolescents.* UK National Guidelines. Royal College of Surgeons Publications. Available at www.rcseng.ac.uk/fds/publications- clinical-guidelines/clinical_gui delines/documents/di scolor.pdf.

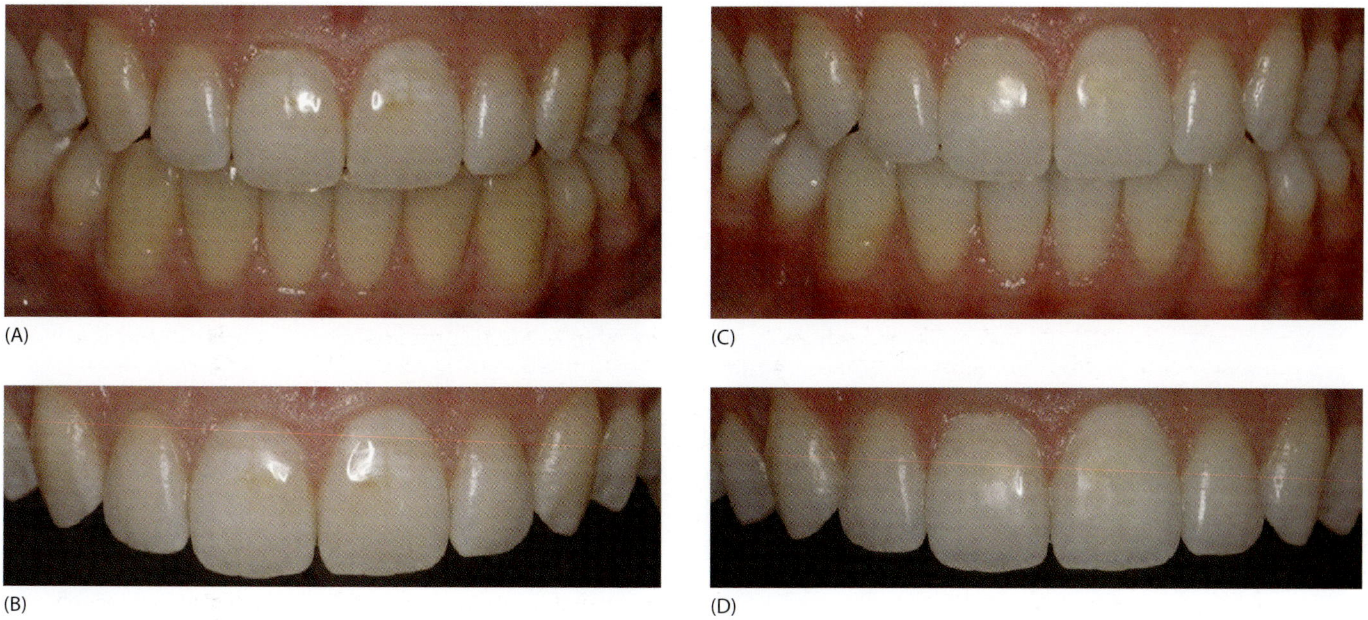

Figure 22.1

(A) At age 15 this patient had multiple brown and white marks on the teeth from a variety of causes including trauma and high fever. (B) Retracted contrast view of upper six anterior teeth before treatment. (C) The result after treatment with whitening, microabrasion, and resin infiltration. The lower teeth had much deeper discoloration than the upper and took 6–8 weeks to whiten under parental supervision; the upper tooth took 4 weeks. (D) Retracted contrast view of upper six anterior teeth after treatment.

23

MANAGING AND DEVELOPING A SUCCESSFUL WHITENING PRACTICE

Linda Greenwall

INTRODUCTION

Tooth whitening has become one of the treatments most requested by dental patients. Dentists should ensure that they are knowledgeable about the full range of whitening treatments available to patients and should know how best to deliver these. Now that the legislation on whitening has been amended, it is very clear which whitening treatments can be undertaken in an effective way. Furthermore, tooth whitening is the practice of dentistry; therefore only dentists and their trained teams may undertake this treatment for patients, after performing a thorough assessment of the suitability of the patient to undergo the whitening treatment. This chapter will explore ways to develop and manage a successful whitening practice in which whitening is the beginning of the treatment plan and further minimally invasive treatments can be undertaken. This knowledge will help dentists run and manage a successful whitening practice with the full dental team engaged to assist with all aspects of whitening.

Developing and managing a successful whitening practice (Table 23.1) can be achieved with the use of 15 strategies (Table 23.2).

STRATEGY 1—LISTEN

"First seek to understand, then to be understood" (see Covey 2004).

Before undertaking any form of esthetic treatment, it is essential first to understand what the patient is requesting (see Figure 23.2 and Table 23.3). Patients who have seen television makeover shows may think that chairside treatments can be undertaken in 20 minutes during a lunch break. Many of the treatments take much longer, and patients need to fully understand what is required to achieve a significantly lighter shade. A commitment from the patient is essential. Some patients may have unrealistic expectations of the desired outcome. There exists a quest for unrealistic white shades such as the Hollywood white shade, which may be impossible to achieve with home whitening, and this should be carefully explained to the patient before the start of treatment. Full explanations should be given to the patient once he or she has clarified the request for whitening treatment.

STRATEGY 2—CLASSIFY THE WHITENING TREATMENTS (SEE TABLE 23.4)

There may be several reasons for the discoloration that the patient is experiencing. It is essential that the dentist diagnose the reason for the discoloration because this will affect the outcome and the length of time that it will take to complete the whitening treatment. Not all whitening cases are the same. Classifying whitening treatments based on patient need will help with planning, staging, sequencing, and fee setting for the different types of discoloration and whitening treatments. It will help with determination of the correct appointment lengths and types. Once the procedure analysis of the whitening appointments is completed, then appropriate fees can be set.

Treatments need to be classified because the treatment times and fees are different for a basic case versus an intermediate case versus an advanced case. More whitening materials will need to be supplied for advanced whitening cases. A basic whitening case requires no restorative dentistry and will take about 4–6 weeks to achieve a B1 shade. An intermediate whitening case normally involves two whitening treatments, such as internal and home whitening (see Table 23.4). An advanced whitening case involves extensive discoloration, such as fluorosis or tetracycline discoloration, and/or requires complex restorative dentistry. Whitening treatments in this category will take longer owing to their complex nature, so the planned sequence of treatments will take longer and the associated fees will be higher.

STRATEGY 3—UNDERTAKE EXCELLENT WHITENING TRAINING

Undertake training for yourself and the entire dental team. There is a vast body of scientific literature demonstrating the effectiveness of the whitening treatments that have been presented in this book (also see Greenwall 2001). It is essential that the dentist and the team understand the process of whitening and how it works and whitens inside the tooth. Tooth whitening has a scientific basis, and we need to further understand what the research demonstrates. Ensure that you are well trained in whitening techniques. Attend seminars and obtain hands-on training on whitening.

Table 23.1 Factors to plan when creating a whitening practice your vision is to develop a practice that offers excellent whitening services.

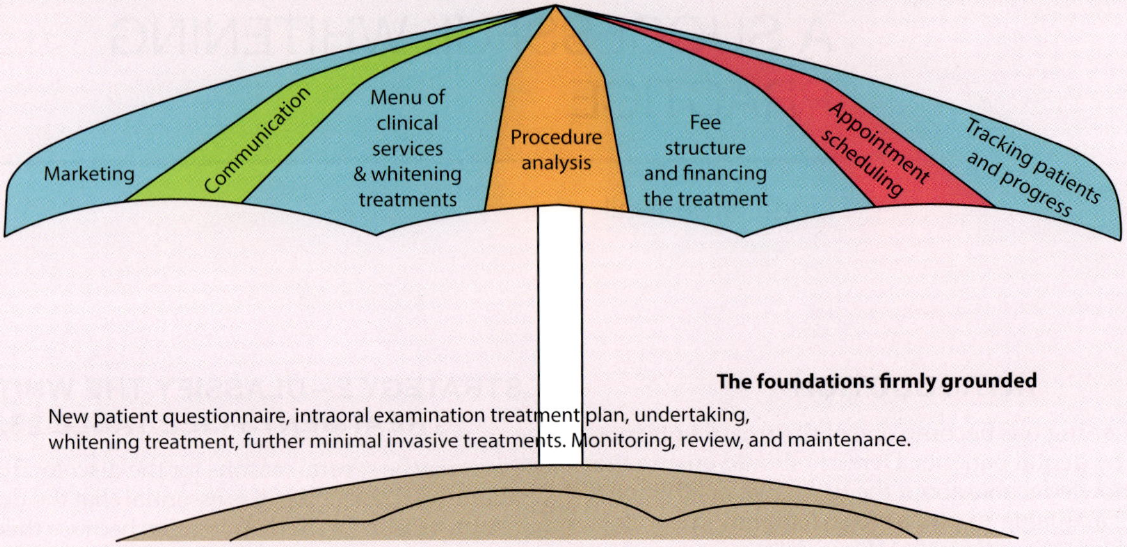

Table 23.2 Fifteen success strategies for whitening

1. Listen to the patient and understand what the patient is requesting (see Figures 23.1 and 23.2; Greenwall 2012). Is the whitening treatment that the patient is requesting realistic or unrealistic treatment?
2. Classify the type of discoloration. Classify the whitening case (Kwon et al. 2009).
3. Undertake excellent whitening training for yourself and the entire dental team.
4. Continually update your knowledge of whitening as regulations change and new whitening materials, technology, and innovations are introduced.
5. Learn to plan whitening treatments effectively so that they remain sustainable and long-lasting (see Figure 23.5C).
6. Manage complications and sensitivity issues that patients may experience (see Chapter 20).
7. Supply excellent professional whitening materials that have been carefully researched (see Chapter 4).
8. Ensure that patients have written instructions and have given written consent when undertaking the treatment so that patients know exactly what to expect and what will happen and what will not happen.
9. Train your entire team on whitening techniques and programs so that everyone will be on board with the treatment that you are offering.
10. Undertake tooth whitening for yourself and your team to demonstrate the benefits of esthetic dentistry and to allow them to empathize with the patient and offer advice on how to treat any problems with sensitivity.
11. Develop an excellent whitening program that includes whitening and whitening and hygienist maintenance (see Chapter 5).
12. Tooth whitening is a behavior-changing experience for patients; ensure that patients complete the treatment effectively, and capture the excitement that the patient experiences when he or she has a beautiful whitened smile. This is good for further marketing.
13. Develop marketing materials. It is useful to have whitening leaflets and a patient newsletter to continually market the whitening services to existing and new patients.
14. Obtain whitening testimonials. It is useful to ask the patient to complete a whitening testimonial after successful whitening treatment. With the patient's permission, it is useful to add these testimonials to your website; such testimonials, along with a gallery of before and after smiles of patients who have undergone successful whitening treatment, are an excellent inspiration for new patients to schedule appointments for whitening.
15. Develop a whitening smile book of before and after photographs of your patients (see Figure 23.2).

STRATEGY 4—CONTINUALLY UPDATE YOUR KNOWLEDGE OF WHITENING

Update your knowledge as the regulations change and new materials and technology are introduced. It is essential to keep up-to-date because many new products enter the market with different modes of action and treatment times.

STRATEGY 5—LEARN TO PLAN WHITENING TREATMENTS EFFECTIVELY

Plan treatments effectively so that the results remain sustainable and long-lasting. The protocols that were established by Haywood (2003) have been shown to be effective. Patients cannot be given the whitening trays and gel and then be left alone. They need constant

Table 23.3 Understanding patient requests involves understanding the new patient journey and the sequence of events that needs to take place in order to help the patient to realize what is involved in achieving a whiter smile. It is essential for patients to understand the timing of the appointments and the patient's financial responsibility.

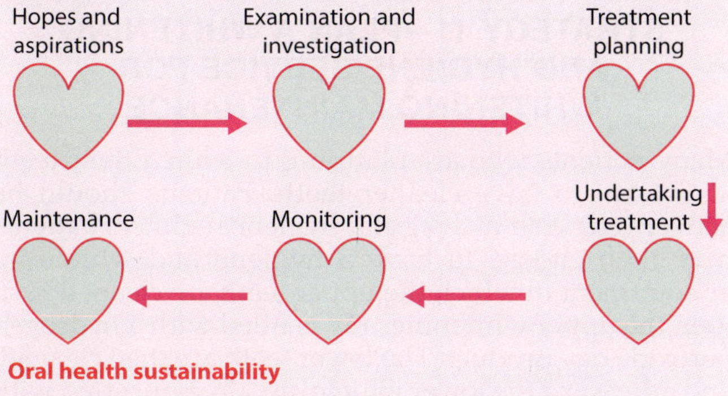

Table 23.4 A classification of whitening treatment based on patient need

Basic

- No restorative dentistry required
- Home whitening: 4–6 weeks to achieve B1

Intermediate

- Some restorative dentistry required
- In combination with two whitening treatments (6–8 weeks to achieve B1)

Advanced

- Complex discoloration
- Advanced restorative treatment (may require prolonged treatment for existing sensitivity)
- Whitening (8–10 weeks to achieve whitening to shade B1)
- Patients with existing sensitivity (whitening treatment may be more complex; apply soothing gels in the bleaching tray prior to commencing whitening)

Modified from Kwon et al. 2009 and Greenwall 2012. With permission

monitoring and motivation to continue the treatment effectively. It is essential that the home whitening treatment be broken down into small, manageable stages so that the patient can comply with the treatment recommendations and the dentist and hygienist-therapist can monitor the patient well.

When planning all dental procedure for patients, it is important to categorize the type of procedure that will be undertaken and to assess whether this is a primary, secondary, or tertiary appointment. A primary appointment is one with a high value in terms of revenue (Tables 23.5 and 23.6). A secondary appointment is one that has a lesser value but still involves essential dentistry. It can be important and urgent. It covers a lesser fee in terms of production than a primary appointment. A tertiary appointment is the lowest value

Table 23.5 Tooth whitening and associated procedures that are categorized as primary, secondary, and tertiary appointments (Greenwall and Jameson 2012)

Primary appointments	*Secondary appointments*	*Tertiary appointments*
Whitening treatments Restorative dentistry Minimally invasive esthetics Crown and bridge, prosthodontics Implants Esthetic dentistry, porcelain veneers	More than two restorations Endodontic treatments Extensive periodontal treatment	Easing a denture Patient reviewing Crown fit Whitening final appointment

Table 23.6 Whitening treatments categorized into primary, secondary, and tertiary appointments categorization allows efficient scheduling to help the practice improve its whitening services and efficiency.

Primary whitening	*Secondary whitening*	*Tertiary whitening*
Power whitening Whitening stage one Microabrasion Nonvital whitening	Examination for whitening Whitening impressions Desensitizing teeth before whitening	Review appointments Treatment planning discussion with patient Planning treatment (including evaluation of radiographs, pictures, intraoral camera photographs) Answering patient's questions about whitening

appointment; it is still important. It is a shorter appointment and does not normally command a fee. These appointment categories are preblocked into the schedule for the year so that every day, primary and secondary appointments can be scheduled. This helps with efficiency, stress management, and planned practice production.

STRATEGY 6—MANAGE COMPLICATIONS AND SENSITIVITY ISSUES THAT PATIENTS MAY EXPERIENCE

Up to 85% of patients experience some type of sensitivity during the whitening treatment. This may be a result of the material penetrating the pulp within 5–15 minutes of gel application or tray pressure, the application of the higher strength materials, or toothbrush abrasion. Sensitivity is a major side effect and should be well managed (Browning et al. 2007) so that the patient knows what to do if he or she experiences it.

STRATEGY 7—SUPPLY EXCELLENT PROFESSIONAL WHITENING MATERIALS

There are excellent professional whitening materials on the market for dentists to supply to their patients. Many of these products have been carefully researched to show safety, effectiveness, and the long-lasting effect of the materials. Many advanced cases of severe discoloration such as fluorosis can be effectively whitened using low-strength whitening gels such as 10% carbamide peroxide materials (see Figure 23.6). Nonvital whitening can be undertaken only with use of 16% carbamide peroxide or no more than 6% hydrogen peroxide; dentists need to know how to apply these materials into the canal properly, how to place the intracanal dressings, and the length of time between visits.

The new regulations state that with each cycle of use the dentist should first examine the patient to ensure that treatment is appropriate for the patient. The receptionist can no longer supply whitening materials to patients for touch-up or maintenance treatment. Each cycle of use requires that the dentist perform an assessment first. This is to protect patient safety.

STRATEGY 8—ENSURE THAT PATIENTS HAVE WRITTEN INSTRUCTIONS

Patients must be given written instructions and must give consent when undertaking the treatment; they must know exactly what to expect, what will happen, and what will not happen (see Figure 23.5C). Explain the instructions verbally and follow up with written information so there is no miscommunication with the patient. This helps the patient to understand what is required of him or her and how to comply with the home treatment instructions. It is essential that patients know what they can expect in terms of the whitening result—what is likely to occur and what expectations are not realistic (see Figure 23.7).

STRATEGY 9—TRAIN YOUR ENTIRE TEAM ON WHITENING TECHNIQUES

The entire team should participate in training and programs so that everyone will be on board with the treatment that you are offering. Each member of staff can be involved in a different aspect of the whitening treatment. The receptionist needs to know which appointments to schedule for whitening and the cost and the time allocation for each whitening appointment. Every team member needs to help with the whitening treatment. Each team member also needs to know how to set up the tray for each stage of whitening and which materials to place on the tray. Team members can also help with marketing the whitening program to existing and new patients.

STRATEGY 10—UNDERTAKE TOOTH WHITENING FOR YOURSELF AND YOUR TEAM

It may be beneficial for yourself and your practice team to undertake the whitening treatment. It is essential that the team members, including the dentist, have a good white smile, which demonstrates the benefits of esthetic dentistry, especially when talking to patients. All staff members need to experience the whitening treatment themselves. If they experience sensitivity, they can empathize with the patient and offer advice on how to treat the sensitivity. This helps with management of the whitening program and communication with the patient.

STRATEGY 11—PLAN A WHITENING AND HYGIENE SERVICE FOR WHITENING MAINTENANCE

Many patients who are planning to whiten their teeth also want to have cleaner teeth. Patients should be actively engaged in a regular hygiene regimen. Patients may then choose to have a hygiene and whitening appointment in which the upper teeth are cleaned first, then the upper whitening tray is filled with a hydrogen peroxide day product. The lower teeth are then cleaned, and afterward the lower whitening tray is inserted with whitening material. That way the patients can undergo initial whitening or maintenance whitening and teeth cleaning during the same appointment. There are several different types of this service that can be designed. In addition, research has demonstrated that tooth whitening materials improve the gingivae (Firat et al. 2011) and reduce swelling, so a regimen can be undertaken that incorporates both treatments. In the study by Firat and colleagues, home and chemically activated whitening systems were found to be safer for tooth whitening and maintaining gingival health than a light-activated whitening system, which might lead to increased proinflammatory cytokines (interleukin [IL]-1β). Many patients would benefit from the use of whitening trays (renamed *therapeutic trays* when used for the purpose of not only whitening but also improving oral health for certain patients) and oral hygiene. Use of the whitening trays has demonstrated an improvement in the oral health of patients, including elderly patients (Haywood 2007) and special needs patients (Lazarchik and Haywood 2010).

STRATEGY 12—TOOTH WHITENING AS A BEHAVIOR-CHANGING EXPERIENCE FOR PATIENTS

Tooth whitening is a practice builder. The behavior of patients changes as they see the benefits of the whitening treatment. Patients are normally delighted with the results. They are walking advertisements for your practice. Ensure that all patients who have completed successful whitening treatments are given practice cards to give to their friends and business colleagues for referral.

When patients report how delighted they are with the results, give them a patient testimonial sheet to complete. Ask the patients for permission to put their testimonials on your website to further promote your whitening. This is very powerful to read for prospective patients looking to have whitening treatment.

Tooth whitening treatments can change patients' lives and how they feel about themselves. Be part of the journey. It is a great experience and brings joy back into dentistry!

STRATEGY 13—MARKETING WHITENING SERVICES

Because whitening is one of the services most requested by patients, dental practices need to be prepared for questions from patients about whitening treatments. It is a good idea to prepare marketing literature, information leaflets, and answers to commonly asked questions about whitening so that patients have information to take away with them. Be ready to answer patient's questions about whitening; this is a way to build the dental practice and expand the range of services. Special days can be allocated for whitening with the hygienists and dental therapists, such as Whitening Wednesdays. Special rates can be applied if a whole wedding party wants to whitening their teeth. It is essential to draw up a marketing plan for this service and all esthetic dentistry.

STRATEGY 14—WHITENING TESTIMONIALS

Patients really enjoy seeing the process of their teeth getting whiter. They are normally delighted with the results of having whiter teeth. They often express their delight with the shade of their teeth on the second visit during the whitening review appointment. It is a good idea to ask the patients to complete a whitening testimonial sheet. With their permission, this can be posted onto your website. My experience is that these testimonials drive patients to the practice, especially when they see the before and after gallery photographs.

Always give the patients extra practice business cards, because many of their friends and colleagues may compliment them on their new whiter smile, and the patients can be walking advertisements for your practice. Whitening teeth is a good way to build your esthetic dentistry practice and expand these services for your patients.

STRATEGY 15—SMILE BOOK

It is a good idea to collate a smile book of your before and after photographs, which should be standardized, showing a portrait of the patient before and after and a close-up of the smile before and after. You should obtain a signed photo release consent form from your patients so that these photographs can be used for marketing services and publication. If you are planning to put these on your website, you should use a special online publication consent form.

DEVELOPMENT OF A THRIVING WHITENING PRACTICE TAKES PLANNING

The dental practice should set a goal of improving its whitening services to patients. The patient's journey should be fully understood before any planning meetings are conducted (see Table 23.3). Hold a team meeting so that whitening appointments can be planned. Whitening procedures should be documented and a procedure analysis form completed for all whitening appointments. Evaluate all whitening treatments that can be offered, and introduce some new whitening treatments as new techniques are offered. Plan each team member's role in the whitening treatments provided by the practice; that way the dental team takes ownership of the new initiative.

GETTING STARTED WITH WHITENING

The aforementioned strategies should be planned in a systematic manner, then goals and plans should be established and activated according to schedule (Table 23.7). First, create the vision of how to deliver excellent whitening treatments for patients by developing an action plan.

It is important to ask existing patients open-ended questions, such as how do they feel about the color of their teeth, so they can discuss any concerns about their tooth shade (see Figures 23.2 and 23.4). Another way is to take current shades of the patient's teeth at the examination appointment. This can lead to a discussion of tooth shade; the patient can be shown the normal tooth shade guide so that he or she can see where the existing shade falls (see Figure 23.5A). The existing shade should be documented in the patient's clinical records.

Most patients would prefer lighter teeth. At the next appointment the patient may ask if the teeth have darkened, and this can be measured.

If new whitening services are introduced at the practice, information leaflets can be given to patients who ask about whitening services. A wide range of treatments is available for patients requesting whitening. Such patients may include adolescent patients who have noticed that their teeth have darkened after orthodontic treatment, during which there was food accumulating around the braces. In addition, patients who have just completed orthodontic treatment may require some minor esthetic treatment—for instance, improvement in the esthetics of peg-shaped laterals (see Figure 23.8). This needs to be carefully planned with the orthodontist. In fact, orthodontists may be an excellent source of referral for whitening treatments. Send your newly created smile book to 20 local orthodontists. That is an excellent way to receive new patient referrals.

Table 23.7 Ten tips for excellent whitening internal marketing

1. Take care of patients.
2. Provide high-quality care and excellent customer service.
3. Define team member job descriptions and responsibilities.
4. Ensure that an excellent new patient telephone call leads to an appointment.
5. Send new patients welcome packs.
6. Schedule a smile evaluation.
7. Greet the patient on arrival at the practice.
8. Ensure excellent photography during whitening treatments.
9. Plan internal marketing campaigns.
10. Suggest that patients with whom you have developed a rapport refer friends to you.

Adapted from Greenwall and Jameson 2012, with permission.

For some patients it is the existing sensitivity that the patient is experiencing that leads him or her to request further professional help. Once the teeth are desensitized, then whitening treatment may begin. This can be followed by further esthetic treatment (many patients request further esthetic treatment after whitening; see Figure 23.9).

Send your patients a whitening newsletter

A whitening newsletter is very effective and can show excellent before and after photographs of different whitening cases. The whitening newsletter should have information about all types of whitening that are provided, as well as a time-sensitive offer for the first 25 patients responding to the newsletter. The newsletters can be sent to patients by direct mail or via an email marketing service such as MailChimp. These whitening newsletters can be sent at special times of the year—for example, to promote summer whitening or a "winter white smile."

Photography

It is useful to build a library of before and after whitening cases. See Chapter 4 for further details on photography for whitening. The photographs can be inserted into a PowerPoint presentation for treatment planning discussions with patients, and they can be inserted into photobooks that are supplied via the Internet. These photobooks of cases should be in every surgery so that all members of the team can use them to discuss the process of tooth whitening and to answer patients' questions. Patients find the photobooks interesting; they can see a similar case to their own before they start their whitening treatment. It is important to get patients to sign a photo release form so that their photographs may be used for education purposes for other patients (see Figure 23.3).

Table 23.8 Nonvital tooth whitening: what is involved

- Consultation
- Radiographs, photographs, intraoral camera shots
- Diagnosis
- Treatment planning
- Repeated root canal treatment, if necessary
- One-month waiting period for teeth to "settle"
- Impressions for whitening trays
- Barrier preparation—cleaning the access cavity and preparing the root canal and pulp chamber
- First-stage whitening dressing
- Second-stage whitening
- Third dressing change
- Placement of final restoration

Table 23.9 Procedure analysis for nonvital whitening of a single tooth and whitening of all the upper teeth afterward

Clinical procedure	*Clinical time required*	*Time interval afterward*	*Administration time*
New patient consultation	1 hour	2 days to 1 week later	10 minutes
Diagnosis	10 minutes		0
Treatment planning; evaluating radiographs, photographs, and other images and data	15 minutes		15 minutes to complete the written treatment plan or PowerPoint presentation
Treatment planning discussion	15-minute clinical discussion	1 day to 1 week later depending on patient's schedule	15–30 minutes to discuss professional fee, make financial arrangements, and complete and sign paperwork
Repeated root canal treatment	90 minutes		
	One or two appointments	1 month later	10–15 minutes; with the procedure form, all appointments can be scheduled with the correct timing and intervals
Barrier preparation; clean cavity and place whitening gel and glass ionomer provisional dressing	40 minutes	1–2 weeks later	5–10 minutes
Fit sectional whitening tray; demonstrate to patient how to place whitening gel into labial part of the tray			
Change dressing; supply more whitening gel for labial placement; review shade; review gingival irritation	30 minutes	1–2 weeks	5–10 minutes
Change dressing as above (if necessary); commence rest of upper whitening treatment using second full-arch upper whitening tray	30 minutes	1–2 weeks	5 minutes
Remove dressing; clean access cavity; place glass ionomer using lightest shade as permanent restoration; review whitening of rest of upper teeth; measure shade	30 minutes	1 week	5 minutes
Review appointment	15 minutes	6 months	5–10 minutes

Appointment scheduling for whitening treatments

It is important to complete a procedure analysis form for each whitening procedure. This helps with time management and efficiency during the appointment. If the correct time is allocated for the procedure, the dentist and hygienist are less stressed and more able to focus their skills on providing the best treatment in a calm environment.

The analysis should be used to determine the primary, secondary, and tertiary whitening appointments (see Tables 23.4 and 23.5) and then all other appointments necessary for treatment. Tables 23.8 and 23.9 show the analysis for a nonvital tooth whitening treatment, listing all the appointments required to achieve a good outcome.

CONCLUSION

Tooth whitening treatments have been available for 25 years, and during that time it has been shown that these treatments are safe, predictable, and effective. Patients can achieve whiter teeth in a minimally invasive way, along with beautiful smiles. Being organized as a practice to deal with patient inquiries about whitening, and thus deliver excellent whitening treatments, is essential. Using the management strategies listed in this chapter will enhance the delivery of better treatments for your patients.

REFERENCES

Browning WD, Blalock JS, Frazier KB, Downey MC. (2007) Duration and timing of sensitivity related to bleaching. *J Esthet Restor Dent* **19**(5):256–64.

Covey S. (2004) *The 7 habits of highly effective people.* New York: Free Press.

Firat E, Ercan E, Gurgan S, Yucel OO. (2011) The effect of bleaching systems on the gingiva and the levels of IL-1β and IL-10 in gingival crevicular fluid. *Oper Dent* **36**(6):572–80.

Greenwall LH. (2001) *Bleaching techniques in restorative dentistry.* Martin Dunitz: London.

Greenwall LH, Jameson C. (2012) *Success strategies in aesthetic dental practice.* Quintessence Publishing: London.

Haywood VB. (2003) New bleaching considerations compared with at home bleaching. *J Esthet Restor Dent* **15**(3):184–7.

Haywood VB. (2007) Bleaching and caries control in elderly patients. *Aesthet Dent Today* **4**:42-44.

Haywood VB. (2012) Pre-bleaching exam vital for optimum whitening. *Compend Contin Educ Dent* **33**(2):72–3.

Kwon SR, Ko J, Greenwall LH. (2009) *Tooth whitening in esthetic dentistry.* Quintessence Publishing: London.

Lazarchik DA, Haywood VB. (2010) Use of tray-applied 10 percent carbamide peroxide gels for improving oral health in patients with special-care needs. *J Am Dent Assoc* **141**(6):639–46.

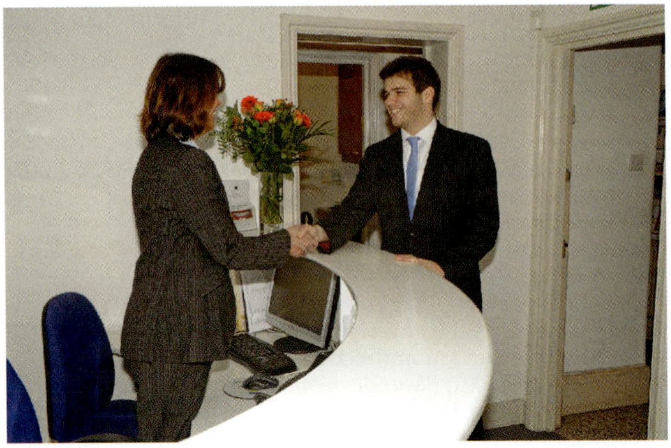

Figure 23.1

The patient should be greeted with a warm welcome on entering the practice. Patient management is really key in establishing and growing an excellent whitening practice.

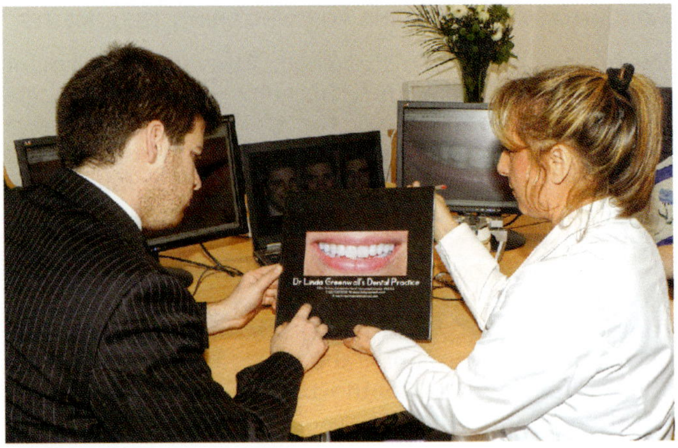

Figure 23.2

Patients are seen in a consulting room, which is separate from the dental surgery, so that they can discuss their concerns face to face. It is important to establish good communication with patients right from the start of the consultation. Patients are asked several open-ended questions about how they feel about the color of the teeth and their hopes and aspirations for their teeth and their smile. In this figure the patient is shown a smile book with images that have been compiled from similar whitening cases of other patients so that the patient can see what is possible with whitening.

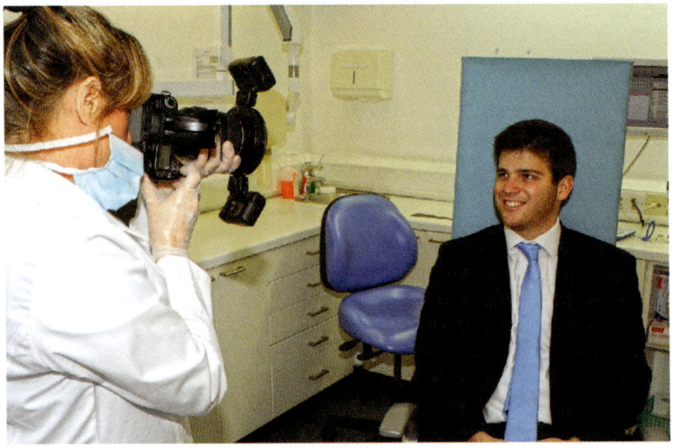

Figure 23.3

After the initial consultation, the patient is taken to the clinical environment and a full clinical intraoral and extraoral examination is conducted. After the patient assessment, photographs of the patient are taken.

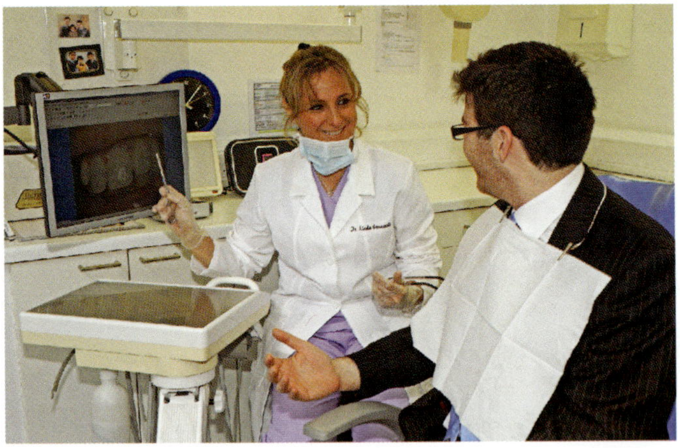

Figure 23.4

Digital intraoral photographs are taken to fully assess the details of the status of the teeth. The patient is shown some of the photographs on-screen to draw attention to any urgent issues discovered on the clinical examination.

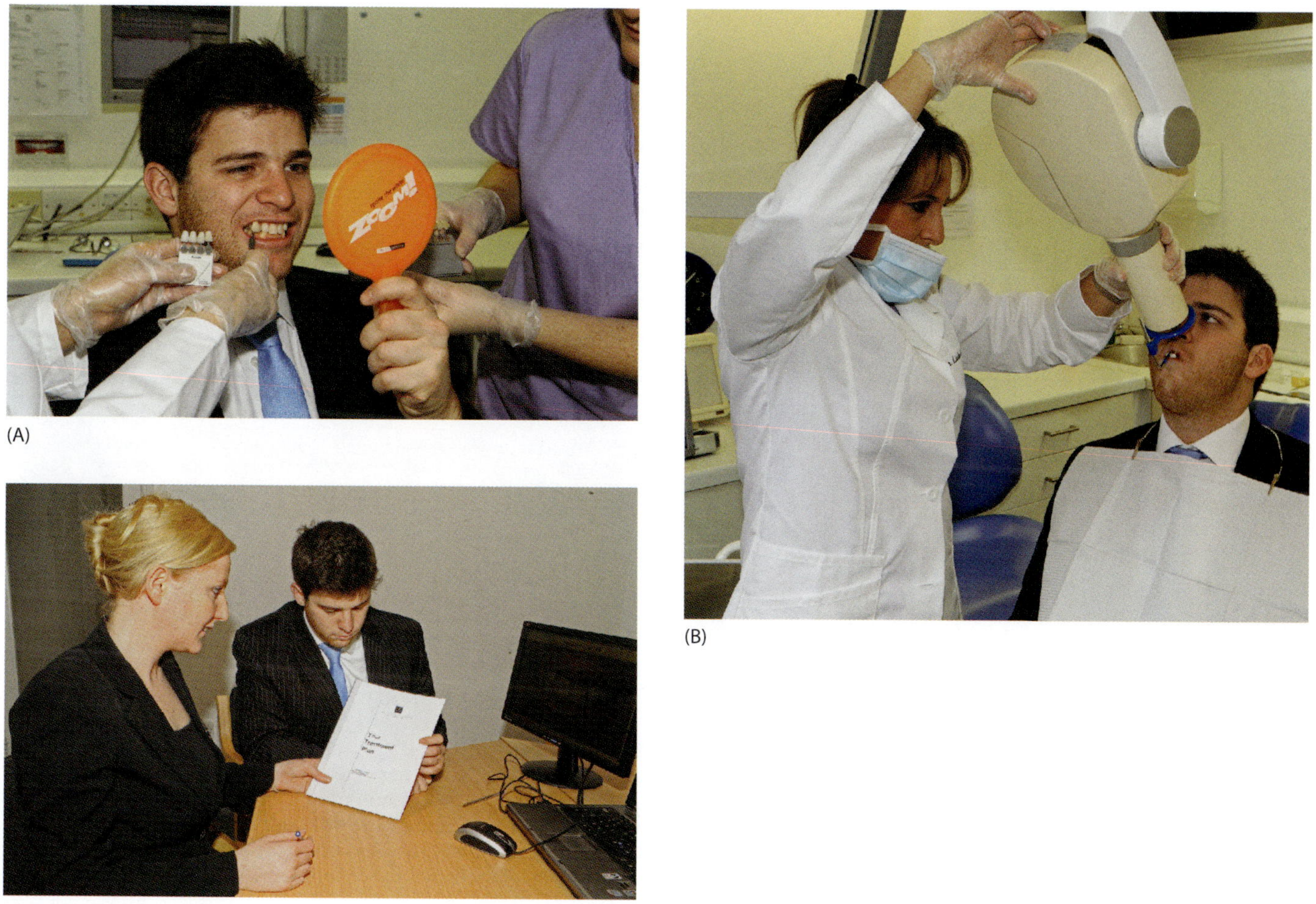

(A)

(B)

(C)

Figure 23.5

(A) The shade of the teeth is assessed at the initial visit. The patient participates in the shade assessment so that he or she can see the existing shade in the mirror, together with a shade guide matching the existing shade and the new potential shade. This shade assessment shows only a possible shade. No guarantees are made as to the amount of lightening that will be achieved. The expectations of the patient regarding the shade are lowered and defined very specifically so that the patient is not disappointed with the final result of the whitening. (B) Digital periapical intraoral radiographs are taken of any discolored teeth. It is important to ensure that there are no undetected existing periapical lesions. (C) Treatment planning appointment with the patient. All clinical data, radiographs, photographs, and digital photographs are assessed at a treatment planning session. This is done at an allocated time in the dentist's schedule each week. The treatment coordinator meets with the dentist to discuss the treatment plan. The treatment coordinator types the treatment plan into a report, which includes photographs and radiographs. The patient is invited back to the surgery for a treatment planning discussion. The patient is shown a tour of his or her photographs and radiographs. The treatment plan will then be discussed with the patient. Patients need to have options for treatment, and these are written down together with the advantages, disadvantages, benefits, and risks of all the dental treatment that is proposed, particularly the whitening treatment. Patients need to know the options and the consequences of not going ahead with any treatment. The dentist explains the clinical treatment, and then the treatment coordinator can explain the financial aspects and the appointment schedule.

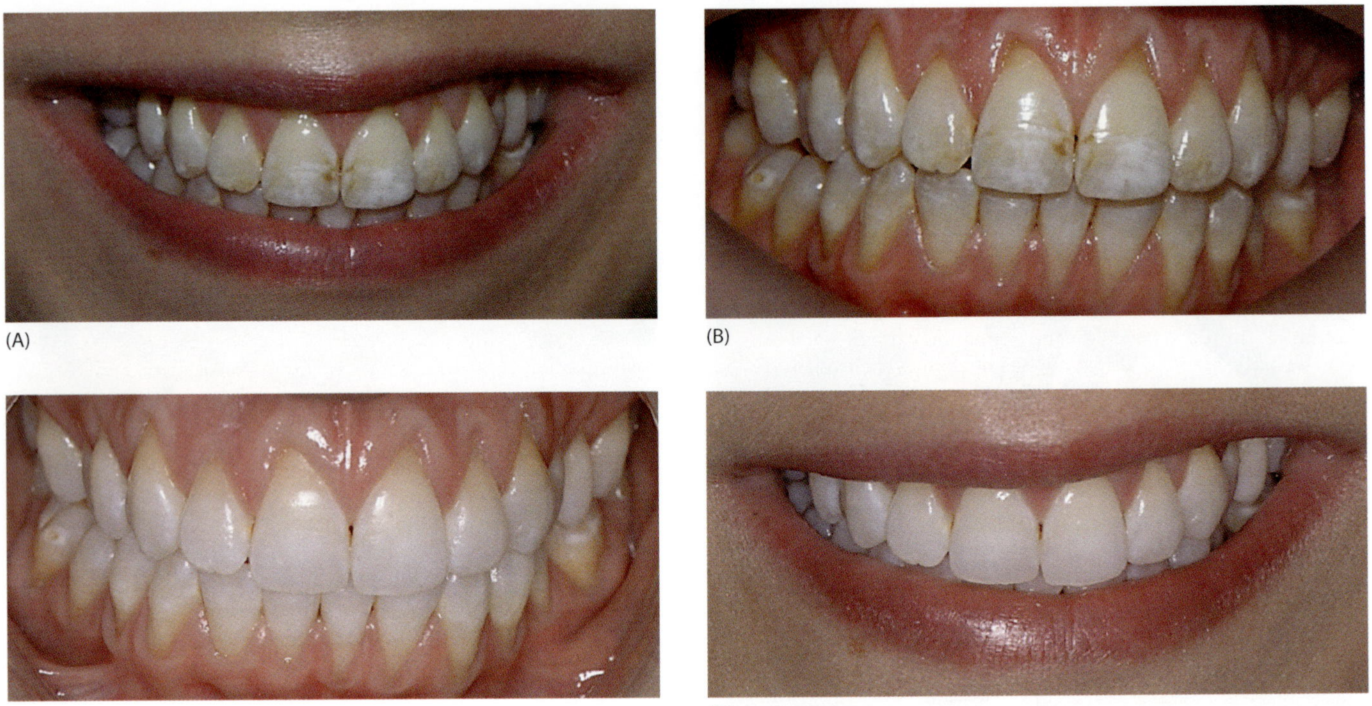

(A) (B) (C) (D)

Figure 23.6

(A and B) Advanced discoloration gives the teeth a mottled appearance. Even though the patient has extensive recession, this was not visible when the patient smiled and was not of concern to her. The patient was given soothing gel (potassium nitrate and fluoride gel [Sooth, SDI—Southern Dental Industries, Bayswater, Melbourne, Australia]) to use for 1 week before whitening to ensure that she did not experience sensitivity. (C) Results after whitening and microabrasion (retracted view). (D) Smile view. The treatment that was undertaken for the patient was 8–10 weeks of home whitening using 10% carbamide peroxide. This was followed by two sessions of microabrasion using 6.6% hydrochloric acid and silica carbide (Opalustre paste (Ultradent Products; supplied by Optident).

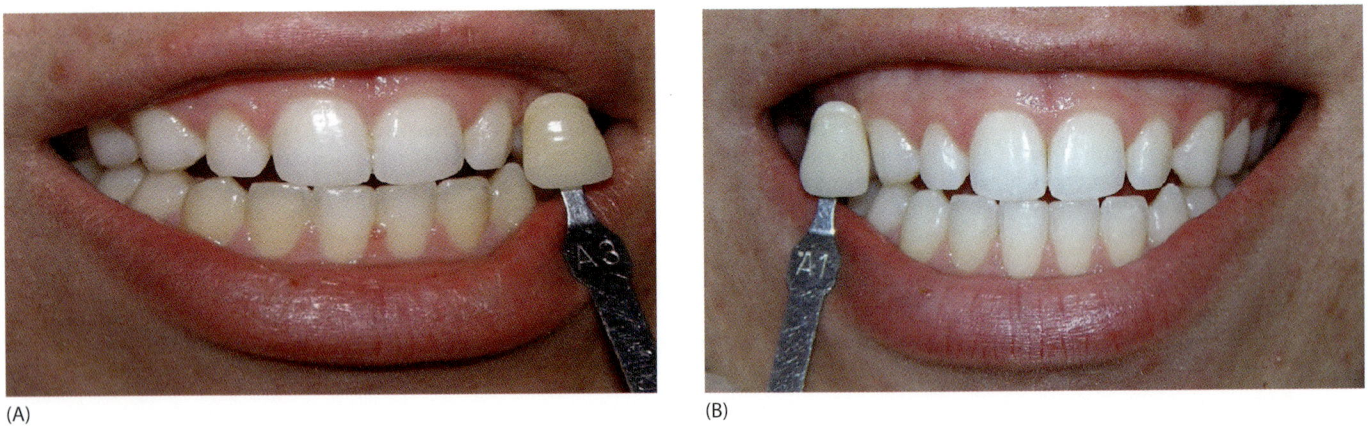

(A) (B)

Figure 23.7

(A) What can patients expect with whitening? Patients often ask what they can expect when they undertake their whitening treatment. It is important to be realistic regarding what shade may be possible, and to not overpromise the results of the whitening treatment, which could cause the patient to be disappointed. Excellent observational skills need to be honed for examining patients' teeth. This figure shows the appearance of the teeth before whitening. Note that the lower teeth are darker than the upper teeth. It is essential that the dentist explain this to the patient so that the patient is fully aware of the implications of this. Upper teeth whiten more quickly; lower teeth take longer because of the washout effect of the mandibular salivary glands. Regarding the treatment protocol for this patient, it may be better to whiten the lower teeth first to match the upper teeth. (B) The results after basic home whitening treatment. The upper and lower teeth are now matching in whiteness and have whitened to shade A1. It is important for the patient to whiten the teeth using a specially designed protocol. Normally the upper teeth are whitened first because it is quicker and results in less sensitivity. But for this patients, who has significantly darker lower teeth, the lower teeth were whitened first and then the upper teeth.

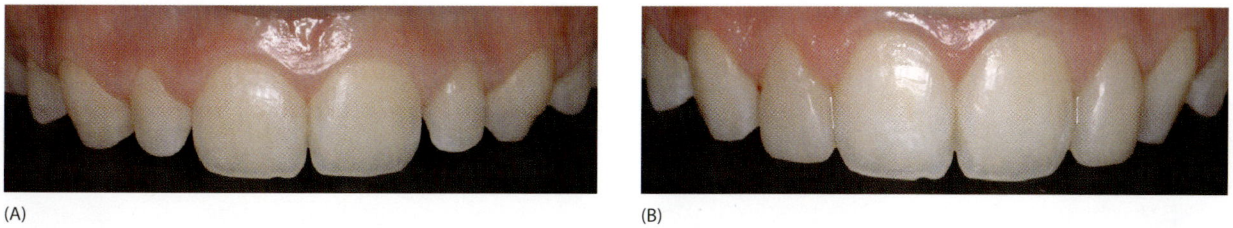

Figure 23.8

(A) Patient management is essential with this young patient. This involves discussions with the patient's parents and the orthodontist managing the braces. Timing and sequencing of treatment are essential, including the whitening treatment, which in this case was best undertaken after removal of the braces. This patient had her braces removed and needs to have restoration of the peg-shaped laterals before placement of the final palatal retainer, which was bonded onto the teeth. The teeth were whitened using the patient's rigid blowdown retainers (Essix orthodontic retainers). This figure shows the result after removal of the braces and some minor whitening. (B) Result a week after placement of preformed Edelweiss veneers. After whitening treatment, a period of time elapsed before the veneers were placed, so that the bond strength of the enamel could be re-established. The veneers were placed, contoured, and shaped before final cementation.

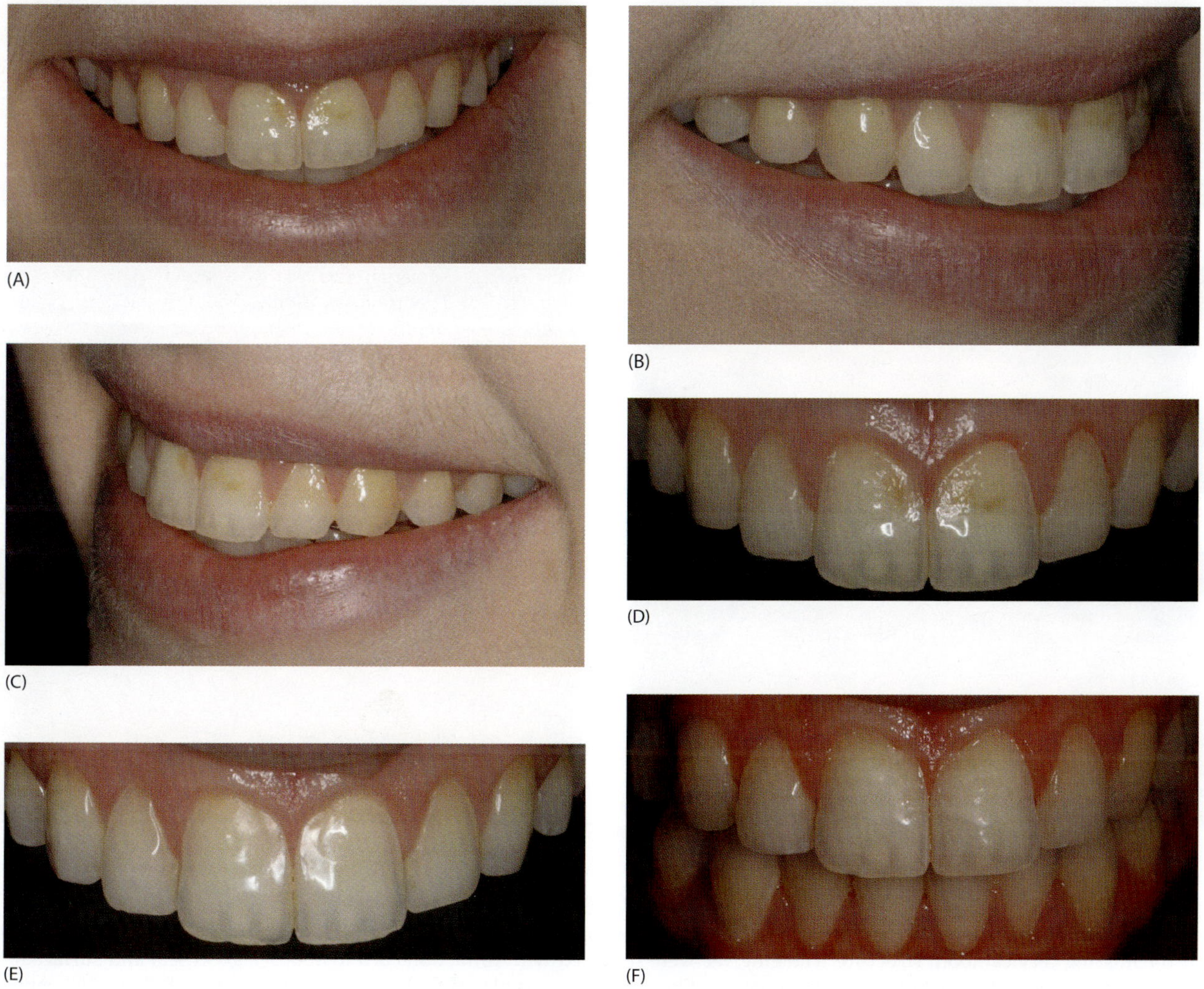

Figure 23.9

(A) This patient needed careful treatment planning because her teeth were very sensitive. As a result she was unable to clean her teeth, and so a cycle of inflammation set in—the gingivae became sensitive and inflamed and the patient could not brush her teeth efficiently. The treatment involved making upper and lower whitening trays. The patient was instructed in how to place the desensitizing material inside the whitening trays. The patient first placed the gel in the tray of the upper teeth and then the lower teeth. The patient was also instructed to use an ultrasoft toothbrush and a desensitizing whitening toothpaste. The patient changed the brand of the desensitizing toothpaste every 2 weeks to make the desensitizing effect more effective. (B) Right lateral view before treatment. (C) Left lateral view. (D) The result after desensitizing using the whitening trays. Staining is still present, but the teeth are no longer sensitive. (E) The result after a professional prophylaxis treatment to remove the staining from the teeth. The teeth appear cleaner and healthier. The oral hygiene and gingival health are considerably improved. (F) Improvement in the gingival health and sensitivity levels.

continued on the next page

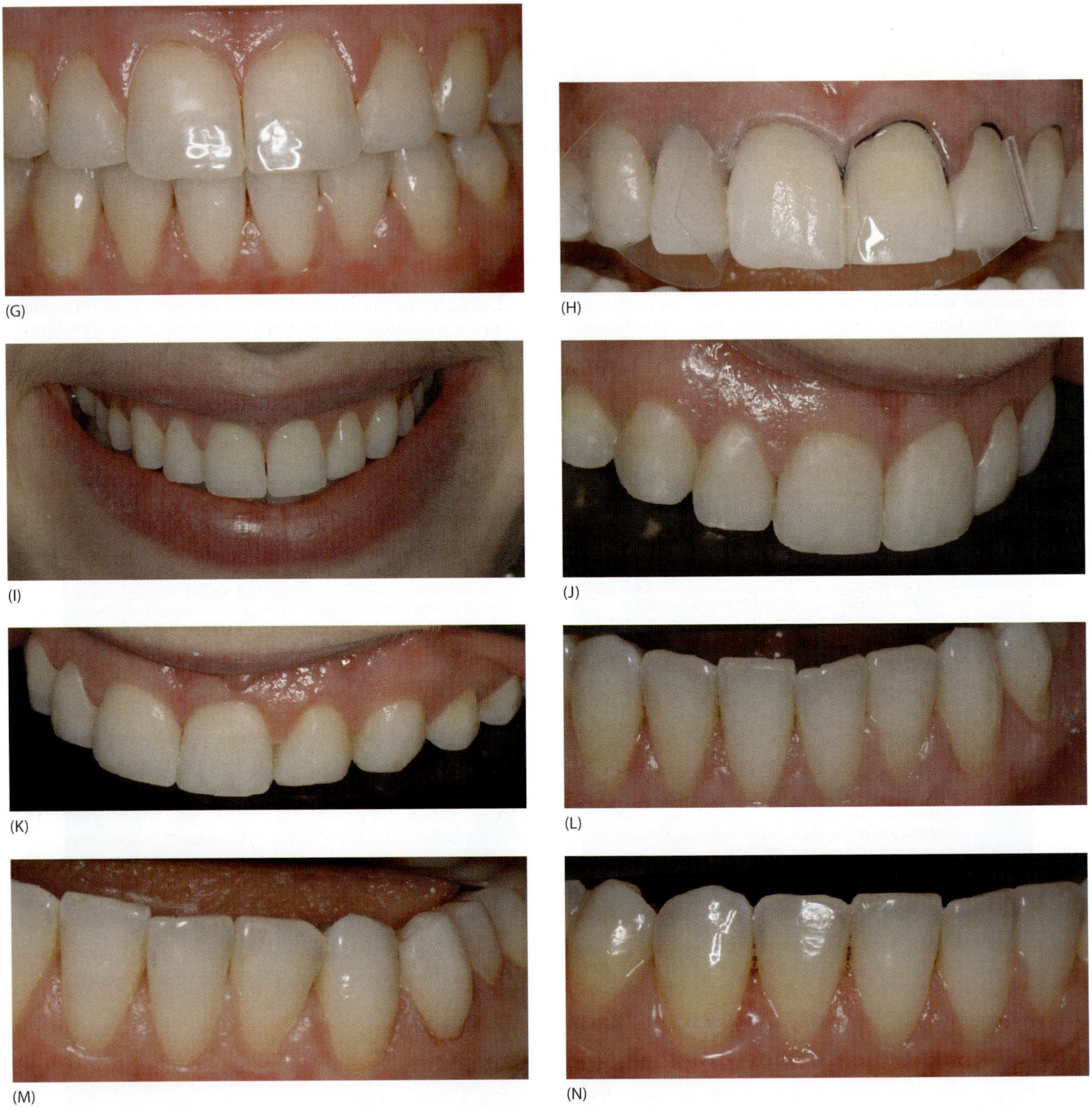

(G) (H) (I) (J) (K) (L) (M) (N)

Figure 23.9 continued

(G) Result after whitening treatment. (H) After whitening treatment, restorative treatment using composite layering techniques was undertaken to repair the missing cervical tooth structure. The gingivae were retracted with retraction cord to obtain a good seal and surface for direct bonding. The three-stage technique was used after bonding. Flowable resin was placed first, then dentin composite, followed by enamel composite, which was more translucent. Owing to the location of the stain in the middle of the tooth and the erosive defects in the middle of the tooth, the enamel layer was bonded over the entire tooth to get a better surface finish for the entire tooth. Here, composite has been placed, layered, and anatomically contoured on the upper right central incisor; the upper left incisor has not had the composite placed. (I) The smile view after the completion of the esthetic treatment. (J) The right lateral view of the completed treatment. (K) The left lateral view of the completed treatment. (L) After completion of the whitening treatment of the lower teeth. (M) Result after completion of the composite bonding treatment to repair cervical defects on the necks of the lower left first premolar and canine. (N) Whitening result on the lower teeth from the right lateral side. The patient has some demineralization on the cervical part of the lower right canine. This patient will need ongoing maintenance treatment and observation. The whitening tray can be used as a therapeutic tray to deliver amorphous calcium phosphate and fluoride to encourage remineralization.

24 WHITENING, THERAPEUTIC ESTHETICS, AND ORAL HEALTH IMPROVEMENT
The Future

Linda Greenwall

INTRODUCTION

With the success of tooth whitening treatments, several health benefits have emerged that can improve patients' oral health (Li and Greenwall 2013). Many people do not know that whitening treatment offers these oral health benefits, which can be harnessed for patients at different times of their lives. It is now essential to make use of these health benefits—to develop them further and create a program to improve patients' dental health throughout their lives. The purpose of this chapter is to elaborate on the benefits of introducing a program of therapeutic esthetics as part of an oral health maintenance program and helping patients to gain health sustainability.

WHAT IS THERAPEUTIC ESTHETICS?

Therapeutic esthetics is the process of sustaining a patient's oral health while improving and maintaining the esthetic health of their teeth. The whitening tray can be transformed to a therapeutic tray to deliver chemicals to help the patient achieve a sustained health gain throughout his or her life (see Figures 24.1 and 24.2 and Table 24.1). The trays are used for different purposes throughout a patient's life (Table 24.2)—for instance, to treat high caries susceptibility at a young age (see Figure 24.3) or to treat dry mouth in an elderly patient who is taking multiple medications (see Figure 24.2A). The trays are worn to undertake a therapeutic use, be it to reduce caries, to reduce the high-risk classification of a caries exposure, to reduce root caries, or to assist with protecting the mouth during and after radiation treatment.

THE MATERIALS USED FOR TOOTH WHITENING

The two main tooth whitening materials are both derived from hydrogen peroxide. Hydrogen peroxide–only products are used as a day product in the tray. When the hydrogen peroxide product is placed in the tray, the material, once mixed with the saliva, releases water and oxygen, releasing effervescent bubbles. The oxygen penetrates into the enamel and dentin and reaches the pulp within 5–15 minutes. The flow of the material is multidirectional in three dimensions. The material also tracks into the gingival crevice and gingival pocket. The liberation of oxygen into the gingival crevice changes the bacterial environment to remove the Gram-negative bacteria, cleanse the pocket, and stimulate healing. All the oxygen is released within 1 hour, so there are no further benefits to using the material for longer than an hour. However, the day products will also improve the health of the gingivae.

Carbamide peroxide is a slower release material. The breakdown of carbamide peroxide is biexponential (Matis et al. 1999). After 2 hours, more than 50% of the active agent in carbamide peroxide whitening gel is available in whitening trays, and 10% is available after 10 hours (Matis et al. 1999). A greater-than-expected degradation occurs during the first 5 minutes.

The carbamide peroxide gels contains Carbopol, which allows the oxygen to be released slowly over a period of 8–10 hours. The carbamide peroxide material breaks down into urea and ammonia. The urea elevates the pH in the mouth. This stimulates healing. Reduction of caries is thought to occur by elevation of the pH above the level at which the caries process can occur, in addition to debridement of the teeth and improvement in gingival health. Carbamide peroxide heals the soft tissues and gingival areas. The effect of the oxygenating agents on the supragingival plaque has been equivocal, but recent data indicate that a stable agent that provides sustained active oxygen release is effective in controlling plaque (Gaffar et al. 1997).

The ammonia and carbon dioxide are released as well, but these are considered to be byproducts. Most of the home whitening materials also contain fluoride or potassium nitrate to act as soothers. These help to reduce the likelihood of sensitivity and reduce areas susceptible to caries. Within 5 minutes of the application of the material in the tray, the salivary pH is elevated for a period of 2 hours. The pH in the tray remains raised for 2 hours (Haywood 2007).

The most commonly used formulation is 10% carbamide peroxide; however, a lower concentration formulation, called Carbamide Plus, e.g., Novon Mild, has

Table 24.1 Materials that can be placed into therapeutic trays

• Potassium nitrate
• Fluoride gel
• Carbamide peroxide
• Hydrogen peroxide
• Amorphous calcium phosphate
• Amorphous calcium phosphate in combination with fluoride
• Corsodyl Dental Gel (chlorhexidine gel)
• Hydrocortisone for patients with severe lichen planus
• Prostaglandin gel for patients experiencing menopause
• Antibiotics
• Other medications according to the patient's needs (e.g., dry mouth gel)

Table 24.2 Who can benefit from the therapeutic esthetic approach?

• Those with special needs
• Those at high risk of tooth decay
• Patients with dry mouth and root
• Elderly patients (Kelleher et al. 2011)
• Chemotherapy patients
• Patients undergoing radiation therapy
• Patients with gingival and periodontal conditions
• Patients whose teeth have white spots
• Patients who are immunocompromised
• Patients with eating disorders or acid reflux
• Peri-implantitis patients
• Patients who have undergone periodontal surgery such as crown lengthening and pocket reduction surgery; the tray can be used to encourage healing

been developed. Its concentration of carbamide is 5%, and it is a three-component system. It contains hydrogen peroxide, urea, and sodium tripolyphosphate (Hyland et al. 2015). It is postulated that this increased whitening efficiency is the result of a marked increase in local pH on dilution, which destabilizes the hydrogen peroxide and expedites the whitening process.

BENEFITS OF TOOTH WHITENING

Teeth

- Whitens and lightens the teeth.
- Reduces stain build up on teeth.
- Preserves tooth structure.

Gingivae

- Reduces gingival inflammation.
- Reduces gingival swelling.
- Reduces plaque formation.
- Reduces extrinsic stain buildup.
- Reduces plaque adherence to teeth.
- Reduces gingival bleeding.
- Improves gingival index scores.

Soft tissues

- Improves health of soft tissue, healing of soft tissue lacerations.
- Improves wound healing in the mouth.

Oral health

- Improves oral hygiene as the patient looks in the mirror to see the whiter teeth.
- Whitens, brightens, and lightens teeth.
- Reduces caries formation (Lee et al. 2005).
- Reduces root caries formation (Haywood 2007).
- Cleaner-feeling teeth as a result of improved oral hygiene.

Psychological and related effects

- Improves patients' self-esteem.
- Improves patients' sense of self-worth.
- Patients smile more.
- Patients become "walking advertisements" for the practice.
- Patients help to market the practice as they show off their beautiful white smiles.

Other effects

- The tooth whitening materials have antibacterial properties, which help to heal the mouth (Lazarchik and Haywood 2010) (see Figures 24.1, 24.2A, and 24.4A).
- Reduction in oral malodor (DeVizio 2008).
- Carbamide peroxide was originally used as an oral antiseptic.

HISTORY

Over the last century, hydrogen peroxide has been used as a treatment for reducing gingival inflammation. Initially patients were instructed to use hydrogen peroxide mouthwash on a toothbrush to help reduce gingival swelling and irritation. In 1968, an orthodontist, Bill Klausmier, advised his patients to use 3% hydrogen peroxide mouthwash in the retainers after completing orthodontic treatment. At the 6-month evaluation he noted that not only was the gingival inflammation reduced, but the teeth were significantly whiter. He developed and used this technique over the next 40 years and wrote a retrospective report about this technique. He wrote that in the 40 years of using the orthodontic retainer to apply the mouthwash to reduce the inflammation and also to whiten the teeth, nobody lost a tooth, needed a root canal, or damaged a tooth as a result of using this technique. Since then, the whitening gels have changed significantly and have become much thicker and more viscous, thus adhering to the trays more in order to deliver the materials.

MATERIALS THAT CAN BE USED IN THERAPEUTIC ESTHETICS

- Carbamide peroxide
- Hydrogen peroxide
- Amorphous calcium phosphate (10% casein phosphopeptides and amorphous calcium phosphate [CPP-ACP] cream)
- ACP plus fluoride (10% CPP-ACP cream plus 900 ppm fluoride)
- Fluoride gel, paste, varnish
- Corsodyl
- Other medications

THE TRAY AS A VEHICLE FOR DELIVERING MATERIALS

Using the tray as a delivery vehicle, various chemicals can be placed to deliver sustained health benefits to the teeth over a chosen period of time (see Figure 24.4) according to the effectiveness of the material as it is released. The placement of the tray helps to keep the material in situ even if it may come into contact with the saliva. The tray can be made of flexible material such as Evacryl or a rigid material such as that used for Essix orthodontic retainers. The various materials are applied in the trays. The concept is that the tray remains in place overnight while the materials are soaking into the teeth or gingivae.

THE TRAY AS A DIAGNOSTIC AND ASSESSMENT TOOL

It is thought that in the future the whitening tray with the material inside will be used for further diagnostics and assessments, such as the salivary flow; pH of saliva; elevation of the PH; rate of remineralization; rate of decalcification; rate of repair of enamel, dentin, and root dentin; rate of whitening; rate of penetration of the whitening gel; and salivary and whitening kinetics. These whitening trays will have microchips inside to measure the rate of bruxism and tooth clenching and to gather further data, much like the wrist bands that are commonly used to measure fitness.

DESIGN OF THE TRAY FOR THERAPEUTIC USE

The tray design for therapeutic use can be varied and multipurpose depending on the material that is being placed in the tray. However, a scalloped tray around the papillae is a useful design. That way it does not impinge on the gingivae. The tray margins are cut just next to the gingival crevices. An orthodontic aligner can be used as a therapeutic tray as well as a retainer.

TRAY TYPES TO BE USED FOR THERAPEUTICS

A variety of tray designs can be used and modified for therapeutic use. The following is a list of trays that can be used for the purpose of therapeutics:

- Aligners
- Retainers such as an Essix retainer
- Whitening tray
- Specially designed tray similar to a whitening tray using a thicker strength material for extended wear time

USE OF THE THERAPEUTIC TRAYS THROUGHOUT THE PATIENT'S LIFE DEPENDING ON HEALTH NEED

There are times in a patient's life when he or she may have additional health challenges. This puts the patient at risk for tooth decay, root decay, gingival inflammation, and dry mouth.

WHO CAN BENEFIT?

- Those with special needs
- Those at high risk for tooth decay
- Patients with dry mouth
- Elderly patients (Kelleher et al. 2011)
- Chemotherapy patients
- Patients undergoing radiation therapy
- Patients with gingival and periodontal conditions
- Patients whose teeth have white spots (see Figure 24.3)
- Patients who are immunocompromised
- Patients with eating disorders or acid reflux
- Peri-implantitis patients (see Figure 24.4)
- Post–periodontal surgery patients (e.g., crown lengthening, pocket reduction surgery).

Elderly patients

Many elderly patients take multiple medications that can cause dry mouth. This polypharmacy can result in reduced saliva. Some patients suck mints to relieve their dry mouth, which exacerbates the condition. Saliva is protective for the mouth, and the lack of saliva can cause the patient to be more susceptible to root decay and to have increased decay around the margins or crowns. Some frail elderly patients have poor oral hygiene owing to lack of motor skills because of arthritis or to caregivers who do not help the patient to brush the teeth. There is a direct link between poor oral hygiene and pneumonia. There is a direct effect of the oral bacteria on respiratory infection in the frail elderly (Scannapieco 1999). Haywood (2007) has shown that use of a nightly whitening tray with carbamide peroxide reduces root caries susceptibility. The whitening material kills caries bacteria and reduces plaque adherence to the teeth. Elderly patients who have difficulty holding a toothbrush may find it easier to apply the carbamide peroxide gel and place this in the mouth overnight. These effects will help patients achieve successful long-term health gains and improve their oral health. This chemotherapeutic approach enhances oral health.

Special needs patients

In a study undertaken by Lazarchik and Haywood (2010), the authors found 10% carbamide peroxide delivered in a custom-fitted tray to be an effective treatment for caries in patients with compromised oral hygiene. Plaque suppression and caries control result from a carbamide peroxide–induced increase in salivary and plaque pH caused by carbamide peroxide's urea component, and from possible antimicrobial action via physical debridement and the direct chemical effect of hydrogen peroxide.

Patients with high risk for decay and white spot lesions

There are many people in this category who can be helped by the use of therapeutic trays, including patients who have poor oral hygiene and cannot maintain a clean mouth, patients with a high-sugar diet, and patients who are immunocompromised. Some patients who have eating disorders or who have reflux and acid regurgitation problems can also be helped by the use of a therapeutic tray. These patients would use carbamide peroxide gel to help reduce the plaque and also could place ACP into the tray to help elevate the pH further while restoring the oral environment to a neutral pH.

A concentration of 10% carbamide peroxide kills lactobacillus, one of the bacteria that causes tooth decay. Chlorhexidine (CHX) kills *Streptococcus mutans* bacteria, which are also responsible for tooth decay. A recent in vitro study testing the use of a 1.1% fluoride (NaF) toothpaste containing 5000 ppm, MI Paste, and MI Paste Plus noted that the sodium fluoride (NaF) was the most effective at reducing the white spots (Oliveira 2014) The results showed that a 1.1% NaF dentifrice (5000 ppm) demonstrated greater remineralization ability than the CPP-ACP topical tooth cream and that the addition of fluoride to its formulation seems to enhance remineralization. Saliva also has the ability to exert an important remineralization effect over time.

White spot lesions after orthodontic debanding are a common occurrence. These can be treated with a therapeutic esthetic approach by using either the therapeutic tray or the orthodontic retainer to apply various fluoride gels or ACP combinations (Heymann and Grauer 2013; see Table 24.3). In addition, patients with white spot lesions after orthodontic treatment may benefit from the use of MI Paste or MI Paste Plus in their orthodontic retainers to heal these lesions. A study showed that it may be more effective to combine this strategy with microabrasion to improve the fluorescence (i.e., the mineral content) of the enamel. A CPP-ACP paste alone does not significantly improve the fluorescence value of white spot lesions. Within the limitations of this in vitro study, microabrasion treatment with or without CPP-ACP improved the fluorescence and thus reduced white spot lesions.

Patients with small clinical root lesions can be given therapeutic trays to place ACP inside. Some patients may undertake whitening treatment first because whitening treatment using carbamide peroxide has been shown to reduce the appearance of root lesions. After the completion of the whitening treatment, the patient is instructed to use the trays for therapeutic purposes to deliver ACP with fluoride twice weekly (see Figure 24.6).

Table 24.3 Options for management of white spot lesions Patients in all categories—normal risk, high risk, intratreatment management, and postorthodontic treatment—can use therapeutic trays.

Normal risk

- Tooth brushing with fluoride toothpaste, 1000 ppm two or three times per day
- Prophylaxis every 4 months
- Fluoride varnish every 4 months
- 0.5% NaF daily at bedtime

High risk

- Tooth brushing two or three times
- Fluoride toothpaste 5000 ppm before bedtime
- 1000 ppm at other times using mechanical brush
- Prophylaxis every 3 months
- Fluoride varnish every 3 months
- Xylitol chewing gum (3–5 pieces per day, at least 10 minutes per chew)
- Chlorohexidine rinse, 2-week regimen (30-second rinse before bedtime)

Intratreatment management

- Tooth brushing, modified technique (5000 ppm)
- 1000 ppm at other times
- Prophylaxis every 3 months
- Fluoride varnish every 3 months
- MI Paste plus nightly application
- Xylitol chewing gum
- (If poor compliance, then early removal of appliance)

Postorthodontic treatment

- No treatment
- Monitoring
- Tooth whitening
- Resin infiltration
- Microabrasion
- Direct resin

Adapted from Heymann and Grauer [2013], with permission from John Wiley and Sons.

Patients with peri-implantitis

The incidence of peri-implantitis is increasing as more implants are placed. There is a wide range of treatment options, most of which are unsatisfactory and involve improved oral hygiene techniques around the implant, the placement of CHX gel around the abutment connection, an intense course of antibiotics, removal of the implant, raising a flap for pocket reduction to salvage the implant, and using ultrasonics and air abrasion around the exposed threads and into the pocket. Sometimes the deterioration can be rapid with severe consequences involving bone loss around the implant. A simple maintenance strategy of placing 10% carbamide peroxide in a specially made therapeutic tray may be a sensible strategy to prevent this from occurring. The patient would wear this tray overnight, depending on the severity of the peri-implantitis. The wear schedule can vary depending on the severity of the peri-implantitis. A maintenance regimen could involve use of CHX once per week overnight, or daily nighttime placement of 10% carbamide peroxide or nightly use if there is suppurative exudate from the pocket. The problem with the standard treatment (i.e., CHX gel or mouthrinse) is that patients can develop a resistance to CHX over time. In addition, allergy to CHX has been reported in the literature to be increasing. For maintenance treatment, patients are shown in detail how to apply the gel and place the tray in the mouth with the gel in place. A specific wear routine will be given to the patient to improve maintenance (see Figure 24.5).

In a recent in vitro study undertaken by Yao et al. (2013), the antibacterial effect of carbamide peroxide on oral biofilm was evaluated. This study compared the effects of carbamide peroxide and CHX on oral biofilm in vitro. Collagen-coated hydroxyapatite disks were inoculated with subgingival plaque. After 3 weeks, the emergent biofilms were subjected to 1-, 3-, and 10-minute exposures of a 1% CHX gel, a 5% carbamide peroxide gel and rinse, and a 10% carbamide peroxide gel and rinse. Subsequently, the biofilms were stained using a two-color fluorescent dye kit for confocal laser scanning microscopy, and the volume ratio of dead bacteria to all bacteria was analyzed. Compared with an untreated gel control, the active agents killed bacteria on all the disks, with higher concentration and longer exposure times killing more bacteria. The rinse form disrupted the biofilm more quickly than the gel form. Overall, 10% carbamide peroxide showed more disruption of biofilm and a greater proportion of killed bacteria than 1% CHX ($P < .05$).

For patients with exposed implant threads, it may be advisable to place a block-out resin interproximally to prevent tearing of the impression material when the impression is taken. That way a therapeutic tray can be placed over the undercuts of the long implant fixtures.

Periodontal patients

A recent study showed that the adjunctive use over 3 months of 1.7% hydrogen peroxide gel, locally administered using prescription customized trays, in the treatment of subjects with moderate to advanced periodontitis demonstrated statistically significant clinical improvements in pocket depths and bleeding when compared with scaling and root planing alone (Putt and Proskin 2012).

SALIVARY CHANGES INSIDE THE TRAY

The research from Leonard et al. (1994a,b) showed that when the saliva comes in contact with the carbamide peroxide, there is an elevation in the pH to about 8 as a result of the liberation of urea. The urea and ammonia are byproducts of the breakdown process of the carbamide peroxide. The hydrogen peroxide breaks down to water and oxygen. The critical pH for demineralization is 5.2–5.5 for enamel and 6.0–6.8 for dentin (Leonard et al. 1994a).

SUMMARY

The use of carbamide peroxide in a whitening tray has additional benefits to help patients improve and maintain their oral health. Dentists are advised to consider this therapeutic approach to improve esthetics while improving health sustainability for many patients. Many patients can benefit from this approach.

REFERENCES

DeVizio W. (2008) The efficacy of a new dentifrice with caries, plaque, gingivitis, calculus, tooth whitening, and oral malodor benefits. *J Clin Dent* **19**(3):79–80.

Gaffar A, Afflitto J, Nabi N. (1997) Chemical agents for the control of plaque and plaque microflora: an overview. *Eur J Oral Sci* **105**(5 Pt 2):502–7.

Greenwall LH. (2014). Therapeutic aesthetics. *Besthet Dent Today* **May**:9–12.

Haywood VB. (2007) Bleaching and caries control in elderly patients. *Aesthet Dent Today* **October**:47–9.

Heymann GC, Grauer DJ. (2013) A contemporary review of white spot lesions in orthodontics. *J Esthet Restor Dent* **25**(2): 85–95.

Hyland BW, McDonald A, Lewis N, Tredwin C. (2015) A new three-component formulation for the efficient whitening of teeth (Carbamide Plus). *Clin Oral Investig* **19**(6): 1395–404.

Kelleher MG, Djemal S, Al-Khayatt AS, Ray-Chaudhuri J. (2011) Bleaching and bonding for the older patient. *Dent Update* **38**(5):294–6, 298–300, 302–3.

Lazarchik DA, Haywood VB. (2010) Use of tray-applied 10 percent carbamide peroxide gels for improving oral health in patients with special-care needs. *J Am Dent Assoc* **141**(6): 639–46.

Lee SS, Zhang W, Lee DH, Li Y (2005) Tooth whitening in children and adolescents: a literature review. *Pediatr Dent* **27** (5):362–8.

Leonard RH, Austin SM, Haywood VB, Bentley CD. (1994a) Change in pH of plaque and 10% carbamide peroxide during Nightguard Vital Bleaching. *Quintessence Int* **25:** 819–23.

Leonard RH, Bentley CD, Haywood VB. (1994b) Salivary pH changes during 10% carbamide peroxide bleaching. *Quintessence Int* **25:**547–50.

Li Y, Greenwall LH. (2013) Safety issues of tooth whitening using peroxide-based materials. *Br Dent J* **215**(1):29–34.

Matis BA, Gaiao U, Blackman D, Schultz FA. (1999) In vivo degradation of bleaching gel used in whitening teeth. *J Am Dent Assoc* **130**(2):227–35.

Nathoo S, Mateo LR, Delgado E, Zhang YP. (2011) Extrinsic stain removal efficacy of a new dentifrice containing 0.3% triclosan, 2.0% PVM/MA copolymer, 0.243% NaF and specially-designed silica for sensitivity relief and whitening benefits as compared to a dentifrice containing 0.3% triclosan, 2% PVM/MA copolymer, 0.243% NaF and to a negative control dentifrice containing 0.243% NaF: a 6-week study. *Am J Dent* **24**(Spec Issue A):28A–31A.

Oliveira GM, Ritter AV, Heymann HO, Swift E Jr. (2014) Remineralization effect of CPP-ACP and fluoride for white spot lesions in vitro. *J Dent* **42**(12):1592–602.

Pliska BT, Warner GA, Tantbirojn D, Larson BE. (2012) Treatment of white spot lesions with ACP paste and microabrasion. *Angle Orthod* **82**(5):765–9.

Putt MS, Proskin HM. (2012) Custom tray application of peroxide gel as an adjunct to scaling and root planing in the treatment of periodontitis: a randomized, controlled three-month clinical trial. *J Clin Dent* **23**(2):48–56.

Scannapieco FA. (1999) Role of oral bacteria in respiratory infection. *J Periodontol* **70:**793–802.

Yao CS, Waterfield JD, Shen Y, Haapasalo M. (2013) In vitro antibacterial effect of carbamide peroxide on oral biofilm. *J Oral Microbiol* **Jun 12:**5.

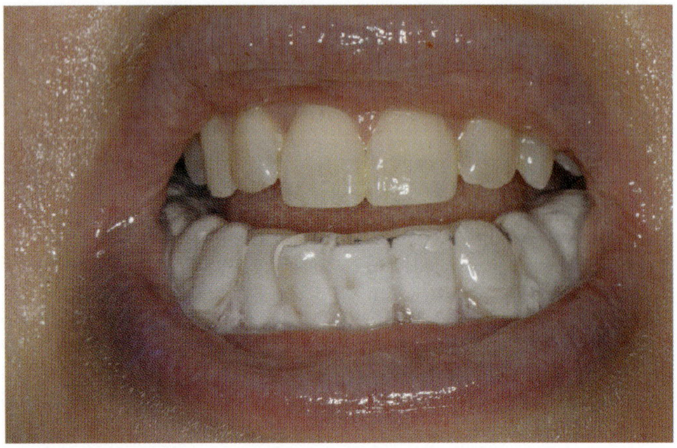

Figure 24.1

This patient had recently completed restorative treatment. She had small defects on her enamel from previous areas of decalcification. She underwent minimally invasive treatment that included air abrasion, bonding, and repair with glass ionomer and flowable composite into the microdefects. This maintenance treatment involved making therapeutic trays for the patient; the patient placed the amorphous calcium phosphate, which included fluoride, into the areas to strengthen the enamel, heal the white areas of decalcification, and stabilize the oral health. The first line of defense in treatment of patients with white spot lesions caused by decalcification is improvement in oral hygiene, reduction of sugary food, and the use of the therapeutic tray with fluoride gel inside to reduce the appearance of the white spots that are caused by demineralization.

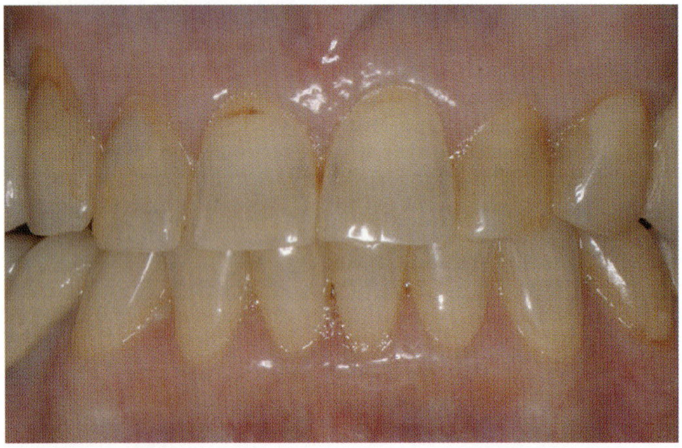

(A)

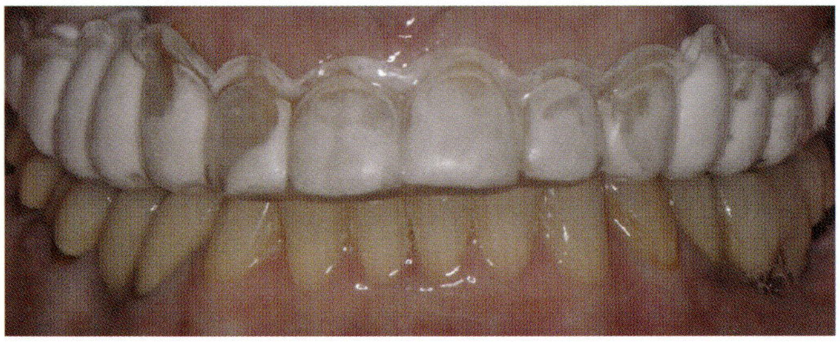

(B)

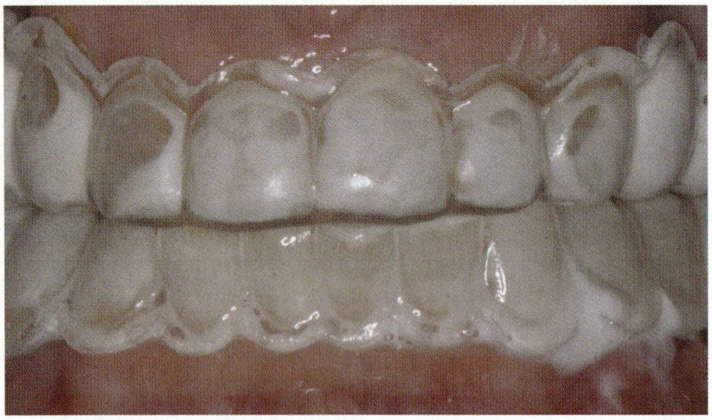

(C)

Figure 24.2

(A) This elderly patient had undergone extensive restorative dentistry 15 years previously. The treatment had included implant reconstruction on the posterior teeth including extensive crown and bridge work. Although the patient was seen on a regular basis for hygienist and maintenance treatment, it was noted that early root lesions were developing. It was decided to make a therapeutic tray for this patient so that amorphous calcium phosphate and fluoride could be administered to prevent further decay as the patient ages. (B) Upper therapeutic tray seated in the patient's mouth. (C) Both upper and lower trays were made for the patient. This figure shows the patient wearing the upper and lower trays at the same time. A regimen of alternate nights was used for the upper and lower therapeutic trays to improve compliance.

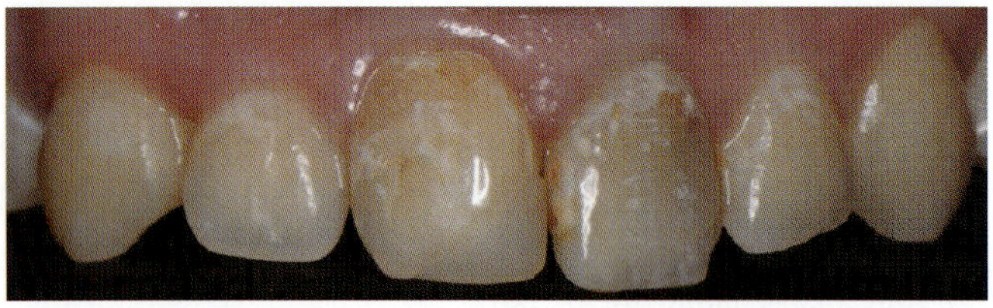

Figure 24.3

This patient had extensive white spot lesions on the anterior teeth because of poor oral hygiene. After oral hygiene instruction, the patient received whitening trays, which were used for therapeutic purposes to administer fluoride gel to reduce the appearance of the white spots. After the fluoride gel had been applied to the upper teeth for 2 weeks, whitening gel was applied to improve the color. The patient also underwent nonvital whitening of the upper central incisor teeth using the same tray. After whitening was completed, the tray was used for maintenance to reduce the other white spots.

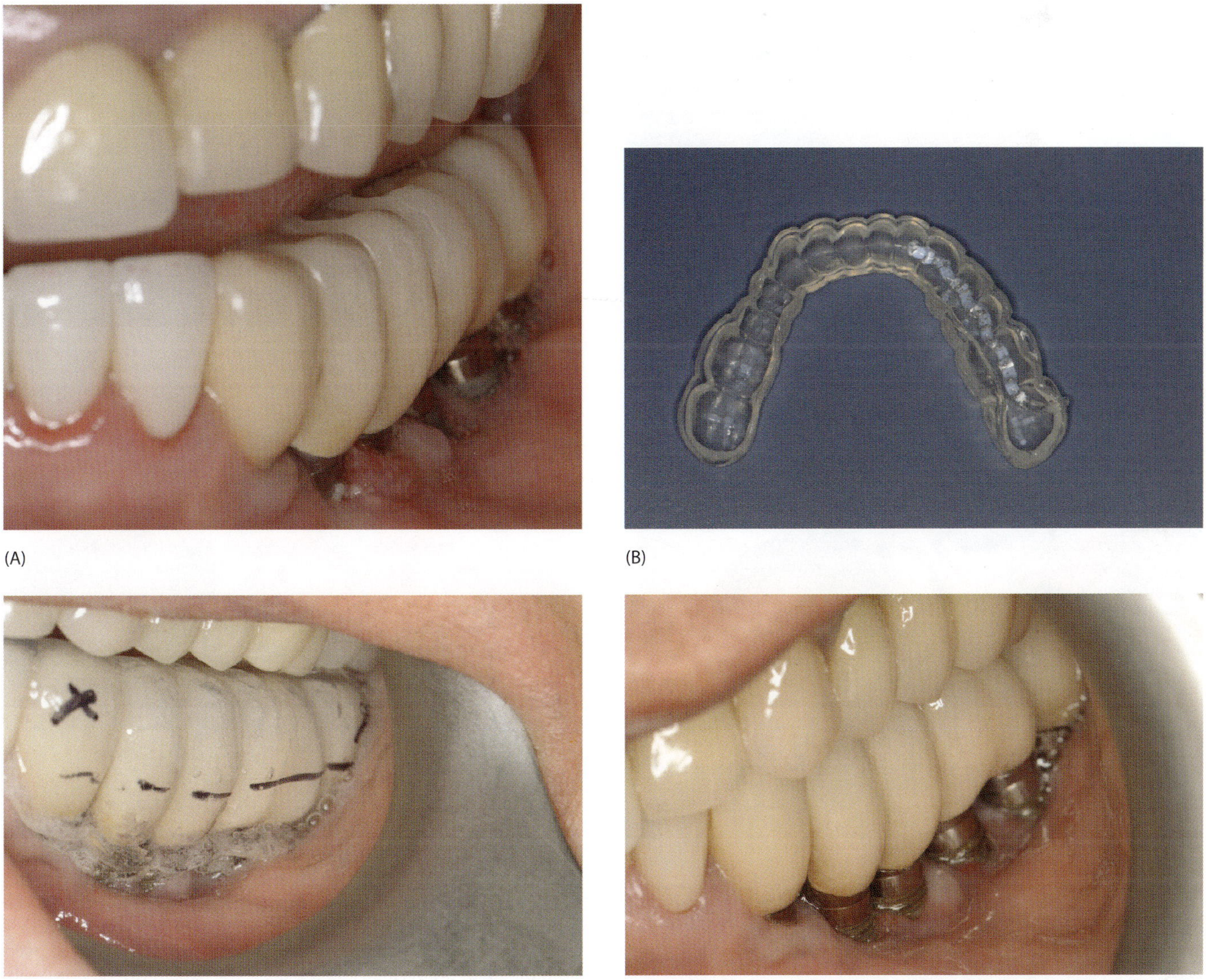

(A) (B) (C) (D)

Figure 24.4

(A) This patient had implants placed 10 years previously. The patient developed peri-implantitis around the implants, and it was decided to make a therapeutic tray to help heal the gingivae around the implants. (B) The patient was instructed to place the 10% carbamide peroxide into the lower left part of the tray. (C) The tray is worn in the mouth; the marking pen shows the patient exactly where to place the whitening gel. The tray is extended slightly to reach the gingivae in order to place the materials in contact with the inflamed gingivae associated with peri-implantitis. (D) The appearance of the gingivae after 2 weeks of wearing the tray. There is good healing of the papillae.

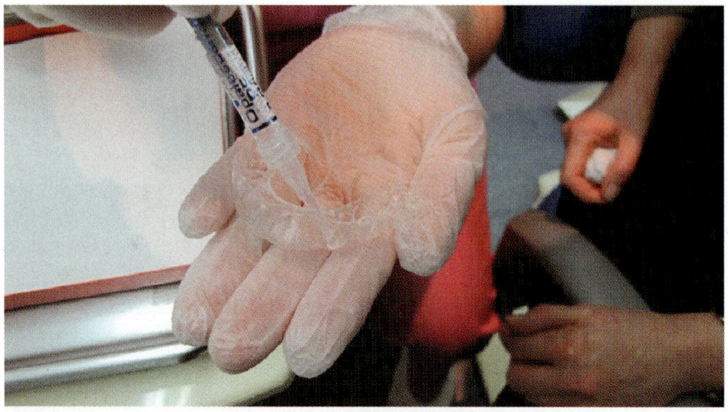

(A)

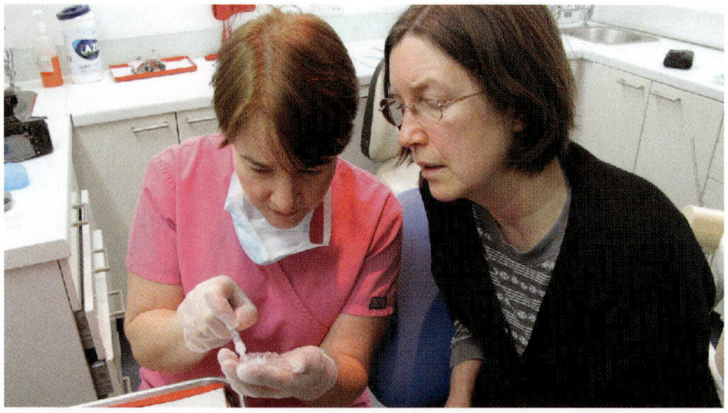

(B)

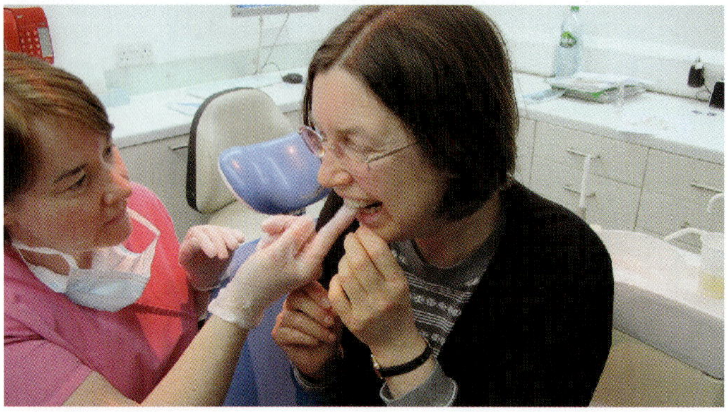

(C)

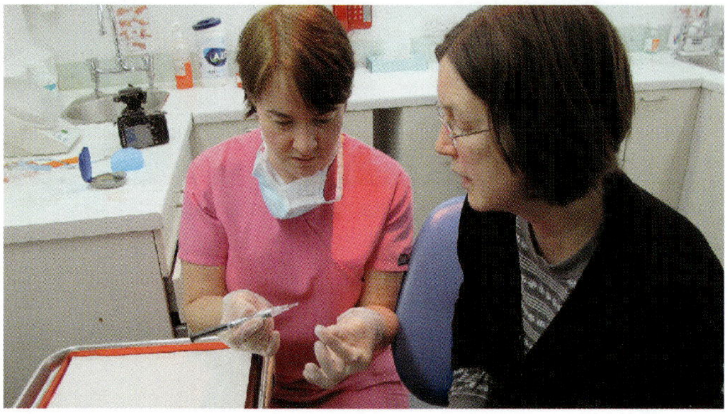

(D)

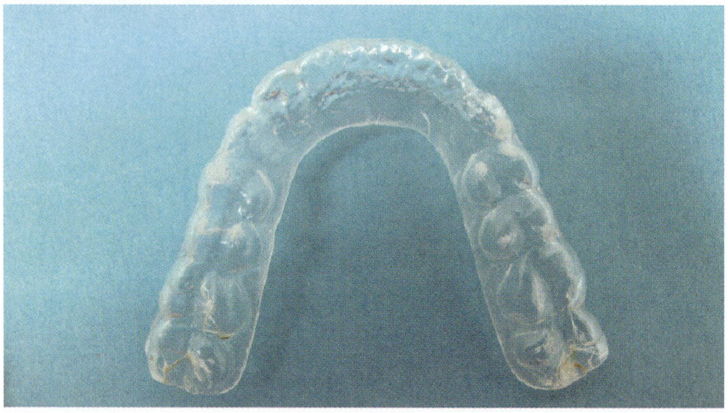

(E)

Figure 24.5

(A) The patient is instructed on how to use the tray and place the material into the tray. The patient's orthodontic retainer is used for this maintenance treatment. (B) It is helpful to demonstrate directly to the patient. (C) The tray is placed with the material inside so that the patient can feel how it should fit and how much material should be placed. (D) The patient is shown exactly how much material to place in the tray and is told that one syringe should last for 3 to 4 nights. The lid is removed from the tip of the syringe and replaced; the patient can do this easily at home as part of the home care. Because this patient had had implants placed 15 years previously and orthodontic treatment, good maintenance was essential. This patient placed the carbamide peroxide in the mouth once a week for maintenance treatment for improved healing of the gingivae around the implants and reduction in root decay. (E) Maintenance tray that the patient used to apply the gel.

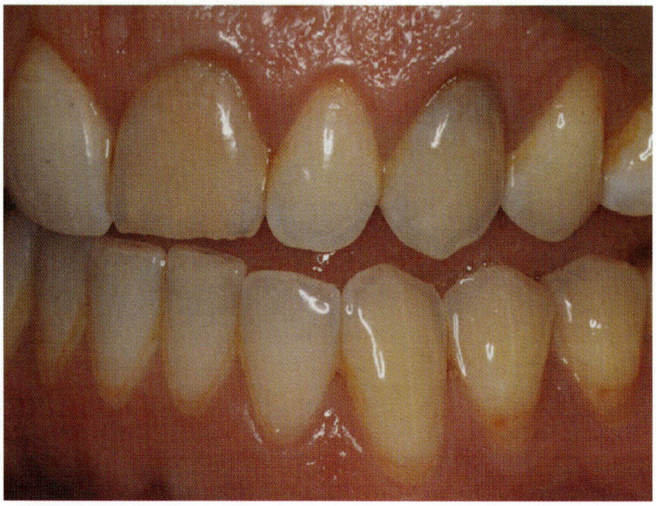

Figure 24.6

Early root caries in a patient who also wanted to whiten his teeth. Note the early root decay on the lower left first and second premolars. The patient's brushing techniques were revised. After completion of the whitening treatment, which included internal whitening of the upper left central incisor and the upper left canine, the upper and lower teeth were whitened. The patient continued to use the tray twice a week, placing amorphous calcium phosphate with fluoride inside to reduce the demineralization of the root surfaces of the lower teeth.

INDEX

U

V

W